THE VITAL BALANCE

KARL MENNINGER

with Martin Mayman and Paul Pruyser

Widely acknowledged as a basic work, *The Vital Balance* offers a new, unitary concept of mental health and illness which dispenses with the old and confusing labels and substitutes a method of diagnosis and treatment in which all disturbed states of the mind and the emotions are seen as stages in a single process. It marks the culmination of a complete revolution in the outlook of psychiatry —from helpless resignation to active hope and assurance.

KARL MENNINGER is Chairman of the Board of Trustees of The Menninger Foundation. His books include *The Human Mind, Man Against Himself, Love Against Hate, The Theory of Psychoanalytic Technique, A Psychiatrist's World*, and *The Crime of Punishment*.

MARTIN MAYMAN, Ph.D., is a member of the Department of Psychiatry at the University of Michigan. PAUL PRUYSER, Ph.D., is director of the Department of Education at The Menninger Foundation.

THE VITAL BALANCE

The Life Process in Mental Health and Illness

THE VITAL BALANCE

*The Life Process
in Mental Health and Illness*

KARL MENNINGER, M.D.

with Martin Mayman, Ph.D. and Paul Pruyser, Ph.D.

The Viking Press, New York

VIKING COMPASS EDITION

ISSUED IN 1967 BY THE VIKING PRESS, INC.

625 MADISON AVENUE, NEW YORK, N.Y. 10022

DISTRIBUTED IN CANADA BY

THE MACMILLAN COMPANY OF CANADA LIMITED

LIBRARY OF CONGRESS CATALOG CARD NUMBER: 63-17075

THIRD PRINTING JANUARY 1969

PRINTED IN U.S.A.

TO MY BROTHERS

Contents

THE VITAL BALANCE

The Life Process in Mental Health and Illness

CHAPTER I

The Name and the Nature

Every standpoint is what it is by virtue of its origin from the past and its urge toward the future. . . . No scientific entity—atom, organ, or wave—is *merely* itself, but is constantly evolving in a context of history . . . (William P. D. Wightman, *The Growth of Scientific Ideas*)

S Y N O P S I S : This chapter reviews the origins of the central idea of the book—how nearly fifty years ago the static and essentially hopeless philosophy of psychiatry spurred the senior author into a lifelong protest. This chapter describes the nature of the change that has taken place in the science and how this book proposes to expand and document that change.

FORTY-EIGHT years ago the senior author of this book was sitting one morning in the office of the clinical director of the Boston Psychopathic Hospital. A group of Harvard medical students were being given their first instruction in psychiatry. They had spent two weeks in this famous institution observing the patients and attending staff meetings, and now one student was reporting to his professor, Herman Adler.

"What's the use? After all your examinations and discussion, you give nearly every patient the same diagnosis; they all seem to have dementia praecox. And the treatment for all of them seems to be merely committing them to the nearest state hospital."

Dr. Adler was patient with his presumptuous student, who, however, resolved to eschew the stupid, sterile specialty forever and pursue "scientific medicine." But new discoveries in pharmacology, the brilliant example of Harvey Cushing in neurosurgery, and news of psychiatric needs in the combat zones of World War 1 led to my spiraling (upward, I trust) back to the Boston Psychopathic Hospital, and to a fresh view of psychiatry under Ernest Southard.

Could things have changed so much in three years, or was it only I that had changed? "Dementia praecox" had disappeared; it had become "Schizophrenia" (which in turn changed later into "the schizophrenias" and still later into "schizophrenic reactions"). But it was not only that mental illness had changed its names. The observers had begun to change.

1

This trend of change has continued ever since, and this book is an effort to describe it in process and in consequence.

In the early part of the century the object of psychiatry was primarily to identify and distinguish the forms and evidences of mental illness, so little suspected and recognized in their minor manifestations and so vastly feared in their larger appearances. We dutifully employed historic designations and historic concepts associated with them. Today these concepts have been largely replaced by more dynamic, pragmatic notions. Our concern now is not so much what to call something as what to do about it. The old point of view assumed that most mental illness was progressive and refractory. The new point of view is that most mental illness serves its purpose and disappears, and does so more rapidly and completely when skillfully understood and dealt with.

Instead of putting our emphasis on different clinical forms of mental illness, we tend today to think of all mental illness as being essentially the same in quality, although differing quantitatively and in external appearance. My teacher was right when he said that each case was different; and I was right, more so than I realized, when I reproached him for calling them all "dementia praecox." We don't call any of them that today, nor do we regard the symptoms of mental illness as so malignant and so inevitably progressive. But we know there is a possibility for human beings to lose their moorings, to become confused and disturbed. Usually this condition disappears more or less promptly; sometimes it grows worse.

Let us imagine that one could set up a kind of scale or yardstick to measure the success of a life—the satisfactoriness to the individual and his environment of their mutual attempts to adapt themselves to each other. Toward one end of such a yardstick positive adjectives like "peaceful," "constructive," "productive" might appear and at the other end such words as "confused," "destructive," "chaotic." These would describe the situation in general. For the individual himself there might be at one end of the yardstick such terms as "healthy," "happy," "creative," and at the other end "miserable," "criminal," "delirious." There would be a large area on our imaginary scale where there would be no marks; the moving finger might veer sometimes toward one pole and sometimes toward the other. There would certainly be no mark labeled "Success" and none labeled "Failure"; we must "treat these two impostors just the same." But there might be some zones with practical labels such as "too comfortable," "help needed," or "danger zone."

This is just a fantasy, of course, to get the reader in a frame of mind to think in terms of process and change rather than in the conventional terms of state and condition. It may shock him at first that we propose to dispense with all names for mental diseases and to learn that some even go so far as to suggest that there are no mental diseases. We know that there is mental illness or something that has been called that; we know that there are apparent failure and faltering. We know that such problems engage the attention of clergymen, judges, lawyers, doctors, hospital administrators, psychologists, and all sorts of people who *profess* a wish to be helpful. The members of these professions must communicate with one another and with the patients to be effective; and they can communicate only if they and the laymen with whom they work speak a language understood by them all.

In accounting for the appearance of this book I had first intended to ascribe its inception to the year 1943, when my brother Will, then assistant to the Surgeon-General, was wrestling with the difficulties caused in the Army medical service by the incompatibility of medical facts and nosological traditions. He appealed to psychiatric colleagues over the nation to assist him in undertaking a revision of our inconsistent psychiatric nomenclature and classification.

In connection with his studies I began the collection of all the psychiatric classifications available in English, German, and French. This was a hobby at first, and then became almost an obsession. I was ably assisted in this at various times by George Devereux, the late Helen Sargent, Henri Ellenberger, E. Stengel of London, and others. The original format of this book was to have been a presentation of these classifications with some conclusions regarding the trend of the changing lists. This collection now constitutes our Appendix.

I recognized even while I was collecting these taxonomic lists that the seeds of my interest in it had been sown long before. At the time of his death in 1919 my teacher Ernest Southard was preoccupied with the problem: "Perhaps I believe that the world can get forward most by clearer and clearer definition of fundamentals. Accordingly, I propose to stick to tasks of nomenclature and terminology, unpopular and ridicule-provoking though they may be." [1] *

I have often recalled these words, with consolation. Southard was indeed ridiculed for his efforts; ** there was little doubt in anyone's mind at

---

* Reference notes begin on page 491.
** Said one of his closest associates, himself a leader at the time: "No adequate reason for classification of mental disease for any other than statistical purposes has ever been advanced. . . . They do not contribute anything of value whatever to our knowledge of symptomatology, diagnosis or treatment. Practically the only point

that time regarding the validity of our standard Kraepelinean "diseases."
But the great influenza epidemic of 1918–1920 gave us pause; it seemed
to precipitate all sorts of psychiatric conditions. Among these were many
cases of "dementia praecox." These were given a bad prognosis, of course,
and stowed away in various state hospitals, presumably to spend the rest
of their lives in apathy, delirium, and dementia. But five years later a
research check of a sizable sample of those we had seen showed that most
of them had recovered and gone home. The reader should remember that
in those days the "Discharged recovered" rate (in one Massachusetts
hospital at least) was 5 per cent of all admissions.

And so the designation "schizophrenia" began to appeal to us as less
ominous-sounding than "dementia praecox," and we began to think in
a heretical way of the possibility of reversibility in mental illness, that
perhaps schizophrenia was not so malignant as we thought but a process
that might in some instances be reversible.* These were radical thoughts
in those days. Mental illness was not supposed to go that way. And young
psychiatrists were not supposed to think that way.

These experiences all came back to my mind in 1945 when my brother
and the Surgeon-General sent five of us to the European front to observe
the psychological demoralization which produced so many casualties and
incapacitations. Some of our findings appear later in this book; one of
them pertinent here is that the classical psychiatric designations do not
correctly describe what happens to soldiers (or anyone else) under accumulating stress. All people are under some stress and some people
are under much stress, and react to it like soldiers. These reactions can
be named. But the names come and go, as our Appendix beautifully demonstrates. Some of these reactions are what we call mental illness, which
is not "a thing" at all but an aspect or quality of life at a particular
time under particular circumstances.

My colleagues and I therefore began to formulate a simple model of
the personality in states of relative health and states of recognized illness, defining our terms as we went and aiming at a dynamic description.

---

on which the writers of our textbooks agree is that there is no one fundamental
principle upon which a satisfactory classification can be based. It is unfortunate that
tradition seems to demand the serious consideration of a problem which many believe admits of no solution and which would mean little or nothing to the future of
psychiatry if it were solved." (May, James. *Mental Diseases*. Boston: Badger, 1922.)
* "Between the mildest attack of simple delirium and the most profound dementia
of late schizophrenia, there is a progressive gradation, not in the intensity of symptoms
present (since these are variable products of little prognostic significance), but in
the degree of reversibility." (Menninger, K. A. "Reversible Schizophrenia." *Am. J.
Psychiatry*, 1:573, 1922.)

We sought for terms which would enable us to dispense with the pretentious, meaningless jargon and name-calling which have so long pervaded psychiatry and impaired its prestige in the eyes of many. Psychiatry should, we believe, provide a better understanding of human beings in trouble—yes, and human beings out of trouble—without pejoratively labeling them.

It is very important, this matter of speaking the common language. For an expanded psychiatry must keep in touch with men and women operating at various levels and in various areas, each with special terminologies and local argot. Psychiatry used to have its own argot—still does, I'm afraid. But if it is to be helpful in law, in criminology, in political science, in economics, in business management, in the school, and in the church, psychiatrists' descriptions and designations must be couched in the universal language, and not in an esoteric jargon. This is part of what is meant by the "unitary concept." For a holistic, humanistic, unitary concept of mental illness makes unnecessary many technical terms which used to have to carry prodigiously condensed but ambiguous information.

It is this view of mental illness as personality dysfunction and living impairment which is presented in this book. It sees all patients not as individuals afflicted with certain diseases but as human beings obliged to make awkward and expensive maneuvers to maintain themselves, individuals who have become somewhat isolated from their fellows, harassed by faulty techniques of living, uncomfortable themselves, and often to others. Their reactions are intended to make the best of a bad situation and at the same time forestall a worse one—in other words, to insure survival even at the cost of suffering and social disaster.

We disclaim any pretensions that this viewpoint is original or uniquely held by us. Many colleagues seem to be coming to the same conclusion. The trend toward a unitary concept of mental illness is clearly apparent in psychiatric history. It follows contemporary trends in other branches of science. Some colleagues have even gone so far, it would seem, as to dispense altogether with case study and diagnosis. The patient's feelings are the best evidence that he needs help, they say, and for the help he needs no elaborate analyses, no effort at identifying the sources of irritation or analyzing the nature of the inexpedient reactions is necessary. The symptoms indicate the treatment needed and it should be begun immediately. A colleague, Paul Goolker, has put it well, thus:

> The . . . difficulties of differential diagnosis contribute to an impatience [on the part of psychiatrists] to start with therapy, i.e., help. The

emphasis in descriptive psychiatry on diagnosis . . . used largely as a labeling device . . . brought about a reactive trend in extramural psychiatry against rigid classification. In addition, the historical shift of emphasis to dynamics and understanding of the individual patient tended further to discourage formal diagnosis. In the twenties and early thirties one could often hear leaders in psychotherapy excoriate their colleagues for wasting time in diagnosis instead of studying the patient as an individual with problems.[2]

A medical school professor is quoted as having uttered these timid cautionaries in October 1958: "It is suggested that [the physician] formulate a tentative specific . . . diagnosis . . . *prior* to the administration [of an antibiotic] . . . and that he give such a drug only when [its effectiveness is] . . . indicated [by the diagnosis]." It is not the sense of these words but their diffidence and their implications which shock us. "Why," inquires John Lear, "is such a pointed exhortation called for in these days when the rawest medical student is assumed to accept the primacy of accurate diagnosis?" [3]

Why, indeed? We, the authors, vigorously oppose the view that treatment, other than first aid, should proceed before or without diagnosis. On the contrary, we feel that diagnosis is today more important than ever. The very fact that psychiatric designations have become so meaningless by conflicting usage makes it more rather than less necessary that we approach the specific problem of illness with a cautious, careful scrutiny and appraisal that has characterized the best medical science since the early days. It is still necessary to know in advance, to plan as logically as we can, what kind of interference with a human life we propose to make.

In the course of teaching young doctors to become psychiatrists we constantly renew these old conflicts. Fresh from medical-school training, where they have been taught to identify diseases, they come into psychiatry, where they see illness and hence expect to find diseases. They want to apply labels. They seek, then, to rid the patient of this—his disease. They can scarcely wait to begin treating the patient and observing his "improvement" under their ministrations. This is heartwarming in a way because these young men are distinguished from the majority of their fellow medical students in possessing the belief that something can be done for the mentally ill. And they are anxious to get at it.

But they have to be taught that there are many forms of treatment and many ways of administering it, and that even more important than the treatment is skillful diagnosis. But this means diagnosis in a new sense, not the mere application of a label. It is not a search for a proper name by which one can refer to this affliction in this and other patients. It is diagnosis in the sense of understanding just how the patient is ill and how ill the patient is, how he became ill and how his illness serves him. From this knowledge one may draw logical conclusions regarding how changes might be brought about in or around the patient which would affect his illness.

Diagnosis in this sense requires a different kind of technical approach, a different diagnostic procedure. To be sure, the classical formula of

History + Examinations → Diagnosis → Treatment

must be followed; but then what? What does one do with these data? And just which data are selected to draw just what sort of conclusions?

Such considerations led us to the writing of a textbook on psychiatric case study.[4] It was put together chapter by chapter on the basis of actual teaching experience with hundreds of psychiatric residents. Its thesis is that the patient and the physician must form a compact of mutual service, that the physician must retain his objectivity and at the same time endure some of the patient's sufferings. An understanding of the patient's relationship to the environment and vice versa must conclude with an analysis of the effects of this life experience upon the patient's present endeavors to carry on. It must analyze his potentialities to improve himself and to improve his world, as well as his propensities to destroy himself and to destroy his world. One can then derive logical principles for planning a treatment program. Thus case study comes first, case study for the purpose of diagnosis, and diagnosis for the purpose of treatment.

This *Manual* describing the procedure of making the case study soon revealed many defects in our assumptions and application of theory. We had already started the present book as a systematic presentation of our thinking, but its development was interrupted several times by the discovery from practical experience of the necessity for revising and reformulating some of our ideas. Today we know, as we should have known long ago, that it can never be brought to any degree of completion or even of consistency. Psychiatry—like the world—is on the move; it is *becoming*. Our aim is only to try to describe its present phase and trace its presumptive orbit.

For psychiatry continues to expand. It is no longer the private, esoteric wisdom of a few physicians. It is a discipline served by doctors, psychologists, lawyers, judges, clergymen, and welfare workers; indeed, by all social scientists, theoretical and practical. In Southard's day it was strictly an intramural affair; it was Southard himself who first suggested the possibility of a psychiatric outpatient department.

It would belie our notion of things to say that psychiatry had arrived. It would be better to say that psychiatry is known of now and that much has been given to it and hence much is expected from it. It has been given the great gift of an increasing public confidence; the people have paid it homage and money. They need its help not for the custody of the hopeless, as used to be the case, but for the guidance, support, and redirection of the frail, the faltering, and the failing. Some of these are in hospitals, offices, or clinics; some of them are in jails, and some of them walk the streets. Many of them cling precariously to their niches in the workaday world, bravely masking their sufferings. Wherever they are, they are doing the best they can with what they have and with what they know and with what they are able to will.

But they *can* be helped. This is our gospel. They, and hence those about them, which means us, can be helped by our efforts. They can be helped to help themselves. They can be given what they lack; they can be taught and with this new knowledge helped to will differently and do better. This is psychiatry as we view it.

Like Rip Van Winkle, psychiatry has emerged from a long sleep. Leaving the hospital, with a new haircut and a shave, stretching his arms and legs, he walks across the courtyard square, pausing for a moment in the courthouse where he used to spend so much time. He proceeds on across to the market place, where he is welcomed by neighbors who used to shun him in his vagabond days. He visits the church, the factory, the medical clinic, and the general hospital. He stops in the nursery school and the grade school and the high school. He visits the prison and the detention home. In each case he makes his call and his suggestions and takes his leave—a kind of twentieth-century general practitioner who has awakened from a long sleep and gotten busy helping his neighbors, having given up his childhood dialect and learned to speak English.

CHAPTER II

The Urge to Classify

SYNOPSIS: There are many ways to organize miscellaneous data, and classification is one of the basic devices for bringing order out of chaos both in the universe and in our own thinking. Logically enough it has been a method used by psychiatrists from the earliest times to attempt to understand the mystery of mental illness. Many classifications were composed which endeavor to explain different mental illnesses and relate one to another and all of them to other types of illness. Details of these efforts are given in the Appendix, but we list a few of them here. Each classification, however, seems to provoke ardent adherents and ardent objectors. Several of the more conspicuous revolts are mentioned—the clinical, the rationalist, the pragmatic, and the positivistic. Most of these were European. Several American classifications are discussed.

From a study of these it seems to the authors very evident that there has been a steady trend toward simplification and a reduction of the categories from thousands to hundreds to dozens to a mere four or five. We have carried this forward to the logical implication that perhaps there is only one class of mental illness—namely, mental illness. We propose that all the names so solemnly applied to various classical forms and stages and aspects of mental illness in various individuals be discarded. But in doing so we do not forget the dangers implicit in simplification and reduction. We shall bear these in mind in striving for greater simplicity, greater clarity, greater usefulness.

MANY DRY river beds in central Arizona are filled with pebbles and rock fragments of infinite variety, resulting from earth-crust disturbances centuries ago. Once in such a spot I watched a little girl playing with attractive specimens selected from the millions of stones around her. She made little piles, first of all the white pebbles, then the red pebbles, the black pebbles, the multi-colored pebbles. But many were left which were of no dominant color. So she started again; she put the sharp-cornered pebbles in one pile and the round pebbles in another. Then she tried putting all the longish stones in one pile, the flat ones in a second pile, the chunky ones in a third pile. But this didn't work either, and by this time she was tired of playing and went into the house.

Of course the little girl had no objective purpose in her classification;

she was merely trying to comply with some inner demand for order which, like hope, seems to spring early as well as eternal in the human breast. Perhaps, too, she was attempting to gain some understanding of these little pieces of the universe by discovering classes in which individual specimens had membership. She was using common-sense methods to do this, and she was having the same difficulties which a more sophisticated person using scientific knowledge would have had. She knew nothing about mineralogy, or she might have sorted out the quartz, the obsidian, the calcite, the granite, the conglomerate; but she would still have been overwhelmed by the complexity of her task.

One can imagine that another little girl, coming upon the incomplete piles of stone which her predecessor had left behind, might have continued the game with the help of the relics left by the first little girl. With the accidental discovery of a few quite different stones—let us say some amethysts—perhaps she would have made a more comprehensive and slightly more pretentious schema. Then we can imagine her calling her mother or some other child to see what she had done, to admire, perchance to criticize or scorn or imitate! They might seek to further the process of piling and identifying and classifying. But in time, like those who had preceded, they would fall asleep, leaving behind them little heaps of similar pebbles.

Such are one's reflections in looking back over the arches of the centuries to read the records left by our colleagues in their efforts to bring order out of the chaos of the phenomena of madness. The pictures of broken or inept living are symbolized in tens of thousands of designations, classes, orders, and groups, painstakingly put together only to be taken apart, rearranged, and ultimately discarded by later generations. These names read like the epitaphs on tombstones, to be read with the same sober reflections that life is short and art long, that our grasp of human phenomena is limited and narrow and our concepts are changing and unclear.

The correlating of general knowledge with particular knowledge in the interests of helping a patient is the essence of diagnosis. Diagnosis always relates more to the patient than to the disease, either to *his* disease or *the* disease in general. The need to particularize regarding the affliction of the individual patient is paralleled by a need to generalize, from the afflictions of this and other patients, regarding pathology and illness in the abstract. Such abstractions make up the substance of medical science.

The making of logical abstractions and deductions from observations is one of the methods of science, as is the process of classification. These are ways of bringing order into our thinking about large numbers of particular data. Our Appendix amply demonstrates how taxonomy and nosology have occupied the attention of psychiatrists, who resemble the little girl grouping and regrouping her pebbles. I myself, the senior author, must confess participation in this attempt to better define, label, and classify psychiatric syndromes. Someone has suggested that this is almost an avocation—a veritable addiction—of psychiatrists, this defining new syndromes and reordering them. A month never passes but what a few new psychiatric syndromes are announced in the literature, and yet they are not really new.

A famous colleague [1] once wrote a textbook of psychiatry in which he listed 2400 species of mental diseases! But three years later, after additional clinical experience, he republished the book and had reduced these 2400 to four main ones! It suddenly occurred to me that perhaps something like this happens in the life of every young psychiatrist. At first every patient is completely *sui generis*. Each one seems to be the first case of its kind ever seen on earth. But then the doctor begins to see some similarities to others in a category of illness to which a name has been ascribed. Gradually the common thread becomes more apparent and individual differentiations less important.

And just as this characterizes the experience of the individual psychiatrist, so it has characterized the entire history of the science, as the lists in the Appendix demonstrate. The phenomena of mental illness were always puzzling and mysterious. And one must bear in mind too that they were ominous. No one expected a person afflicted with mental illness to recover, although, of course, it was known that they sometimes did. This was mysterious also. But our preoccupation with treatment could scarcely be imagined in the earlier days when the symptomatic phenomena were so variegated and complex and the essential nature of mental illness so little understood.

It is logical therefore that scientists approaching the data of mental illness adhered to the basic method of science and perhaps one of the basic methods of all human thought. They felt obliged to bring some kind of order into the apparent chaos. Driven by this urge, and greatly stimulated by the pattern set by Linnaeus, they sought to understand this puzzling face of nature.

It is not merely pebbles or symptoms or leaf buds that we classify. All data, all the facts in the universe, can be classified and indeed have been. Over thirty years ago a news item caught my eye regarding a classification offered by Professor Harlow Shapley which "placed" in an order everything in the known universe, based essentially on size. Beginning with a hypothetical "something" pervading the universe, smaller than anything else and to which a rank of −7 is given, the Shapley system was:

−7 (*Something pervading all?*)
−6 *Corpuscles*
    (A something here?)
    Quanta
    Protons
    Electrons
−5 *Atoms* (hydrogen to uranium)
−4 *Molecules* (1 to infinity)
−3 *Molecular Aggregates*
    Crystals
    Colloids
−2 *Colloidal & Crystal Aggregates*
    Inorganic substances (e.g., minerals, meteorites, clouds)
    Organic substances (vegetable and animal worlds)
−1 *Meteoritic Associations*
    Comets
    Meteor streams
    Diffuse nebulae
0 *Satellitic Systems*
    Earth-moon type
    Jovian type
    Saturnian type

+1 *Planetary Structures*
    (Earth belongs here)
    Stars, with corona & meteors
    Stars, with planets, comets, etc.
    (The Sun belongs here)
    Stars with nebulous rings or envelopes
+2 *Double & Multiple Stars*
+3 *Galactic Clusters*
    (e.g., "The Milky Way")
+4 *Globular Clusters*
+5 *Star Clouds*
+6 *Galaxies*
+7 *Super-Galaxies*
+8 *Groups of Super-Galaxies*
+9 *The Cosmoplasma*
    Interstellar gas
    Interstellar electrons & protons
    Radiation
    (Loose energy?)
+10 *The Universe*
    (Einstein's space-time complex)
+11 (*Something enveloping all?*) [2]

I wrote to Professor Shapley about this recently and he very kindly sent me a "revised edition," a tentative offering for the "classification of material systems." Size is still the basis of the first grouping, and subsequent groupings vary. The basis of the subdivisions is indicated by the symbols used in their ordinal list. Thus Greek letters indicate that the differences between classes are largely dependent on differences in basic nature. Arabic numerals indicate differences largely dependent on size or mass. Roman numerals stand for differences largely dependent on structure, and English alphabet letters for differences largely dependent on the position of the observer. I submit this classification as the work of a master and an illustration of the compelling urge of a great scientist who has himself added much to human knowledge.

−5 . . . . .
−4 *Corpuscles* (*Fundamental Particles*)
    α . . . . ζ . Positrons
    β . Radiation quanta η . Mesons, 1 to x
    γ . Electrons θ . Neutrinos
    δ . Protons ι . Antineutrinos ?
    ε . Neutrons κ . Negatrons

−3 *Atoms*
o to 100 +

−2 *Molecules*
1 to n

−1 *Molecular Systems*
    I. Crystals
    II. Colloids

  o *Colloidal and Crystallic Aggregates*
    α . Inorganic (minerals, meteorites, etc.)
    β . Organic (organisms, colonies, etc.)

+1 *Meteoritic Associations*
    1. Meteor Streams
    2. Comets
    3. Coherent Nebulosities

+2 *Satellitic Systems*
    I. Earth-Moon Type
    II. Jovian Type
    III. Saturnian Type

+3 *Stars and Star Families*
    α . Stars with Secondaries
        I. With Coronae, Meteors, and Comets
        II. With Nebulous Envelopes
        III. With Planets and Satellites

    β . Stars with Equals
        I. Close Pairs (or Multiples)
          a. Eclipsing
          b. Spectroscopic
        II. Wide Pairs (or Multiples)
          (α) Gravitational
          [(β) Optical]
        III. Motion Affiliates

+4 *Stellar Clusters*
    α . Open
      [a. Field Irregularities]
      b. Associations
      c. Loose Groups
      d. Compact Groups
      e. Dense Groups
    β . Globular
        I. Most Concentrated
        II. . . . . . .
        . . . .
        XII. Least Concentrated

+5 *Galaxies*
    A. Bright
        I. Irregular (I)

    II. Spiral (S)
       α . Abnormal (Sp)
       β . Barred (SB)
           (I) Open (SBc)
           (II) Medium (SBb)
          (III) Concentrated (SBa)
       γ . Regular (S)
           (I) Arms Very Wide (Sd)
           (II) Arms Wide (Sc)
          (III) Arms Close (Sb)
          (IV) Arms Very Close (Sa)
    III. Spheroidal (E)
       a. Most Elongated (E_7)
       b. Less Elongated ($E6$)
       . . . .
       g. Least Elongated (E_1)
       h. Circular Outline (E_0)
  B. Faint (Bruce classification)
    Concentration and Shape
    a_1 a_2 a_3 . . . . a_{10}
    b_1 b_2 b_3 . . . . b_{10}

    . . . .
    f_1 f_2 f_3 . . . . f_{10}

+6 *Galaxy Aggregations*
    1. Doubles
    2. Groups
    3. Clusters
    4. Clouds
    [5. Field Irregularities]

+7 *The Metagalaxy*
    α . Organized Sidereal Bodies and Systems
       1. Meteors   4. Stars
       2. Satellites   5. Clusters
       3. Planets   6. Galaxies
    β . The Cosmoplasma or Matrix
       (α) . *Interstellar Particles*
           1. Cosmic Dust and Meteors
           2. Diffused Nebulosity (dark)
       (β) . *Interstellar Gas*
           1. Corpuscles
           2. Atoms
           3. Molecules
       (γ) . *Radiation*
       (δ) . . . . . .

+8 *The Universe: Space-Time Complex*

+9 . . . .

The Functions and Fallacies of Classification

Classifications owe their existence, as Riese has neatly put it, to an economizing principle of the human intellect. "Indeed," he said, "if we were to renounce classifications and deliberately restrict our descriptions and actions to individual experiences, we would not only at the same time denounce science as an articulated whole, thus as a system of experiences, but we would also condemn ourselves to treat every new experience as the first one, not using previous experiences of the same or of an analogous kind. Our intellect would be overburdened by an ever-renewed start *ab ovo*, and increase in knowledge would be at a very slow rate. Since individuals of the same species have very much in common, an analysis of our experiences on exclusively individual grounds would mean endless repetitions and reiterations denounced already by Aristotle." [3]

But there are many pitfalls, fallacies, and sources of error implicit in the irrepressible work of classification. These have been of particular interest to our colleague Henri Ellenberger, who suggests that the kinds of classes established with the grouping of phenomena may be unconsciously determined by factors quite other than some objective facts intrinsic in the data classified, for example, by social traditions or assumptions inextricably impressed in the classifier's view of the world. Again, these social determinants may be apparent in prevalent customs or in prevalent philosophies or even in the language itself. Language is already in *itself* a form of classification because of the categories of thought implied in grammar and syntax. It is not by chance that grammar and logic were founded in India and Greece by thinkers who were using two of the most perfectly structured existing languages: Sanskrit and ancient Greek.*

---

* We cannot here follow the multiple implications of psycho-linguistics for classification and will content ourselves by mentioning only one instance: In a remarkable paper published in 1916, Ernest Southard proposed that the delusions of mental patients could be expressed in terms of the grammatical categories of our language. Delusions of grandeur represent the first person singular, passive voice. Significant differences were found in the delusions if they corresponded to the second or to the third person (in the former case they had a greater intensity and dramatic quality). Very important differences were connected to the "moods" (indicative, imperative, subjunctive, optative) of the verbs. (Southard, E. E. "On the Application of Grammatical Categories to the Analysis of Delusions." *Philosophical Review*, 25:424–455, 1916.)

One has to concede that many classifications are worse than useless. Too often names and classifications seem to have served only to rationalize the attitude of one group of individuals toward another. The roles of classification in the bloodshed of the Christian-infidel, Catholic-heretic, Aryan-Jew, colored-white controversies might be recalled. These classifications seemed real, valid, even scientific in their day, and were defended just as vehemently as "criminal psychopath" and "process schizophrenia" are defended by some today.

A new classification can be very fruitful, therefore, if it helps put old observations in a new light and generates new questions for research. But no classification can be any better than the classifier's knowledge and understanding of the observations he is classifying.

Ancient Classifications of Mental Illness

While the Children of Israel were still in Egypt and the Greeks three hundred years away from their Trojan exploit, classifications of mental derangement were being recorded in India; seven kinds of demoniacal possession were distinguished. The Old Testament records of six or eight centuries later contain various descriptive accounts of mental illness, and madness began to appear frequently in the mythical tales of the Greeks. Hippocrates recognized four—possibly six—syndromes. (See page 420.)

Less cautious observers both preceded and followed Hippocrates, and religious and mystical explanations of mental illness persisted for many centuries. Studies of many primitive disease concepts suggest that there are probably only five main types: sorcery, soul loss, taboo breach, and either spirit or object intrusion.[4] Plato recognized two broad categories of illnesses: those of natural origin and those of supernatural (divine) origin. Four hundred years later Celsus and Galen tried to replace religious and mystical explanations of disease with somatogenic concepts or, as we would say today, physio-chemical concepts. They systematized the medical knowledge extant at the time and listed all the known syndromes, classified anatomically. A classification into acute and chronic diseases had been used by Soranus and Caelius Aurelianus.[5]

A millennium later, in the famous *Malleus Maleficarum* (*The Witches' Hammer*, 1489), a catalogue of witchcraft appeared. The hands of two zealous but misguided Dominicans with political and ecclesiastical authority soon displaced the humoralism, solidism, systematic description, and other explanations in favor of superstitious demonology. Some of these *stigmata diaboli* were still pointed out by instructors while I was a student in medical school (1917). "Satanic fugacity" was not given a psychological explanation, according to Zilboorg,[6] until Bernheim explained the phenomenon in terms of suggestion (1885). Demonism was destroyed scientifically in 1563 by the courageous Swiss Johann Weyer [7] in his famous *De Prestigiis Daemonum* (*On the Trickery of Demons*), in which he sided with the accused witches, as it were, and described them as sick. It was a big step forward when Weyer began to reconsider the various forms of strange behavior as illness, as the Greek and Roman physicians before him had done, and to name them anew, however fantastically. It was a move away from superstition, even though disease names came to be regarded almost as were the witches before them, with a kind of awe, unquestioning acceptance, and undying persistence.

But it was two hundred years after Weyer before psychiatry in the modern sense began to be a regular part of medical science. It seems to have become such partly from the continual shuffling and reshuffling of symptoms into various tentative syndromes and proposed disease entities, and partly from an arising sense of public concern leading to the extension of humane principles even to the mad, and partly from the continued dilemma regarding the nature of the lesser forms of psychiatric illness for which William Cullen, Professor of Medicine at Edinburgh, coined the term "neuroses" in 1769.[8] Cullen and Hughlings Jackson, who followed Cullen, believed that "our concern as physicians is simply to get to know what is wrong with the nervous system. . . . Our concern as medical men is with the body. If there is such a thing as a disease of the mind we can do nothing for it." [9] *

But physicians were supposed, and indeed believed themselves, to be able to distinguish one condition of madness from another. Once the witch theory, which led to the slaughter of hundreds of thousands of afflicted ones, was at long last dispelled, physicians began to coin other names for the varying pictures of queer behavior, partly to master their own fear and partly to serve as a kind of communication and classification

---

* This view, as Stengel ("The Origin and the Status of Dynamic Psychiatry," *Brit. J. Med. Psychol.*, 27:193–200, 1954) has said, was "shared by most of Jackson's colleagues, even by those more intimately concerned with mental illness than himself, for instance, Maudsley (1867)." And these views are still held by most neurologists and some psychiatrists today. The contrast between them and those held by modern psychiatrists, whatever their attitude to psychoanalysis, is evidence of what Zilboorg and Henry called "the second psychiatric revolution." Curiously enough, as Stengel has shown, Jackson had a profound influence on Sigmund Freud, who, of course, had precisely the opposite conception.

device. In this way many magical designations were invented, some of which still persist, carrying with them the old connotations.

Through the subsequent centuries, thousands of names were proposed for the various forms of "madness," "lunacy," "insanity," "psychosis," "dementia," and "mania." Various pictures of disturbed existence were described by doctors in various parts of the world, usually with some administrative significance in mind, e.g., the decision whether to confine the victims or not. It was important to recognize which patients were dangerous, which merely helpless, which likely to die soon. Some might perchance "come to" quickly and be themselves again.

The Clinical Revolt

Until the middle of the seventeenth century observers were restricted in their thinking by preconceived theories, by firmly entrenched traditions of thinking and procedure, and by much metaphysical speculation. Thomas Sydenham (1624–1689) brought some order out of chaos by forcefully adopting a simple, fresh, consistent view of illness. He rejected all the speculations of the humoralists, who proposed that disease was the expression of various mixtures of body fluids, and of the solidists, who held that disease was due to laxity and tension in bodily organs. There were also groups called systematists, rationalists, and others. Sydenham became a vigorous advocate of clinical empiricism and of specificity in the concept of disease. He believed in the existence of large numbers of diseases and touched off an enthusiastic search for them. He advocated careful description and classification, in a way anticipating Linnaeus, who came nearly a century later, in emphasizing the relationship later to be known as genus and species.

In this way Sydenham put an end to the Galenic tradition in medicine, which had become stultifying, and successfully broke its grip upon medical thinking and research. He inspired a new surge of investigation by careful, unprejudiced observation which earned him the name of the modern Hippocrates. But this new impetus was still pathetically lacking in any useful etiological concepts (Sydenham deprecated "concepts" and "hypotheses") and was almost predestined to get stuck in the obsessional morass of nosological complexity which took hold of nineteenth-century psychiatry. The nosologies which evolved following Sydenham became increasingly differentiated, empirical, and sterile.

The Rationalist Revolt

The impetus behind the rationalist movement in taxonomy came from the great philosophical and cultural movement of the Enlightenment. The best representative work of this movement was the famous French encyclopedia published by Diderot and d'Alembert. Several articles on mental disease in the encyclopedia organized mental illnesses according to an essentially psychological system: weakness or diminution of understanding and memory, confusion of reason, delusion without fever or fury, delusion without fever but with fury, acute mental disturbance with both fever and fury, and complete abolition of the reasoning faculty.

One of the last of the leaders of the Enlightenment, and its most famous, was the philosopher Immanuel Kant. In 1798 he published a kind of compendium of philosophical psychology under the title *Anthropology in Pragmatic Regard*. In it, as a rather supplementary chapter, is a short treatise on "the weaknesses and sicknesses of the soul in regard to its faculty of cognition." His classification of disorders in that chapter referred to total weakness in the *cognitive faculty* such as is found in idiocy, and partial weaknesses such as lack of wit, of judgment, of comprehension, of attention, lack of ability to distinguish between the valuable and the worthless, and offensive foolishness. Under sicknesses *of the soul* he included hypochondria, disturbances in mood, and melancholia, which he defined as "a delusion of misery created by the gloomy person." Finally, as distinct from disturbances in mood, he identified disturbances of *Gemüt*, including "amentia," "dementia," "insanity," and "vesania." The rationalists offered a more comprehensible system, but an essentially logical-psychological scheme without any etiological pretensions, and their devotion to logic was necessarily accomplished at the expense of careful empirical nosography.

The Pragmatic Revolt

Some physicians had little stomach for either the classical theoretical speculations or the Sydenham empiricism and collecting. One of them, Joseph Daquin (1733–1815), was a physician, a naturalist, and a librarian, and at the age of fifty-four became the medical director of an asylum full

of patients whom he knew little about but was determined to handle
well. He studied them actively and later published a book, *The Philosophy of Madness* (1791). In this he made the following highly practical
if unsophisticated classification:

1. Madness which requires restraints   4. The stupid and silly
2. Madness which is quiet   5. Imbeciles and cretins
3. The whimsical   6. Dementia

Philippe Pinel is perhaps the best example of this pragmatic reaction
in nosography. While still a professor, he constructed an elaborate sys-
tematization of the mental and physical illnesses, following the ideas of
Boissier de Sauvages, a physician and botanist who had bettered Linnaeus
and classified all diseases into 10 classes with 295 genera and about 2400
species. One of these 10 classes included mental diseases and was subdivided into 4 orders and 23 genera. This system was published in 1798.

Three years later, following his appointment as superintendent of a
large psychiatric hospital, Pinel came forth with an extremely simple
nosology consisting of only *four* fundamental clinical types! One can
scarcely imagine a more prompt revisionist reaction to ivory-tower theorizing. (See page 443.)

"In spite of his classificatory tendencies, he advocated the study of the
undisturbed, i.e., natural, course of disease. This was true Hippocratism.
In fact, Hippocratic medicine had no use for disease entities and diagnoses. That Pinel, when facing the insane [man], as an *individual*, deprived him temporarily of his diagnosis or his *nosologic* stigma, was a
masterstroke. He then experienced him simply as a human being in distress, excitement, anxiety, hostility, humiliation." [10] *

A contemporary of Pinel's in Italy, Chiarugi, reduced the types of
mental illnesses to three, and a successor, Esquirol (1772–1840), extended
them merely to five. Most observers went in the opposite direction, impressed by the wide variety of symptoms, and so extending and complicating the list of mental diseases. The great names of psychiatric history
are all associated with special nosologies, each expressing certain em-
phases or concepts. The reader is recommended to consult at this point
pages 424–464 of the Appendix in order to gain a more accurate idea of
the extent and variety of these classifying activities.

Concerning this essentially "unitary" concept of mental illness, which
Kahlbaum, Rush, Griesinger, and others echoed, we shall have more to

---

* Ilza Veith makes the point that as a matter of fact Pinel's classification was in
part inspired by his desire to enhance his patients' recovery by grouping them in
separate lodgings according to their illnesses. (Veith, Ilza. "Philippe Pinel and the
Moral Treatment of Insanity." *Modern Medicine*, 28:212–216, September 1960.)

say presently; these early "flirtations" with it were ineffectual and forgotten until the nineteenth-century tide of pluralism had run its course. The search for specific diseases with specific causes touched off by Sydenham had gained momentum with the new discoveries in the laboratory. This search was to dominate psychiatry for another hundred years and culminate in a therapeutic nihilism from which psychiatry is only now emerging.

The Positivistic Revolt

Sydenham was so convinced of the specificity of illness that the bacteriological discoveries nearly two centuries after his death made him seem like a great prophet. The late renaissance in medicine seemed to center about this proposition that illnesses were the specific products of specific events. Then, in psychiatry, three other nineteenth-century discoveries fanned the hopes that a search for specific connections was on the verge of a major break-through in this still darkened area of medical science. These were the discovery by Paul Broca that certain forms of aphasia were correlated with definite loci of cortical injury, by Bayle that general paresis was indeed a brain disease, and by Richard von Krafft-Ebing that syphilis was related to this syndrome. The enthusiastic positivistic spirit of the nineteenth century imbued many scientists with the conviction that only in the search for the tangible could science free itself from the metaphysical speculations of the philosophers. And brain lesions were *tangible* and tangible things could be classified.

Medicine Becomes a Science

For hundreds of years medical dogma could not be altered. "Galen knows everything, has an answer for everything. He confidently pictures the origin of all diseases and outlines their cure. He is the incarnation, perhaps for the first time in history, of the physician who regards himself as omniscient and whose attitude of authority emanates from every act and every word." [11] Whitehead [12] has described the seductive tendency to assume that "mankind has consciously entertained all the fundamental ideas which are applicable to its experience [and that] human language, in single words or phrases, explicitly expresses those ideas." Once there *was* "a perfect dictionary" of medical matters; it lasted for a thousand

years, a millennium during which the average life expectancy of p
was about thirty-five years! When Galen's formulations were replace
empirical diagnosis, the way was opened for the creative studies that h
helped to bring the average life expectancy to nearly seventy years.
a way one might say that the basis of this great success lay in the discarding
of the fantasy of the perfect dictionary. Instead, the scientific method of
collecting, correlating, classifying data was introduced into medicine. The
construction of hypotheses was made for the purpose of testing them
and, if necessary, rejecting or altering them.

The great advance of medical science in the eighteenth and nineteenth
centuries can be attributed to this development of the scientific method,
including classification, to the general intellectual awakening, and to
mechanical discoveries. A few new instruments for treatment procedures
were invented, but the big advance was in diagnostic tools. The microscope,* the stethoscope, the clinical thermometer, the ophthalmoscope,

---

* It is a curious historical fact that the serious use of the microscope in medicine
was delayed for many years after its discovery by Zacharias Hanssen in 1590. Five
great seventeenth-century microscopists—Malpighi, Swammerdam, Hooke, Grew, and
Leeuwenhoek—remained without effective followers until the nineteenth century.
This long lag is a remarkable fact awaiting adequate explanation.

One reason for the lag appears to have been an intellectual resistance of rather
complex composition. Sydenham (and his friend John Locke) opposed Francis
Bacon, Robert Boyle, and Robert Hooke in regard to the basis of effective medical
practice. Sydenham and Locke held that little acquaintance with anatomical structure was required.

"Sydenham's humoral theory of disease is the other important reason for his
damnation of microscopy.

" 'By diligent research during dissections, and by careful scrutiny, we may attain
to the knowledge of those larger organs by which Nature conducts her more visible
operations. . . . *What, however, neither human eye will see, nor microscope disclose*, is the origin and primary cause of such movements. What microscope, however exquisitely elaborate, shall make visible those minute pores by which . . . the
chyle passes from the intestines to the chyliferous vessels? Or what microscope
shall exhibit those ducts through which the blood, conducted by the arteries, is
passed onwards to the orifices of the veins?' (Latham, R. G. *The Works of Thomas
Sydenham* (2 vol.). London: The Sydenham Soc., 1848–1850, Vol. 1, p. 171.)

"Sydenham asked these questions *two decades after* Malpighi had described capil-
laries with his microscope, an observation of such theoretical importance that it
alone might have insured the continued use of that instrument in biological investigation, in the absence of intellectual resistance. It took an electron microscope to
'make visible those minute pores by which . . . the chyle passes from the intestines to the chyliferous vessels.' "

Said Sydenham: "Now it is certaine and beyond controversy that nature performes
all her operations on the body by parts so minute and insensible that I thinke noe
body will ever hope or pretend, even by the assistance of glasses . . . , to come to a
sight of them . . . and though we cut into these inside, we see but the outside
of things and make but a new superficies for ourselves to stare at." (Wolfe, David E.

and all the appurtenances and procedures of the chemical laboratory were added to the diagnostic armamentarium of the physician. A little later came the X-ray, the electrocardiograph, the electroencephalograph, and the Wassermann test.

In addition to these technical instruments, the expanded business of publishing and the growth of libraries greatly improved communication between living scientists and provided readier access to the recorded wisdom of predecessors.

From this hasty survey of medical advances in the nineteenth century one can see that most of the great discoveries in the medical field were not therapeutic measures but diagnostic procedures. Diagnosis began (again) to be important, but diagnosis of a new sort. It was now much more a matter of studying the individual and less a matter of classifying his kind of sickness.

The effort to arrive at a conclusion of some sort regarding a particular illness had always been an essential part of medicine. But it had become obscured by so much humbug, ignorance, uncertainty, and futility that to a considerable degree diagnosis was for a long time perfunctory.

SGANAREL: Here quick, let physicians be got, and in abundance; one can't have too many upon such an accident. Ah, my girl! My poor girl! . . .

LYSETTA: What will you do, sir, with four physicians? Is not one enough to kill any one body?

SGANAREL: Hold your tongue. Four advices are better than one.

LYSETTA: Why, can't your daughter die well enough without the assistance of these gentlemen?

SGANAREL: Do the physicians kill people?

LYSETTA: Undoubtedly; and I knew a man who proved by good reason that we should never say, such a one is dead of a fever, or a catarrh, but she is dead of four doctors and two apothecaries.

SGANAREL: Hush! Don't offend these gentlemen.

LYSETTA: Faith, sir, our cat is lately recovered of a fall she had from the top of the house into the street, and was three days without

---

"Sydenham and Locke on the Limits of Anatomy." *Bull. Hist. Med.*, 35:193–220, 1961.)

We cite this illuminating history of the lag in the use of the microscope and the illogical rationalizations for its neglect in order to show how the concept of illness in exclusively "process" terms could lead to error just as egregious as the errors made by an exclusively structural view of illness. In this volume we explore the advantages and the merits of a process orientation to mental illness but in no sense intend to exclude from consideration the equally significant structural, psychodynamic, and genetic viewpoints regarding illness discussed so effectively by Rapaport and Gill ("The Points of View and Assumptions of Metapsychology." *Int. J. Psa.* 40:153–162, 1959).

either eating or moving foot or paw; but 'tis very lucky for her that there are no cat doctors, for 'twould have been over with her, and they would not have failed purging her and bleeding her.

SCANAREL: Will you hold your tongue, I say? What impertinence is this! Here they come.

LYSETTA: Take care. You are going to be greatly edified; they'll tell you in Latin that your daughter is sick.[13]

Diagnosis ex Machina

But, by the end of the nineteenth and the beginning of the twentieth century, diagnosis once again became a cult. Interest in medical treatment had reached a low ebb. Scientific skepticism and therapeutic nihilism were regnant; it was unscientific and rather obvious to pretend to treat illness. But diagnosis was now a scientific pursuit of high esteem, worthy of the best medical minds.

Typical of the spirit of the time is a handbook—small in its first edition in 1915 but later much enlarged—in which diagnosis is declared to be the most important part of the art of medicine. "He who would excel in it," continues the author, "must be well equipped both mentally and physically." The reader—presumably a young doctor—is then warned of the fallacies of diagnosis. Patients, we are told, fall into four classes: the pessimistic, the optimistic, the complacent, and the mendacious. These temperaments affect diagnosis. Let the doctor especially beware the Fallacy of Suggestion. Let him beware the Fallacy of Antecedent or Concurrent Disease, the Fallacy of Obsession (i.e., in the doctor's psychology), the Fallacy of too little or too broad Perspective, the Fallacy of Malingering, the Fallacy of the Personal Equation, and the Fallacy of Variations within the Normal! (The nature of the fallacies referred to may be inferred from the titles.)

After these cautionaries, the author lists in column after column the different conditions (i.e., diseases) in which various individual symptoms may occur. A soft and compressible pulse is to be found in anemia, aneurysm, aortitis, asphyxia, asthma, broncho-pneumonia, cholera, delirium tremens, diphtheria, glanders, and many other diseases; a full or large pulse is to be found in aortic regurgitation, cerebral concussion, erysipelas, pericarditis, and acute rheumatic fever. In such fashion the book proceeds through a list of approximately two thousand symptoms.[14]

The logical extension of this kind of thinking is to the use of mathematical devices. If the patient has, let us say, five symptoms, one can look up each of these symptoms and find which disease is so characterized under all five headings. Then, *voilà!* the diagnosis! This has been worked out in a practical(?) way by a number of people; for example, a British surgeon has invented what he calls a Logoscope, or a slide-rule "Grouped Symbol Associator." [15]

Other colleagues have derived "an equation of conditional probability . . . to express the logical process used by a clinician in making a diagnosis from clinical data. Solutions of this equation take the form of a differential diagnosis. The probability that each disease represents the correct diagnosis in any particular patient may be calculated. Sufficient statistical data regarding the incidence of clinical signs, symptoms, and electrocardiographic findings in patients with congenital heart disease have been assembled to allow application of this approach to differential diagnosis in this field. This approach provides a means by which electronic computing equipment may be used to advantage in clinical medicine." [16] And an editorial in the *Journal of the American Medical Association* inquires: "Is it possible that the training of large numbers of expert diagnosticians may be unnecessary in the future and that the general practitioner, trained to collect information accurately from his patient and to administer certain forms of treatment expertly, may, with the help of a computer (as accessible as his telephone), handle the bulk of medical practice again?" [17]

This trend in diagnosis *away* from the concept of understanding the afflicted individual and back *toward* the goal of identifying and tabulating "the disease" seems regressive and archaic to us. It implies a precision of findings and a conformity of pathology which do not—in our opinion—exist.

From this long excursion into the history of development of the concepts of illness in general medicine, let us return to the province of psychiatry, with which we are primarily concerned. Let us see how the developments of its diagnostic procedures and concepts of pathology parallel those of general medicine.

When psychiatry was at long last gingerly allowed standing room in the temple of medical science, its practitioners adhered faithfully to the orthodox dogma of the parent body. They were neurologists, specialists in the structure and functions of the nervous system. They sought to discover disease entities corresponding to brain lesions of various kinds and loci. They applied names to their discoveries. Even more than in general medicine, an official label became the chief end of diagnosis. It gave a sense of definiteness and partial security in an area of great strange-ness and mystery. Only a poet would dare ask, "What is true madness but to be nothing else but mad?" Scientists must know what madness is; they must call it by name. Physical suffering could occur in silence, or even if noticed could lead to medical attention, but madness was apt to be both conspicuous and untreatable—and above all, incomprehensible.

One of the more influential advocates of this positivist philosophy was Griesinger, who left his mark on all German psychiatry. With his slogan that "mental diseases are brain diseases" Griesinger declared war against the survivors of the old philosophical and psychological schools of psychiatry. For him and his successors, such as Meynert and Wernicke, brain anatomy was the one firm basis for psychiatry. Where brain lesions were not demonstrable under the microscope, vascular, nutritional, or other functional disorders of the brain were to be assumed.

This proliferation and direction of research in psychiatry in the nine-teenth century reached its zenith in the monumental achievements of Emil Kraepelin. Most of the nosologic systems of his contemporaries and successors were derivatives of Kraepelin's system. By insisting on the case-study method, a careful study of the course of each mental disorder in each individual case, Kraepelin succeeded in integrating psychiatry into the field of general medicine, an achievement which had been the goal and ideal of psychiatric workers since the time of Hippocrates.

In the Appendix will be found the changing classifications offered by Emil Kraepelin in the nine successive editions of his textbook. These came to influence the official classifications used in many countries, but by no means all of them. Neither the French nor the British psychiatrists were so impressed by them as were the Americans, to whom Kraepelin's system was introduced by Adolf Meyer. But Meyer came to repent of this and himself developed and offered a nosology based on a unitary principle of *ergasia*. The various classical syndromes he considered to be various "reaction types," various patterns of misdirected energy. His holistic personality theory (unfortunately christened psychobiology) was supported by the eloquent psychiatric leader William Alanson White, and these two systems developed in American psychiatry side by side—the specific entity concept of Kraepelin and the unitary concept which Meyer [18] developed. (See pages 457–468.)

Opposition to Kraepelin's system came also from Ernest Southard, who protested that its genera and species were poorly organized, illogically related, and unrealistically detailed. He ridiculed the idea of a hundred or more diagnostic entities, which the American Psychiatric Association had felt obliged to reduce (in 1917) to twenty-one principal types. South-ard proposed reducing the major groups of mental illnesses to eleven categories, arranged in the order of our then definitive diagnostic knowl-edge of them. Southard's untimely death prevented his pushing this move toward simplification, and the American Psychiatric Association *increased* its list (in 1934) to twenty-four main groups with eighty-two subdivisions!

A definite turning of the tide in the direction of simplification came from the work of my brother, William Menninger, in the Surgeon General's office of the Army (1945). The official 1934 classification of the American Psychiatric Association had led to confusion and incon-sistent handling of patients, which in the armed services was a matter of national concern. My brother conferred with many colleagues regarding a new classification which would be consistent, practical, and in line with the newer (Freudian) theories of personology and psychodynamics. The classification proposed had to run the gamut of military and civilian concurrences, with the result that many compromises and modifications were introduced. As it finally emerged [19] it included five main groups of psychiatric illness:

1. Acute, amorphous states of *disorganization*
2. Psychotic *reactions*: schizophrenic, paranoid, affective, and organic
3. Neurotic *reactions*
4. Personality *deformities*
5. *Defect states* (mental retardation, feeble-mindedness, infantilism)

At first sight it may seem as if the real issues of psychiatric taxonomy had been evaded, since it was the subdivisions of the "psychotic" group which mainly preoccupied the older psychiatrists. But that was precisely the virtue of my brother's innovation. It put the extreme phenomena of clinical psychiatry into a position relative to other clinical pictures. Furthermore, it emphasized the fact that some phenomena were sympto-matic *reactions* rather than disease *entities*.

Perhaps of all the fine achievements of the Psychiatric Division of the Surgeon General's office during World War II, nothing exceeded in its long-range importance the introduction of this new nomenclature and classification. Imperfect as they were, they represented an enormous advance over those in use prior to 1945. Many years had been required for the Kraepelinian system to become established, but, once established, it had seemed as immovable as the mountains. Yet within two or three years following the adoption of my brother's classification by the Army Medical Corps in 1945, it was in general use throughout the country, having been adopted by the Veterans Administration in 1946 and by the Navy in 1947.*

The Trend from Pluralism and Ontology to Monism

Looking back, then, to the days of Hippocrates and since, we see how psychiatric nosology, after modest beginnings, gradually expanded and increased in differentiation until it reached gigantic proportions, then reversed the trend and progressively contracted to shorter and shorter length. What is needed, of course, is not a list which is "long" or "short" for arbitrary reasons, but one which is adequate. We argue, in the remainder of this book, for a simplified, indeed a unified "list," on the ground that it does two things better than the old nosologies: (1) it better corresponds to the nature of all illness; and (2) it does more justice to the intricacies of the particular psychiatric afflictions in the particular individual.

In each generation since Paracelsus there have been a few who caught a glimpse of mental illness as a process in flux rather than as a motley collection of bizarre entities. We propose to follow these visionary predecessors, abandoning the old names and listings, not because some of them do not have a certain usefulness in communication but because they are based on obsolete concepts of the human personality and of the vicissitudes which have been called illness.

Many classical designations were of course practical, administrative descriptions rather than scientific concepts. But it is always difficult to free ourselves from the misleading implications that become attached to labels, not necessarily put there by their originators, but often added

---

* My brother began work on this enormous task almost immediately after taking over the psychiatric responsibilities in the Surgeon-General's office, using some material that he and I had developed at the Menninger Clinic. Nomenclature was of crucial importance to the armed services because the diagnostic terms had direct implications for discharging men from service. After many meetings of his staff, drafts were submitted to nearly two hundred colleagues, most of whom replied with various suggestions and minor criticisms but in the main strong endorsement. Nevertheless, the classification encountered vigorous opposition at first in the American Psychiatric Association. It was not until 1948 that the Committee on Nomenclature and Statistics and subsequently the American Psychiatric Association approved and adopted it. Since then the Committee on Nomenclature and Statistics has made numerous improvements. A fuller discussion of my brother's classification and its vicissitudes is given in the Appendix, pages 474–476.

gradually by their users. This is true even when the old label is replaced with a new model or the concept revised. Here the principle of psychological inertia seems to act.

"Nothing seems to be more refractory and more resistant," wrote Riese, "than the ontological * view of disease. While it was true that nobody believed any longer in spirits and demons as invaders of the diseased individual, very few resisted (and still resist) the temptation of isolating in their thought the disease from the individual himself. Ontology, an offspring of magic and demoniacal medicine, reappeared in the new shape of disease entities." [20]

The notion that there were disease entities which could be discovered and defined and delimited and confirmed by various tests—this notion set psychiatrists off on one kind of wild-goose chase. One name after another was applied to the special proprietary delimitations of some highly articulate or compulsive describer. A hundred names have been applied throughout the ages to the same syndrome; what was called by one generation "hebephrenia," "catatonia," or "onirical delirium" was called by the following generation "dementia praecox" and by the next generation of psychiatrists "schizophrenia." Some of us hope that this generation will solve its name-calling problem by substituting for these appellations the categorical term "mental illness." The failure to recognize the essential characteristics of mental illness persisted in spite of a succession of categorical name changes. "Possession" (demonologic) became "bewitchery," "bewitchery" became "madness," "madness" became "lunacy," "lunacy" became "insanity," "insanity" became "psychosis," a word many of us feel to be no more scientific than the word "bewitched." **

During the second half of the nineteenth century the discoveries of bacteriology, pathological anatomy, and genetics seemed to bring irref-

---

* "Ontology" is a word with somewhat shifting meanings. As here used it implies the notion that a disease is a real and special thing—not a state of being or a state of the organism or a phase of existence or an aspect of functioning or a reaction of the organism but a thing in itself, a concretely demonstrable invasion by some alien force or substance or entity.

** If a patient is poor, said Janet with tongue in cheek, he is committed to a public hospital as "psychotic"; if he can afford the luxury of a private sanitarium, he is put there with the diagnosis of "neurasthenia"; if he is wealthy enough to be isolated in his own home under constant watch of nurses and physicians he is simply an indisposed "eccentric." (Janet, Pierre. *La Force et la faiblesse psychologiques.* Paris: Maloine, 1932.) Janet devoted an entire chapter to a sharp criticism of the current psychiatric classifications. He himself distinguished only two large groups: the organic and the functional. Sometimes, he said, a car stops because the machinery is broken, sometimes because it is out of gasoline. Essentially Janet was a unitarian.

utable confirmation of Trousseau's famous declaration: "The principle of specificity dominates all medicine." [21] The unitary concept of mental illness seemed to be forgotten.

The Unitary Concept

But even while the systematists were elaborating their hundreds and even thousands of orders, classes, genera, and species of mental illness some colleagues strove for simplification and consistency. Georget, Guislain, Zeller, Griesinger, Arndt, Rush, Chiarugi, Esquirol, Heinroth, Morel (in his *first* classification), Pinel (in his *second* classification), Kraepelin, and Adolf Meyer deserve mention for their efforts in this direction.*

Heinrich Neumann was the most outspoken and definite of them all. He felt and declared (in his textbook of 1859) that psychiatric classifications of all kinds were not only artificial and illusory, but directly dangerous. "Rather no classification," he said, "than a false one. The lack of any classification at least leaves free space for investigation, whereas a false classification leads directly into errors! . . . Diagnosis is not simply the designation of a group of symptoms but the key to the comprehension of the case. . . . We [i.e., I] consider any classification of mental illness to be artificial, and therefore unsatisfactory, [and] we do not believe that one can make progress in psychiatry until one has resolved to throw overboard all classifications and declare with us: *there is only one kind of mental illness. . . .*" [22]

Neumann, like the present writers, conceived of a progressive and developmental tendency in mental illness; a first stage of sleeplessness, hypersensitiveness, inattention, and allied symptoms might (or might not) proceed to successive and more severe stages, perhaps on to *Verwirrtheit* (confusion) or even to *Blödsinn* (dementia). But these, he emphasized, were different stages, not different things. (See page 445.)

Almost contemporary with Heinrich Neumann was Hughlings Jackson, "the father of British neurology." Jackson was not only a neurologist but,

---

* It is of historical interest to note that as a part of the reaction against Sydenham's systematicity and the multiplication of syndromes there was a return to the unitary theory of a common pathological state in all forms of illness. One leader in this was Benjamin Rush, who, although an advocate of solidism, held that all disease was due to tension or a lack thereof in bodily systems. This was in 1830. "He was hailed by many as having brought order out of the chaos of nosologies. A long poem to this effect is preserved in the Rush MS in the Library Company of that city." (Shryock, R. H. "Benjamin Rush from the Perspective of the Twentieth Century." *Trans. & Stud. College of Phys. of Phil.*, 14:113–120, 1946.)

in spite of his modest disavowals, he was also a psychiatrist of deep perception, although his ideas "never became part of the recognized teachings of psychiatry, even in Britain." [23] His great influence upon psychiatry was exerted, as Stengel has shown, through Freud. "The close resemblance between Jackson's and Freud's dynamic theories, which has astonished a number of writers (Jones, Grinker, M. Levin, Ey, Angel, and others), can be understood as the result of Freud's encounter with the ideas of Hughlings Jackson."

Jackson has been thus emphasized by us because as far back as 1874 he proposed two types of classification, one for practical purposes, the other for scientific purposes. "He advocated [says Stengel] the ordering of mental diseases according to the degree of the dissolution of functions, i.e. of regression, similar to what Karl Menninger has recommended more recently. . . ."

This unitary view has been consistently supported in the twentieth century by Henri Ey [24] in a form which has been called Neo-Jacksonianism. Ey regards mental illnesses not as disease entities but as syndromes or "pathological reactions" resulting from a multiplicity of factors. He considers these to be the expression of various degrees of dissolution, in Hughlings Jackson's terms. Llopis [25] also concurs in this concept and has recently contributed a history of the unitary concept.*

Concerning a particular syndrome one colleague wrote:

> Much confusion arises from indecision and evasion regarding the name of the syndrome. To my mind, the following designations are more or less synonymous: atypical, prepsychosis, ego deviant, seriously deviant child, infantile anaclitic depression, preschizophrenic, autistic, symbiotic, brain-injured, incipient schizophrenia, pseudo psychosis, pseudo-neurotic psychosis, abnormal child, schizoid personality, impulse-ridden character, and oligophrenia. All are conditions of serious ego disturbance. Indeed, among the large group of nonorganic childhood intellectual retardation or so-called idiopathic mental deficiency, many are also probably symptomatic expres-

---

* Similarly Arndt (1835–1902), whom Bartolomé Llopis of Madrid calls the last defender of the unitary concept in Germany, held that every mental illness follows the same course of evolution, a stage beginning with neurasthenia or melancholia, followed by stages of mania, stupor, and finally dementia. He called this cycle *vesania typica*, and tried to explain this typical evolution of mental illness by Pflüger's "basic biological law" which holds that "feeble stimulations activate vital processes, stimulations of intermediate intensity accelerate them; violent stimulations inhibit and finally paralyze them." Thus, in mental illness, Arndt said, the initial feeble stimulation determines conditions of neurasthenia or melancholia, when the stimulation increases, the conditions turns into mania, and its further increase results in inhibition (stupor) and paralysis (dementia). (Llopis, Bartolomé. "La Psicosis unica." *Arch. de Neurobiol.* 17:1–39, 1954.) The reader will later see how strikingly this anticipated our modern concepts of stress.

sions of early ego maldevelopment. . . . Nevertheless, I favor the straight-forward designation childhood schizophrenia for all these states of ego dis-organization, which is the essence of schizophrenia.[26]

Blau's adjective "straightforward" is not quite the *mot juste* unless one takes the position of colleagues in Research in Schizophrenia Endowment. As an example of something really forthright, listen to this from a personal letter from the director, Stanley Dean: "Unfortunately, the public at large is unable to identify [itself] with 'mental illness' as an omnibus term, and since identification seems to be a necessary psychological concomitant to participation, I selected schizophrenia as the most widely known and most compelling nosological focal point about which to rally public opinion." In other words, "schizophrenia" is used as synonymous with "mental illness." It is clear that we have the same notion, namely, that *severe* mental illness is "schizophrenia" and lesser degrees of mental illness may become greater (i.e., severe) degrees.

This idea that there is but one general category of mental illness is paradoxically corroborated by Szasz, who holds that there is no such thing at all! Mental disease is, he believes, a myth which, like all myths, had certain value and expressed a certain understanding at one time. It was derived by analogy from bodily disorders, long the province of the medical practitioner, and called disease. When the evidences of social and psychological maladjustment in individuals began to come within the purview of physicians, the word "disease" was borrowed for something actually different in nature.[27]

We disagree with Szasz on technical and epistemological grounds. We insist that there are conditions best described as mental illness. But instead of putting so much emphasis on different kinds and clinical pictures of illness, we propose to think of all forms of mental illness as being essentially the same in quality, and differing quantitatively. This is what is meant when we say that all people have mental illness of different degrees at different times, and that sometimes some are much worse, or better. And this is precisely what recent epidemiological studies have demonstrated.

For example, a very careful research project recently completed analyzed the population of a representative sample of American people living in New York City.[28] The area was roughly 200 blocks; the population roughly 175,000. Of these, only about 32,000 (18.5 per cent) showed no symptoms of mental illness. Over 58 per cent gave evidence of mild to moderate mental illness; 23.4 per cent showed marked or severe mental illness. Bear in mind that all individuals under twenty, that is all children, and all individuals over fifty-nine, that is all older people, and all individuals of African or Puerto Rican origins were excluded from the survey. In other words, no one can say that most of the mentally ill were maladjusted adolescents (although there are plenty of them), or confused seniles, or frustrated Negroes or struggling Puerto Ricans. If the troubled individuals in these groups had also been included, the statistics would no doubt have been even more startling.

Gone forever is the notion that the mentally ill person is an exception. It is now accepted that most people have some degree of mental illness at some time, and many of them have a degree of mental illness most of the time. This really should not surprise anyone, for do not most of us have some physical illness some of the time, and some of us much of the time?

The unitary concept does not dispense with the descriptive designations. These we must have if they can be cast in a form that will not deny the essential unity of the process or obscure the understanding of the adaptation difficulties of the patient. The object of the process of diagnostication is not the collecting and sorting of pretty pebbles (although even this may be of some scientific value in large-scale epidemiological studies). It is, rather, to provide a sound basis for formulating a *treatment* program, a planned ameliorative intervention.

For this purpose current nosologies and diagnostic nomenclature are not only useless but restrictive and obstructive. *This does not mean the discarding of useful terminology or syndrome appellations.* To refer to a constellation of symptoms as constituting a schizophrenic picture is very different from referring to the individual presenting these symptoms as a victim of "schizophrenia" or as being "a schizophrenic." Some *symptoms* are by definition "schizophrenic," but no patient is. The same patient may present another syndrome tomorrow.

We do not forget the danger implicit in efforts at simplification. Our friend Benjamin Rush, previously referred to, announced in 1789 that he had "found all schemes of physic [medical treatment] faulty" and sought to evolve "a more simple and consistent system of medicine than the world had yet seen." Seven years later he propounded to his students a system reducing all diseases to one, which of course greatly simplified therapy.

"I have formerly said that there was but one fever in the world," said Rush. "Be not startled, gentlemen; follow me and I will say that there is but one disease in the world!" [29] (See page 444.)

"Unfortunately," comments Norwood, "many physicians . . . accepted [Rush's] theory and went about their professional duties imposing the heroic treatments of purging and bleeding . . . to reduce 'convulsive action' by a process of 'depletion.' " [30]

Here the weakness was not so much the unitary concept of illness proposed, unsound as that was, but the illogical conclusion regarding the indicated therapy. If our efforts to overhaul the concept of mental illness were to result in some unitary blanket therapy, it would be a most deplorable and paradoxical outcome. But it is unlikely.

But, in proposing such a unifying principle for psychiatric nosography, we shall not forget, either, the advice of Alfred North Whitehead: "Distrust the jaunty assurances with which every age prides itself that it at last has hit upon the ultimate concepts in which all that happens can be formulated. The aim of science is to seek the simplest explanations of complex facts. We are apt to fall into the error of thinking that the facts are simple because simplicity is the goal of our quest. The guiding motto in the life of every natural philosopher should be, 'Seek simplicity and distrust it.' " [31]

We shall take this advice—both parts of it. We shall strive for greater simplicity, greater clarity, greater consistency, greater usefulness. But while offering our proposals and formulations for what they may prove to be worth, we shall ourselves not cease to question them nor to listen earnestly to the objections of our critics.

CHAPTER III

The Evolution of Diagnosis

SYNOPSIS: Diagnosis has evolved from its earliest uses in distinguishing and naming individual members of a class to the complicated procedure involved in identifying a classical syndrome in a particular individual. Many of these syndromes, however, appear to have changed so that the old labels no longer fit. Diagnosis has gradually become a matter less of seeking to identify a classical picture and give it a name than of understanding the way in which an individual has been taken with a disability, partly self-imposed and partly externally brought about.

Medicine has made steady advances since the period of the Enlightenment, although the pendulum has tended to swing back and forth between the different methods of diagnosis, since these were based on conflicting concepts of illness.

This is true not only of medical illnesses in general but of psychiatric illnesses. But most of the tendency has been away from name-calling toward an effort to understand and describe the process in a way useful in the rational prescribing of treatment.

PSYCHIATRY IS a branch of medicine, and its methodology was borrowed from medicine, including its diagnostic approach. It will be helpful, therefore, to review the way in which diagnosis and the concept of diagnosis have evolved over the years in the mother specialty and then in psychiatry.

Different forms of sickness were no doubt matters of common knowledge early in human history. No physician was needed to distinguish hemorrhage from fever or skin eruptions from tumorous growths. But the ways in which human beings suffer or falter must have seemed numberless, quite beyond organization or classification. Nevertheless, from a combination of superstition, fantasy, experience, trial-and-error, and finally systematic research, certain distinctions gradually became established. Knowledge about the human body and its afflictions slowly accumulated, at an incalculable cost in dedication and diligence, in suffering and sorrow. There was much "knowledge" that was false, much that was foolish, much that did not survive the trial of the years.

But there was also a core of truth which slowly grew into the great edifice of modern medical science. That life is today longer and safer and fuller, that pain is lessened for millions and death deferred for millions more, that lasting health is the rule rather than the exception (in favored countries)—all this is to be credited to practices and preachments emanating from the shrine of Aesculapius.

The word "edifice" does scant justice to the growing, moving, living body of medical science. As an area of human concern, it is constantly enlarging its scope and its content. As a science, it is subject to continuous change. Its most precious dogmas and its best-established practices are constantly being reviewed, revised, rejected. Each new discovery requires the abandonment of much that was once considered precious. Scores of old remedies are discarded for each new one discovered. Older techniques of prevention seem quaint and trivial when superseded by better ones. They too change, as do the methods of diagnosis. It is this evolution of diagnosis that occupies our attention in this chapter, and the next.

Just what is diagnosis? Is it not a basic process, the essential nature of which has not changed since its earliest use? To diagnose is to differentiate, to distinguish, to designate. It is to recognize, to have knowledge of, or to come to an understanding of. How can this procedure change except to grow sounder and surer? This, indeed, it has done, we believe, but it has grown sounder and surer partly through a change in concepts. This is reflected in the language of diagnosis, the verbal expression of the understanding arrived at.

Naming has long been a feature of diagnosing; giving a name to something implies an acquaintanceship with it. This can be very misleading; an acquaintanceship may be shallow or deep, and there is no easy way of telling which it is. Furthermore, giving a name to something implies a degree of mastery over it. "And Jacob was left alone; and there wrestled a man with him until the breaking of the day. . . . And he said unto him, What is thy name? And he said, Jacob. And he said, Thy name shall be called no more Jacob, but Israel: for . . . thou . . . hast prevailed."

Thousands of names have been given to the various forms of illnesses which people have observed in themselves and their friends or which physicians have observed in their patients. For a long time people have suffered from conditions called colds and fevers, measles and mumps, cancer and pneumonia. There are many names which no one hears any more, such as the sweating sickness, ague, and typhilitis. Medical science has mastered many diseases not by giving them names but by coming to understand their nature. We have many drugs now which quickly control the development of various infections. Preventive medicine and the whole program of public-health measures have made vast reductions in the incidence of illness.

Yet sickness does not seem to disappear. Diseases keep disappearing, but sickness remains. Except during epidemics, doctors were never so busy. Patients keep coming. Hospitals multiply, and they are all full of sick people. But the roll of diseases grows shorter.

What does this mean? If diseases are disappearing, with what illnesses are present-day sufferers afflicted? What has taken the place of those potent enemies which new discoveries have slain or preventive medicine has kept at bay? Has medicine been reduced to a contest with the relatively few remaining diseases which have not yet been brought under control? What are people sick with today? What are the diagnoses?

The great paradox is that the patients who today crowd the physicians' offices and fill the hospital beds suffer, for the most part, from conditions to which no simple labels can be given. Their afflictions do not fall into the classical categories of illness painstakingly delineated by our predecessors. They do not correspond to the paradigms in the textbooks. Established names of diseases often seem not to apply to the forms of illness that people are sick with.

These people are sick—there is no question about that. They are weak, they run fevers, they suffer pain, they sleep poorly, they lose weight, they feel miserable. All these and many other symptoms the doctors understand, and go about relieving with a high degree of proficiency and effectiveness. What the physician can't do, the surgeon often can. Infections, obstructions, inflammations, dislocations, paralyses, hemorrhages, growths —all these we know, and what to do about them we know.

But are these diseases? Illnesses, yes, but if they are diseases, what are their names? What are the diagnoses?

The fact is that these afflictions do not have simple names because they are not simple things and because diagnosis is no longer a matter of naming diseases.* It has come into its fuller meaning of understanding

---

* In a review article on reliability studies of psychiatric diagnosis, many inadequacies of classification, nomenclature, and taxonomy are exposed. One conclusion of the author is: "The traditional class model . . . implies that a given patient has one and only one psychiatric syndrome. The designation of a specific syndrome automatically excludes all others for that patient. The polydimensional model, on the other hand, does not require that the individual syndromes be mutually exclusive, but assumes that more than one syndrome (e.g. anxiety state, depressive state, paranoid state) may be present in a patient at the same time." (Beck, A. T. "Reliability of Psychiatric Diagnosis: 1. A Critique of Systematic Studies." *Am. J. of Psychiat.*, 119:210–216, 1962.)

the nature of a particular illness which is never quite the same in any two people.

Diseases without Names

Visit a hospital with me and you will see what I mean.

Consider this man lying here in a bed in room 417. He is thirty-six years old. He has always been a frail chap, but since leaving high school he has supported his widowed mother, with whom he lives. He works— or has worked—very hard in a small department of a large organization, immersing himself in the details of a tedious and complicated clerical job. From eyestrain perhaps, or from sheer weariness, he developed in- tense headaches and incidental to these lost time from work on several occasions. The recommendation of an efficiency expert led to payroll deductions for such sick leave and, while they did not amount to very much in cash, the procedure gave rise to worry and sleeplessness. He began to vomit after eating and hence to lose weight. Finally his frantic mother importuned him to go to the hospital, and now here he is. The doctors have examined him; they found inanition, leucocytosis, and an enlarged spleen—nothing more. He seems to be improving. Clearly he has been ill, but with what disease? How shall we name it? What—in the older sense—is the diagnosis?

In another room in the hospital is a middle-aged, strait-laced school- teacher, a little older than the first patient. She had come to the doctor's office after school and waited her turn. Although frightened and tense, she described haltingly the frequent intrusion of unpleasant thoughts which so occupied her mind as to impede her teaching activities. She re- ported living alone, having almost no friends or social contacts. Her principal had spoken to her about her depressed, worried appearance, and in fear of losing her job she had even considered suicide. She came here to the clinic without telling anyone. The X-ray examination of her lungs shows suspicious shadows. What treatment will help this woman recover? And the diagnosis? Is her disease pulmonary?

Or look at this school child, who has been running a fever for weeks and who has suddenly lost the power of speech. It may be that she has also become deaf. Her parents are not certain just when she became ill, because they were both away from home for an extended period, leaving the child with an aunt and uncle. The uncle had become sick and had so occupied the wife's time that she had paid little attention to her niece. There was some rumor of an unpleasant situation in the school. But from what disease does the little girl suffer?

Or take this young sailor who has been here three months. Until recently he was a useful member of the United States Navy. For some careless performance of duty many months ago he had been reprimanded, which greatly hurt his pride. He was described then as being sulky and "sorry for himself." He had reported on sick call because of a rash which broke out on various parts of his body. In spite of treatment, it progressed to be an itchy, scaling, disfiguring eruption; his entire face was involved. He was placed in the hospital bay of his ship, where he was restless during the day with inactivity, and sleepless at night from the itching. He joked grimly about "scratching out of the Navy." In a kind of nightmarish frenzy he several times disturbed other sick sailors and so was confined more closely. He ate and drank little. He became feverish and delirious. By the time his ship arrived at port he was almost dead. But of what?

Or consider a case recently reported by George Engel.[1] A loud, coarse, intelligent, but uncouth man suffered constantly for twenty-eight years from two severely painful lesions—a peptic ulcer and a vascular tumor beneath the nail of one of his toes. In spite of them he worked hard and achieved great success. He consulted many physicians and was highly contemptuous of their impotence. When these afflictions were finally relieved, he rapidly disintegrated.

The man's childhood had been a hard one; he arose at four in the morning and worked until late at night, helping and submitting to his strong, aggressive, industrious father. In school he was industrious and a leader, but frequently engaged in fighting. His father disapproved of his fighting as a waste of time, but beat him if he lost a fight. Weakness in any form was not to be tolerated.

At the age of eighteen, just out of high school, he was drafted into the Army, from which he was discharged because of an accidental injury to his hand, which "caused" him continuing pain. This led to a "nervous breakdown"; he was in a hospital for some months and emerged free of his depression but suffering repeated attacks of excruciating pain in his foot and from a peptic ulcer. In spite of them he entered the field of industrial engineering and made a very successful career of it. He married, had three daughters, was divorced, and married again. His increasing business success and fame reached a peak during World War II.

When first seen by Dr. Engel in 1946, the patient was forty-eight years old. The tumor on his toe, which had caused him so much pain for many years, had finally been removed surgically. He was delighted with this result but distressed by the worsening of his ulcer. Surgery was recommended and a vagotomy was performed, to which he reacted badly. During convalescence he reproached the doctors and nurses as having been neglectful. But the ulcer healed and the symptoms from this source permanently disappeared. For the first time in many years he was free from pain.

But now he began to have many new complaints—fatigue, backache, discomfort in other parts of the body, bloating, diarrhea, and sexual impotence. He began to use alcohol to excess and had episodes of confusion. The gastrointestinal symptoms were cured with another surgical operation. When these symptoms improved, the depression and drinking increased and he wrecked his car, causing a cerebral hemorrhage and necessitating another operation.

"More than ten years have elapsed since the fateful accident. He lives quietly on a farm with his wife, who helps support them with an egg business. . . . He is vague, detached, inattentive . . . but enjoys excellent health and has no complaints, and has had no need for a physician . . ." (Engel).

These patients are not exceptional beyond the point that every patient is an exception. Hospitals and clinics are full of suffering and disabled people whose symptoms do not add up to the simple, clear-cut disease entities described in the books on the practice of medicine. Diagnostic labels, "while commonly appearing in case reports, do not exist in patients. . . . They do not enable us to understand the subtle qualities which lead to recovery in one and to death in another patient apparently suffering from the same 'entity.' " [2]

The same ambiguity applies to the identification of many common indispositions, some of which every reader has experienced: ill-defined exhaustion, a persistent sense of uneasiness, recurrent digestive disturbances, morning headaches, chronic backache—these and scores of others. For such conditions there are no adequate diagnostic labels. These have no proper names. They are symptoms of illness but of no disease.

Some afflictions are given diagnostic labels which are almost nicknames. This man has "a back," this one "a heart," that one "an ulcer," "a disk," "a virus." This is a kind of jargon which does not attempt a precise diagnosis. Its very vagueness is an indication of the change that is occurring in diagnosis and especially in diagnostic labels.

Changing Diagnoses

Diagnosis is changing because we are changing our concepts of illness and disease. Fifty years ago we thought we knew the etiology, the pathology, the life history, and in some instances the effective treatment of scores of definite diseases. Today we are not so sure about some of these "known" things. We have more specific remedies for certain conditions, but we are less certain about etiologies. Illnesses seem to be more complicated than we used to think in the days when we could speak so definitely about various disease entities. Illness is seen less as an ugly visitor falling upon hapless victims by chance than as an altered state of being which has come about in an individual from the interaction of many factors. Some of these factors may, indeed, be bacteria; some may be guilt feelings or desperation or self-destructive drives. It was neither a virus nor a cancer that brought King Lear low; Parsifal's King Amfortas sustained an unhealing wound which was manifestly more than a chronic suppuration; it was more than a combination of pneumococci and alcohol that ended the life of Edgar Allan Poe.

What, then, is disease?

About a hundred years ago the great pathologist Rudolf Virchow declared that the proper objects of therapy are not diseases but conditions: "Disease is nothing but life under altered conditions."

More recently Romano put it this way: "Health and disease are not static entities but are phases of life, dependent at any time on the balance maintained by devices, genetically and experientially determined, intent on fulfilling needs and adapting to and mastering stresses as they may arise from within the organism or from without. Health, in a positive sense, consists in the capacity of the organism to maintain a balance in which it may be reasonably free of undue pain, discomfort, disability or limitation of action, including social capacity." [3] To this Engel added, and we agree: "Disease [we would prefer the term *illness*] corresponds to failures or disturbances in the growth, development, functions, and adjustments of the organism as a whole or of any of its systems." [4]

But it is very difficult to rid our thinking and our language of the old entity concept of illness. We often speak in figurative terms of "fighting the disease," "facing it," "resisting it"; of having a cancer, of suffering from arthritis, or of being afflicted with high blood pressure.

This argot reflects the tendency to go on thinking of all disease as a *thing*, a horrid, hateful, alien thing which invades the organism like a snake crawling into a dove's nest.* And to free someone of his symptoms one does not so much treat the person as attack the disease. To be sure, there are a few well-known models for this—tapeworm, cancer, septicemia, multiple sclerosis, syphilis. When the presence of one of these dread visitors is detected, it does seem like an invasion, and a possession. This is, indeed, one kind of illness.

But one truth which has to be learned, and relearned, and relearned again, because we continually forget it, is that two apparently opposite things can both be true. It is sometimes *true* that disease is an invasion; in other instances it is just as true that disease is *not* an invasion. To observe in oneself or a loved one the insidious but implacable development of a carcinoma is to have no doubt as to the invasive nature of some afflictions, despite our intellectual realization that it is *our* cells, our own cells turned cancerous, which now destroy us. But even in such invasions as the bacterial and virus infections there is the degree of lowered resistance and heightened susceptibility to consider. Illness is in part what the world has done to a victim, but in a larger part it is what the victim has done with his world, and with himself.

My teacher Richard Cabot (1868–1939), author of an early classic on clinical diagnosis,[5] did a spectacular and justly celebrated thing when he began comparing systematically the findings made by clinicians with the autopsy findings of the pathologists. In so doing he was only repeating the dramatic innovation of Andreas Vesalius four centuries before him. But Cabot worked with the benefits of a thousand discoveries, discoveries which had tended to obscure the simple correlations which Vesalius had sought. His work was not only magnificent teaching but important scientific research. It rebuked our complacency and presumptuousness; it justified the warnings of Leftwich regarding the fallacies of diagnosis. For Cabot showed that most disease diagnoses, even when made in the very best of hospitals with the most modern equipment and the most excellent professional staff, were proved by the autopsy findings to be incorrect or incomplete or both.

Of course such embarrassing demonstrations were met with all sorts

---

* Engel has suggested that "to be able to think of disease as an entity, separate from man and caused by an identifiable substance, apparently has great appeal to the human mind. Perhaps the persistence of such views in medicine reflects the operation of psychological processes to protect the physician from the emotional implications of the material with which he deals." (Engel, George L. "A Unified Concept of Health and Disease." *Perspectives in Biology and Medicine*, 3:460, 1960.)

of explanation, indignation, and refutation, but the plain facts continued to stare us all in the face—i.e., all who would look at them. They emphasized the necessity of still further improving our techniques of diagnosis, but they also hinted at, and helped to hasten, changes in our concepts of the nature of disease, changes which a few colleagues seem to have forgotten—or to ignore.

Great distances have been covered since the days when patients were "seen" by a doctor, listened to briefly, asked to protrude a tongue, and then "treated." Today a patient is not only seen and heard; he is questioned and tested, inspected and probed. He and those who know him are asked for descriptions of his former ways and states of being, and of the alterations that have occurred in his personality, behavior, or comfort. Not only his recent disability but his entire life passes in review before the examiner. The historical data making up a longitudinal view of a patient are gathered from birth up to the present moment. They are compared with *observed* data from the here-and-now, the results of the inspections, palpations, percussions, auscultations, and laboratory investigations which make up the complete medical examination. An examination of psychological structure and functions, once so completely ignored, is now included to some degree in all comprehensive examinations, since the patient's ways of perceiving, thinking, speaking, behaving, and relating his needs and purposes to the environment are features of his life no less than are his viscera. In psychiatric case study this psychological examination is, of course, pre-eminent.

Case study of this sort is the basis of diagnosis in modern medical practice. We probably acquire today a hundred times more data, more pieces of specialized information about any particular patient, than did our medical forebears of even two generations ago. We know more about the body, the mind, and the interaction of human beings with one another; we know more about our world and our universe.

Pejorative Labeling

It is of the utmost importance, however, that the conclusions of psychiatric case study, the diagnosis made by the doctor, be conveyed in terms that are understood by all those concerned. As we shall discuss later in this book, psychiatric treatment is carried out by many people in addition to the doctor. The cooperation of the members of the family is often urgently needed. All these people must understand the words and the meaning of the doctor's diagnostic conclusion, and his treatment recommendations. Merely giving incomprehensible names to psychiatric conditions is somewhat reassuring in that it gives the impression that the condition is recognized and understood by *someone*. But it does not assist in the dispersal of this understanding. Furthermore, it introduces a new kind of fear, fear not of the actual condition as it exists but of the condition which is implied—usually incorrectly—by the exotic name.

The very word "cancer" is said to kill some patients who would not have succumbed (so quickly) to the malignancy from which they suffer.[6] The effect of some psychiatric words can also be terrifying. Or, if not terrifying, they may be offensive in other ways. Many colleagues have written about this, none more eloquently than Henry Davidson:

"From our residents' lounge, the other day, came a mish-mash of morbid words: anal . . . aggressive . . . guilt . . . acting out . . . genitals . . . hostile. The psychiatric lexicon is indeed loaded with words which make the ordinary fellow blush or bristle. Sometimes the patient must think we look down our noses at him. How else is he to react to words like 'infantile' or 'aggressive'? . . .

"Whatever meaning they convey to the sophisticate, these are scolding words to the average man. To say that a thought is unconscious is, to innocent ears, an insult. The word 'ego' may be a technical noun to some, but to the uninformed it means 'conceit.' Such terms as 'death wish' and 'sadistic' may be everyday currency in our residents' lounge, but they sound positively morbid to the unschooled. To the cognoscenti, a tincture of homosexuality is universal. But to the uninstructed, this is indecent. Too lightly we toss off such words as 'erotic,' 'incestuous,' and 'castration'; these terms, indeed, have become so shopworn that they have long since lost their impact.

"What a strange vocabulary we psychiatrists have! Probing the depths of the mind should surely reveal wellsprings of idealism, courage, and nobility. If lower than angels, we are higher than beasts—using those adjectives 'lower' and 'higher' in the conventional sense. Yet somehow the idiom of psychiatry seems to the average man to be overloaded with words of insult, reproof, or gloom. How odd it is that we who should be the keepers of the richer life, we who should hold the keys to the door of happiness and the answer to the mystery of adjustment, we, of all people, should have so unattractive a glossary!"[7]

To call our technical language unattractive is almost a euphemism. Diagnostic name-calling may be damning. Applicants for college enrollment, life insurance, club membership, officer candidacy, graduate training, and other special privileges, can be quickly blacklisted by such labels as "psychopathy," "character disorder," and "schizophrenia." The applicant's appearance and his record of achievement are lost sight of. Nor does qualifying these damning labels with such adjectives as "latent" or "potential" or "borderline" undo the damage.*

Nor is the patient, or ex-patient, the only sufferer from this situation. An entire family can be hurt by the diagnostic label attached to one of its members, because of the various implications such labels have in the minds of the various groups of people with whom that family comes in contact.**

Need all labeling be pejorative? the reader may ask. And, if a label is correctly applied, is the doctor responsible for its implications? These are certainly sensible questions, and I can illustrate them. An attractive-looking baby is thought by his parents to develop slowly, to show strange lack of response to light. Neurological study shows him to be afflicted with Congenital Amaurotic Idiocy, or Tay-Sachs Disease. This label says that such cases of blindness and idiocy have been observed many times; they do not recover; we have no remedy. The label is pejorative, indeed. So is the condition. Do we now imply that these deplorable realities should be masked with euphemistic evasions?

The answer is an emphatic no. But there are few psychiatric conditions in which we are able to make so definite and final a pronouncement as we can in the case of Tay-Sachs Disease—fortunately a rare condition. Actually Tay-Sachs disease is not a very good example of what we are trying to show. What we are objecting to is the inference so easily drawn that the diagnostic labels in common use to describe psychiatric conditions are as definite and constant as those of Tay-Sachs disease.

---

* An able young colleague of my acquaintance suffered from an episode of some anxiety and indecision. After he consulted a professional friend, who was very helpful, he recovered promptly. Unfortunately, a "tentative" diagnosis of "schizophrenia" got abroad—I don't know how—and my colleague's professional career was thereby seriously damaged.

** Baruk in France has denounced the "destructive prognoses of psychiatry." "What psychiatrist cannot list scores of such experiences as that of a young college graduate whose family was led to assume that it was useless to ever come and visit him? Patients often recover in spite of this, of course, but they always bear the scars. More serious are the desperate radical treatment programs sometimes instituted as soon as the fatal diagnostic label has been attached. What psychiatrist does not know patients who were rushed into irreversible neuro-surgical procedures? On the other hand, what psychiatrist does not know of recoveries, even in those damned by the diagnosis of schizophrenia and relegated to the chronic 'treatment' of hopeless atmosphere and custodial aim? We have all seen them recover, even after five and ten and fifteen years—in spite of this." (Baruk, Henri. *"Les pronostics destructeurs en psychiatrie."* *Anns. Med. Psychol.*, 109:63–65, x 1951.)

The pragmatic point in the whole matter hinges upon the effect that such labeling is apt to have upon those who might bring about improvement in the patient were they not deterred by the implications of the label. This means not only the physicians but his relatives and friends, the community at large, and even the patient himself. Giving a dog a bad name and hanging him has been too long an easy but false solution for psychiatric problems.

Judge Bazelon was sharp but yet more than charitable when he said: "Usually psychiatrists attached to public mental institutions are the only ones who see the indigent defendant. Understandably, they are oriented in the use of what may be characterized as a dispositional diagnosis. In such quick work, labels, based on more or less patent symptoms, are employed to describe patients for the purpose of institutional classification —admissions, releases, types of ward assignment, shock treatment, and such. This special language, which may be worth something administratively—that is, if people must be treated as merchandise—is then applied to legal purposes; but is considerably less than adequate as a means of conveying information to a jury.

"The big terms of a psychiatrist's discourse under any rule are large ominous-sounding words which no one else in the courtroom really understands and which, as time goes on, clever lawyers are becoming quite adept at proving that the psychiatrist himself does not fully understand." [8]

Having mentioned the discovery of a few disease entities, I have digressed to say how much harm the names applied to these syndromes have caused us in recent years. But for a century they served a good purpose. They brought order into a field of utter chaos. They enabled that psychiatry of today to emerge. Kraepelin and others who devoted themselves to the empirical study of the patients confined so faithfully and futilely to state hospitals dignified clinical observation and vividly portrayed characteristic clinical pictures. Kraepelin lived in the golden age of "causal" diagnosis. The "cause" of typhoid fever had just been identified, and that scourge was being eliminated. The "cause" of syphilis had been discovered and effective treatment soon followed. The "cause" of diphtheria had been identified and that dreadful affliction stayed.

The suggestion that every illness had its "cause" was irresistibly exciting, and the etiology concept of diagnosis and of treatment naturally spread to the etiological basis for classifying diseases. Kraepelin admitted that he could not *find* the "causes" for the mental disease syndromes which he defined, but he was convinced that the conditions which he had identified *had* causes which would some day and in some way be found; then the disease could be eliminated.

He was disappointed, as everyone knows; the treatments which have been so dramatically effective in psychiatry have had nothing to do with either a discovered or a theoretical etiology, for the most part. But it can easily be seen why a half a century ago the precise identification and labeling of a syndrome or of a disease was the basis for a logical search for its etiology and hence for its cure.

For the moment we shall end on this negative note. We disparage labeling of all kinds in psychiatry insofar as these labels apply to supposed diseases or conditions of specific etiological determination. We deplore the tendency of psychiatry to retain its old pejorative name-calling function. Patients who consult us because of their suffering and their distress and their disability have every right to resent being plastered with a damning index tab. Our function is to help these people, not to further afflict them.

And well-intentioned as our efforts at nosological naming were, the whole business has turned sour. The chances are very considerable that the reader of these lines, like the authors, has behaved on certain days and even for periods of time in a way which could be described as "schizoid" or even as "schizophrenic." Many millions of people have done so and are doing so at this moment. But this does not entitle anyone to label them as being afflicted with a *disease* called schizophrenia.

In a study of "Contradictions in the Concepts of Schizophrenia" [9] our Dutch contemporary Rümke has attempted to sum up the most outstanding contradictions and differences of opinion. Thus,

Schizophrenia is a nosological entity.—Schizophrenia is a syndrome, a particular mode of reaction.

Schizophrenia is characterized by primary symptoms.—There are no genuine primary symptoms of schizophrenia.

Schizophrenia is an organic disease.—Schizophrenia is a psychogenetically determined condition.

Schizophrenia is not curable.—Schizophrenia is curable.

There are no fluent transitions between schizophrenia and the normal state of mind.—Transitions are fluent.

Psychodynamics are of greatest importance in the study of schizophrenia, but are not the decisive issue.—The knowledge of the psychodynamics involved will finally bring about the solution of the problem; psychodynamics *are* decisive.

Genetic factors are decisive in the development of the disease.—The role of genetic influences is a minor one.

The enigma or secret of schizophrenia is a secret of form.—The secret of schizophrenia is more a secret of content.

In the realm of schizophrenia description is in its very beginning.—In schizophrenia description has failed.

The so-called pharmaco-psychopathological "models" of schizophrenia have nothing to do with real schizophrenia.—The "models" are true experimental schizophrenia.*

The identification of classical illness pictures is important in the diagnostic process. But there is far more to the task of diagnosis than this. Diagnosis must examine and identify and describe the nature and course of the illness in such a way that effective treatment can be instituted. Designations are necessary, and later in this book we shall say precisely and in considerable detail how we think instances of mental illness can be referred to and described in a shorthand way for convenient reference. It will not be by means of any of the obsolete handles which have been so long used, arranged, ordered, rearranged, reordered, disputed, and at last, we hope, discarded.

In the next chapter we shall examine the way in which treatment was determined throughout history, not so much by the name of the special form of illness as by the general concept of illness to which the profession subscribed at the time.

---

* Rümke does not regard all these contradictions as irreconcilable. But he does not face up to the basic fallacy of attempting to identify a thing, a disease, which will embrace all these contradictions and theories. The connection between symptoms, or even symptom patterns, and an eventual psychiatric label, old-fashioned diagnosis as a verbal label, has been examined by Zigler and Phillips. From their studies they declare that the magnitude of the relations between symptom and diagnosis is so small that membership in a particular diagnostic group conveys only minimal information about the symptomatology of the patient. In a later publication these authors contend that "so long as diagnosis is confined to broad diagnostic categories it is reasonably reliable, but the reliability diminishes as one proceeds from broad, inclusive class categories to narrower, more specific ones." (Zigler, E., and Philips, L. "Psychiatric Diagnosis: A Critique." *J. Abnorm. & Soc. Psychol.*, 63:607-618, 1961.) We prefer to go further than this, having considerable doubt also about the broad categories, since these too are contaminated by untenable assumptions. Indeed, these authors themselves point out that Kraepelin excluded recovered dementia-praecox patients because he assumed irreversibility as a criterion for this disorder.

CHAPTER IV

The Evolution of Treatment

SYNOPSIS: Patients whom we now call mentally ill were treated in olden times by extrusion from the social mass, subsequently by cruelty and gross neglect and futile confinement. Gradually humanitarianism, and very recently science, began to be applied to the understanding and proper treatment of these afflicted ones. In part this treatment has been determined by the prevalent concepts of personality; depending on whether one takes an ontologic or dynamic concept of illness, one will chiefly decide to fight the enemy or support the patient. When mental illness was regarded as the infestation of the devil or of evil spirits or, at the very best, of sinful thoughts and sinful acts, the logical treatment was abuse, cruelty, neglect. And this is what the afflicted got.

Various notions of the nature of human personality were entertained by our forebears. Perhaps the oldest was a chemical concept, i.e., that the human body is a chemical mixture contained in a sac, fed from above and drained from below. Later the physical concept of the organism began to gain some dominance over the chemical one; and this was reflected in the growth of physical modalities to remedy illness, now conceived in physical, structural terms. In a later, more sophisticated sense these concepts might be symbolized on the one hand by the bloodstream and the various body juices, and on the other by the cell and the various organs and structures.

To this day the model of personality which prevails in the minds of most physicians is a kind of combined physical and chemical one. The introduction of psychological factors into personality concepts came late, came slowly, and came with great difficulty. Once included, they permitted a holistic concept of personality, a psycho-socio-physio-chemical concept. This is the one the authors subscribe to.

THE DIFFERENTIATION of illness was probably a preoccupation of man in the earliest stages of civilization, and as it became a professional prerogative it was determined by the concept of illness held by the physicians. This concept rather than the diagnosis also determined treatment. Thus the early demonic concept of mental illness dictated treatment by cruelty; the incurable afflictions concept dictated treatment by humanitarian concern or by its opposite, callous neglect; the chemical concept of personality dictated treatment by medication; the physical concept dictated treatment by surgery and other manipulations; the psychological concept which succeeded these two led to treatment by psychotherapy and by placebos.

But to some extent also our ancestors must be given credit for trying to do something not only for themselves but also for the afflicted ones. Mercy was not altogether lacking. Furthermore, some of the "treatment" undoubtedly achieved good results, or seemed to. It is inconceivable that no patient ever got well under those cruel regimes. The patients of that day undoubtedly shared the beliefs of those who were treating them; even now many patients believe that they deserve punishment, and sometimes events which they construe as punitive may have a beneficial effect upon them. Today science regards this concept of illness as a delusion, but where it was the generally held concept it justifies forms of treatment based chiefly on the infliction of pain, which were—as we *now* realize—grossly ineffective and hence extravagantly costly. Remember, this was considered better treatment than mere heedless neglect, which was even more common.

Treatment by Cruelty

It is difficult for us to realize today the extraordinary amount and variety of torture that was inflicted upon these unfortunate ones. Some reports are more than incredible; they are unreadable. Starving, freezing, cramping, and terrifying were routine procedures, and one of the least cruel methods was just plain beating, beating with clubs, whips, wires, chains, and fists.* The familiar expression, "beating the devil out of" someone, reflects a well-established, now fortunately obsolescent, concept of mental illness. But patients were also starved, drenched, whirled, immersed suddenly in cold water, frightened with snakes and pistol shots.

" 'We lock these unfortunate creatures in lunatic cells, as if they were criminals,' exclaimed Reil *in 1803* [italics ours], 'we keep them in chains in forlorn jails, near the roosts of owls in hidden recesses above the gates of towns, or in the damp cellars of reformatories where no sympathetic human being can ever bestow on them a friendly glance, and we let them

---

* Even George III of England, who had ample means to pay for it, was given treatment in a private sanitarium where his attendants made no secret of the fact that from time to time they slapped the king's face or struck him to the floor. One can imagine what happened to the average citizen, to say nothing of the poor man, under similar circumstances.

rot in their own filth. Their fetters scrape the flesh from their bones, and their wan, hollow faces search for the grave that their wailing and our ignominy conceals from them.' " [1]

Rivaling chains in popularity was the lash. Müller related that in the Juliusspital attendants were generously provided with many restraining and punitive devices—chains, manacles, shackles, and efficient, leather-encased bullwhips. They made ample use of these instruments whenever a patient complained, littered his quarters, or became recalcitrant or abusive. "Thrashing was almost a part of the daily routine," he concluded. Lichtenberg explained that thrashings were often better for lunatics than anything else, and that they helped them to adjust to the harsh realities of daily life. Even Reil, the enthusiastic champion of mental care for the insane, noted that the strait jacket, confinement, hunger, and a few lashes with the bullwhip would readily bring patients into line.

Even to this day abuse is regarded in many places as the appropriate measure to take with certain troublesome individuals. Even when the ideas of possession by devils or by sinfulness were (partially) abandoned, the old "therapeutic" principles and methods—based upon outmoded assumptions regarding the nature of illness—were retained.

By the nineteenth century even psychiatrists had taken over some of the moralistic excitement which the authors of *The Witches' Hammer* had exhibited several centuries earlier.[2] For example, Heinroth (1773–1843) repeatedly declared that psychic disorders arose from the voluntary pursuit of evil, and he constructed a psychiatric classification partly based on different kinds of consequences for different kinds of sins. He declared that "faith penetrates to the very roots of our earthly existence, fortifying and strengthening us. As long as it permeates our bodies it affords protection against all mental disorders and temptations. It is the one sure defense identified by our search." [3] And Burrows began his book (in 1828) on mental disorders thus: "Insanity is the scourge brought down on sinful men by the wrath of the Almighty." [4]

But it is unfair to imply that the idea that physical punishment would make sick people act in a more seemly way developed only after the spread of Judaeo-Christian morality. Celsus, an early Roman physician in the time of Julius Caesar, advocated chaining, flogging, and starving as a treatment regimen (but he also employed music, sports, reading aloud, and swinging in a hammock, and notes some recoveries!). Soranus a century later stands out for having opposed the prevalent practice of flogging and chaining. Rather, said he, "the patient should be kept quiet in moderate light and temperature—beds should be low or on the floor. If they are so violent that they can only be given a bed of straw it should be picked over and made as soft as possible. . . . Try to check their digressions in such a way as not to excite them, not to be too lenient but let them see that their faults have been observed, give them sometimes limited freedom . . . only in rare cases bonds or ties must be used but only with great precautions . . . for methods of repression used without discrimination only cause the madness to start up with increased vigor." [5]

Treatment by Neglect

It was the gradual emergence of latent humanity rather than increased diagnostic perception which began to substitute *holding* for *hurting* as a program. For the stupid, the bewildered, the witless, and the bereft, no less than for the aggressive, the recalcitrant, the rebellious, the remedy came to be one of detention, usually in jails.*

While the Europeans were searching for witches or punishing wickedness or coining new names for new entities, the Moslems, under the inspiration of Avicenna, went ahead with the "invention" of hospitals for the mentally ill and introduced some rational therapeutic regimes. They were imitated, according to Tuke,[6] by the Spaniards, who established the first *European* institution exclusively for the mentally ill in Valencia in 1408. An asylum was built in Amsterdam in 1562; it was over a hundred years before France followed with Avignon (1681). One was founded in Florence, Italy, in 1645; in Warsaw, Poland, in 1728; in Springfield, England, in 1741; in Austria at Salzburg in 1772; in Copenhagen in 1766; and in Upsala, Sweden, the same year. But these institutions were little more than dumping grounds for raging, incurable derelicts; there was small hope that any of their inmates would ever recover. Autenrieth observed as late as 1807 that only incurable patients were taken to the public asylums, 'where no one tries to effect cures,' while others had to be taken to private doctors who might undertake to cure them either through compassion or through ambition. He added that doctors were easily dis-

---

* "Many people do not know or have forgotten, if indeed they ever happened to discover, that imprisonment as a *penalty for a crime* is very modern and was probably introduced into penology in America. Formerly the detention was merely incidental to the trial or to some notions of public safety or personal prejudice. It was isolation in a sense just described. It was not considered painful and punishment had to be painful, such as whipping or hard labor or mutilation. But it gradually dawned on social consciousness that just being locked up could be painful and hence punitive, and holding began to be substituted for hurting all over the world." (Lewis, Nolan D. C. A *Short History of Psychiatric Achievement*. New York: Norton, 1941.)

couraged 'by the prospect of having to engage in activities of this kind for an inordinate period of time.' Haindorf explained in 1811 that under the conditions which then prevailed in public asylums in Germany, 'only a few can be cured by science unless fate works miracles.' " [7]

Treatment by Kindness and Education

Now and then, in all ages and at all levels, exceptional individuals appear who rise above current concepts, who seem to be actuated by higher principles and greater humanity. Perhaps such individuals are outstanding in that they refuse to accept the commonly held basic assumptions. In every age there has been a Soranus, an Avicenna, a Pinel, a Tuke, a Dorothea Dix—individuals who disavowed and denounced neglect and cruelty as methods of treatment. They refused to concede that the mentally ill had no souls and no sensations, that they were wicked and devil-possessed, that they were hopeless and incurable. They held to the contrary, in the face of public and professional opinion, and they acted in accord with their beliefs. They were ignored, threatened, ridiculed, and denounced as sentimentalists, reformers, and fanatics. Even Charcot and Freud were ridiculed, it will be recalled, for presuming to treat neurotic illnesses, which "everybody" knew were incurable, and Mesmer was officially declared to be a charlatan. Sneering references to "the cult of curability" and to the claim that mentally ill persons could be cured did not deter them.

Dorothea Dix addressed the Senate of the State of Illinois on January 11, 1847, urging that care and treatment be provided for the mentally ill.*

Recent cases, except there be a positive *organic* disease, are curable under judiciously directed hospital treatment.

Dr. Bell, the eminently distinguished and successful physician and superintendent of the McLean hospital at Somerville, Mass., shows that the records of that institution "justify the declaration that *all cases certainly recent*, recover under fair trial." This is the *general* law; the occasional instances to the contrary, are *the exceptions.*

Dr. Earle, the intelligent physician of the Bloomingdale hospital, N.Y., remarks, in his annual report of 1844, "it is satisfactorily *proved* that, of cases where there is no constitutional weakness of intellect, and where the proper measures are adopted in the *early stages*, no less than eighty in every hundred have been relieved in that institution"; and adds, "*there are few acute diseases from which so large a percentage* of the persons attacked are restored as from insanity."

---

* The italics throughout are hers, not ours, although had she neglected them it would have been our temptation to supply them.

Dr. Kirkbride, in his reports of the Pennsylvania hospital, continually urges "*early* and *prompt removal* to suitable hospitals, by which large numbers are restored to health, and to usefulness in society, who otherwise would remain a burthen to themselves and their friends." [8]

Back in Massachusetts, where Dorothea Dix began, the "state lunatic hospital" in Worcester had received its first patient in January 1837. Samuel B. Woodward, to whom we refer later in this book, was its first superintendent. Woodward had a sense of social idealism and warm humanitarian concern which "led him to accept an obligation to improve the conditions of his fellow citizens. Imbued with an ardent social consciousness, he could not conceive of a life devoted merely to the pursuit of material goods. Instead he believed that he had a religious obligation to better society and be of service to his fellow man." [9]

Woodward's hospital became world-famous. He demonstrated that the mentally ill could be treated kindly, that they could be helped, and that they could recover. "Woodward's primary contribution to American psychiatry had been his popularization of the idea that insanity was a curable disease, given early enough hospitalization and properly directed treatment." [10]

The very assumption that the individual mentally ill patient should receive *any* treatment other than punitive was novel and exciting. Despite often discouraging results, many techniques of effecting change in afflicted individuals were tried out, and some widely employed, which went far beyond the "moral" treatment regimes of Woodward, Ray, and others. "Tranquiling" and restraining devices, physical and hydrologic methods, many drugs and various surgical operations had their day, and their advocates. Indeed, the method of treatment seems to have depended, as in general medicine, upon the concept of the human organism currently held by the profession at the time or place.

The Chemical Concept of Illness: Treatment by Medicine

The earliest notion of the human organism would seem to have been essentially a simple one; it saw the human being as a rather complex chemical mixture contained in a sac, with orifices. It could be fed from above and drained from below. Whatever went into its mouth became a part of the organism. Its contents were in constant ferment and might change color or consistency or fluidity under various influences. These could be restored by putting a corrective into the intake tube. A pinch of salt, or of Epsom salts; some treacle or some pulverized crocodile dung;

hot drinks, cold drinks, poisons and placebos, various mixtures of exotic and nauseous substances—all these and a thousand others were believed to effect changes in this fleshy bag of chemical instability. That one can take into his mouth a few particles of a substance like aspirin or opium or strychnine—an amount less than one millionth part of his total body weight—and feel so *utterly* different lends convincing subjective support to this chemical concept.

The earliest "chemicals" used to bring about a remedial change in the human organism were plants. The *materia medica* of Dioscorides (first century A.D.) lists six hundred medicinal plants, which is more than twice as many as mentioned in the Hippocratic writings. Later the Arabs added many more. Chemicals in the ordinary sense, usually minerals, were one of the special achievements of Paracelsus. He used not only the plants and chemicals but such miscellany as jewels, mummies, and old skulls. "He classified diseases according to the remedies which cured them, and thus created a 'morbus helleboricus,' a 'morbus terpentinus,' etc." [11]

The commonest chemical influence over the body is obviously diet. "One is what one eats." In the time of Hippocrates therapeutics consisted above all in dietetics. "The famous work on *Regimen in Acute Diseases* could almost be called 'The book on barley gruel.' The notion of diet includes by the way not only nutritional but other measures, like heat, exercise or rest, baths, psychological influence, etc. The use of medicaments is very limited." [12]

Hippocrates did use some medicinal treatment, as we know from other writers. But the heavy medication programs (along with many other kinds of treatment) were the work of Galen, who talked "nature" but practiced dosing. Probably most medical ministration was based on the chemical concept, and diet, pills, and potion were the mainstay of the physician.*

---

* "An anonymous Sumerian physician, who lived toward the end of the third millennium B.C., decided to collect and record, for his colleagues and students, his most valuable medical prescriptions. He prepared a tablet of moist clay, 3¾ by 6¼ inches in size, sharpened a reed stylus to a wedge-shaped end, and wrote down, in the cuneiform script of his day, more than a dozen of his favorite remedies. This clay document, the oldest medical "handbook" known to man, lay buried in the Nippur ruins for more than four thousand years, until it was excavated by an American expedition and brought to the University Museum in Philadelphia. . . .

"The Sumerian physician, we learn from this ancient document, went, as does his modern counterpart, to botanical, zoological, and mineralogical sources for his materia medica. His favorite minerals were sodium chloride (salt) and potassium nitrate (saltpeter). From the animal kingdom he utilized milk, snake skin, and turtle shell. But most of his medicinals came from the botanical world, from plants such as cassia, myrtle, asafoetida, and thyme, and from trees such as willow, pear, fir, fig and date. These simples were prepared from the seed, root, branch, bark, or gum, and must have been stored, as today, in either solid or powdered form. The remedies

It is difficult for us to imagine today the pseudo-chemical conglomerations which intrigued the ingenuity of the practitioners of the late Middle Ages. What is probably the first medical essay on the therapy of syphilis was presented in poetic form at a medical convention in Salamanca in 1498 by de Villalobos. Contaminated bile was the etiologic explanation for the affection; hence terrific purging "based on reason and experimentation" was the main treatment. Consider these few samples of seventy-five stanzas:

Stanza 53

Cathartics

Put in a vessel clean a measured like amount
Of centaury, anise, fennel and epithyme,
Likewise of bastard saffron, camomile, count
Of raisins, prunes and violets a like amount.
To a laggard boil one must give a little time;
Cool it then and through a fine cloth strain it well.
To this acacia the half of ounces three,
One ounce of rue, honey, salt and common oil.
Swift evacuation one can thus foretell,
'Tis safe, from poisons it will make the body free.

Stanza 54

After This Has Been Used for Eight Days in Succession, a Purging Should Be Accomplished with the Following Decoction

Eight days in line one swallow should this good brew.
For a lesser purge this decoction one should take:
Myrobalan golden one ounce should measured be
Of Indian fruits and chebule fine take three,
Add to this prunes ounces one a sauce to make
Again of epithyme add half an ounce thereto
Of tamarind and lavender a like amount,
Ounces one of raisins and fumeterre add to this brew
And boil in three pounds of water, waste but two.
Upon this method a fine decoction one can count.

---

prescribed by our physician were both salves and filtrates to be applied externally, and liquids to be taken internally. . . .

"In one respect our ancient text is most disappointing. It fails to name the diseases for which the remedies were intended, and we are unable to check their therapeutic value. . . .

"It is interesting to note that the Sumerian physician who wrote our tablet did not resort to magic spells and incantations. Not one god or demon is mentioned anywhere throughout the text. This does not mean that the use of charms and exorcisms to cure the sick was unknown in Sumer in the third millennium B.C. Quite the contrary is true. . . .

"However, the startling fact remains that our clay document, the oldest 'page' of medical text as yet uncovered, is completely free from mystical and irrational elements. . . ." [13]

In ounces six of this decoction briskly stirred
Dissolve a single ounce of cassia powdered fine.
When wakened in the morn by cry o'singing bird
Drink deeply once and twice and even drink a third.
I count this a remedy royal of mine.

Follow this with the syrup aforementioned
Until the faulty humors well digested be.
The purges mild can often be repeated.
If one be not from this firm course desisted
One can of purging make a fine remedy.

Stanza 56

The Signs Indicating That the Humor Is Digested

Stabs the lance no longer, then gentle sleep steals in.
This can only be done when humors are digested.
Vile pustules will no more appear to plague the skin,
The burning pain in liver will no more begin.
Weakness in the arms and leggs will be arrested,
Again the golden stream will flow both light and free,
The palms and soles of hands and feet their crusts will lose.
While standing in the crystal glass no earth will be,
The face again from color dark is drained free,
The belly long abused is freed from all refuse.[14]

It is painful for physicians to reflect how many patients have been killed or injured by medication. Medical historians diffidently confront us with the fact that at many periods in the history of civilization members of our well-meaning medical profession had an effect opposite to their intentions. Doctors themselves have risen up in alarm at this "therapeutic hyperactivity" and polypharmacy, and there have been repeated campaigns to remove noxious items from the pharmacopoeia. Indeed, therapeutic excesses of some aroused the therapeutic skepticism and even nihilism of others. There have been several waves of this. Ackerknecht [15] described the practice of the early nineteenth century as follows:

> [It] remained a mixture of polypharmacy, speculative rationalism, and crude empiricism. It remained heroic. The centuries-old abuse of mercurial preparations is reflected in the fact that anatomists seriously discussed in the 1850's whether mercury was a normal constituent of human bones! In his autobiography James Marion Sims wrote of practice in the 1840's (and every cholera epidemic tended to underline this statement):
> "The practice of that time was heroic; it was murderous. I knew nothing about medicine, but I had sense enough to see that doctors were killing their patients, that medicine was not an exact science, that it was wholly empirical and that it would be better to trust entirely to Nature than to the hazardous skill of the doctors."

The relief brought by French scepticism was but temporary. Therapeutic hyperactivity again became noticeable, encouraged particularly by the many synthetic antipyretica and analgetica which, beginning in the 1870's, the chemical industry threw on the market, yet which had but symptomatic effect and therefore limited value. It is therefore not surprising that large sectors of the population favored "nature healers" like Priessnitz, Kneipp, and Schroth, and some more alert members of the regular profession adopted similar treatment, by diet (Bock), water (Vogler, Braun, Brand), open air (treatment of tuberculosis by Brehmers at Görbersdorf), or gymnastics.

The chemical model of personality, and hence of treatment, yielded ultimately, as we shall see, to physical concepts and modalities, but it did not die. Indeed, it seems to be having a rebirth in our own era. People *still* cling to it, ingesting all sorts of things besides food in hopes of changing their chemical constitutions. And what the people want, the people get; what they believe, the doctors tend to believe. The concept of humors was essentially a chemical one; it was replaced with an elaborate schema based on interacting endocrine-gland secretions.[16] The recent plethora of pharmaceutical products designed to have specific effects upon various states of mind or degrees of motor activity of the body recalls the ancient chemical concept of personality. Some of these have been scientifically arrived at, tested, and proved.

The Physical Concept of Illness: Treatment by Manipulation

With the rise of surgery, orthopedics, obstetrics, urology, and other specialties employing *physical* modalities * and devices, the chemical model of the human individual went into a temporary eclipse. Mechanical methods were long disdained by "ethical" physicians and employed only by tradesmen—barbers, bonesetters, midwives, and others. But reluctantly and belatedly these tradesmen were accepted into the medical profession, simply because their methods were so obviously useful. Pill-peddling and

---

* The medical historian must please forgive us for skipping so swiftly over the complicated interaction of physical and chemical procedures that characterized the post-Hippocratic period. Ackerknecht says that surgery up to the nineteenth century was a primarily conservative art concerned with wound treatment. But it seems to us that bloodletting is in a sense surgical, and certainly there are many crafts in the seventeenth and eighteenth centuries which while not quite surgical were certainly physical therapy. (Ackerknecht, Erwin H. "Aspects of the History of Therapeutics." *Bull. Hist. Med.*, 36:389–419, 1962.)

concoction-feeding faded into the background. Bleeding, blistering, clystering, dunking, and all sorts of cutting took their place of prominence. "Doctors may be divided roughly into physicians who know a lot but can't do anything and surgeons who can do a great deal but who don't know very much." [17]

The physical model of the personality is so tangible and obvious that it may indeed have been the original one. For Hippocrates it was so. Plato and some other critics subsequently distorted this view with the charge that it made the physician into a kind of physical trainer, a trend reflected many years later in the highly developed physical therapy methods of the Scandinavians. But these modalities always lacked the magic mystery of the pill and the concoction and were, for many years, eclipsed. They were reintroduced into medicine in three ways: first, by the increase in surgical skills; second, by the discovery of such ingenious devices as the obstetrical forceps; and third, by the researches of the anatomists and microscopists. Virchow, while endeavoring to show the absurdity of the theory of *sedes morborum* (physical seats of diseases), demonstrated that the cell is the physical unit of the body and can be pathologically affected, constituting, one may assume, a physical site of disease.

Physical modalities were given an unabashed central place in the philosophy of medical treatment espoused by the osteopaths, although to some degree this was a reaction against not only the polypharmacy of "orthodox" medical science but the tendency toward radical and open surgery. The ascendancy of surgery during the nineteenth century came about as the result of the discovery of anaesthesia and of asepsis. These revolutionized surgical procedure and enabled surgery to evolve from a level of heroic and sometimes apparently callous but necessary obliviousness to screams, groans and scenes of horror, to one in which elegant and skillful manipulation dramatically and abundantly saves lives and relieves pain. Even more recently the orthopedists, dentists, and physical therapists have worked miracles in connection with the rehabilitation of traumatically handicapped individuals, as in the magnificent work of Dr. Howard Rusk in the Institute of Physical Medicine and Rehabilitation of New York University.

Surgeons do things which one can see and feel and talk about. The best of them always remember that when the operator has done his work in the abdomen and sewed it up, his work is finished. The work of nature, the process of recovery, has just started. "Nature has to heal that wound, bind it together, absorb the stitches. The surgeon properly collects the fee, but . . . nature does a good share of the work." * Both surgeons and physicians sometimes forget this.

The conflict between physical and chemical concepts has gone on for centuries. An example of this conflict was mentioned in the records of a twelfth-century physician, contained in the memoirs of one of the Crusaders which were rediscovered in the ruins of Byblos.

"The Frankish lord of Mneitri wrote to my uncle, the ruling Emir of Shayzar, asking him to dispatch a physician to treat certain sick persons among his people. My uncle sent him a Christian physician named Thabit."

This Doctor Thabit was an Arab and a leading physician at Sidon, steeped in the learning of Avicenna and Ibn Rhazes and thoroughly indoctrinated with the Quanun of Avicenna. It should be recalled that the writings of Avicenna and Rhazes were borrowed from Hippocrates and Galen; Greco-Roman medicine provided the framework of their medical thinking. On arrival at the crusader castle of Mneitri, Dr. Thabit was shown a Frankish knight suffering from "an abscess of the leg," and a slave girl who was "majnoun," epileptic.

Now, the therapeutics of Arab medicine, like those of the Greeks and Romans, was very conservative and placed great confidence in the healing powers of nature. Thabit of Sidon prescribed poultices and dietary measures for the knight, under which regimen the abscessed leg began to improve. He also prescribed a dietary course for the poor woman suffering from epilepsy. According to Dr. Thabit's diary she was "relieved of her convulsive seizures and was becoming amenable to persuasion, indeed and in fact she was on the way to recovery of her sanity." This conservative medical regimen had gone on for some weeks when a troop of Italian crusaders arrived at the castle of Mneitri, and among them a Frankish physician. The newcomer expressed dissatisfaction with the Arab methods of treatment and asked the knight with the abscessed leg point-blank:

" 'Which wouldst thou prefer, living with one leg or dying with two?'

"The latter replied, 'Living with one leg.'

"The Frankish physician said: 'Bring me a strong knight and a sharp axe.' "

After the wounded knight had duly expired following what Thabit

---

* "It is really ironic that the doctor who tells the mother that her sick child does *not* need an operation only gets paid his small house-call fee. For this he frequently has to spend an inordinate amount of time reassuring the anxious mother, parrying subsequent telephone calls, and then, stimulated by the mother's anxieties, he may end up spending a restless night wondering whether, perhaps, his diagnosis was wrong. On the other hand, the doctor who proceeds on the principle that it is better to remove nine normal appendices than have one rupture (a bad medical principle) lays his magic hand on the abdomen and rushes the child to the hospital for a 'life-saving' appendectomy. For this he gets a substantial surgical fee for a short period of cutting and sewing, a good night's sleep, and is looked upon as a savior. In other words, rescuing a reluctant patient from an unnecessary operation results in much pressure—consumer pressure, so to speak—and a small fee; whereas performing an operation, even when it is unnecessary, makes one a hero and the recipient of an heroic fee." (Bickers, William. "Medicine—East and West." *J.A.M.A.*, 181:149–150, 1962.)

deemed an extremely crude and most unnecessary amputation, the Frankish doctor turned to the convalescing woman.

"This is a woman in whose head there is a devil which has possessed her. Shave off her hair." The Frankish physician ordered a return to the patient's previous diet of "garlic and mustard." Within a few days, according to Usamah's testimony, "her imbecility took a turn for the worse." The Frankish physician then made a cruciform incision upon her scalp into which he rubbed salt. According to the contemporary observer's diary, "the woman expired instantly."

We have at hand the clinical records made by Thabit confirming these details. We also have his diary in which he states:

"I asked them then whether my services were needed any longer, and when they replied in the negative, I returned home, having learned of their medicine what I knew not before." [18]

Psychological Principles Invade Medicine

Classical Sydenham orthodoxy grew rapidly in all branches of medicine during the latter part of the nineteenth century, furthered by the development of methods of staining brain tissue, combined with anatomical and neuropathological studies of many kinds.* It will be recalled that Freud himself entered his professional career through the then popular field of neurophysiology and almost discovered the local anesthetic effects of cocaine. The clinical experiences of army surgeons in the Franco-Prussian War and the American Civil War added greatly to our knowledge of brain localization. Psychiatry was, until about 1920,**

---

* In 1918 my teacher, Ernest Southard, *confided* to me his puzzling observation that only about 50 per cent of the cases of general paresis (brain syphilis) upon whom he had performed autopsies showed brain destruction of a degree corresponding to the "amnesia" and "dementia" found clinically. This suggestion of a "functional" basis for some "organic" symptoms was revolutionary then. But of course we know today that even general paresis, the classical clinical entity of psychiatry, can occur without spirochetal encephalitis, that most syphilitic infections of the brain do not produce the picture of "general paresis," and that the symptoms of paresis sometimes respond to psychotherapy and *not* to spirocheticides. (See two well-documented cases from Topeka: [1] Fellows, Ralph M. "Sodium Amytal in the Treatment of Paresis. Preliminary Report." *J. Mo. State Med. Assn.*, 29:194–196, 1932. [2] Wallerstein, Robert S. "Treatment of the Psychosis of General Paresis with Combined Sodium Amytal and Psychotherapy. Report of a Case." *Psychiatry*, 14:307–317, 1951.)

In short, we know that syphilis alone does not "cause" the mental disorder "general paresis." Syphilitic and other toxins which injure the brain can contribute to the production of a variety of symptoms which in a given culture have a certain general similarity. But this is a far cry from our once cherished and "established" paradigm of a specific psychosis.

** It is true that Jung published *The Psychology of Dementia Praecox* in 1906 and Bleuler *The Group of Schizophrenias* in 1911 and Freud and Braun their studies on *Hysteria* in 1895. But at that time these publications had little influence on general medical practice and thinking.

merely an appendage to neurology, dealing with the epiphenomena of central-nervous-system injury or defect. Mental illness was the expression —one kind of expression—of brain disease.

Then came the revolution. As with most revolutions, the way had been prepared by many widely separated events. William James and Sir Francis Galton and Wilhelm Wundt and Alfred Binet had expanded the scope and depth of the science of psychology. Various psychotherapeutic devices were being tentatively tried. The demonstrations of Mesmer that physical processes could be influenced in a mysterious way by psychological * events—including the command of another person—were so revolutionary, so unbelievable, that they had been officially denounced as fraudulent. But the persistent work of Liébeault, Bernheim, Braid, and Charcot led to reversal of the original judgment and forced the beginning of a revision in psychological and behavior theory. The young neurologist Sigmund Freud began to seek for better methods of penetrating the limits of consciousness and connecting external and internal "events." He reported some observations, some cures, some hypotheses. They were ridiculed, ignored, or condemned.

It's an Ill Wind . . .

Suddenly the catastrophe of World War I occurred. "War is the father of all things," said Heraclitus. Whether or not this be true, it is a fact that again the experience of military surgeons with an infinite variety of demoralized and incapacitated soldiers advanced the science of healing. It brought the issue of the nature and treatment of psychiatric illness to a focus. All over the European theater of combat, on both sides, soldiers had to be withdrawn from duty because of paralysis, fits of trembling, uncontrollable vomiting, senseless screaming, running in circles, sudden speechlessness, and overwhelming terror. After a year or so of fumbling, there was a general and frantic realization by military physicians that neither neurology nor neurosurgery nor all the drugs in the pharmacopoeia were going to be of any help in such cases.

---

* E. B. Holt began his small epoch-making volume, *The Freudian Wish and Its Place in Ethics* (New York: Holt, 1915), with an account of how Immanuel Kant demonstrated to his own satisfaction that conscious psychological processes could be set in motion deliberately which could control real pain. One might have supposed that Kant knew of the common human experience of being fearfully injured under exciting circumstances, such as a railroad wreck or a battle engagement, and remaining quite unaware of pain at the time.

The neurologists believed that these various pictures of dysfunction or demoralization could be ascribed to petechial, perhaps microscopic, hemorrhages in the brain tissue resulting from repeated concussions; the condition was accordingly labeled "shell shock." [19] But psychiatrists (and many other physicians without psychiatric or neurological orientation) were quick to suspect that these symptoms represented not neurological injury but psychological disorganization whereby "subconscious processes" usually kept in abeyance were trying to escape control. The wish to escape from an unbearable situation partially overcame the wish to be obedient, useful, and approved.

The military authorities were sure that this behavior was nothing but "soldiering," an age-old device for escaping duty and danger. Disturbed behavior from the effects of brain injury could be forgiven; syncope, paralysis, and even violence could be understood if they were symptomatic of medical illness. But symptoms which served the purposes of the individual must be highly suspect. To the surgeons it was malingering; to the public, it was cowardice; to the military, it was treason.

Shirking or showing fear or running from danger—these are precisely the things a soldier is taught not to do; they are precisely the things which even children grow out of with the proper rearing. Granted that flesh is weak, that any one of us may have his moments, is it fitting—or good public policy—that such behavior be dignified with the title of an illness? If a man is yellow, shall we let him save face by becoming "sick"? But on the other hand, some of these "shell-shocked" escapists obviously suffered, and greatly; some of them seemed completely demoralized and even "demented." Even when they were returned to places of complete safety the symptoms often persisted in spite of all sorts of treatment. Is this consistent with the "soldiering" notion?

This problem puzzled physicians, even the most practical and concrete-minded. If these were self-preservative devices, they were inefficient and self-injurious. Furthermore, despite the obvious usefulness of the symptoms, in some instances, some of the victims really seemed completely unaware of this aspect. Some of them seemed most convincingly remorseful or regretful that they could not remain with their companions and fulfill the expectations of their commanders. They were not weaklings.

And even when scientific explanation could be offered of why an undoubtedly brave, devoted Achilles should suddenly succumb to a wound in the heel, it was regarded by both physicians and the public as a most ambiguous and unpleasant area of exploration, a concession to the frailty of humankind, something which, like the contents of the abdominal cavity, might need to be explored in the privacy of the operating room but not talked about in polite society.

It was this quandary which Freud's curiosity, courage, and persistence helped us to solve. It was not that Freud worked with war cases; most of his great discoveries had been made long before World War I. But they began to be known all over the world shortly after World War I, and they offered us the key to this previously closed book of unconscious motivation.

Freud's work had been based not on the dramatic incidents of self-preservative demoralization characteristic of the battlefield, but on private casualties from the walks of everyday life. One of the first things exposed in his psychological dissection was the multiplicity of reactions to the prevalent social hypocrisy about sex. The public was quite willing to switch its attention from "subconscious" battle fears to "subconscious" sexual fears as the basis for queer symptoms. The war had ended, and physicians came back from military service convinced that there were many "nervous" afflictions which did not depend upon brain injury. Brain surgery offered no relief for such cases, but some of them seemed amenable to methods not taught in medical school. Some of these physicians were determined to learn more about these cases, and while formal graduate-study programs were not yet organized, a new interest sprang up in scores of centers.

The old ideas of illness were not discarded. It was not to be denied that some symptoms reflect brain lesions, nerve injuries, and somatic dysfunctions of many kinds—inflammations, new growths. All these damages constitute tickets of admission to the doctor's office for "repairs." But not all symptoms are of this kind. Some must be ascribed to mismanaged adaptation, to impaired self-direction and self-control, to over-expensive compromises in the obtaining of desired goals, the maintaining of acceptance, and survival.

Many internists and surgeons recognize the importance of psychological factors in various forms of physical illness, and even venture a little psychotherapy themselves. Often the modalities employed are called by some name other than psychotherapy; perhaps they are not even regarded as therapy but as common sense (psychotherapy being, of course, most uncommon sense). This "common-sense" medical psychotherapy is probably widely used by many physicians. I have seen it most skillfully employed and I have many times urged medical colleagues to use it more, comparing this "minor psychiatry" with the minor surgery which the general practitioner feels competent to do in contrast to major surgery (and "major psychiatry"), which he should not feel competent to do.

Certainly there are conditions such as an attack of influenza or of appendicitis in a healthy young man which do not require any psychotherapy at all. But in most instances of illness in our culture there is some indication of the need for some psychotherapy, whether or not the physician supplies it. There is a medical treatment for iritis, but the anxiety about losing an eye is something which cannot be fully relieved by medicine. A tonsillectomy may seem like a simple operation to the surgeon; it is not simple to the frightened child. In general, physicians and surgeons use what they believe to be the best-known procedures, physical and chemical, for the conditions they observe, forgetting that psychological factors are always present—not the least of which are the patient's reactions to the mode of treatment itself—and the need for some kind and some degree of psychotherapy is rarely absent.

There are some conditions, such as asthma, arthralgia, gastric hyperacidity, vascular hypertension, and some skin diseases, which are successfully treated by chemical methods, by physical methods, *and by psychological methods*. The choice seems to depend upon the skills and convictions of the therapist. Cures are obtained by the use of all these modalities, and, of course, failures have been reported, likewise, by all. But the implications of this complementarianism are rarely thought through. Some doctors see in it good evidence that all psychological phenomena will ultimately be reducible to physical and chemical terms. Others, including the author, read it to mean rather that many conditions now regarded as intractable somatic disorders will ultimately be found capable of relief through psychological means.

The "brain-spot" versus "mind-twist" issue continues to divide psychiatrists to this very day, but there has been a steady shift from the organicist school, to which we all belonged forty years ago, toward the dynamic position held by the great majority of American psychiatrists today and by many Europeans. Many psychiatrists would say that they recognize both concepts as applicable in varying degrees to every case. Unfortunately, the language of many textbooks, the nosological designations in common use, and the stipulations of legal statutes are all couched exclusively in the terms of the older concept of disease, terms which many of us consider obsolete. This explains why it is that flatly contradictory answers can be given in the courtroom by colleagues of competence and good standing who may actually not disagree at all regarding the facts, but who apply designations deriving from two different stages of medical history.*

Meanwhile there have arisen a third and even a fourth position; the Body Fluid concept of personality and disease, which is a kind of reversion to the old chemicalism of antiquity, and the Social Factor school, the ultra-sociological viewpoint, which is sympathetically aware of the interactive processes we have noted but which tends to advocate handling medical history by jumping out of it.

Students of linguistics have learned only recently to what extent our very thoughts and attitudes and feelings are molded to fit the words available for their expression. In psychiatry today we still try to fit our new understandings into an anachronistic terminology. And the old terms carry with them the old preconceptions from which we haven't yet learned to free ourselves. A more adequate language has not yet been developed. We go on putting our new wine into old bottles, carelessly disregarding the consequences. Inevitably, the wine turns sour, and the old bottles fall apart.

It is to this incongruity between our knowledge and our terms that this book addresses itself. In a sense the entire book is an extended definition—a definition of the new view of mental illness, a definition of the diagnostic terms which seem to us more correctly to convey the nature and "causes" of mental illness, with some reference as well to those diagnostic and treatment techniques by which the new terms become operational. In the chapters which follow, especially those chapters which deal with symptoms and syndromes, the new terms may seem to some at first oddly unfamiliar; to others they may seem inadequate in ways which we overlook or dismiss too lightly. But our aim is not to create a new lexicon; it is to contribute in some measure to the development of the new psychiatry into an articulate science of human misery and travail, human failure and triumph.

---

* It is true Hippocrates said: "And men ought to know that from nothing else but the brain come joys, delights, laughter, and sports, and sorrows, griefs, despondency, and lamentation. And by this [the brain], in a special manner, we acquire wisdom and knowledge, and see and hear. . . ."

To this Meduna adds: "Our basic tenet is that the mind and the so-called mental functions are functions of the brain, wherefore a disturbance in these functions must be caused by a physical disturbance in the substance of the brain, and therefore is amenable to pharmacological and other physical treatments." (Meduna, L. J. "Meduna: Pro Domo Sua." *J. of Neuropsychiat.*, 1:63, 1959.)

The Psychological Concept of Illness: Treatment by Psychological Methods

While the tide of the competitive offering of relief to suffering mankind fluctuated back and forth between the physicalists and the chemicalists, the psychological perspective was rarely considered by either. To this very day the physiochemical model of the personality is held by the vast majority of medical men. Physics and chemistry are considered basic sciences; for some curious reason psychology is not. Hence, even after their spectacular developments in the past few decades, psychology and psychotherapy still occupy a small part of medical or surgical thinking, a defect which Hippocrates pointed out to his colleagues twenty-five hundred years ago. And even more serious is the fact that much psychiatry, emulating medicine and surgery, *also* ignores the psychological, clinging instead to the physical or chemical or physiochemical concept of personality and treating patients (relatively unsuccessfully) on this basis. It is no wonder that an exasperated colleague denounces the very notion of mental illness as a myth, referring of course to the classical, deficient medical definition of illness (or disease). Mental illness is NOT a myth, but neither is it in our opinion the *propter hoc* result of a chronic infection, a defective gene, or a poisoned neuron. These "facts" may be found, sometimes, but they neither explain nor define nor describe the mental illness.

So long as the general concept of the human organism was that of a chemical sac, chemical alterations were the logical approach to the relief of *internal* distress. When the anatomy and physical structure of the organism were better understood, physical devices became increasingly used. When psychology ceased to be speculative philosophy and became a laboratory and clinical science, psychological treatment modalities were developed.

Moral Treatment

Psychology was used in psychiatric diagnosis long before it was put to work in therapy. Early in the nineteenth century under the influence of Pinel, Tuke, and others, it became customary for enlightened superintendents of hospitals for the mentally ill to treat their patients more and more like human beings and their illnesses as something which might be expected—at least in some instances—to recover. "Moral treatment" it was called, not in the sense of opposing immorality but in the sense of introducing modalities of treatment derived from the mores, from the culture, from the belief in the effectiveness of education, recreation, and human kindness. It was not a specific procedure, says Bockoven in his excellent essay, "but rather a general effort to create a favorable environment in which spontaneous recovery could take place. This general effort was supplemented by a more specific effort to give whatever psychological help that seemed to be needed." It meant "kind, individualized care in a small hospital with occupational therapy, religious exercises, amusements and games, kind treatment, and in large measure a repudiation of all threats of physical violence and an infrequent resort to mechanical restraint. In brief, the new therapy implied the creation of a healthy psychological environment for both the individual patient as well as the group." (See also Grob,[20] Deutsch,[21] Bockoven,[22] Dain and Carlson.[23])

This "moral treatment" included such things as exercise, studies, recreation, gardening, farming. Bockoven has defined it as "organized group living in which the integration and continuity of work, play and social activities produce a meaningful total life experience in which growth of individual capacity to enjoy life has maximum opportunity."

This, you will say, sounds like the best of modern psychiatric hospital treatment. Listen to it in the words of one of its stanch advocates, Amariah Brigham, written in 1847.

> Many cases we believe cannot be cured or improved, but by a rousing and calling into exercise the dormant faculties of the mind. Hence schools are beneficial, not merely to the curable class of patients, but to the demented and those approaching this condition.
>
> In such, the active state of the disease, which originated the mental disturbance, has passed, and left the brain and faculties of the mind in a torpid state. In these cases, medicine is generally of no use, and they cannot often be much improved, but by exercising the faculties of the mind.
>
> But others also benefitted by devoting a portion of every day to mental improvement. To those who are nearly or quite well, and who remain in an asylum for fear of relapsing at home, or for other reasons, schools afford enjoyment and often means for improvement which are highly valued by the patients themselves.
>
> The melancholy and despairing, and all those suffering from delusions of mind, and those that are uneasy and nervous, that are constantly restless and disposed to find fault and to annoy the attendants and quarrel with all about them, because they had nothing else to occupy their minds,

are frequently cured by mental occupation and exercises of a school, by attending to composition, declamation, the writing and acting of dialogues and plays. . . .

Various are the methods that may be adopted to awaken into activity the dormant faculties of the mind and to dispel delusions and melancholy trains of thought. A *museum* or collection of minerals, shells, pictures, specimens of ancient and modern art and curiosities of all sorts, should be connected with institutions for the insane. The opportunities are abundant for making interesting and valuable collections of this kind by the aid of the patients that have recovered and their friends.

By means thus indicated institutions for the care and cure of those affected by mental disorders will be made to resemble those for education, rather than hospitals for the sick, or prisons for criminals, and when we call to mind that the greater part of those committed to such establishments are not actually sick, and do not require medical treatment, but are suffering from deranged intellect, feelings and passions, it is evident that a judicious course of mental and moral discipline is most essential for their comfort and restoration.[24]

The Decline of Moral Treatment

The words you have just read, written over a century and a quarter ago, represented the theory and the practice of the leaders in psychiatry at that time. It was a group of idealistic young men who believed in this concept of helping the mentally ill recover, who came together in the formation of the first medical organization in America, later to be known as the American Psychiatric Association. The names of Samuel Woodward, Eli Todd, Isaac Ray, John S. Butler, Luther Bell, Amariah Brigham, Thomas Kirkbride, and Pliny Earle should be immortal. They believed that it was their duty and their privilege to minister to the mentally ill. They believed that the mind influenced the body and vice versa. For them the "mind" included, as it still does for a few of us, the expression and expectation of love and hate. Above all, these men believed in the curability of mental illness—a daring, unconventional, unorthodox, and highly unpopular view.

These psychiatric pioneers believed this to be a scientific treatment, and they demonstrated and documented the fact that under this treatment recovery from mental illness was the rule, not the exception! Doctor Todd reported recovery in over 90 per cent of the patients admitted to the Hartford Retreat with mental illness of less than a year's duration. For nearly twenty years Woodward's percentage of cases discharged ran from 60 to 70 per cent, plus another 5 per cent discharged "improved." In 1841 the recovery of "recent cases" at the Worcester State Hospital ranged between 82 and 92 per cent, and in the same period the recovery of what he called "old cases" ranged from 15 to 22 per cent. Then, as now, the sooner the illness was brought to treatment, the better the prospects seemed to be for recovery.

Then catastrophe struck. About the middle of the nineteenth century, after this treatment and this concept of mental illness had been demonstrated for over twenty years, the whole thing collapsed. Moral treatment was abandoned. The psychiatric leaders who introduced it resigned, died, or entered other fields of work. An era of pessimism set in which lasted almost exactly one century.

What had happened? This has been analyzed by Bockoven [25] and by Grob.[26] In part it came about from the sudden influx of millions of immigrants, many of them in deplorable states of mental and physical health, who crammed the hospitals as they did other charitable institutions. In part, it came about through the preoccupation of this country with the Civil War. But in part it came about through the paradoxical effect of the efforts of one of its strong proponents to support it.

Unfortunate events in the life of Dr. Pliny Earle led him to be, although wise and intelligent, a man given to despondency and pessimism. He was perceptive enough to denounce the building of huge hospitals, which he considered to be extravagant shams covering up the neglect of patients. He favored 200-patient hospitals as we do today. He was successful in changing the outlook of the medical profession in his state (New York) regarding the incurability of insanity and was responsible for important changes in the attitude of state administrations regarding state hospitals. He was described as "consecrated" to the care of the mentally ill. He took excellent care of his patients.

And yet this good, this wise, this well-intentioned man so vigorously attacked certain fallacies in the statistics of his colleague Woodward that he convinced the medical profession of what he himself did not believe, namely, that Woodward had lied and that mental illness was incurable! In the vigor of his critique he bungled or misused even his own statistics in proving that Woodward's statistics were wrong. Seemingly arguing that lifetime followups would inevitably disclose recurrences of mental illness, he convinced the medical profession that the prognosis of mental illness was extremely poor, and thereby struck a death blow at moral treatment, i.e., the use of psychology and re-educative techniques in psychiatric treatment.

Within a few years no superintendents had the courage to admit that they had cured more than 5 per cent of their patients! The effect upon legislatures of this change in attitude of psychiatrists can be imagined. In spite of Dorothea Dix, in spite of the protests of Isaac Ray and others, the belief in the curability of the mentally ill declined. Nine of the discouraged pioneers and spokesmen resigned or died, and moral treatment disappeared.

With this collapse of moral treatment, the most pessimistic predictions then came true and mental illness *became* "incurable." *

The moral treatment of the mentally ill is used today in a more ambitious and extensive way than its first proponents could have imagined. In the good psychiatric hospital today there are assignments, there are exercises for the mind and for the body; there are programs of activity and programs of inactivity. Instead of moral treatment it is today called milieu treatment or rehabilitation, which do not necessarily represent an improvement in terms. But the idea back of it is the same, namely, to guide or lead or instruct or induct the patient into a new way of life and then gradually withdraw the instruction and the supports and permit him to take up an independent existence, once more using his own assets and his new techniques. Along with the normative factors in moral therapy go many intangible factors which are largely psychological—the give and take of daily life with others in difficulty, seeing other patients improve, the model of living set by doctors and nurses, the attention given to psychological matters by staff and patients alike. (See William C. Menninger.[27])

Psychotherapy

Until the discoveries of Freud and until the erection of his consistent theory of personality organization, the use of psychology as a treatment method in any form was always a little suspect. To many physicians it still seems to partake of the nature of suggestion, or talking someone out of something. Psychotherapy has been called "the talking cure" by people who have little grasp of how much more is involved.

---

* Around the turn of the century things began to look up again. Charles Page in Connecticut, Henry Hutchings at Utica, William Zeller in Illinois, and William Alanson White in Washington began to revive what was essentially the old moral treatment. The movement gathered momentum when Clifford Beers used his own case to demonstrate the falsity of a current popular and professional belief that mental illness is incurable. Then came J. J. Putnam, Adolf Meyer, A. A. Brill, Smyth Ely Jelliffe, and Ernest Southard, and from across the ocean the influence of a new point of view to support these optimists—the discoveries of Sigmund Freud.

Psychotherapy did not begin with Freud by any means; Mesmer and Quimby both demonstrated long before Freud that the mind could prevail over matter, as it were, and certainly over some disease. And long before Mesmer and Quimby there were uses of psychology in therapy based upon magic, superstition, religious faith, and of course suggestion. But psychotherapy in the sense of the intent to affect an illness favorably by the intent and behavior—chiefly verbal—of a second person really began with what was called at first "animal magnetism," later "hypnosis."

Neither Mesmer nor Quimby knew why they obtained their results. But they did obtain them and they did so without the use of drugs or instruments. Hypnosis ultimately became a recognized procedure of psychology, and still later of medicine. For this we are indebted to a long list of courageous explorers—Charcot, Bernheim, Liébeault, Braid, Hull, and others.* As a result hypnosis has come to be a useful method of psychotherapy employing intensive suggestion and is capable of annulling pain, recalling deeply buried memories, influencing dreams and other psychological processes, and even modifying some physiological processes and physical structures.

In 1919 Pierre Janet, a contemporary of Sigmund Freud, published a book, *Psychological Healing,* which influenced the medical profession all over the world, especially psychiatrists. This was based on the assumption that psychological factors, as well as physical and chemical factors, entered into all illness and could be dealt with therapeutically. Simultaneously Freud was developing his theories of psychoanalysis. From these roots modern psychotherapy developed.**

At the present time psychotherapy is being applied in other than vis-à-vis interview situations (or the couch situation), namely, in small groups of patients from six to ten, presided over by a leader whose function it is to guide the development of the group expression and enlightenment. The ultimate value of the effort to apply psychotherapy to larger groups of people at lesser expense is as yet unknown.

Psychoanalysis remains, in the minds of many including the authors, the supreme paradigm of psychotherapy. It is supreme in the sense that it is the most thoroughgoing, the most penetrative, the most intensive

---

* Various colleagues in The Menninger Foundation under the lead of Brenman and Gill have pursued researches in this field over a number of years. (*See* Brenman, Margaret, and Gill, Merton: *Hypnotherapy.* New York: International Universities, 1947.)
** See, for example, Walter Bromberg's excellent history, *Man above Humanity* (Philadelphia: Lippincott, 1954).

and persistent. Indeed, these virtues are also among its drawbacks, since much time and money is consumed in the process of continuous diagnosis and continuous change which we all wish could be shortened. The special merit of psychoanalysis is that from the painstaking, long-continued treatment of some individuals so much has been learned that is helpful in the shorter treatment of other individuals.

The Holistic Concept

Today chemical concepts, physical concepts, psychological concepts, and social concepts are incorporated into our total personality concept. We see the individual as a unit in a social group which is, in turn, a part of other social groups. These individuals have certain physical, chemical, and psychological equipment with which they interact with other individuals in this society. From time to time one of them shows signs of distress or threatened failure or transgressive nonconformity. This comes to the notice of somebody who cares, and the faltering individual is given help. Not all falterings are called illness; but if the failure or threatened failure is of a sort for which our present medical knowledge and skill are believed to be helpful, the patient is taken to a doctor and his condition is described as illness.

If, on the other hand, his behavior is not of a sort which customarily is treated by doctors he may be lodged in various places of refuge—his home, his church, the city jail, the federal penitentiary. Here he may be examined, and if so the examination should be precisely the same as he would have received in a hospital or in a clinic. The purpose of the examination will be the making of a diagnosis. And that diagnosis will be based on modern concepts of psychology, of personality, of behavior, as well as modern concepts of anatomy, of physiology, and of pharmacology.

Our present-day view of the human being is therefore a holistic one; we are not dominated by solidism, somaticism, or psychologism in trying to make a diagnosis of the difficulty that has arisen in and about this individual. The purpose of that diagnosis is very definite. Someone wants the situation improved. Usually this "someone" includes the subject himself, although sometimes the greatest pressure for therapeutic intervention comes from outside.

In thinking of a presentation of our view which could capture the imagination of the reader, I was reminded of experiences of my own while working evenings in a roller-skating rink during my first year at college. While the music was playing and all the skaters were going round and round, the floor manager was constantly on the alert for collisions. Those of us who patrolled the floor tried to anticipate these disasters as much as possible; if a skater went down, not only might he hurt himself but he was pretty sure to trip some other skaters, and sometimes there was quite a pile-up.

A skater's expectation of falling might be signaled by frantic efforts to maintain his balance, by a squeal, or by a silent plunge. Frequently the skater was able to correct his own disequilibration, or drift uneventfully over to the side of the rink and sit down. Sometimes one of his friends helped him, or one of us was able to get to his side before he fell.

This was not the end of it, however. The music kept on going, and so did a lot of other skaters who seemed to have no trouble—yet. But those who had fallen and some of the other skaters nearest to them had to get back into the current with a slightly altered orbit, after more or less delay incident to a readjustment of clothes, tightening of skate straps, and subsidence of embarrassment.

Now the reasons for these falls and traffic tie-ups are numerous. Some skaters were inexperienced or clumsy; but even skillful ones sometimes fell. A too zealous skater occasionally clipped or crossed in front of an unwary companion, who might also be going too fast. But the reason could also be now and then that a pair of skates was badly worn, a ballbearing defective, or a strap loose. These mechanical matters could be remedied by the skate boys. I hope surgeons will not feel demeaned if we think of some of their very essential repairs as being comparable to the tasks of the skate boys. A most skillful skater will fall if his skate comes off, but many skaters who need education, correction, caution, redirection, or just a little support *tend* to blame it on their skates. And sometimes a little chemistry—a little oil on the skates—solved everything.

Having carried this figure so far, I feel constrained to add another parallel. I remember that many skaters who considered themselves highly competent went swiftly and spectacularly about the rink, contemptuous of those who were having difficulties. Every now and then the unexpected would happen—the misadventure of another skater or a defect in the skate—and pride was followed by the proverbial fall accompanied by chagrin, anger, and above all astonishment that such a thing could happen "to me."

Many people who become psychiatric patients have scoffed at the idea of such a thing ever being possible for them; they have often been at considerable pains to ridicule and denounce psychiatry as the preoccupation of weaklings. When the fall comes, the crash is usually so great that there is no time or strength left for remorse, apology, or recantation.

Where is psychiatry today in its skills, in its concepts, in its diagnostic designations, and in its therapeutic modalities? In the succeeding chapters we propose to answer that question, first by setting forth our hypotheses about the determinants of human behavior, and then by illustrating the kinds of floundering and threatened falls which we observe, grading them as to severity and at the same time endeavoring to explain not so much their production as their function.

CHAPTER V

Toward a Theory of Human Behavior

SYNOPSIS: *This chapter begins the presentation of a holistic theory of personality consistent with the process concept of mental illness, i.e., the disturbance and re-establishment of internal and external equilibria. Four principles are discussed: (1) mutual adaptation and interaction by the environment and the individual; (11) organization or "system" theory, including the principles of homeostasis and heterostasis; (111) regulatory functions; and (1v) motivation.*

The first two of these principles are discussed in Chapter V, the second two in Chapter VI. Other principles of behavior theory will be mentioned.

THE AMBITIOUS title of this chapter might seem to promise more than many chapters could deliver. It is not our intention to present such a theory in full dress, but only to suggest a way of looking at human behavior—especially misbehavior—in a broader continuum than is customary, one which would establish the relationship of psychiatry to other sciences, one which would enable us to discard some of the misleading characterizations and labels which have been applied to phases of human existence and aspects of human personality.

The hypotheses which we shall submit as a basis for subsequent theorizing in this book are not *new* nor are they *ours*, except in the sense that we accept and use them. They have been constructed and used to explain the process of living, especially human living, and human living in a society. In part they are applicable to all life and are in common use not only in medicine and other biological sciences but in some of the non-biological sciences.

Nor can we present all the relevant theories. To be thoroughgoing we could, for example, begin with the phenomenon of protoplasmic irritability. This is undoubtedly relevant and certainly basic. But we shall have to assume some knowledge of it—and other basic principles—on the part of the reader. We shall have to assume some knowledge on his part of the genetic theory of personality, the belief that certain innate capacities in the newborn mature according to a biological timetable and that the injuries of childhood have a relevance to subsequent behavior, even though the scars are invisible to the casual observer. Along with this theory, we assume knowledge on the reader's part of the general principles of psychodynamics worked out so carefully by Freud and his followers, although we shall try to add something in this area.

The four principles which we particularly wish to elaborate as a basis for our study of psychiatric phenomena are as follows:

I. The theory of individual-environmental interaction and mutual adaptation effort; this is often referred to as *adjustment theory*, or *adaptation theory*.

II. A theory of organization, also called *system theory* and *organismic theory*.

III. A theory of psychological regulation and control, called in psychoanalytic terms *ego theory*.

IV. A theory of ultimate motivation, frequently called *instinct theory*.

1. ADAPTATION AND BALANCES

Today in virtually every field of science the pattern of explanatory thinking is shifting from static, classificatory, single-cause analyses to dynamic, process-oriented genetic explanations. Kurt Lewin [1] has called it the change "from Aristotelian to Galilean modes of thought." * In such terms we can define illness as being a certain state of existence which is uncomfortable to someone and for which medical science offers or is believed by the public to offer relief. The suffering may be in the afflicted person or in those around him or both, but a disturbance has occurred in the total economics of a personality which becomes the focus of our clinical attention. The continuous internal and external adaptation to continuously changing internal and external conditions by an organism, which carries the triumphs and scars and hidden weaknesses of many similar prior efforts and failures, has been jolted by something which may take advantage of the consequences of previous battles and their residual scars, and also pre-existent weaknesses. A shift in balance occurs with a lowering of the effective level of living.

Shifts of some kind and degree are going on constantly, and with them constant processes of restoration. But certain events or combinations of events or persistence of events upset the balance beyond immediate right-

---

* Perhaps he might better have called our modern modes of thinking Heraclitean, bearing in mind the emphasis that Heraclitus and Empedocles put upon process, interaction, and conflicting forces.

ing. Then comes a crisis, a state of emergency, and special unusual restorative maneuvers are automatically instituted. It is the totality of these things, including the actual injury suffered and the reaction to that injury or stress, which makes up what we call the picture of illness. It is an imbalance, an organismic disequilibration, and re-equilibration at a lower level of effectiveness and well-being. And if the imbalance is not corrected, it tends to impair the comfort or even threatens the biological survival of the individual. This leads to a search for relief, and the physician becomes a part of the complex of interrelationships. The sufferer becomes the subject of treatment, i.e., a "patient"; his condition, his altered equilibrium, becomes the "illness."

Internal and external equilibrium and the automatic maintenance of certain levels of functioning within the organism by various homeostatic devices were elegantly described by Claude Bernard, and later by Walter B. Cannon, in biochemical and physiological terms. This principle can, and in our opinion must, be extended to include psychological and social factors. Some of the interactions of individual and environment take place in ways that cannot be usefully reduced to physical and chemical terms. Organismic equilibrium maintenance and reciprocation between the individual and the outside world take place with the aid of special symbols, feelings, gestures, thoughts, and acts in patterns that are governed by the same general principles of reciprocity and integration which have been described by these eminent physiologists and others in regard to body tissues and body fluids.[2]

Forty years ago, when Freudian principles were beginning to have their effect upon static psychiatric concepts, the psychiatrist William A. White, the energetic behaviorist psychologist John B. Watson, Adolf Meyer, and numerous other spokesmen offered new formulae for approaching the study of human behavior. The basic model was that of an individual and an environment trying to get something out of each other, perhaps giving something to each other, and, at any rate, getting along with each other. One consequence might be that both of them were relatively satisfied; this was described as "adjustment." But if either was depleted or injured, this was described as "maladjustment." Many modifications of this oversimplified principle were gradually added in the growth of adaptation theory.

The clinical questions asked were: How does this individual gratify and frustrate his environment, and vice versa? This concept of adjustment neglected the fact that the individual himself is always a part of his own environment and is partly responsible for it. The oversimplification led to the rather easy classification of (a) well-adjusted or healthy persons and (b) maladjusted or unhealthy persons. Little was said about the environment. For this psychiatry was sharply criticized, with good cause, by sociologists, who tend to see what a nuisance certain individuals are to the commonweal, while the psychiatrists tend to regard the environment as that unpleasant aspect of the external world which has hurt their patients.

Many years ago, in trying to grasp this problem of the individual interacting with the environment for my own edification, I drew up a diagram [3] showing the continuous efforts of the individual and the environment to get something out of each other and to get along. The result might be that both the individual and the environment were satisfied (adjustment), or that either the individual or the environment was depleted or injured (no adjustment).

Actually the adjustment concept was a step ahead of the more simple notion of injury. Something in the environment had to be blamed. Cassius was very modern in declaring that it was not in our stars but in our selves. In many people's minds it is *still* in our stars that we are underlings. Later it was rather the moon which got blamed, followed by a series of somewhat smaller objects—dragons, werewolves, and witches. The physical size of danger continued to shrink; after lions, bears, and wolves were disposed of, it was rats, snakes, and varmints; then came insects, bacteria, and at the present moment viruses!

But this progressive shrinkage in the size, if not in the number, of external dangers has been accompanied by a greatly increased recognition of the danger inherent in the activities of man himself. And with such internal dangers, each individual is born into this world of external dangers and *opportunities* with certain genetic possibilities and limitations. Beginning with the pumping of the air surrounding him into and out of his bloodstream, and beginning with his mother's womb and breast and hands and face, the individual interacts with his environment, giving to and taking from it, a process which continues until the day he dies and his body is returned to the inorganic matrix of that environment as his last contribution. In the meantime he has interacted with it, given to it, taken from it, altered it, and been altered by it.

These sentences are bound to sound trite. In a way everyone knows this. Everyone accepts the fact that there is such an interactive and mutual process of adaptation between the individual and the world around him. But there are *many* worlds around us, some closer and some farther, and there are variable interactions between them. Very soon the whole thing becomes so complicated that we take refuge in oversimplification. We quote the reference that no man is an island, but we go on describing him as if he were. What has been offered here, has been only a reminder of this coexistence, this mutual dependency, this interaction, as something that can be kept in mind as we leave it now to concentrate upon the function and structure of the individual, the organism.

II. ORGANIZATION

We shall discuss some of the principles governing organization, along lines that have come to be referred to as "system theory." As applied to biological organizations, it is usually called "organismic theory." In every organism, despite constant irritations which provoke local or general reactions, a flexible balance is maintained internally with respect to the relationship of the parts. At the same time, a flexible balance is maintained externally with the environment, to which reference has just been made. Some change is allowed for in both of these flexible balances, and in the balance that exists between the balances, as it were.

The organism must maintain its own uniqueness or integrity, despite these variabilities, internal and external, and it must be able to alter its levels of operation and even of internal organization. Despite its material composition, the organism is able within limits to transcend matter; despite its operation in a lawful order, it may behave in ways which can also be described as free.

These and many other seemingly paradoxical statements contain the substance of modern scientific thinking regarding life and living. They constitute the point of view called organismic, admirably formulated by Kurt Goldstein,[4] which emphasizes process rather than structure, or process through structure. We, the authors, hold to this concept and hope to explain how we have found it useful.

A patient sometimes exclaims, "I feel as if I were going to pieces!" This description is apt to be met with condescending perception by the psychiatrist, who translates it into impressive professional terms such as "anxiety state" or "tension awareness." From the technical standpoint the expressions "falling apart," "getting upset," or "flying to pieces" describe a threatened state of imbalance and possible disintegration more accurately than do the contrived designations which fill the pages of many learned works on the physical and mental miseries of mankind. The man who feels himself "falling apart" or "going to pieces" has some vague sense of the unity and integrity of his personality. He *feels* rather than *knows* this to be a normal or ideal characteristic of life. By "being upset" or "unbalanced" or "going to pieces," he describes by implication an awareness of an equilibrium which we may well call "the vital balance."

Homeostasis

The principle that all organisms react to changing conditions in such a manner as to maintain a relatively constant "internal environment," as Claude Bernard [5] called it, or a "steady state," a term which von Bertalanffy [6] prefers, was introduced into physiology from chemistry by Claude Bernard and supported by many others such as Haldane,[7] Loeb,[8] Henderson.[9] It was most clearly and convincingly presented by Cannon [10] in his book *The Wisdom of the Body*. He wrote: "The constant conditions which are maintained in the body might be termed *equilibria*. That word, however, has come to have fairly exact meaning as applied to relatively simple physio-chemical states, in closed systems, where known forces are balanced. The coordinated physiological processes which maintain most of the steady states in the organism are so complex and so peculiar to living beings—involving, as they may, the brain and nerves, the heart, lungs, kidneys and spleen, all working cooperatively—that I have suggested a special designation for these states, *homeostasis*."

It is difficult to say who first enunciated the principle. Pierre-Louis Mareau de Maupertuis (1698–1759) "considered his own greatest achievement (among many) to be the discovery of the principle of least action (commonly credited to Leonhard Euler, Joseph Louis Lagrange or William Rowan Hamilton). Translated into modern biological terminology . . . Maupertuis' principle is none other than Claude Bernard's principle of the maintenance of the internal environment, Walter Cannon's principle of homeostasis, or Le Châtelier's law of chemical equilibrium: In a system in equilibrium, when one of the factors which determine the equilibrium is made to vary, the system reacts in such a way as to oppose the variation of the factor, and partially to annul it." (Le Châtelier's principle is often condensed to read that "a system tends to change so as to minimize an external disturbance.") But even prior to Le Châtelier,[11] Fechner [12] had developed a concept of stability in which the homeostatic principle was implicit. The monograph in which Fechner formulates this stability principle is extremely rare. His formulation as translated by John

Romano (personal communication) was: "All development progresses in the direction of an always more complete utilization of energy for stationary systems—maximum stability therefore always means maximum utilization of energy." *

Cannon saw homeostasis as a process of adaptive stabilization whereby a physiochemical constancy is maintained, such as the automatic regulation of body temperature, of the pH level of the blood, the maintenance of osmotic pressure, etc. His principle of homeostasis considered the regulations to be largely automatic; it emphasized function and direction in describing how forces act and counteract to bring an unbalanced situation back to a prior state of equilibrium. The following fragment of Cannon's description is typical:

> Note the nice economy of this organization in the body. The contracting muscles which need extra oxygen because of their contractions automatically favor the securing of the needed oxygen by returning the blood which carries it. And the diaphragm, which, as we have seen, is made to pump more vigorously during exercise, not only maintains in the lungs the oxygen supply for loading the oxygen carriers, but also aids to speed up the circulation of the carriers and thereby to augment their delivery of oxygen to the needy tissues.[13]

The principle of homeostasis has been extended by Freeman and others to "higher" levels of organismic behavior. For his own sake man tries to maintain a "steady state" outside, i.e., outside his body, as well as inside.

> The paramecium [remarks Freeman] maintains a beneficent external environment only by migration through food-laden waters. But man, faced with similar needs, improves upon the paramecium and maintains a superabundance of food (or the means of ready access) directly about himself. His . . . activities serve to maintain in the external environment not only a constant supply of food on the pantry shelf, but also the bank account, shelter, union membership, or circle of friends which are safeguards against potential external threats to internal constancies.
>   . . . Although it may sound farfetched at first, we should properly regard complicated total behavior and the maintenance operations of such organs as the liver as both directed to the same ultimate end—internal quiescence, relaxation, and the preservation of essential life constancies. In fact, the organismic energy system is organized so that homeostatic functions are taken over in a progressive fashion from lower to higher levels, as one after another fails to achieve adequate adjustment. [This takes us, by inference, into the fields of economics and sociology.] [14]

The principle of homeostasis as delineated by Cannon had the great advantage that it was very precise; it had denotable content at microscopic and macroscopic levels, and it could utilize the established and under-

---

* For a discussion of Fechner's impact on Freud's thinking, see: Ellenberger, H. F. "Fechner and Freud." *Bull. Menninger Clin.*, 20:201–214, 1956.

standable language of physics and chemistry. The fascination of this concept of homeostasis may lie in the fact that it brought wondrous things into the fold of science and pointed beyond the strictures of its own field and beyond the strictures of earlier concepts which relegated the study of life processes to a rather nebulous metaphysical vitalism. Its kinship to other scientific laws or principles, e.g., to the action of chemical buffer solutions, the principle of least action, the law of chemical equilibrium, and other forms of lawful self-controlling activity,* has been pointed out. It allowed, perhaps because of its daringness, a metaphoric application to ever wider spheres, to subject matters that had traditionally belonged to other sciences which had little direct relation to physics and chemistry. Well-known data, which had hitherto been poorly explained, began to make more sense. Cannon [15] conceived of homeostasis as a device to "release the highest activities of the nervous system for adventure and achievement . . ." From our point of view, these "highest activities" include total organismic government as represented in phenomena of self-regulation, which we regard as of the greatest importance.

Heterostasis

Ali ibn Hazm (994–1064) anticipated many modern psychiatrists when, in search of the "one end in human actions which all men unanimously hold as good and which they all seek," he discovered that all men were constantly escaping anxiety; this, he concluded, was the primary principle (i.e., motivation) of their behavior. He saw that "no one is moved to

---

* Long is the list of names of scientists who, in one field or another, found further application of this principle of homeostasis. Of particular interest for our purposes is the use which psychologists and psychiatrists have made of the homeostasis concept. The work of Orr, Kubie, Lindner, Goldstein, Cameron, Masserman, French, Burrow, Alexander, and many others invoked it. Freeman and Stagner used it as the basis for their psychological systems.

According to Kris, Anna Freud, and Bonaparte, Freud was occupied for years with the principle of the constancy of psychic energy. "In a letter to Breuer of 29.6.1892 he mentions 'the theorem which deals with the constancy of the sums of excitation' as the first of their joint theories, and in the first draft of their 'Preliminary Communication,' which was written at the end of November, 1892, the idea is taken further. The principle of constancy plays an important role in Freud's 'Project for a Scientific Psychology,' 1895 (p. 357) as the 'principle of inertia.' It then developed in the form of the 'pleasure principle' (the tendency of the mental apparatus to maintain a constant tension) and the 'Nirvana principle' (the tendency of the mental apparatus to reduce its tension to zero) into one of the regulative principles of psychoanalysis." (Kris, Ernst; Freud, Anna; and Bonaparte, Marie: *The Origins of Psychoanalysis.* New York: Basic Books, 1954.)

act, or resolves to speak a single word, who does not hope by means of
this action or word to release anxiety from his spirit."

Present thinking revises the wording of this scholar of a thousand years
ago by saying that all human behavior represents the endeavor on the
part of an organism to maintain a relatively constant inner and outer
environment by promptly correcting all upsetting eventualities. This was
worded in just about these terms in the famous essays of Claude Bernard.[16]
Any threat of radical change at any level will mobilize and direct energies,
locally and generally, which can cope with the changed conditions in the
direction of retarding any further change in the former harmony. Bacterial invasions evoke one kind of response, cold air evokes another, thirst
another, sexual stimulation another. Sentinel functions exist on many
fronts, like the elaborate DEW line in the north, which register any
threat or deviation and start a corrective chain of events. This conservative and defensive reaction pattern has been recognized as a primary
determinant of human behavior for a long time. We shall shortly discuss
it further.

But consider some larger pieces of behavior. What about falling in
love, riding a hobby-horse, learning a trade? Is the maintenance of satisfying relationships with the members of one's family or with one's co-
workers guided by the same principles which hold the blood-sugar balance constant? Or are we the victims of a pretty metaphor, a figure of
speech?

When such large-scale molar phenomena are brought under this principle and particularly when long-term adjustment processes are considered, some difficulties arise as to the precise meaning of self-regulation.
For example, as subsumed under the principle of homeostasis, is there a
complete return to the *status quo ante* after some disturbance in an organism? Is the process from disequilibrium to equilibration a circular one?
Can long-term processes such as growth, maturation, and decline be en-
compassed by the principle of homeostasis? Cannon had already devoted
attention to the aging of homeostatic mechanisms, describing the progressive failing of homeostatic regulation. Conversely, it has been seen
by some that homeostasis is also a product of evolution, that the human
infant, for instance, possesses a less perfect set of homeostatic mechanisms
than the adult. Is there, then, growth of homeostatic action and decline
of it? Or is it that when homeostasis at one level falls short, we have to
look at the next higher level of organization to find there a broader system of homeostatic regulation of which the lower level may partake?

It would be one-sided indeed to ignore the fact that there are other determinants of human behavior than merely passive adjustment to it. There is a strong urge within the organism to effect change, to initiate some of the very disturbances which the regulatory processes of the organism are patterned to resist. It is the conflict between the wish for change—newness, variety, opportunity—and the fear of *other* consequences of change which makes for the complexity of human behavior.

We must realize too that organismic regulation occurs in a number of different relationships simultaneously. There is the over-all question of regulated interaction between the organism and other organisms as well as the environment which involves all. And as to internal regulation, there is not only that which takes place between various parts of a system—let us say in the cardiovascular system—there are the interrelations between various complexities of tissues and structure. We speak of the cellular level, the organ level, the psychological level, the social level. This sort of thinking was introduced into psychiatry thirty years ago by Jelliffe and White, who proposed that we think in terms of the hormone as the "tool" of functioning at the physiochemical level, the reflex at the sensory-motor level, and the symbol at the psychic level. A *hierarchy* of levels can be recognized, each with its own mode and means of homeostatic regulation, interrelated by an over-all homeostatic tendency.

A case in point would be the human infant, whose regulation of body heat is poor as compared to that of the adult, but whose mother compensates for the infant's weaknesses by covering and uncovering its body when needed. One danger in this way of thinking is that it tries to explain the applicability or inapplicability of homeostasis by the principle itself. This is partly because there are certain phenomena, such as growth, which more aptly illustrate the entirely different principle of *heterostasis*, i.e., the progressively moving away from the *status quo*, the search for new and unsettled states, in contrast to the automatic return to the comfortable and relatively tension-free previous state of balance. As Freud [17] puts it:

> This is in close agreement with the hypothesis that the life-process of an individual leads, from internal causes, to the equalizing of chemical tensions: i.e., to death, while union with an individually different living substance increases these tensions—so to speak, introduces new vital differentia, which then have to be again lived out. For this difference between the two there must naturally be one or more optima. Our recognition that the ruling tendency of psychic life, perhaps of nerve life altogether, is the struggle for reduction, keeping at a constant level, or removal of the inner stimulus tension (the Nirvana-principle, as Barbara Low terms it)—a struggle which comes to expression in the pleasure-principle—is indeed one of our strongest motives for believing in the existence of the death-instinct.

This can be illustrated with a familiar problem in political science. When certain individuals in society are comfortable under a certain political regime, any proposed change is apt to be seen as a threat. The proposers of such a change are called radicals. If some members of the comfortable society are not quite as comfortable as others and see some possible benefits in some change, they are called liberals. Both they and the stable group regard themselves as conservative. But the radicals, on the other hand, who very much desire some kind of change, because it may benefit many, *including* themselves, regard those who oppose it as more than conservatives, as reacting against proposed progress. The practical fact is that everybody considers himself conservative; those who oppose any change are called reactionary, and those who want to disturb even the good things in the hopes of a better deal at least for themselves are "radicals." The contest fluctuates from one leaning to the other, maintaining a dynamic balance, capable of being overthrown. Corrective devices seem to be implicit in our universe, such that not only cells and organs but individuals and groups are governed by them.*

Servo-Mechanisms

One of many interesting analogues to the concept of homeostasis may be seen in the development of cybernetics, a body of knowledge relating to regulation and organized around the model of electronic servo-mechanisms. The automatic regulation of heat in our homes by means of

---

* As it found wider application in psychiatric and psychological thinking, the concept of homeostasis did not remain what it originally was, and the extended use of it has been criticized by many. A recent article by Toch and Hastorf [18] concludes with the observation that it is no longer a single concept, but really many concepts which have a common denominator in the various present uses of the concept of homeostasis: (1) the formal sequence that a state of disturbance is followed by quiescence; (2) quiescence is seen as the object or as the cause of the behavior initiated in connection with the previous state. The first statement is clearly a matter of mere observation, but the second statement is really a premise. Descriptive and explanatory elements are thoroughly mixed in the present use of the word homeostasis; it is sometimes even seen as a force or a drive. Another major fallacy in explaining behavioral phenomena in terms of homeostasis has been pointed out by Maze,[19] who warns that any observed stability can be the by-product of the many-sided clashes of sectional interests. It remains necessary to study the mechanisms that produce the effect; otherwise the term homeostasis may easily become a mysterious force or a pseudo-concept. Of course, this criticism is directed not against the more restricted use of the concept to explain certain forms of automatic self-regulation in physiology, with a demonstration of the precise mechanisms that are involved, but only against its overextended application where the term becomes a dangerous analogy. Davis [20] issues a similar warning, stating that the term homeostasis often refers indiscriminately to both the end and the means (mechanisms) of consistency maintenance.

a thermostat is a classic illustration. An earlier, purely mechanical fore-runner of such servo-mechanisms can be found in Watt's governor for steam engines. The analogy with the principle of homeostasis is striking: the performance of certain machines is automatically held constant, just as some physiochemical states are kept constant; deviations from some optimum or predetermined type of functioning are recorded by sentinel or signal devices; a chain of events is started to counteract the deviation that took place, and the end result is a return to the original state of balance or a very close approximation thereof. The whole chain of events takes place automatically, without interference by a consciousness, despite its seeming purposiveness.

Could this be another model from which concepts could be derived to better explain the complexities as well as the order of behavior? Several attempts have been made, notably by the originators of the idea (Wiener [21] and Woodger [22]). Stabilizing behavior by means of built-in automatic control devices which derive their energy from within the system that they regulate seems indeed a rather apt description of what happens to persons who get hungry and eat; who get cold and build houses with their hands and the materials which nature provides; who are threatened by an enemy, become angry, and are so propelled into action to remove the intruder by efficient counteraction; or who cope with an anxiety-arousing idea by turning it into an acceptable and comfortable opposite in order to restore the disturbed emotional equilibrium. Many pieces of complicated behavior can be seen as controlled by "feedback" networks. If an upsetting event happens, a part of the energy which caused the disturbance may be "borrowed" to counteract the source of the disturbance and so lead the organism back to its original level of balance.

Concerning the cybernetics model, one may ask the same questions which were raised about homeostasis. Do feedback devices produce a complete return to the *status quo ante?* Is the process circular? Are the mechanics of control the same at every level? Does it apply equally to parts and wholes, to systems, subsystems, and supersystems? Who "sets" the control device at the required limits?

There is one very interesting phenomenon which the cybernetic type of control makes much clearer than does the principle of homeostasis: the very counteractivity which corrects the undesirable deviation often proceeds in an oscillating fashion. Restoration of the original state of equilibrium is not a very smooth process but consists of a series of pulls and pushes, like the swings of a pendulum which gradually approximates the center-of-gravity position. The corrective activity may overdo or underdo the job it is called to do; there may be an overshooting or under-shooting of the mark while the corrective process is going on. This is a very familiar idea to those who study human behavior. In the course of adjustment to changing inner or outer conditions, people are often seen to overdo or underdo their corrective reactions. While the direction is clear, and the activity for it is mobilized, the adjustment may still fail because it proceeds by too much oscillation, which in turn may imply a further deviation from a given optimum. Devices which are meant to cope with anxiety may create new anxieties; anger modified into a forced niceness toward a given person becomes unctuousness but also retains the sting of anger and may be all the more intense because of the con-trast.

McCulloch [23] speaks in this connection of "the intrinsic disease * of negative feedbacks" and describes it in mathematical terms, the gist of which is an interesting analogue to the human situation faced by psy-chiatrists. Even when we think of all human behavior, including symp-toms of illness, as controlled by an inherent purposeful tendency toward self-regulation, do we not also observe that the corrective process may acquire autonomy so that the devices perpetuate themselves and be-come a nuisance? Then this condition in turn will have to be cor-rected.

Vital Balance

The principles of homeostasis and negative feedback, although devel-oped in different disciplines, converge on a sufficient number of points to be taken as valuable interscientific analogues. They can be borrowed from their original disciplines and applied to psychological data, and the result "makes sense." But again we must ask the troublesome ques-tion whether they can do justice to the long-term adjustment processes of life. Can they adequately account for those higher and more complex forms of behavior which show rich variability—creativity, a search for novelty and uniqueness, a continued growth of the organism? Life can-

---

* McCulloch's term "disease of negative feedbacks," though obviously used in a meta-phorical sense, is one of those phrases which point to an inherent difficulty in all attempts to use machine models for the understanding of human behavior. We are always apt to forget that a scientific model is not identical with the more complex, subtle, and less accessible part of reality which it attempts to clarify; the model does not proclaim that man *is* a machine, but only that his doings can be better understood if we consider him machinelike in certain ways.

not be without stability, but is a completely stable life human? How can we account for growth and learning? When the term "equilibrium" is used in human behavior, what do we really mean? What is "the vital balance"?

Further consideration of the idea of equilibrium and constancy has led to the scrutiny of another concept which was once thought to have great potential as an interdisciplinary analogue. It is the physicist's concept of entropy, formulated in connection with the second law of thermodynamics. This law states that energy exchange between two systems at different temperatures occurs in only one direction: from the hotter to the colder body. Other formulations of the law are possible, but the important thing for our discussion is that under certain conditions physical changes occur in one direction which cannot be counteracted from within. Boltzmann saw it as a universal law of nature and gave it the interesting formulation that the accumulation of all such irreversible changes in physical systems is tantamount to increased randomization of particles or a loss of order. A measure of this loss of order is entropy. As entropy increases, nature approaches an entropy-death—forms dissolve into a chaotic disorder governed merely by mathematical probability (thermodynamic equilibrium).

This conception has not failed to stir thinkers in other fields who found in this physical model an interesting parallel to their somber apperception of life as a living-unto-death solely guided by some victorious force of destruction. What is most important to remember, however, is the restriction under which this universal principle is seen to operate: it occurs in closed systems which cannot maintain a free exchange of energy with their surroundings. Can, then, the entropy concept be applied to living organisms, which are—by definition—not closed but open, their chief characteristic consisting in a perpetual exchange of energy with their environment? Quite aside from the probability that nature has very few truly closed systems, major distinctions will have to be made between closed and open systems when one sets out to study the changes, in all varieties, that take place within them.

Parts and Wholes

The considerations just detailed have given rise to a good deal of rethinking of the problems of self-regulation, organismic integrity, constancy maintenance, adaptation, equilibration, and many related matters only hinted at in the preceding pages. While our discussion has been mainly in terms of processes or mechanical action, we have occasionally used the word "system," and it should now be asked what *system* really means, and what kinds of system are most relevant to the phenomena of life and behavior. The structures and functions of life are an organization [24] beyond the layman's description of illness as a going to pieces or a loss of balance. We may ask what it is that falls apart, what the relations are between parts and whole, what balance could have prevailed and what the described state of unbalance implies. There is a considerable literature on these problems from which we would like to select the highly constructive work of the psychologists Köhler [25] and F. H. Allport [26] and the theoretical biologist von Bertalanffy,[27] as being most relevant to our discussion.

As a preamble, let us first consider two contrasting types of thought on the part-whole question.

One can conceive of a living organism as an intricate and specific arrangement of cells, each with its own structural and functional properties, which by addition constitute some totality that can be called organism. For one who has labored a lifetime behind a microscope, such a viewpoint makes sense. There is much in traditional psychiatry that converges with this rather molecular point of view: the assumed existence of an "entity" such as "dementia" that could "invade" an organism from somewhere and shatter it, is one example. A man "possesses" so and so much "intelligence" and "has" this or that temperament, which together "make him" what he is.

But one can also be impressed by the totality of a living organism, not as the product or addition of parts, but as a unit within which "parts" may evolve only by a deliberate and temporary shift of focus in the observer. In this case the observer, even while becoming analytical for a while, remains faithful to his first impression, which was the "entity" of the Gestalt. Köhler has amply documented the validity of this point of view by pointing out how many of such direct and irreducible wholes seem given in our universe.

When we feel that the two camps have ably presented their arguments with the help of empirical data, we may conclude that there is reasonable justification for both points of view to be relevant; it depends on what we see as the major or "true" ultimate purpose of our thinking, which was a factor in determining "what we first saw." What is a part from one point of view may be a whole from another point of view, and on whatever one focuses one's attention, the same "thing" is both part and whole, depending on an upward or downward perspective which one is free to take.* The whole man is a part of his family; his hand is a part of himself as well as a whole to his fingers; he would have never been born if there had not been the pre-existing whole of his parents. And if he is grossly deranged, some people would say that he "has" a "psychosis" and that this is a part of him which one may try to remove or to cure; but one can also say that he, as a whole, "is" psychotic, this being his present mode of total existence.

If one takes a position above the conflict between molar and molecular or holistic and elementaristic doctrines, one might prefer the more neutral term "aggregates." For Allport,[28] who frequently uses this term, it is only a provisional formulation which will receive further specification in terms of theory:

> The complex of elements and events making up an act of behavior, to which we have given the general name "aggregate," has been referred to by theorists under a number of names. It has been spoken of, for example, as a configuration, a pattern, an organized whole, a field, an assembly, or a mechanism. Still another term, one which we have also used on occasion, is "system." The system concept, like the notion of field, has received special development in various areas of science, and both these ideas have attained considerable generality as explanations of natural phenomena.

In other words, there are various wholes with different internal arrangements and different degrees of preponderance of parts (R. W. Gerard).[29] Several more distinctions cut across the ones just mentioned: the spatial-temporal, the static-dynamic, and the structural-functional dimensions. Each of the different theoretical concepts of wholes seems to emphasize a particular choice of these distinctions. If configuration, the preponderance of the whole over the parts, the dynamic equilibrium of a field of forces

---

* In all scientific thought a principle of reduction is at work. Raw experience is too varied, too manifold, too fleeting, too chaotic, and must be "fixed" and "shrunk" by a process of abstraction into a more manageable and orderly set of concepts which allows systematic grouping. Only then are mastery, explanation, control, and prediction possible. But that process also entails, or at least highlights, the so-called part-whole problem. In any scientific observation, small or large, what is taken as the whole and what as the parts? What are parts of? What is comprised by the whole? This leads to further questions about causal connections: does the whole constitute or determine its parts or do the parts constitute the whole? The history of science shows that the answers to these questions depend very much on personal preference of the theorist, the fashions of thought in certain eras, and the culture one belongs to, whereas Gestalt psychology has shown that it also depends on the inherent organization of certain natural phenomena. Therefore we find not only atomistic and holistic *views* side by side, but also atomistic and holistic *patterns of organization* in the things themselves.

and a relative independence of form from matter are emphasized, we obviously speak of a Gestalt; if, however, we stress a fixed arrangement of well-bounded parts which are all geared to forcing events into one predetermined course, we come close to the concept of machine. There is a tendency among thinkers in the behavioral sciences to stay clear of the doctrinaire position that "most wholes" or even "all wholes" with which science deals are of one type, e.g., a mechanism, a field, or a Gestalt (R. W. Gerard).* [30]

Open Systems and Closed Systems

Practically all authors who are concerned with system theory call attention to the distinction between closed and open systems, the latter being characteristic of living organisms. The open system exchanges energy with its environment, its components are materially in flux, and not only does it maintain itself as a whole with a relative degree of constancy, but it may also change to different levels of organization, as an organism does when it grows. The combination of these and other features of open systems have some bearing upon the form of equilibrium that can be attributed to it under the principle of constancy. While homeostatic processes provide the return to an original state as if it were a duplication of the point of departure, and whereas cybernetic constancy maintenance proceeds by oscillation between a fixed range of prearranged mechanisms, the sort of constancy that is maintained by open systems can perhaps better be described as a relatively steady state. Von Bertalanffy [32] is mainly responsible for the designation of "steady state" as a *terminus technicus*.

---

* As Allport points out, there is a general preference among modern biologists for a more generic conception of aggregates under the designation of a "system." A system can be defined in several ways, such as "a recognizably delimited aggregate of dynamic elements that are in some way interconnected and interdependent and that continue to operate together according to certain laws and in such a way as to produce some characteristic total effect." It is "concerned with some kind of activity and preserves a kind of integration and unity; and a particular system can be recognized as distinct from other systems to which, however, it may be dynamically related." The relationship between whole and parts of a system can be quantified as has been attempted by Gerard [31] in his idea of the "cellulation index" which ranges from zero for complete homogeneity to one for complete isolation of the parts. The same author speaks of stability (being) and change (becoming) as properties of the system. Various types of systems can be found in the specific realities with which the sciences deal, but it is also possible and even desirable to elevate the concept of system to a higher and more abstract plane.

The steady state is not static in most respects: the "parts" are in constant flux, there are perpetual intake and expenditure of energy, a state of complete rest is never reached, but a settling is constantly aimed at. ". . . A system, to perform work, however, must not *be* in equilibrium but continually on the way toward attaining it." [33] *

The closedness or openness of systems is a matter of degree, and open systems such as living organisms also contain internal arrangements in subsystems which provide equilibria of the homeostatic and cybernetic type. The organization of living organisms is so complex that both structural arrangements and various types of functional processes can be recognized at multiple levels, with different modes of integrity, degrees of cellulation, partial autonomy, constancy, division of labor, morphological and functional specialization, etc.

The concepts developed by the theory of open systems thus go well beyond the simpler models of self-regulation of homeostasis and feedback. Dynamic adjustments to changed conditions are not mere returns to a *status quo ante*, although they certainly act "to minimize an external disturbance," as Le Châtelier observed in the much simpler chemical systems. The very general principle of constancy maintenance, implying the ideas of integrity and regulation, pertains to all varieties of systems. Around this principle a number of specific models and theories have been built, each pointing to a particular mode of regulation and type of integrity. At certain levels we can find evidence of near-reversibility of change with an almost complete return to the point of departure; at other levels we find evidence for irreversible changes which produce variability itself as the consequence of special modes of constancy.

Man can be seen as an intricate combination of all these levels and modes of change: his temperature remains almost perfectly constant despite great changes in surrounding conditions, and his behavior patterns

---

* In a lucid article, Köhler describes the dynamic production of steady states in open systems by contrasting it with the fixed pathways of a machine, which exert control by constraints:

"It is true that certain anatomical arrangements force processes to take a course which helps the organism to survive. But what is the nature of such arrangements? Are they really comparable to the rigid constraints which we find in inanimate machines? In a most important sense, they are not. The very way in which they exist differs widely from the way in which constraints exist in machines. For the most part, such constraints consist of solid objects; they are composed of permanent materials which have been given one shape or another depending upon their particular purpose. On the other hand, no part of the anatomy of an organism is a permanent object. Rather, any such part must be regarded as a steady state, only the shape of which persists, while its material is all the time being removed and replaced by metabolic events." (Köhler, Wolfgang: *Dynamics in Psychology.* New York: Liveright, 1940.)

repeat themselves with discouraging monotony. But as a curious animal he also shows the possibility of new variations by seeking adventures, by creating new things, making new friends, and developing new theories. In other words, he is "discovered" somewhere between absolute closedness and complete openness.

Thus it may create confusion to speak of man's integration, for is not the gist of the foregoing that he has all sorts of integrations? The inevitable fact is, however, that the different levels of organization within a system are not separate entities but just so many ways in which it functions. There are levels integrated with each other and within the system. Their mere juxtaposition is no organism—it is recognition of different levels of organization, implying the idea of hierarchy, which makes organization.

Gerard [34] suggests that the degree of integration of an organism is that of the top level: "Highly integrated units could be present in a poorly integrated org [organism]; although societies are made of men, perhaps the most highly integrated orgs at the individual level, most of our societies are the equivalent of the flatworm or sponge stage, on the biological scale."

Of the criteria of integration Gerard holds that: (1) the more integration, the greater the differentiation of the units composing it; (2) the more the interaction between the units and their interdependence, the sharper the boundary of the organism; (3) the more powerful its buffer or homeostatic mechanisms, the stronger the influence of the whole on the units as compared to the influence of the units on the whole, and the greater the cohesion.

Indeed, when we wish to find out how well Mr. X is integrated, we do not check his performance randomly at any odd level and leave it at that, but we try to formulate an organized statement about his over-all functioning with an ultimate emphasis on his topmost performances: how he gets along with other people, how "whole" he is, how well he can adapt himself to the demands of the day, how well he can master his inner and outer environment to the benefit of himself and society. In our statement, however, we do take into account, e.g., the existence of a poorly integrated subsystem of locomotion due to a crippled leg, or the pressure of an almost autonomous and whole-disrupting unit called "carcinoma," or the energy-absorbing process of mourning over a loved one. The integration at the top level is what it is, sometimes despite and sometimes because of whatever we find in the subsystems.

Need for Multiple Observations

The foregoing considerations, abstruse as they may sound at first reading, are basic to the philosophy of modern psychiatric case study, the object of which is to examine and describe the degree and nature of a disturbing imbalance.

We cannot rely upon a patient to tell us just what is wrong or wherein his integration is failing, just where or when the boiler will burst or the lid fly off. No apology is offered for this mixture of metaphors; all of them are close but none of them is right. A person's relationship with the outside world has begun to fail, and this failure is related to his internal integrations, which ought to be able to manage things, but can't. If he loses his job, he may lose his wife; if he loses his wife his heart may break. If he keeps his job he may develop an ulcer, and if he develops an ulcer he may strike down his neighbor and go to jail.

Such is the complicated and delicate network of interdependencies. The dismay and discouragement of the young student of psychiatry are understandable. How will he ever grasp all this? he wonders. How can he discover all the patterns of internal integration and of external integration operating for his patient, or which did once operate, only to break down? How relate the sensations the patient describes with the sensations experienced by the patient's relatives?

There is always the easy way out of the perplexity, consisting of looking for classical landmarks and traditional forms. There still *are* doctors who refer glibly to the "praecoxes" they are caring for, or the "manics" or the "neuros" or the "psychotics" or the "psychopaths." It is not only the vulgarity of such designations that one deplores; it is rather the low level of comprehension of mental illness they betray. These users forget that the "manics" of yesterday are not here today, nor are the witches or the wolf-men or the swine-infesting evil spirits.

We think it is better to teach young psychiatrists to endure the bewilderment of complexity for a time, to make observations at all levels, and to learn to think in polydimensional terms in regard to integration. They must see this integration as both external and internal, the integration of the individual in the outside world (which has been called adaptation) and the integration at the various levels of organismic function under the aegis of homeostasis. Integration in a total sense implies, of course, methods of self-regulation and the proper maintenance of the vital balance.

This is more than three-dimensional thinking; it is thinking in five dimensions. There are the external relationships; there are the internal relationships; there are the reactions of the one set to the other. Then there is the effect of time and of growth; nothing ever remains what it was at the moment it was observed. Thus one has to begin to think in terms of trends and directions and total changing forms. All these are related to intricate, interrelated balances which go to make up the total picture.

There is, thus, in the thinking of behavioral scientists a broad trend toward accepting a unitary formulation for the data studied in the separate disciplines. In a way this is an attempt to arrive at a "common sense" of all the sciences which might serve as a much needed correction for the tyranny of words, which is so ready to take over when the conceptual framework of a given discipline expands. Moreover, although the layman's opinion cannot be a court of last resort, scientific formulations must keep in touch with the visions and feelings of the common man concerning whom it has so much to say. To the extent that psychiatry deals with suffering, the ultimate verification of its technique must depend for a large part on people who know "what it feels like" as well as "what it looks like" to suffer. To many it feels like falling apart, going to pieces, or losing one's balance, and we now propose to view it that way, systematically and at some length.

CHAPTER VI

Toward a Theory of Human Behavior

(CONTINUED)

III. CONTROL

THE PHYSICAL parts of the total human organism or "personality" are maintained in relationship to one another by intricate anatomical and physiological processes, but there are also psychological functions which act as parts relating themselves to each other and to the whole or total personality. Freud assumed that the instinctual drives of the human organism are controlled and directed by another group of psychological parts or functions called the ego.

Colloquial uses of the word "ego" often carry accusatory overtones of selfishness or vanity, perhaps through association with the derivative concept of egotism. In scholastic philosophy the term ego denoted the integration of body and soul which affords distinctness and uniqueness to a personality. In metaphysics ego denotes the subject of experience in distinction to the content of that experience. In psychology the term ego retains some elements of these older meanings. Stressing unitary cohesiveness and organization of various mental states, the term "ego" is used to designate that part of the personality which experiences, perceives, reflects, suffers, and decides. Inevitably this abstraction is often concretized and comes to be thought of as a kind of invisible ruler of the brain. In part this can be attributed to language; the functions of the ego tend to be projected into a thing or subject behind the action referred to by the verb. But the problem is not entirely one of language, for there is a structure responsible for most functioning, and function and structure are, indeed, interdependent.* Rapaport endeavored to harmonize the structure-

---

* Biology offers many examples of organismic functions which alter the structural properties of the whole and give rise to new structures, such as the linear and sagittal leaves developing under different conditions in *Sagittaria sagittifolia*. It conversely may be found in many instances of tissue atrophy after disuse. On the other hand, gross alteration in structure is possible without noticeable impact on functioning, as was demonstrated by Driesch in the dissection of cells from *Echinus* larvae. The induction processes of "organizers" in transplants, the phenomena of polarity between proximal and distal parts in botany and zoology, and the general biological concept of equifinality, all refer to a demonstrated reciprocity between function and structure.

function dichotomy in psychology by describing psychic structures as "processes with a slow rate of change." [1]

The history of psychoanalytic writings reflects this ambiguity in respect to the functional and structural attributes of the ego. In earlier publications, insofar as it was given any status at all, the ego often appeared as a poor helpless manikin buffeted about by the powerful forces of the instincts, the prime organizers (it might seem) of the personality. In later writings the ego appeared more and more as a harassed monarch governing a complicated household of institutions and forces.

Sometimes it would seem to be the ego which gives personality its firmness, its boundaries, its articulation and delineation; but, if instinct theory is overemphasized, it would appear as if the ego were an executive, appointed by all-powerful instincts. Sometimes the term ego is equated with personality or character structure. Sometimes the ego is described as having special functions of its own; sometimes as merely having a subservient role (e.g., seeking objects for the satisfaction of instincts).

The genesis of the ego has been a subject of much speculation and research; [2] opinions are divided as to whether the ego is a product of differentiation of instincts, an epiphenomenon of drive-dynamics, or whether it was always there, at least in embryonic form, with its own potential structure, its autonomy, and its primal reality.

It has often been described as an emergent entity, the product of conflict, and yet at the same time it is assumed by many theorists to antecede conflict, being present in embryonic form, as it were, prior to birth as a bio-psychological *Anlage*. In other words, psychoanalytic theory ascribes to the ego a role of organizer in the process of growth and at the same time views it as an appendage to a special group of instinctual functions over which it acquires a certain modifying or controlling dominance.

Freud [3] postulated an accessory or "super" ego serving as an adviser, admonisher, encourager, and threatener to the ego and as a judiciary body, acting in accordance with a rule book inscribed during the infancy and early childhood periods. So aptly did these concepts fill the needs of psychiatric thought that, in their wide acceptance, the ego and superego became frequently referred to as if they were organs, lodged somewhere within the body like the medieval "soul."

Light is thrown on this problem by reference to system theory as discussed some pages above. The question is not whether the ego is master or servant, whether it is controlled or a controlling agency, whether it is a (mere) drive-appendage or an independent institution. [4] Let us change the form of the questions somewhat. We know of systems in general that they have parts, although the mere juxtaposition of parts does not of itself make the system. We know that systems have a hierarchical order of substructures which are more or less delineated and which relate to one another in specific ways through more or less permeable boundaries. We know that systems tend to a division of labor, giving rise to specialized functions for certain parts, but that despite this they preserve their over-all unity in varying degrees. We also know that systems maintain some degree of stability despite undergoing constant change. We know, in short, that systems are systems in that they maintain a certain degree of integrity, identity, and stability by economic self-regulation.

And so, with respect to the ego, we may ask questions like this: What kind of subsystem is the ego, and what special functions does it have as a subsystem? What is its degree of independence or autonomy? How does it fare in the division of labor and how does it further this process of division? How is it related to the integrative tendencies of the total system? What role does it play in that process? What does it regulate, and by what is it in turn controlled? If it is a product of differentiation, what role does it play in preserving the unity of the system? What role does it play in the adaptive capacities of the system? How does it serve the goal and processes of constancy maintenance for the system as a whole? Does it add to the "openness" of the system or does it tend to make the system more closed? Is it an advocate of constancy or of change and versatility?

Several of the functions traditionally ascribed to the ego are performed at "lower" (physiological and chemical) levels of organization. Constancy maintenance is also observed in simpler systems which do not have sufficient differentiation and division of labor to fall within the purview of what psychologists call "ego." Adaptation is found throughout nature, and self-regulation is a characteristic of all systems.

There is no denying, however, that the ego concept is particularly applicable to the bulk of processes employed in the self-regulation of human behavior. Typical ego functions as conceived by Freud include such processes as perception, control of voluntary movement, management of memory, production of adaptive delay between perception and action, decisions between "fight" or "flight," the channelization of instinctual action tendencies, the selection of needs to be gratified or to be suppressed, the judging and evaluating of internal and external conditions, etc. The balance between assimilation and accommodation, in which Piaget [5] sees the essence of the adaptation process, must also be mediated and implemented by the ego. Many other functions have been added to this list.[6] All these functions perhaps have primitive and simple forerunners with other names in simpler organisms where there is no reason to postulate an ego proper, such as the nucleus of a living cell, the "organizer" in transplants. Thus, for the very reason that the ego is defined by these functions, it may be considered as an advanced subsystem in organisms, a product of differentiation, a part of the process of division of labor, and a means to the ends of the total system. Among these ends are such items as constancy maintenance, adaptation, self-preservation, growth, and procreation.

Many of our previous questions about how the ego arises must await further research, but research is bound to be more wholehearted when it is guided by belief that the ego does have some degree of autonomy and that it cannot be explained by complete reduction to the antecedent drive conditions. The parts of a system are most usefully defined by their structural delineation from other parts, by their functional specialization, by their dynamic relations with other parts, and above all, by the tendencies, tasks, purposes, etc., of the whole system and the "fitting" of that system into the larger systems in which it pursues its vital interests.

Psychic Topography

Freud [7] approached the structural delineation of the ego by means of a topographical analysis of the total person. He thought of the ego (and the superego) as the most clearly bounded of the main subdivisions of the personality and the id as a permeable buffer zone which also represents one border of the ego, but the other delineations of the id were vague and unspecified, or even nonexistent. The ego, however, was assigned fairly clear boundaries, also, with respect to the outside world, with which it maintained contact by means of its perceptual and motor apparatuses, and with respect to the super-ego. Freud saw the mature ego as a well-developed, well-delineated, fairly autonomous subdivision of the personality system. A similar thought must have guided those theorists who take the firmness or sharpness of ego-boundaries as an indication of ego strength and good over-all functioning of the organism.[8]

From an evaluative point of view the well-functioning ego is also seen as a "highest level" or "ultimate achievement," a goal of therapy.

"Where id was, there shall ego be." [9] This presupposes that the ego strives to acquire as much autonomy as is consistent with the larger goals and aims of the system.*

The ego cannot act solely in the service of the instincts. Ego and instincts are two intra-organismic subsystems which have to come to terms with each other, both working toward the larger organismic goals, and therefore both defined, in part, by those goals.** The ego's importance depends upon its functions of self-regulation, steady-state maintenance, and integrity preservation. This is exactly what Freud described when he gave formal status to both the instincts and the ego, each with their relative autonomy and their own mode of regulation: one obeying the pleasure principle and the other obeying the reality principle. The term "primary process"—though it is sometimes poetically described as a "seething caldron"—describes a kind of regulation intrinsic in instinct organization, while "secondary process" stands for the regulations typical of ego functioning. There has been an unfortunate tendency to slip into the error of assuming that "primary process" means chaos, disorderliness, maladaptation, and, in the strict sense of the word, absence of any regulatory principle. For Freud this was obviously not so, since his work has consisted for a large part in showing how lawful and well regulated the vicissitudes of instincts are. His dualistic instinct theory in itself (to be discussed in the next section) contains the possibility of dynamic form and order in that opposing tendencies are pitted against each other. From an organismic viewpoint, it would be more correct to assume that instinctual functions and ego functions represent different levels of organization and activity which interact with each other for the sake of the whole. [10]

---

* One consequence of this is that the ego must be placed high in the hierarchical order of the system, playing an exceptionally important role in the system's general work. For this reason the degree of integration of a person is usually stated in terms of the organization of his ego, which is, after all, a subsystem, and this seems entirely in line with Gerard's contention that the degree of integration in any system must be formulated in terms of its highest level.

** Division of labor within a system does not necessarily mean that the functions of one part are totally different from the functions of another part so that the parts become functionally incomparable; more often than not it amounts only to a specialization in, or a proportionally greater emphasis on a certain task or type of work. It may even be rather a difference of style in the performance of something that is necessary for the whole. If the human organism is one specimen of the open system, we must then envisage the possibility that instincts are not just forces that may become a nuisance and that should be by all means controlled or dampened, but that they, in their own style, may participate in the processes of regulation, constancy maintenance, and many of the other tasks and goals of the whole organism.

Our present aim is to focus on the relationships between the ego (including the superego) and the instincts with respect to self-regulation and constancy maintenance of the organism. Given the task to regulate, to integrate, to maintain and repair, to create the highest degree of organismic order, how do the ego and the instincts relate themselves to each other? What reciprocal relationships do they maintain under various conditions; which are the power relations between the ego on the one hand, and the constructive and destructive action tendencies of the organism on the other hand?

The Functions of the Ego

We ascribe to the ego first of all the function of orientation and detection. Like a monitor or a periscope it constantly scans the environmental horizons for possibilities and necessities, threats and opportunities. Simultaneously it remains in constant contact with the internal situation; it "listens" to many voices. It is aware of instinctual needs and urges, of states of somatic functioning, of standards and stipulations of the conscience and of various internal autonomies, including its own. The conjunction of internal and external details makes an infinite kaleidoscopic pattern; pressures sometimes coincide and sometimes conflict. An infinite number of reconciliations is achieved, most of them without any strain or stress. Like our breathing, the ego acts for the most part automatically. But circumstances can accelerate it or slow it or distress it to the very threshold of extinction.

In accounting for the mechanisms or processes used in personality government, Freud described something that is in some ways analogous to what we have described above as cybernetic feedbacks. Energies derived from the great reservoir of instinctual impulses, capable of direction toward the outside world (in response to opportunities and dangers), become organized, so to speak, into a functional device which serves to counsel delay or modification in the instinctual response to outside stimuli in favor of more adaptive, i.e., more selective and guarded, releases. The anxiety-perceiving functions of the ego constitute another element found in cybernetic control: the signal function. It is thus that the ego can be described as organizing the investment of the instincts, by permitting or not permitting the outflow of their energies. The energy needed for this mode of control is derived from the energies of the instincts themselves. But the ego also seems to *direct* the investment of the instincts, by selecting * their objects and determining in what form they are permitted to emerge; it also evaluates and chooses between the opposing instinctual tendencies and often attempts to combine these in a particular configuration.**

In order to perform its adaptive function of discrimination (as a prelude to instinct direction and release), the ego must perceive and appreciate reality. It must make tests and distinctions and it must make decisions on the basis of experience. The latter term implies access to a memory storehouse—foreconscious memories, conscious memories, unconscious memories—the complicated structure and management of which constitute much of the technical material of psychoanalytic investigation. In dealing with external events, the ego must be able to appreciate opportunities for satisfaction and situations of excessive stimulation as well as situations of insufficient gratification for instinctual needs, or threats of danger and loss. It may bring about appropriate modifications in the external world, or in the relations of the organism to that external world, in order to gain the maximum advantage. It can, in other words, initiate intermediary activity or behavior, the function of which is to bring about a situation in which organismic satisfactions may occur.

But the ego must have more than an external orientation; it must also

---

* "The intact, normally functioning, awake organism operates in a milieu from which a dynamic flux of input stimulation is continually received. Adaptive organismic accommodation to this input entails: 1. A receptor system for external stimuli; 2. A receptor system for internal stimuli including those from muscle, joints, and viscera; 3. A system for filtering the diverse sensory input and integrating and interpreting it; 4. An effector system involving autonomic and volitional motor acts; and 5. A chemical energy production system necessary for the adequate evocation of reactions in each of the separate systems mentioned." (Luby, E. D., et al. "Model Psychoses and Schizophrenia." *Am. J. Psychiat.* 119:61–68, 1962.)

** When such selective functions of the ego are taken into account, and particularly when it is recognized that the relative autonomy of the drives themselves has a reverberating effect on the ego's selectivity and choice, the model of cybernetics seems no longer tenable as an adequate analogue to the psychological process. We are then at a level of thorough interaction of variables giving rise to dynamic patterns, with a type of causality which Jordan described as a "pantocepter relation" and with processes described by von Bertalanffy and Köhler as "dynamic regulations." The latter are typically found in open systems with a high degree of internal and external exchange of materials and energies. The recognition of more flexible and selective (or, in the words of cybernetics, nonbinary) ego functions imposes a restriction on the suitability of the feedback model for psychological analysis; but there is no reason, particularly when one recognizes the coexistence of many different levels within the same organism, to exclude any form of regulation from one's conceptual repertoire. The gist of the matter is that all three classical forms of self-regulation—homeostasis, cybernetics, and dynamics—are found in the complex open system that the human organism is. As mechanics and processes of open systems, they serve the ends of the system by promoting its stability as well as its versatility, its integration as well as its differentiation, its rise and fall.

be perceptually sensitive and discriminating in an internal direction, i.e., toward the demands, on the one hand, of the instinctual forces in their qualitative and quantitative aspects, and on the other hand toward the internalized psychological representations of external reality through the development of the "superego" and "ego ideal." The latter have their beginnings in relation to the social situation present in the developmental stages of the individual, the demands and ideals to which it was exposed and to which it aspired.

With all this information, the ego is in a position to select the most expedient program for dealing on the one hand with the instinctual urges and on the other hand with reality. The various ways in which it does this have been the subject of innumerable psychological and psychoanalytic studies and reports. While it is exposed to a variety of forces on different sides, the ego is, however, not merely the arena of these forces but also their mediator and arbiter. It has an autonomy of its own and it also has energy of its own; it is not only a means to the ends of drives and reality, but it poses its own development as an end, to the extent that this is compatible with the over-all well-being of the organism. Various ego devices have been discovered by psychoanalytic studies, such as repression, suppression, acting to alter, taking flight, identifying with the enemy, and sublimation. We must assume that the reader is already familiar with these basic activities of the ego. Our emphasis is now upon the ego's use of all these devices in the interest of the maintenance of a steady state for the organism, allowing in that concept for the inclusion of constructive shifts in the level of organization and functioning to permit growth, development, and the realization of potentialities. This will lead us to a consideration of the ego's methods of dealing with those adventitious disturbances which come from a combination of external trauma and internal instincts and which may effect shifts of adaptation in a retrograde direction.

For our purposes, then, the ego may be described as a controlling agency which recognizes, receives, stores, discriminates, integrates, and acts by restraining, releasing, modifying, and directing impulses. It may be conceived of as an expression (and product) of basic biological tendencies toward organismic unity, synthesis, integration, and steadiness. At the same time the instincts, which are also expressions of biological tendencies toward survival and adaptation, are among the pressures which the ego has to mediate and manage. Thus the ego is the guardian of the vital balance.

The Ego and the Body

In order to make our theory applicable not only to psychological be-havior and interpersonal relationships, but also to the organism's relation to matter needed for the maintenance of life, we include among the pres-sures which the ego mediates those deriving from physiological processes, including homeostatic regulations of the sort described by Cannon. When physiologists say that the maintenance of physiological homeostasis is automatic, what they presumably mean is that it takes place without a preponderant participation of consciousness: we know when we are thirsty, or cold, even if we do not know when we are deficient in calcium. Over a wide range the ego continues to recognize and deal with the or-ganism's needs for oxygen, for water, for certain minerals, for warmth, for rest and other biological necessities. Murray [11] aptly calls these the viscerogenic drives (the word drive is here used as a hypothetical con-struct denoting a force and felt by the individual as tension) and lists twelve of them.

What we call ego functions include several which are also present in the single body cell. Since in ontogenesis and phylogenesis the ego emerges within the organismic system, it retains certain qualities of the system and must maintain relations of similarity, analogy, and perhaps even identity with other parts and functions of the system, in addition to its specific differences. Because of its emergent nature, the ego must have a whole range of relations to the body.[12] The effects of hormones on dreams, which Daniels,[13] Finley,[14] Benedek,[15] and others have demon-strated, suggest that all biological needs are registered and regulated by the same governing "apparatus" which registers and mediates in more specialized form the psychological needs. Automatic activity does not exclude ego participation; in many cases, the ego is certainly able to interfere with automatic activity. Conscious interference with such reflex activities as respiration and eyeblinking is possible, and voluntary starva-tion is not uncommon. We see no reason, therefore, to exclude any of these physiological processes from the same formula which has been outlined for the psychological ones—or perhaps the clauses in this sen-tence should be reversed, since the concept of homeostasis antedates the present search for concepts of psychological self-regulation. The span of human attention and comprehension is limited, and hence there may be practical advantages to restricting our discussion of ego functions to what is usually called organized behavior. But there are also practical reasons for not doing so, and we have in mind now the whole sphere of so-called psychosomatic medicine.[16] One could say that psychosomatic medicine is a practical clinical effort to make piecemeal applications of the hypothesis of total organismic steady-state maintenance to processes which should never have been excluded from it. It is astonishing to see how often in our prevalent concepts of the human personality the body and its processes seem to have been forgotten or only treated as some necessary, but not quite relevant substratum.

Recapitulation

We have had much to say about control, and little so far about the forces which challenge or disrupt controls. Before we turn to a discussion of these, let us recapitulate what has been said so far. We have submitted that all behavior, that of cells and organs and the total organism, may be defined as a continuous attempt to preserve or enhance organismic integrity by some degree or type of adjustment to disturbed balances. We must define the steady state in a broad sense, not just as physiological constancy or just as psychological steadiness, but as the integrated operation of all constancy-maintaining partial systems of any kind comprising the total personality, and even the environment in which it moves. Changes in the balance of one partial system may reverberate throughout the system and may sometimes grossly affect the steadiness of other partial systems. One has only to review the literature of experimental and accidental isolation (Hebb,[17] Lilly,[18] etc.) to see what striking imbalance can be produced by such seemingly "simple" changes as stimulus deprivation of one sort or another. We would also call attention to the production of experimental psychoses by various drugs, and its converse, the influence of ataractic drugs on ego functions. There is probably also a hierarchy of integrative processes, whereby one process is more autonomous than another, or takes precedence over another.* Within the hierarchy many processes shade easily into one another. As for the mech-

---

* In a recent paper, Teitelbaum called attention to the relationship between "simple mobilization processes" which regulate "automatically" the constancy of body temperature, and the "motivation process" which they activate after failure, as when one takes off one's coat and prepares a refreshing drink. (Teitelbaum, H. A.: "Homeostasis and Personality." *Arch. Neurol. Psychiat.* 76:317–324, 1956.)

anisms involved, and their possible impact on the hierarchy of maintenance processes, there is much fascination in the researches of Penfield [19] et al on the centroencephalic system and of Magoun [20] and his co-workers on the reticular activating system. Several investigators have made attempts to relate the experience of anxiety and the personality's defenses against it to the neurophysiological processes in the reticular activating system.

And now we can refer back to one of our opening statements, which was that the ego is the name for a group of functions and not a thing. While still thinking that this is valid for the ego as a concept, we may nevertheless say that subjectively the ego is often experienced as thing-like. In many respects this seems a result of the close connections between the ego and the body.

Our broad concept of organismic self-regulation is that it produces or strives for a state of balance by a reconciliation of all the demands (physical and psychic) operating upon and within the organism, whereby maximum satisfaction is achieved at minimal cost, in a variable outer and inner environment. Effecting this reconciliation, maintaining this physio-psycho-social balance, is one of the most specialized functions of the ego. In this sense the integrating work of the ego (representing a very high level of organization within the total system) may be taken as an index of the over-all integration of the whole system.

IV. MOTIVATION

When a scientist makes assumptions or working hypotheses, he recognizes them to be tentative and is prepared to abandon them if they prove unworkable or when more useful ones develop. In a sense all science is the searching for more useful hypotheses that may become explanatory principles or "laws." In this presentation we have made many assumptions; most of them are in current use and favor.

One group of *moot* assumptions which we make has to do with the ultimate motivation of behavior. Nothing is, on the surface, more completely a matter of common sense than why we do what we do, and nothing upon investigation proves to be more abstruse and controversial. When a child or a prisoner before the bar is asked why he did a certain thing, the answer that infuriates us most is: "I don't know." If he says, "I know but I won't tell you," he gets more respect. If he gives an explanation we don't understand, he at least challenges our perspicacity.

If he palpably lies, he does no more than use a universal human defense measure and we forgive him. If he offers an explanation that doesn't hold water he may be pitied and punished but he will not be abused. But for him to be totally unable to explain his own behavior suggests a kind of departure from the modes and customs of the human race and we abhor it—and him.

Medical science traditionally has never been much concerned with motivation, while religion and philosophy—and later psychology—have long had a proprietary attitude toward it. The right, the wrong, the reason, the need, the wish, the fear, the intention, the stimulus, the inhibition—all these things existed, of course. They were known to doctors as to everyone else. But who could bring order and structure to the whims of the human heart?

Freud could, and did. He was almost the first physician even to try, and his attempt came about unexpectedly. Educated in a strict biological, organic, neurological tradition, he disclaimed any competence in religion and philosophy. He had little training either in psychology or in psychiatry, except for a period of study with Brentano. But his neurological practice brought him face to face with clinical paradoxes that forced him to erect hypotheses regarding motivation, particularly motivation lying *behind* consciousness. Instinctual forces of various kinds had long been assumed to play a part in human behavior. What Freud did was to construct a comprehensive theory to relate these instinctual forces to the kinds of dealing with objects and events in the environment which occur, and to show how the whole process is partially governed and directed by what he called the ego.

Watching the behavior of any of the lower animals impresses one by the activities that seem clearly to be dictated by physiological needs—nutritional, reproductive, life-preservative, pain-avoiding. Actually these needs overlap; a need to avoid freezing to death can pretty much modify an animal's "need" to reproduce. Then there are many "needs" which we do not understand at all—certain kinds of antics, certain migrations, certain antipathies. The animal seems driven to do certain things beyond the gratification of a need. In other words, the motivation seems to be in the nature of a push rather than a pull. And thus we gradually begin to attribute to the animals something more basic than a mere set of "needs," namely, some kind of internal motivation.

When we turn to human beings, the situation becomes more complex and yet more clear. Many more needs are recognized, and yet the striving and propulsion from within are even more obvious. Not only can we make the same observations we make on laboratory rats, but we can also "feel" them in *ourselves* and inquire about such feelings in others. Body needs present themselves to us with great urgency and often persist until measures for their satisfaction have been taken. Feelings of love, pride, anger, lust, and envy hover gently over or rise to a high pitch and lead to all sorts of action. Thoughts and fantasies come and go—sometimes fleetingly as in reverie, sometimes sharply focused on a problem. Moreover, when we are in each of these different states the world outside us will take on a different significance or appear in a different light: to a man in a rage the furniture of his room will become "things to be smashed up," while to the same man in love the same furniture may appear as "something to recline on."

Traditional psychology focused its primary attention upon sensation, perception, memory, and cognition rather than upon motivation. As E. B. Holt [21] put it in his classic presentation, *The Freudian Wish*, Freud's discoveries led to the substitution in psychological theory of the *wish* for the *sensation* as the unit of experience. It was with neurological studies of sensation that Freud began his scientific career, and his research work led to the discovery of the local obliteration of sensation through injected chemicals (cocaine, etc.). When he then turned to clinical work, the phenomena of blocked sensation were of particular interest to him, as they appeared in "hysterical" patients, and in experiments with hypnosis. But as Freud watched the demonstrations of Charcot in this field, he kept asking himself, Why? Why do they accept the suggestion *not* to feel? What is their reason? What need of theirs is thereby fulfilled? What is the motive? And how can it produce the clinical result?

It is easy to see how this shift in Freud's preoccupations from the sensation to the motive was interpreted by his colleagues as an abandonment of proper scientific thinking and a turning toward the mystical. When the English (later American) psychologist McDougall—although far removed from Freud in his basic concepts—had the temerity to describe *instincts* as the primary sources of human motivation, he too was denounced; the behaviorist Watson cited it as evidence that "Professor McDougall returns to religion!" [22]

Scientists—especially physical scientists—impose a strict taboo on poorly defined or ambiguous words. They feel that if it is to live up to its rules, science should confine itself to the "what" and "how" of behavior, to the detailed processes that can be observed, recorded, produced, or repeated. But psychologists cannot stop asking about the "why" of human behavior; psychiatrists even less. They are directly confronted by people who come to them either with the question itself, or with proposed answers, or with both. Patients ask anxiously, "Why do I have this symptom?" Or they give all sorts of reasons *why* they come to the psychiatrist and *why* they think they need help and *why* that need arose. What they say is often a mixture of self-justification and embarrassment, with very little explanation and very unsound reasoning. Yet the search for an explanation of the symptoms, the maladjustment, the moves and countermoves remains a valid one. We all *think* we can explain why we do what we do.

Furthermore, there is an obvious fallacy in the assumption that the question "why" as applied to behavior is answered by listing "reasons," unless one understands by the word "reasons" more than merely the "reasoning" of the individual. We want to believe that man is a rational creature, but there is so much evidence that he is not. No one can know all the reasons for his behavior, and yet almost anyone can give *many* reasons for specific acts. Over and beyond the reasons he gives, there are many reasons which he doesn't give. There are reasonable but unmentioned reasons and there are unmentioned and unreasonable reasons, reasons depending upon emotions or biological processes of which the individual has no full knowledge.

In everyday life it is common practice to explain a small piece of one's behavior, or even a large program, in ways that pass muster. Such explanations are the very bulk of our social intercourse. We tell a child why we send him to school, why we put him to bed early, why we do not want him to run in the street. We envisage health, education, growth, safety, and other such goals. We acknowledge in our children and ourselves such motives as greed, pride, envy, and the like. We feel convinced that these are parts of the why. But we also know—even without being psychoanalyst or psychologist or philosopher—that there is more to it. We know that behavior is not determined solely either by these external necessities and forces or by the simple one-phase answers or purposes. Even in the earliest infancy, human activity is individualized and is determined in part by innate internal factors or pressures. The infant is not a *tabula rasa*; it is active as well as reactive. Furthermore, its activity is selective and implies a recognition of built-in mechanisms, of dispositions which lead to specialized rather than random behavior.

When we say of an organism that it is driven or motivated to do something—whether we express it broadly as "instinct" [23] or narrowly as "wish"—we imply that it is making determined efforts to move in a certain direction for a "reason that makes sense" to us. By "a reason that makes sense" we are only saying that the steps in our explanation follow logically upon one another. If a mouse "wants" a grain of wheat we think it is logical that he translate this want into muscular contractions of his legs so controlled that they take him in the direction of the grain of wheat. We also assume that this attraction which the grain of wheat has for the mouse is something different from the attraction which a magnet has for a bar of iron, or vice versa. But when we try to say just wherein lies the difference we have to use words which according to strict scientific usage are not permissible. We have to speak of purpose, or wish, or goal, or intention and we have to distinguish between conscious and unconscious wish and intent.

Freudian Drive Theory

Freud's thinking about motivation underwent many changes during the course of his very active life. He abandoned the effort to relate behavior to physiological stimulus and response, to need-fulfillment and inhibition. He went gradually from the short view—the need, the wish, the goal, the intention—to the long view of unconscious basic drives. First he tried to catalogue and classify wishes, conscious and unconscious. But more and more he tended toward an abstraction. To account for all the variable "little wishes" he sought to postulate a great and pervading *vis a tergo*—the *Trieb*, the drive, the impulse, the instinct. He sought to emphasize its urge or energic character. In line with Fechner's ideas, he used the concept of essential energy and systematized it.[24] Motivation for Freud was intimately connected with the Latin root *motus*—being moved, propelled, put in motion. This does some justice to the subjective experiences of urge, tension, and driveness which strong motives give us. When we are very hungry and without possibility of satisfying our need for food, the feeling becomes a desire and the desire becomes a craving which may overrule many other wishes and considerations, even our sense of reality. Its reign may become so supreme that it breaks the integrity of judgment, reasoning, and perception, inducing us to hallucinate food where there is none, despite repeated disappointments, from which little learning seems to proceed.

Under the impact of the clinical problems with which he was confronted, Freud focused at first on one impulse of major importance: the sexual impulse. Stepwise, he discovered that certain links exist between such diverse phenomena as thumbsucking, the love of one's own body, or deep interest in parts thereof, attachments to persons, competitive games, genital relations with persons of the other sex, romantic love, artistic production, play, etc. From certain similarities between these activities he inferred that they must have a common root and that some of the differences could be explained as developmental variations on the same theme. Hence came the conceptual differentiation of drives from partial drives or drive derivatives.

Freud sought to distinguish between impulse, aim, object, and source and intensity of the basic drive. Impulse or impetus indicates the strength of the drive, which is usually thought of as fluctuating, according to but not necessarily parallel with the presence or absence of possibilities for satisfaction. There may also be individual biological differences in impulse or drive strength. The aim of a drive is always toward discharge or diminution of tension * (but the word "aim" has also come to mean, at times, the way in which the aim is achieved). Drives have also objects, i.e., the person, thing, or activity that serves to reduce the tension of the impulse. The object that satisfies hunger is food; the object that satisfies sexual desire is ordinarily a person of the opposite sex.

A speculative aspect of drive is its source, by which is meant the totality of presumably physiochemical or glandular processes which generate the drive energy. Obviously this aspect of drive is no longer psychological, but biological, involving many unknowns which it is hoped will ultimately be solved or clarified by other disciplines such as neurophysiology, chemistry, etc.

There are still many different theories of motivation. Strict behaviorists tend to assume, at best, "drives" or "action tendencies" as mere hypothetical constructs, without specifying their nature, and treating them merely as "intervening variables" between the stimulus and the response which can be observed and recorded. Psychologists with biological interests tend to be more specific about their theoretical constructions and will deal with certain glandular or other somatic processes as the "basis" of motivation, sometimes in great detail. Others treat motivation without reference to the body, or anything internal, but speak of "goal-seeking behavior" or "end situations." A theory of motivation may

---

* On this point there has been much misunderstanding. Some have argued that a drive's aim is to discharge all tension; others have felt that optimal tension maintenance, which means on occasion a reduction of tension, or an abolition of excesses, is closer to the truth. Freud developed his ideas in close connection with Fechner's principle of constancy, which is a stability principle, but obviously was of two minds on this subject. (See: Ellenberger, H. F. "Fechner and Freud." *Bull. Menninger Clinic.* Freud, S. *Beyond the Pleasure Principle* and *Studies on Hysteria.*)

start out as a purely psychological one but become broadened into a much more general one, dealing with goals and ends, values, purposes, and ultimate causes. Some of this is uncomfortable to those who have been brought up with a materialistic and mechanistic model such as prevailed in physics in the second half of the last century. From their point of view, a discussion of "purposive behavior" in biology is an atavism or an anomaly; for vitalism, *élan vital*, emergence, and purpose are to them mere words, with a dangerous similarity to a God-creator or Aristotle's entelechy. Such a viewpoint is correct when it expresses the conviction that theology and science proceed from different assumptions and obey different rules. But we must add that theologians have also little use for biological vitalism or for Bergson's *élan vital*. And there is still a difference between the "causes" of which science approves as suitable for its purposes, and all possible causes that a responsible and disciplined scholar can think of. W. K. Clifford [25] stated nearly a century ago that the word represented by "cause" has sixty-four meanings in Plato and forty-eight in Aristotle! Recently the psychologist MacLeod [26] has argued that science since the Renaissance has focused almost exclusively on only two of Aristotle's four causes: it has dealt with material and efficient causes but has tended to shrink away from formal and final causes. He questions whether the biological and social sciences can be pressed into the narrow framework without sacrifice of their subject matter. And he points out (correctly, we think, and without feeling shock about it) that such principles as homeostasis, steady states, and perceptual constancy, and even the conception of the ego defending itself against threats are very close to what Aristotle would have subsumed under formal causes. They imply optima, with a purposive striving toward their attainment. But does that make them mystical notions, or poetry, or take away their explanatory power? We believe not; such concepts are still a far cry from taking refuge in a deity, and few theologians, philosophers, or moralists would be satisfied with them.[27] Aristotle also said somewhere that poetry is truer than history, and his contemporaries agreed with him. Then we went through many centuries of credulous skepticism, and once more we begin again to agree with Aristotle.

One very important part of the psychoanalytic theory of motivation is that it is also the cornerstone of a theory of conflict. A drive creates tension within the person; its inherent tendency toward discharge presents a problem to the administrative, executive, or regulatory functions within the person which we have earlier described as the special task of the ego. The ego is impelled to respond to the urgent pressures of drives seeking satisfaction; but the ego is also impelled to regard the possibilities, threats, demands, and norms of the environment. So, between the two sources of pressure, it must establish a compromise. Certain satisfactions are possible at some times; but never are all satisfactions possible at all times. Life is thus a succession of more or less wide swings in the disturbance of equilibrium of internal and external systems which must be brought into an ecological balance that is inevitably a fleeting, dynamic, and unstable one—Bertalanffy's steady state. The vital balance is thus a perpetually unstable restabilizing.

The Dual Instinct Theory

The fact that the psychoanalytic theory of motivation contains also the core of a theory of conflict is no accident. Freud was both a theoretician and a clinician; his practice confronted him with people who obviously suffered from conflict, i.e., from incompatible wishes, painful compromises, costly experiments in "having your cake and eating it." He was impressed by the ubiquitousness of sexual difficulties and, at that time, the conspiracy of silence and neglect which prevailed even in scientific circles regarding sexual behavior. This contrast appeared as, and was felt by his patient as, conflict: a conflict between personal and social goals, between a biological function and social custom or rule.

As time went by, this view broadened to the conception of the *process* of man's sexual life: its genetic beginnings and early manifestations, its different phases of development, its "life history" with all the modifications and distortions, departures, deflections, changes of aim and objects under the impact of social necessities (or the person's interpretations of social circumstances). Gradually Freud changed the concept of a persistent biological need, felt as a fluctuating yearning in specific directions, to the still broader conception that it was related to (but not identical with) the need for establishing positive relationships with other human, and non-human, beings in the universe. He resisted the suggestion that what he had called sexual drive thus became a social instinct, not so much because he denied the social meaning of it as because he feared the hypocritical implication of separating the ideas once more into a "sacred" and a "profane" love. And he also wanted to explain, not merely describe, human events.

Freud made still another and final shift in his concept of drive. As his theory began to win support and demonstrate its fertility and clinical usefulness, he took a new look at his hypotheses and revised them. He certainly never said these *words*, but he may have followed some such train of thought as indicated by these sentences:

"My critics have said that I overemphasize sex. In a sense they are right: I concentrated upon what I saw my fellow physicians ignoring, the suffering incurred by man in his unsuccessful attempts to reconcile his childhood misconceptions, his adult biological needs, and the hypocritical standards of his culture. Some of my critics may be laboring under this very difficulty in opposing my point of view; others, however, are right when they feel that the theory of sexuality is not enough to explain the major themes of human behavior. There *is* more: the afflictions of mankind flow *not* from the frustration of his sexual drive—as I, at first, thought—but from man's ineradicable aggressiveness, his destructiveness, his persistent malevolence. I have called it malevolent and destructive, and so it certainly appears when not sufficiently cloaked or fused with those loving and constructive tendencies which also motivate us. I see the sexual life, the erotic feelings, the love of human beings for one another and for their children, homes, pets and hobbies and possessions as manifestations of a fundamental constructive force, opposed by driving impulses toward a radically different goal, destructiveness." *

This, briefly, is the revised formulation of Freud's theory of motivation and conflict, the so-called "dual-instinct theory." It assumes the coexistence of two forces, or drives, with opposing purposes or directions, and always more or less fused with each other. This view doubles the possibility of conflict: man is not only torn between demands from within and demands from the outer environment; his inner environment itself is also torn between opposing tendencies, with very different qualities which, if satisfied in unadulterated form, would lead to widely different responses of the environment. The words "purpose" and "direction," as used in this connection, have a variable meaning, depending upon how narrow or broad one's focus of attention is. Freud's focus became ever broader: he was later taken with the speculative no-

---

* This sudden and belated discovery of evil is a psychological phenomenon Freud never analyzed. Its most famous exemplar was Gautama Buddha, from whom—according to the story—the sight of evil was artificially hidden until the day of his enlightenment. The British philosopher C. E. M. Joad, who long held to the hypothesis of a single life force, recorded his similar insights thus: "Then came the war, and the existence of evil made its impact upon me as a positive and obtrusive fact. All my life it had been staring me in the face; now it hit me in the face. . . . I see now that evil is endemic in man. . . ." (Joad, C. E. M., in *The Faith of Great Scientists*. New York: Hearst Publishing Co., 1950.)

tion that life as we know it is a temporary abnormal disturbance in the even flow of the universe, a biological occurrence out of keeping with natural entropy processes, a brief flash of existence in a dark, cold continuum. And in philosophical terms he reasoned that the creative, synthesizing, reproductive, erotic, agapic tendencies or principle in human behavior oppose temporarily the destructive, regressive, disintegrative tendencies or principle. At this level of speculation, lifelessness is seen as the normal state, and from it, under the influence of a temporary ascendancy of the "life instinct," each individual makes a brief ascension into the stratosphere, sparks another "abnormal event" like himself, and disappears again into the matrix of the so-called inorganic.

One does not have to subscribe to this enlarged metaphysical view in order to use the dual-drive theory; yet Freud's speculations have didactic value.* They show lucidly the impressive analogy that exists between his theory of motivation and conflict, and the common human wisdom of many civilizations. Many significant opposites of human life experiences have been paired by various people:

life	death	
good	evil	(Mani)
love	hate	
Eros	Neikos	(Empedocles)
Eros	Thanatos	(Freud)
libido	mortido	(Federn)
forces of light	forces of darkness	(Zoroaster; later the Essenes, *et alii*)
Yang	Yin	(ancient China)
assimilation	accommodation	(Piaget)
synthesis	disintegration	(Spencer)
diastole	systole	(Harvey, Goethe)
anabolism	katabolism	
constructiveness	destructiveness	

---

* Freud's rather long argument for a death instinct in *Beyond the Pleasure Principle* (London: Hogarth, 1922) and its simplified version in "Anxiety and Instinctual Life" (*New Introductory Lectures on Psychoanalysis*, New York: Norton, 1933) place great emphasis on the phenomenon of repetition compulsion. This is a purely psychological concept, needed to account for clinical data which seem to indicate a seeking of unpleasure, e.g., the reliving in dreams of a traumatic situation. Chein has argued that such phenomena do not run counter to the pleasure principle but are rather a special case of it ("The Genetic Factor in Ahistorical Psychology," *J. Gen. Psychol.*, 36:151–172, 1947). Freud's interpretation of it as a belated, partial discharge of unbearable tension suggests the same. At a different level of conceptualization,

The dual-drive theory is an inference from clinical and normal data (including observations of developmental stages) leading to the proposition that much of human behavior can be explained in terms of two original drives which are subject to mutual and separate modifications in aim, object, and modality. They are psychological constructs, but also contain a reference to a source, which is as yet unknown, but believed to be of somatic origin. They lead to goal-striving, purposive behavior. Though they are isolated as constructs, the complexity of observable behavior is such that they always appear in fusion. They represent the mainsprings of action, giving rise to derivatives which may obtain a certain degree of autonomy. They are subject to learning. Moreover, they show considerable analogy to certain biological, and even to some widely recognized philosophical principles. Such motives as curiosity, hunger, rhythm, envy, the need to be active, and so on are partial instincts or, better, derivatives. The same can be said of the sort of behavior in animals which used to be called instinctual, such as nest-building and migration. If we assume that there are two basic instinctual trends, we do not necessarily assume that there are no other comparably basic and fundamental instinctual trends, but it is difficult for us to imagine what they would be. It is easier to assume that hunger, for example, is not a drive at all but a cybernetic signal of a water deficiency. Others in such a list could similarly be explained as not drives or instincts in the Freudian sense at all. Still others could be explained as derivatives from the two basic instincts fused in varying proportions and directed to various specific objectives.

One of the merits of the dual-drive theory is, then, that it provides a very useful conceptualization of conflict and conflict solution. Yet it may not quite explain the whole of human motivation. It is certainly possible to postulate other drives and propensities, less visceral in nature, without reducing them to the primary drives of libido and aggression or without seeing them as products of sublimation. Cognitive impulses, the urge to know and expand knowledge and to master one's world conceptually not only for survival, but for *improved* survival, or even for improvement

---

however, Freud nearly equated repetition compulsion (then no longer a psychological concept) with the physicist's concept of entropy, and derived his death instinct really from the latter. The repetition compulsion was related to a purely speculative thought, namely, the general principle that living matter, by an inner impulse, seeks its return to a previous, non-living state, i.e., death, as a goal. This makes repetition compulsion a cosmic principle; it ceases to be an instinct, which by definition must be a property of living matter, related to typical life processes such as memory, etc. Freud's logic is strained at this point, and his use of Weissman's germ-plasm theory seems fallacious. The organism never was "dust"; if it dies it becomes dust but does not *return* to it.

per se, have often been singled out as a special and potent source of human activity. Our colleague Gardner Murphy [28] has eloquently pleaded for a consideration of curiosity as an extremely important motive [29] in men and animals.*

Freud's hypothesis of an aggressive, destructive, or disintegrative drive (under the perhaps too poetic name "death instinct") has proved to be a stumbling block to many theorists, practitioners, and laymen. Few people deny that there are aggressive behavior patterns, but few have the candor to hypothesize, with Freud, that aggression is a fundamental characteristic of the individual, the race, the species, indeed the universe. Such denial often leads to a play with words, to word substitutions, to an attempt to establish basic differences between words that have an overruling similarity of content. This is well illustrated in a cartoon in *The New Yorker*, showing a counselor or a psychiatrist saying to the mother of a misbehaving boy: "Mrs. Minton, there's no such thing as a bad boy. Hostile, perhaps. Aggressive, recalcitrant, destructive, even sadistic! but not *bad*." The reader will recall the ironic refrain, "We are sick," from "Gee, Officer Krupke," the song of the gang of adolescents in *West Side Story*.[30]

In striking contrast to this attitude is the unabashed admiration and even adoration of aggression in some individuals, some cultures, and some subcultures. Many individuals of this sort will come to the reader's mind. A subculture (street gang) has already been mentioned. And for a broader illustration, consider the comment of Margolin in a study of American Indian value systems. Margolin [31] finds that "the Utes put a high premium on aggression. The more aggression a man is capable of the more he is respected. This is a little like certain kinds of adoles-

---

* Such considerations involve the difficult problem of the classification of instincts. How many and which instincts is the theorist to recognize? Shall he assume just a very small number of primary instincts and explain the enormous diversity of behavior by the added assumption of partial or derivative instincts? Or shall he recognize many primary instincts and run the risk of fragmenting the organism? What importance shall he attach to the criteria of economy and elegance in theory-building?

These questions may lead to diverse answers. A recent study on instinct in man (Fletcher, R. *Instinct in Man, in the Light of Recent Work in Comparative Psychology*. New York: International Universities Press, 1957) discusses various possibilities and favors a pluralistic view, postulating ten different instincts, of which some have several subdivisions. The exigencies of the psychiatric situation, however, require an explicit emphasis on *conflict* and *developmental continuity* which predisposes us to the assumption of two broad, encompassing, generic, and complex tendencies which can explain both the diversity and the unity of human behavior. If, moreover, as Fletcher suggests, the conative and affective aspects of instinctual experience in man are of central importance, we find all the more reason to consider the dynamics of love and hate of overruling impact and to conceptualize all instincts accordingly.

cent societies in our culture—certainly not like adults in our culture."

Words have so many and often conflicting implications that it is understandable that Freud's original designation "death instinct" may have been an unfortunate one. He explicitly included in his hypothesis that the death instinct was never visible in its naked form; there was always some turning outward from self-destruction toward aggressiveness, and there was almost always some mingling with this externally directed aggressiveness and constructiveness, some—perhaps ever so slight—neutralization. This essential dualism disturbed some people, who persist in a kind of ideal monism according to which aggressive and destructive tendencies emerge from unfortunate social experiences and become differentiated from the primary stream as adventitious elements. But for Freud and for the present authors aggressive, destructive tendencies are not adventitious but essential, native "givens."

From our point of view, the varying attitudes men take toward the recognition of aggression as a drive reflect variations in temperament and psychological make-up. Whether seen as defect, as sin, as destruction, or as error, it can be emphasized or de-emphasized. Thus, these words, including the more generic term "evil," have a great similarity of content or referents, although they belong to different categories and represent different levels of conceptualization. Moral, aesthetic, and religious biases give rise to selective attention and inattention, for example in the counselor whom we just quoted.

One can arrange a kind of scale of attitudes toward evil and aggression:

1. There are those who see only evil in man, taking with Hobbes the view that it is man's most distinguishing characteristic. Man is the wolf of mankind. Man's aggression is the origin of the political state: with the feeble light of reason people may escape extinction by subjugating themselves under a benevolent tyrant, who channelizes their aggression into orderly political action.

2. A nearly equal emphasis on good and evil is represented by the Zoroastrian conflict of Ahura Mazda and Ahriman, virtue and wickedness, love and hate, anchored in all creation—the race, the species, and the individual. Two basic cosmic principles or forces of opposite intent struggle with each other. This is essentially equivalent to Freud's dual-drive theory, and to Empedocles' cosmogony: [32]

> For even as Love and Hate were strong of yore,
> they shall have their hereafter; nor I think
> shall endless Age be emptied of these Twain.

3. A partial de-emphasis on evil, a partial denial of it, is represented by the frustration-aggression hypothesis widely held in social science today. It deals with evil reluctantly, excusing aggressive behavior in the individual as a provoked response, the responsibility for which is to be sought elsewhere—in a frustrating parent, an uncooperative spouse, or just "out there" in the social conditions. "There are no bad boys, only bad parents."

4. An even stronger de-emphasis on, or denial of, evil is to be detected in the social theory of evil expounded by Rousseau and others: man is naturally good, but culture and technology have spoiled him. In this view there are not only no bad boys, but no bad parents, no bad grandparents, no bad anybody—just bad society. Such humanistic optimism lies at the heart of Fromm's contemporary writings.

5. And, finally, there is the radical denial of evil, according to which everything is good except the attitude of some erring people who *think* they see evil. Hear no evil, see no evil, speak no evil; it doesn't exist.*

In these attitudes there is a variable mixture of the psychological processes or mechanisms which we describe as denial, as fantasy substitution for reality, as reaction formation with forced niceness, limited vision, prettiness, and Pollyannaism. The notion that evil (or its analogues) is present only in others could be a projection of the unacknowledgeable evil (or aggression, destructiveness, etc.) within us and the convening to the scapegoat of sins that are then no longer ours.

From our point of view the de-emphasis on evil is as unrealistic as the pessimistic conclusion that man is all evil. The dual-instinct theory

---

* "Why, the instinct of self-preservation is the normal law of humanity. . . ."

"Who told you that?" cried Yevgeny Pavlovitch suddenly. "It's a law, that's true; but it's no more normal than the law of destruction, or even self-destruction. . . ."

"An artful and ironical idea, insidious as a larding-needle!—but a true idea! For you, a worldly scoffer and cavalry officer (though not without brains), are not yourself aware how true and profound your idea is. Yes, sir, the law of self-destruction and the law of self-preservation are equally strong in humanity! The devil has equal dominion over humanity till the limit of time which we know not. You laugh? You don't believe in the devil? Disbelief in the devil is a French idea, a frivolous idea. Do you know who the devil is? Do you know his name? Without even knowing his name, you laugh at the form of him, following Voltaire's example, at his hoofs, at his tail, at his horns, which you have invented; for the evil spirit is a mighty menacing spirit, but he has not the hoofs and horns you've invented for him. . . ." (Dostoevski, Feodor: *The Idiot*, Constance Garnett, tr. New York: Macmillan, 1948, pp. 366–367.)

makes evil neither an unconquerable, pervading monster nor a mere nuisance and irritant. It recognizes aggression and destructiveness as a potent drive, not to be minimized but to be dealt with; not to be denied but to be converted; not to be hated but to be harnessed.

Some recent studies of brain functioning in animals and man strongly suggest the existence of two opposed neural mechanisms important for the organization of instincts. Stimulation of one system produces pleasurable sensations and activities and provides rewards in learning, whereas the other system underlies the experience of punishment, anger, and painful sensations (J. P. Lilly).[33]

Because of their daily contact with it, medical men are not likely to scotomatize destruction, or fail to recognize the conflict of antagonistic forces in all biological phenomena. Biologists, botanists, and chemists are familiar with processes in molecules, in ecology, and in solutions which are analogous. It is axiomatic that both anabolism and catabolism are required to produce the proper metabolism. On the one hand there are such processes as autolysis and decay; on the other such processes as reproduction and proliferation. The disintegration of tissue is necessary to its replacement with more and better tissue, and hence to growth. To be sure, adventitious and exogenous elements continually complicate the picture so that trauma or bacteria, for example, may accomplish some of the destruction which would otherwise have to be accomplished by internal lytic processes.

In such fields as histological pathology the mechanical evidences of a destructive process are clearly visible; similarly, with the aid of proper stains and other methods, the evidences (i.e., results) of the reparative process are visible. Biologists can, therefore, concentrate upon the detailed manifestations of the process which they can *see*, without having to speculate regarding the implied forces or principles behind it, which they cannot see. Psychiatrists and psychologists, on the other hand, study material in which the details of the destructive (and reintegrative) processes are less denotable. There are no visible psychological equivalents of fibroblasts and fibroclasts, leukocytes and fibrin. The processes both of destruction and of integration have had to be inferred, on the one hand from the behavior of the total organism (which, of course, is visible) and on the other hand from the patient's verbalizations of subjective experience (which are audible). Thus most biologists, having been able to see the immediate evidence of steps in the process, have been less concerned with the explanation; the psychiatrists, who, unable to see the processes, have had to infer them, have gone further and have assumed or inferred the probable energic determinants.

In clinical psychiatry destructive trends may be observed in both internal and external directions, and the more such tendencies can be controlled by fusion with or neutralization by the integrative tendencies or by being directed in ways least likely to harm the individual, the better for the organism and for its environment. In *Man Against Himself* [34] are outlined some of the forms in which imperfectly controlled aggression manifests itself clinically. I was largely concerned there with the damage to the subject, that is, the ways in which such aggressiveness, insufficiently controlled, becomes again self-directed. Externally directed aggressiveness is for the most part not regarded as clinical, unless accompanied by some internally directed aggression. Indeed, social tolerance of aggression varies considerably. In a few instances, such as acting in self-defense or in fighting for one's country or for one's friends or one's family, aggressiveness is actually approved and rewarded. Commercial and political competition, as well as some types of sports, may become very aggressive indeed without social condemnation. Perhaps these dual standards which societies apply toward aggression are themselves a form of evidence that it is an active force which cannot be reasoned away or dispensed with. The reality of its character has been seen by generations and is to us most conspicuous in clinical material.

Applying the instinct theory to the organismic point of view, we can visualize personality in all its complexity and in each of its developmental phases as being at the point of convergence of antagonistic drives. It is largely propelled by their force; its activities are led by the goals inherent in constructiveness and destructiveness or any combination thereof. Its reaching out for environmental relations is determined by a search for those objects or situations which would best gratify the quality of its urges. Action and inaction of the organism depend on the drive status at any given time; its stability or instability relates to the play of instinctual forces within its relation to the environmental context. Not only all the common acts of behavior which we can easily understand, but also the puzzling sequences of activities which we find hard to decipher, must be consistently explained as manifestations of basic drives. Freud emphasized over and over that according to the dual-drive theory there could be no such thing as pure destructiveness or pure constructiveness but that these were fused in the motivation of every act in different proportions, so that in one instance the resultant might be highly creative behavior and in another instance essentially destructive, criminal behavior. The balance is probably constantly changing, and sometimes the change is progressive from what we might describe as bad to worse, or vice versa.

But personality is not merely the resultant of drives. Organismic theory holds that the system as a whole is enclosing or containing; the parts must "fit into" it. No drive can be conceptualized without an enveloping organism. A complete autonomy of drives could not exist; using Gerard's concept, we can say that complete autonomy of drives would yield a cellulation index of one, which would terminate the organism. It is therefore unsound to speak of such regulatory processes as homeostasis, feedback, or steady states as if they were simply a direct accommodation of forces to each other, automatically keeping themselves in balance. Neither is it necessary to think of organismic constancy-maintenance as the result of a special "homeostatic instinct," as proposed by Orr,[35] or by any other special regulatory *force*. We consider steady states, homeostasis, etc., to be words describing characteristic conditions or "states of being" of living systems. They are explainable in terms of general properties of organisms, and these properties are not those which account for the energy utilized by the organism. They cannot be understood without recognition of the essential role played by *opposing* forces or directions of energy. From the conflict of these opposing forces as well as from the conflicts engendered by them between the organism and the environment derives our interest in the maintenance of relative stability as a biological requisite. But stability would quickly become stagnation and death were it not for the constant change impelled by them, which is equally characterisitic of life. The Heraclitean adage that "everything is change" has little value unless it is contrasted with another truth at times more conspicuous, namely that everything remains approximately the same.*

Recapitulation

This concludes a brief review of some of the basic hypotheses employed in the clinical and theoretical discussions to follow. The general principles of individual environment-adjustment and adaptation are now an ac-

---

* It has been correctly pointed out by Maze that in many applications of the concept of homeostasis the emphasis has been exclusively on steadiness, while the idea of opposing forces has been neglected. (Maze, J. R. "On Some Corruptions of the Doctrine of Homeostasis." *Psychol. Rev.*, 1953, 60:405–412.)

cepted tenet of all the behavioral sciences. In presenting organismic theory, we have tried to show that principles of organization, interaction, homeostasis, heterostasis, steady-state maintenance, adaptation, modification, and regulation may be applied to the psychology functions or aspects of the human being in the human situation. We have offered a definition of the ego in its special role of system-regulator and organization-maintainer. And finally we have presented the dual-instinct or dual-drive theory of motivation, with the corollary assumption that the aggressive drive is the dangerous and disturbing one, to the environment, to the organism, and to their essential interrelation.

CHAPTER VII

Coping Devices of Everyday Living

SYNOPSIS: The basic principles and personality theory presented in Chapters V and VI are here applied to the everyday human life, with discussion of stress and a list of some of the ordinary ways of coping with it, with minor fluctuations in adaptation and adjustment. The phenomena incident to steady-state maintenance of this degree do not constitute illness in the popular vocabulary, but every regulatory device costs something in energy expenditure. If the objective is not achieved, a higher price will have to be paid and devices of a more expensive kind will have to be called upon to maintain the vital balance.

IN THE previous chapters we spoke in broad general terms about the processes of organization, interaction, motivation, and control, especially as they apply to the human organism. These principles comprise the essence of a theory of personality and of human life consistent with the simplified or unitary concept of mental illness announced in the first chapter.

We proceed now to an exposition of how these principles appear in action in the daily lives of people—ourselves, our friends, our patients. We can begin by quoting some incomparably clear, simple sentences set down by a layman—a novelist, indeed—nearly one hundred years ago:

> All our lives long, every day and every hour, we are engaged in the process of accommodating our changed and unchanged selves to changed and unchanged surroundings; living, in fact, is nothing else than this process of accommodation; when we fail in it a little we are stupid, when we fail flagrantly we are mad, when we suspend it temporarily we sleep, when we give up the attempt altogether we die. In quiet, uneventful lives the changes internal and external are so small that there is little or no strain in the process of fusion and accommodation; in other lives there is great strain, but there is also great fusing and accommodating power; in others great strain with little accommodating power. A life will be successful or not, according as the power of accommodation is equal to or unequal to the strain of fusing and adjusting internal and external changes.[1]

Why does this sound so new, so fresh, so modern? Is it because static concepts tend to obliterate dynamic and process concepts, as being more stable and tangible? For Butler's insights were not shared by the scientists of the day. It took an Einstein and a Freud and many others to convince us. My own father, however, while still a young physician in general practice, committed to paper the following lines three years before I was born:

> Life in all of its forms, physical and mental, morbid and healthy, is a relation; its phenomena result from the reciprocal action of an individual organism and of external forces. Health is the consequence and the evidence of a successful adaptation to the conditions of existence . . . while disease marks a failure in organic adaptation and leads to disorder, decay and death. The harmonious relation existing between the organism and its environment, which is the condition of health, may be disturbed either (1) by a cause in the organism, (2) by a cause in the environment, (3) by a cause or causes in both. . . . Great mistakes are often made, even by men of culture, in fixing upon supposed causes of disease in particular cases. A single event is selected as in itself effective to explain the whole disaster, when that event alone was merely one of a whole train of causes. A series of external events in concurrence with steadily operating conditions within—but not a single event—an accident, a sorrow, or need, or adversity—can all be regarded as adequate cause for insanity . . .[2]

What Butler called "accommodation" and my father "adaptation" we now refer to more often as "interaction." This refers, as the quotations make clear, to the individual in constant, dynamic interactive relation with the other organisms and organizations and facts and fictions of his environment. These outside units also "adjust" and "adapt" and "accommodate" themselves to one another and to this individual, each in its own way.

Just how is this process accomplished, in terms of the theories of the preceding chapter? Given an organism, an individual, launched into a world full of other individuals *like* and *unlike* himself, many of them driven by the same drives and seeking the same ends—what happens?

What happens is that he pursues his ends, seeking to express his intentions and fulfill his needs as he perceives them and as he finds opportunity. He tries to survive, with minimal pain and maximal pleasure, including the pleasures of achievement, of pride, and of loyalty to principle. All this requires an infinitude of doing, of trying and failing, of trying and succeeding, of trying and partially succeeding and having to compromise. It involves going ahead, stepping aside, stepping back, perhaps even running away. It involves fights and embraces, bargains and donations, gestures and conversations, working and playing, reproaches, rewards and retrenchments.

This is the uncomplicated process of living, with all major contingencies, including those of growing older and feebler, temporarily left out of consideration. But, as we all know, there are contingencies. The unexpected is always happening. Emergencies are constantly arising. The "mis"-behavior of other individuals, the occurrence of disruptive events, the change in certain situations—deaths, births, accidents—all sorts of things happen which may strain the capacity of the individual for easy accommodation. His comfort, his gratifications, perhaps even his growth or safety are threatened. Such a challenge stimulates extra or renewed effort, and he puts up the best battle he can for the best possible bargain under the changed circumstances of the new situation.

Forgive us a shift to another illustrative metaphor, and think of a man paddling a canoe downstream. By skillful balance, by holding back his canoe at certain moments, by choosing the most likely channel and using the current where he can, he achieves his purpose and he remains alive and comfortable. He encounters sharp turns, overhanging branches, threatening rapids, but by skillful adaptive steering and paddling he passes them safely.

But for some things ordinary maneuvers will not suffice. A half-submerged log suddenly looms up. A parcel falls from the boat and must be retrieved. His paddle, caught on a rock, snaps in two. The canoe springs a leak or goes aground. For such emergencies special *ad hoc* steps have to be taken. The time may even come when he has to have help. This need may be apparent from the shore, if anyone is looking, or he may have to spend some of his energy running up distress signals.

The strength or the unexpectedness or the peculiar nature of an external event may upset the relative steady state which was being maintained. Sometimes this is because of special vulnerabilities—a thin spot in the boat, a paddle weakened from an earlier exigency. The boatman's extra exertions tire him; they diminish his comfort; they reduce his efficiency. They may exhaust him. He may have to pull over to the shore and temporarily discontinue his voyage; he is "laid up."

But on the other hand, if by special efforts he can rather quickly correct the difficulties and keep going, if he can shortly resume his old efficiency and speed and confidence and pleasure, we would never consider this minor episode pathological. It was an emergency situation, quickly settled by an emergency maneuver.

Life is made up of just such slight departures from the normal state of affairs with more or less prompt correction, plus the occasional major interruption. Minor episodes occur constantly and everywhere and all the time; they are the very fabric of life. From each one of them we learn more about reality and about our own potentialities. We develop better and better techniques of dealing with external and internal pressures. Certain patterns of work and play, certain things and persons loved, certain aversions and avocations are developed as a part of the life pattern or way of living.[3] These must provide for a considerable amount of shock-absorption for the inevitable bumps and twists and twinges. These may be slightly unpleasant, but they will not noticeably increase internal tension when the ego has mastered devices for dealing with them. A somewhat larger shock may occasion brief pain, but it too will usually be absorbed and a comfortable equilibrium restored.

But we may assume—and we know from personal experience—that such capacity for varied adaptation requires a continuous alertness. A certain optimum tension must be present in the organism in order to insure the detection—as far in advance as possible—of the necessity for special maneuvering. This tension must be at an optimum level; if it is too high, it will be painful; if it is too low, functioning will be impaired. If the boatman in our illustration is too tense he will be inefficient and unskillful. If his state of inner tension is too low, he will fail to see dangers quickly enough and may capsize.

There have been many attempts to be more scientifically precise about the nature of this ego tension, but we are still tied to the use of various metaphors. For the past few years the word "stress" has been popular. The boatman in our illustration certainly is under some degreee of stress. Then he encounters events which are said to be stressful, and these stresses evoke more internal stress. Stress is, therefore, a most ambiguous term used both for that which produces a certain state and for the state which is thus produced. We must assume that there is always *some* stress present in all fluid relationships; an increase in external stress in turn arouses an increase in internal stress. If stress causes stress, when does stress become so stressful as to be distressing? (One is reminded of the old joke: What kind of noise annoys an oyster most? Answer: A noisy noise annoys an oyster most.) [4] When does stress become strain?

Stress and Tension

There are many current discussions of psychological stress in scientific writing, with no generally agreed upon definition. Various authors have given up the attempt to define stress in favor of classifying it. One of them suggests that mild stresses be considered those the effects of which last from seconds to hours, such as insect stings or missing a train; moderate stresses those with effects lasting from hours to days, such as overwork, a gastric upset, the visit of an unwelcome guest; and severe stress that which results in effects lasting for weeks, months, or even years, such as the death of a loved one or drastic financial loss.

Engel [5] offers this practical definition: "Psychological stress refers to all processes, whether originating in the external environment or within the person, which impose a demand or requirement upon the organism the resolution or handling of which requires . . . activity of the mental apparatus before any other system is involved or activated."

Thus he applies the word "stress" to the initiation or producer, not to the effects. This avoids the ambiguity, providing we adhere to the definition, which in common parlance we often fail to do. For our purposes we accept Engel's definition, and we refer to the internal state of increased activity and pressure aroused by stress, as "tension."

"Tension" is also a metaphor, one based on several different models—hydrostatic, mechanical, chemical. The operations of these various models are not identical, and the inferences tacitly made in psychological writings are sometimes difficult to follow, but perhaps there is a value in this vagueness. Tension has the value of connoting even to a layman the notion of increased internal activity and pressure. It also has subject confirmation. Every individual, many times in his life, has been aware of something within him which he can describe as feeling "tense." As we declared earlier in the book, we take seriously these metaphorical words used by the uninformed to describe their feelings. This is often a muscular tension, of course, but there is more to the internal tension feeling. It is a sense of something's not being quite right, a mild uneasiness, a "worried" feeling, a kind of psychic discomfort, although scarcely pain.

Through a mistranslation of the German word *Angst*, which Freud used, psychoanalysts got into the habit many years ago of calling this uncomfortable tension awareness "anxiety." In her classic book on the subject Anna Freud [6] described various symptoms as measures of defense erected against this *Angst*. Her idea was not that the tension was dangerous, but that it was brought about by conflicts and that it stimulated certain emergency remedies. Something analogous occurs when the body becomes somewhat dehydrated; the fluid imbalance is perceived as thirstiness, and this feeling excites remedial action not for the sense of thirst, but for the bodily dehydration.

Similarly, tension awareness seems to impel the ego to take action. More strictly speaking, the internal tension and stress automatically mobilize the ego in a special maneuver designed to relieve the tension. The ego undoubtedly settles many problems for the organism without our conscious participation or even our previous awareness of increasing tension.

There are many things the ego can do. It may stimulate action to alter the situation, to remove the threat, to fill painful need, to arrange a compromise, or to otherwise deal with the exigency in a way to reduce external and internal tension. This costs energy; it costs effort; it may cost more than that. The use of the word "cost" introduces the economic model or principle or frame of reference upon which we shall lean heavily in our subsequent discussion. The mastering of difficulties, the averting of threats, the making of a special exertion for the achievement of a goal, the restoration of a disturbing loss, all require energy investment as a price or as a *quid pro quo*. There is a price or cost for reducing tension and maintaining the equilibrium. And it is expedient always to pay the least price necessary and keep the cost of living as low as possible!

Adaptational disruption, however slight or however great, is always bilateral. It is easy to fall into a way of thinking of the organism as sitting peacefully on a garden bench, taking the air and the sun, occasionally beset by bees which have to be brushed off or run from. We lose sight of the fact that the organism itself has beelike qualities and is constantly pursuing goals of its own, some of which involve the displacement, the disturbing, and even the demolition of other individuals. An encounter with the bees is likely to have been preceded by designs on "their" flowers, "their" living space, or "their" honey!

Illustration of Emergency Management

It might be helpful to submit an illustration of an unexpected event's giving rise to stress reactions, equilibrium disturbance, and ultimate resolution. The incident to be described actually happened to the senior author some years ago, and it may remind the reader of similar events in his own life which will assist in visualizing the details.

My wife, my four-year-old daughter, and I were going in our car to my father's home for a family supper. The car just in front of us suddenly reduced speed and stopped. To avoid hitting it I automatically applied the brakes of my car sharply, acutely alarmed lest we crash into the rear of the offending car. My little daughter was thrown forward against the instrument panel and windshield. She bumped her head and began to cry. Our car did not touch the car ahead, and fortunately there was no car behind us, so that this was the end of the *physical* event.

But now began a chain of *psychological* events. My original fright about an impending collision was quickly replaced by the fear that my daughter had been injured. Inspection proved this not to be the case. No collision, no injury, no further danger or cause for concern. All's well that ends well.

Only it did not end. After a momentary time lapse, my brief alarm gave way to a surge of aggressive feelings, thoughts, and actions. "What kind of irresponsible, incompetent driving is this?" I thought. I glowered fiercely at the other driver, who had by this time gotten out of his car and come toward us to see if the baby's cries meant serious injury.

To this considerateness I responded angrily that she was not hurt seriously, that this good fortune was not *his* fault and no credit to his style of driving. In embarrassment and relief, no doubt, he laughed. This greatly intensified my anger and I felt impelled to do something to change his arrogant, callous, unrepentant manner—hit him, perhaps. This being both imprudent and impossible, I asked in a tone of forced calmness for his name and address. He refused to give it, retorting that the incident was my fault, and it was just luck that I had not damaged his car. This, insult added to injury, excited in me a painful degree of suppressed rage, plus mortification at my helplessness to express it effectively. Yet there was nothing to do but to note down his license number and drive on in silence.

Well, scarcely silence. Driving along, acutely uncomfortable, I recited the entire event to my wife (who, of course, had seen and heard it all). I emphasized the recklessness of the man's driving, saying nothing about the fact that I was obviously driving too close behind him for safety. (I kept myself completely oblivious of this fact for some time, and even when my wife suggested it a little later, I rebutted it vigorously.) I proclaimed the danger of sudden slowing in traffic. I formulated various retorts that I should have made to the man when he accused *me* of being careless. I repeated over to myself several times his license number, which I had noted, and resolved to call the state Vehicle Department to get his name, despite his refusal to give it. I would "do something about it." Fantasies of *what* I would do raced through my mind: I would find out all about him and prove that he was an incompetent, scurrilous ne'er-do-well who ought not to be permitted to have a car, let alone a license. I would report him to the police. I would write him a vitriolic letter.

Evidently these Walter Mitty fantasies of direct action had relieved the tension somewhat by the time we had arrived at my father's house. I described the event at supper, passing over the unpleasantness lightly. It did not seem quite so important now. It recurred to my mind, however, several times during the evening as we were playing cards, and I noticed that I felt a little shaky and uneasy. That night I did not go to sleep immediately, and a few more fantasies returned, but when I did fall asleep I slept well. (I may have dreamed about the episode, although I do not recall doing so.)

The next morning it all seemed amusing. But it was obviously still on my mind. I told several people about it as a joke on myself—how I had averted an accident by skillful driving only to be accused of having almost caused one! Gradually other matters claimed my attention more completely, and I ceased to think at all about the event. Then, an evening or so later, while I was engaged in teaching a psychoanalytic seminar, the whole thing suddenly popped into my mind as an example of something we were discussing and seemed *most* apropos!

Some tension remained, even after this controlled distribution of the aroused aggression, and various well-known means of tension-reduction were employed such as talking out, repetition, humor, and intellectualization. We shall shortly discuss these systematically. Afterward the incident rapidly paled in importance and vividness for me, and only at the insistence of my co-authors is it used in this chapter, because it now seems almost unreal.

The incident illustrates how, in addition to the innumerable minor compromises incident to every hour of daily living, there are also occasions when the ego is temporarily overwhelmed, or at least *threatened* with being overwhelmed, by the upsurge of aggressive drives stimulated by some event. The ego presumably senses the amount of stimulation and the strength of the reaction and the available power of suppression and diversion in these incessant internal and external adjustments. Presumably this sensing is not painful except when sudden imbalance occurs, and then the increment of pressure is experienced as unpleasant, and a more vigorous effort is made to control the aggressions which are threatening to emerge. Curiously enough, the discomfort itself may be experienced as a danger and call for further defenses.[7]

This discomfort may be of short duration. Faced with an increased task of adjustment and sensing the increased tension, the ego seems capable of *over*exerting itself. It makes special efforts, and it has at its disposal many techniques for solving the problem and diminishing the tension. It can suppress, it can repress, it can permit some gratification or effect more sublimation. It can direct some behavior toward altering the external circumstances, perhaps focusing some aggressive energy directly against the threat or danger; it can sidestep the issue, or it can provide some antidote. It can direct a withdrawal of the personality from the danger situation, or it can invoke help from external sources.

Coping Devices for Minor Emergencies

Just which of these many devices for living will be selected in a particular instance will certainly depend partly upon external circumstances, partly upon the suddenness and strength of the disturbance, but largely upon the predisposition of the ego, a phrase used here to imply that many such disturbances have occurred before *this* one, the one we are now considering. Certain patterns and styles of reaction have been established. The series of "one damned thing after another" which is said to constitute life refers to those successive irritations, changes, traumata, and emergencies which have been successively met with varying degrees of success in the course of one's development. In childhood, when knowledge was more limited and the regulatory system less developed, the lasting effects of certain traumata were greater and more determining with respect to subsequent reactions to similar traumata. Hence comes our psychiatric dictum that the reactions of today represent the painful experiences of yesterday, meaning the long ago of childhood and infancy.*

---

* In a recent study of patients suffering from the severe stress of poliomyelitis residuals the observer commented that "in many patients, we observe a kind of defense-in-depth. Such patients employ not a single means of protecting themselves against the noxious developments in the course of their illness, but rather a set of related thought-and-action processes that provide a reserve measure for dealing with stressful experiences. Frequently we see an interlocking or alternation of protective strategies. If coping pattern A does not work, then pattern B is brought to bear on the problem. If A and B together do not work, then pattern C is brought into play; and so on. . . . Such coping strategies appear to be formed and employed at every level of consciousness. They are sometimes developed in a largely automatic, unthinking way and yet can be brought

For the purposes of exposition we shall assume that we are describing a relatively healthy and intact ego, one whose "elasticity" is not reduced more than the average by scars and weaknesses and tender spots and blind spots. Such an ego will have established a system of relationships with love objects, a network of intercommunication, a program of life involving work satisfactions and play satisfactions. A person with such an ego will have learned to channel his aggressiveness in the least harmful directions and toward the most suitable objects. He will have found ways to be creative within the limits of his talents. He will have developed a love-and-let-love attitude toward the universe.

But even so, the ego of our relatively healthy-minded individual will have to make some choices and resort to some expediencies. For even this normal individual has his limits of tolerance, his unexpected and disturbing encounters, his hard-to-bear disappointments and his unconsolable griefs. As John Cowper Powys [8] says, "even the toughest and strongest among us may be sent howling to a suicidal collapse."

But we are not yet ready to speak of collapse. There are always those everyday events which disturb us a little bit, but for which the ego is able to make relatively prompt readjustments, so that no one thinks of calling the disturbance illness. For some years Dr. Lois Murphy [9] of our Foundation has been observing and collecting the various "coping devices" by which children manage to "get along" in the face of difficulties, including devices used under conditions of minor stress as well as those arising merely from growing curiosity and ingenuity.

No doubt the earliest method of relieving stress is a very familiar anaclitic method, turning to mother or to something resembling mother, and hence getting protection and comfort. The original situation is a realistic one; the mother's arms and breast and voice are identified with her functions of nursing, soothing, and protecting. In time mother is replaced * by many other figures, animate and inanimate—friends, spouse, house, automobile, bank account, and so forth.

The comfort of *touch*,[10] *rhythmic movement* (rocking, patting) and the *soft, reassuring voice sounds* [11] is probably always sought by the ego in times of stress, even when more sophisticated adjustments become possible. These were the primitive ways of establishing or strengthen-

---

into focus without too much difficulty; and they sometimes operate entirely outside awareness." (Visotsky, H. M., et al. "Coping Behavior under Extreme Stress; Observations of Patients with Severe Poliomyelitis." *Arch Gen. Psychiat.*, 1961, 5:423–448.)
* The brilliant experiments of Harlow with monkeys have taught us much concerning this transfer. (Harlow, H. F. and Margaret K.: "The Effect of Rearing Conditions on Behavior." *Bull. Menninger Clinic*, 26:213–224, 1962.)

ing *ad personam* cathexes, i.e., supportive interpersonal relations which absorb hate or love. "Misery loves company" because internal distress always evokes the infantile need to look for help from fellow creatures. To give love is to get love, and to get love is to be reassured of one's lovableness and of the protecting attitude of those who prize us even in time of danger and error. The soothing of the troubled child finds its counterpart in numerous more subtle interpersonal gestures in adult life, including various group associations and other forms of companionship.

As the child grows older, the soft touches and sounds of infancy take more specific forms. They may become reassurances of various kinds: "Don't be afraid." "It can't hurt you." "I won't leave you." Or they may convey merely sympathy and comfort: "Don't cry. I know it hurts." Such consolation is so much a part of the everyday social intercourse that its economic function is often overlooked.[12] Instead of words, the sounds may become organized as formal music, and the lullabies of the nursery are replaced by the symphonies and chorales of adult life.

The total experience of the infant's interaction with the mother (food, warmth, touch, being held, etc.) is, of course, the original great basic reassurance. Some believe that all our concepts and notions of loving and of being loved stem from this early ecstatic experience. Innumerable clinical observations by internists and psychiatrists confirm the psychologically restorative effects of eating food, and even of taking into the mouth food substitutes such as thumbs, pipes, cigars, and chewing gum. Only part of the effects can be credited to an increase in blood sugar; Jonathan's spirit was lifted by eating some honey for reasons other than merely chemical (I Samuel 14:27).

The psychological value of eating is intuitively so well known to everybody that it is apt to get passed over in scientific considerations just because of its obviousness. Lunching together, dining, banqueting, supping, feasting, the family meal, the Thanksgiving dinner, the Communion service, the Seder, the coffee break—these and scores of other examples will come to mind as instances in which that which is absorbed by the stomach is probably much less important for the total well-being of the individual than that which the process of eating and of eating together accomplishes psychologically. The search for excellent food, fine restaurants,* and epicurean dishes or menus reflects the search

---

* "No, sir! there is nothing which has yet been contrived by man by which happiness is produced as by a good tavern or inn" (Samuel Johnson).

for a re-creation of that perfection of delight which occurred for a few happy moments every day during the first year of life (I. A. Mirsky).[13]

Perhaps the very fluidity of *alcoholic beverages* makes them better symbols of the primal food than something solid. When one adds to this the chemical effect of the alcohol, a diminishing sharpness of reality-testing and an elevation of the general feeling tone, one can easily see why alcoholic drinks come to be so commonly employed as an adjuvant to the control of minor disturbances of equilibrium. Alcohol's very effectiveness here is its great menace; it works too well—up to a point. For it also misleads, reduces adaptability, impairs judgment, loosens controls, and becomes habit-forming. Larger and larger "doses" are required. There are other substances long known to us yet seldom used in our culture. I have no knowledge about the effects of chewing betel nut, or of the cocoa used by the people of the Latin American countries. But I am informed that they have more effect than our tea and coffee. Peyote is highly esteemed and reverently used by some of the Pueblos and Navajos in this country, and Aldous Huxley[14] has suggested the taking of lysergic acid for the removal of minor states of discomfort, to replace the present widespread use of alcohol and nicotine, the former achieving a closer approximation to a state of happiness without any of the deleterious affects of alcohol and nicotine. There are numerous other chemical substances which can sharply affect one's sense of well-being—restore it temporarily, enhance or modify its character. Numerous synthetic drugs are now being investigated.

In all such self-administered "treatments," the individual has the satisfaction of thinking that he has done something by and for himself, without recourse to the anaclitic dependency upon the mother (or her substitute). This is an illusion, of course, as are all narcissistic inflations, but it may, nonetheless, serve a purpose. Denied the mother's nipple, one can always do for oneself and substitute a thumb—one's own thumb —and it is only a short step from the thumb to other objects. By trial and error a vast panel is constructed of the desirable and undesirable, the pleasant and unpleasant, the tasty and the repulsive, the good and the bad. There is an established evolution in the selection of such objects, the natural history of which Freud[15] gave to the world first in the *Three Contributions to the Theory of Sex.*

In time the investment in the breast and thumb is transferred to the playmate, the comrade, and the teacher. Attitudes based on oral modalities, later anal modalities, and, still later, phallic and genital modalities, determine the qualities of the gradually strengthened net of interrelation with other human beings. The total life pattern of every individual depends upon this matrix of relationships. Feelings of stress can lead to an increased drive toward making contacts and linkages with people, being or talking with someone. But the opposite also occurs: relationships are broken off, with a tendency to regression toward isolation and self-solace.

One of the commonest of stabilizing devices is the use of stern *self-discipline*. Self-control ranks high in our social value system, but not nearly so high as in the value systems of some Indian tribes, such as the early Iroquois, or as in those of the ancient Stoics. There is a game played by adolescents and adults in many countries, known in the South of our own country as "The numbers" or "The dozens." In it one player tries to incite the other to anger and physical reprisal while maintaining his own self-control in the face of similar insults.[16] Just as one must learn in the course of growing up that some impulses must be suppressed, some temptations resisted, some frustrations and renunciations endured, so one can learn to exert special efforts to master and conceal the uncomfortable increase in tension arising from other situations. If being proud of oneself for doing so helps—and for some people it does—let us not discount it but at the same time not fail to note that it may result not in decrease but in increase in ego tension.

Allied to pride in one's suppressive and repressive efforts is the device of *"laughing it off"*—discharging some of the tension in the form of humor, either at one's own or at someone else's expense. Freud [17] was the first to show convincingly how wit and humor have their pleasant effect just because of their tension-relieving capacity. "A wit is an angry man in search of a victim. A witticism is his way of releasing repressed hostility. . . . Laughter . . . as it provides a permissible release of unconscious aggressions, is one of the best safeguards of mental health." [18]

"Crying it out" is probably almost as common, even if not as enjoyable; the economic principle is the same. "We must concede great importance to weeping as a warding-off function even from the moment of birth, for it indicates the beginning of the reality sense and, therefore, the existence of positive and negative object relationships immediately after birth." [19]

The close association of laughing, weeping, and swearing has often been noted, in that all three tend to bring about a sense of relief from a state of tension. *Swearing* may serve this purpose.[20]

> Swearing is like pimples, better to come out; cleanses the moral system. The person who controls himself must have lots of terrible oaths

circulating in his blood. Swearing is not the only remedy. I suppose you prefer the gilded pill of a curate's sermon; I prefer pimples to pills.[21]

"Small curses . . . upon great occasions," quoth my father . . . "are but so much waste of our strength and soul's health to no manner of purpose." "I own it," replied Dr. Slop. "They are like sparrow-shot," quoth my Uncle Toby (suspending his whistling), "fired against a bastion." "They serve," continued my father, "to stir the humours, but carry off none of their acrimony; for my own part, I seldom swear or curse at all—I hold it bad, but if I fall into it by surprise I generally retain so much presence of mind . . . as to make it answer my purpose, that is, I swear on till I find myself easy. A wise and just man, however, would always endeavour to proportion the vent given to these humours, not only to the degree of them stirring within himself, but to the size and ill-intent of the offense upon which they are to fall." "Injuries come only from the heart," quoth my Uncle Toby.[22]

Hughlings Jackson said oaths and ejaculations in general were all parts of emotional language which, when uttered by healthy people, restored equilibrium to a greatly disturbed nervous system. He quoted the following passage from an unsigned review:

The value of swearing as a safety-valve to the feelings, and substitute to aggressive muscular action, in accordance with the well-known law of the transmutation of forces, is not sufficiently dwelt on. Thus the reflex effect of treading on a man's corn may either be an oath or a blow, seldom both together. The Scotch minister's man had mastered that bit of brain physiology when he whispered to his master, who was in great distress of things going wrong, "Wad na an aith relieve ya?" It has been said that he who was the first to abuse his fellow-man instead of knocking out his brains without a word laid thereby the basis of civilization.[23]

Swearing is a device easily and often abused. If it becomes a habit, it loses its usefulness as an escape-valve device and may even become a symptom.[24] This is less likely to occur with the safety device of *weeping*, perhaps the most human and the most universal of all relief measures.

Weeping, by lowering the general feeling-tone of the body, breaks or reduces the shock of the stimulus, and keeps the subject less intensely aware of it, meanwhile exerting a distinctively soothing effect upon the mind until, by allowing the painfully induced and temporarily dominant energy of the shock to be worked off gradually, a return is made to the state of normal feeling-tone. In the adult, as well as in the child, this not infrequently declares itself in a distinct sigh of relief.[25]

Children often relieve chronic apprehensiveness and insecurity by resorting to *big talk* and "tall" tales. A fantasy is always more satisfying and credible if someone else can be made to believe it; hence the narration. Uncomfortable fear and inferiority feelings diminish if one can excite astonishment or envy. This explains some of the boasting and lying of young children, but it also describes the similar behavior of some adults.

Some of the more "infantile" methods have already been mentioned; to these should be added withdrawal with *sleep*. Whereas most people find sleep more difficult in the presence of increased tension, some individuals react to bad news with somnolence. Sleeping has a relief value for many people and beyond its physiologic functions.[26] On the island of Bali, reports Margaret Mead,[27] accused prisoners often fall asleep. Some people are able to drop into a kind of waking sleep in the form of apathy, i.e., emotional withdrawal, which accomplishes the same thing.[28]

Tension relief is found by many people, perhaps by all of us to some extent, in *"talking it out."* This is so simple, so everyday, so universal, that its complex nature might easily be overlooked. In the first place, talking implies the establishment and the maintaining of a contact of sorts with another human being. The Ancient Mariner *had* to tell his story and he had to be listened to. He had to be assured that someone still accepted him as a human being and as a penitent one. This is not the only kind of emotional language implied by a talking session, but it is a typical one. In addition, certain ideas emerge; new viewpoints may be arrived at and conflicts solved just by hearing one's own statements spoken aloud. There is always the possibility that the friend may say something helpful. But this is a dividend, not the basic phenomenon.*

Talking it out, and being listened to, are a basic modality of human interrelation and, not surprisingly, the medium of most psychiatric therapy. We shall therefore return to a discussion of it later. But for the present we must be content merely to list it among other widely used devices for "everyday use."

Quietly *"thinking through"* a problem related to increased tension is a form of "talking it out," but to oneself or some imagined listener. It is a device which intelligent people like to think they use most fre-

---

* The celebrated experiments in the Western Electric plant in Hawthorne (Roethlisberger, F. J., and Dickson, W. J. *Management and the Worker*. Cambridge, Mass.: Harvard Univ. Press, 1939) were not the first demonstration that employees felt better and worked better after having a chance to talk freely to a non-critical listener. The experiment has been re-evaluated (Landsberger, Henry A. *Hawthorne Revisited*. Ithaca, N.Y.: Cornell Univ. Press, 1958), but there is no discounting the relief achieved by talking it out. See also a more recent work of our own colleagues: Levinson, Harry, et al. *Men, Management and Mental Health*. Cambridge, Mass.: Harvard Univ. Press, 1962.

quently. The primary model of thinking [29] is a mounting tension from certain drives, absence of an immediately available drive object, a "hallucinated" conception or image of the object. This process provides a release of ego tension in addition to its effectiveness in problem-solving. Intellection may thus be considered as a continuous normal tension-relieving mechanism. It may easily become "rationalization," i.e., false reasoning. This often does relieve tension and probably much of the self-deception is relatively harmless.

More direct than either talking or thinking it out or laughing it off is the device of *working off* excess (aggressive) energy by means of the neuromuscular systems. After all, this is our primary function, this moving and doing and going; thinking serves only to direct and inhibit it.[30] Stone has speculated on the relative adequacy of these various channels for the release of aroused excitation: [31]

> Speech, since it provides some degree of externalization of energy, may be regarded as standing between musculo-skeletal behavior (i.e., action) and thought, and is also a manifestation of partial motor inhibition. The degree of availability of these modes of cortical expression to the instinctual [arousal] levels is in direct proportion to the degree of motor inhibition because of diminishing external risk, yet the degree of relief of instinctual tension depends on the degree of sheer motor component in the expression. Thus action gives the greatest relief, thought or phantasy the least. But instinctual action carries with it the gravest external threat and thought the least grave. Speech stands midway between them in regard to both considerations, and is thus a singularly happy medium of expression. The symbols, the phantasies, with which the patient occupies himself represent a constant effort to translate the physiologic energies of instinct into a form adequate for cortico-spinal expression, or at least into the dissipation of pure thought.

Increased muscular activity is most efficiently relieving when it is directed toward changing the situation. Thus the wasteful, exuberant, or protestant flailings and plungings of infancy gradually come under more and more discipline as we acquire the knowledge and skill to "*act to alter*" in an intelligent and effective way. "For God's sake, do something!" has become a phrase to characterize people who get relief from a common danger by begging *others* to alter the situation. Acting which does not alter anything except the inner tension of the actor is seen in *pointless overactivity* of various kinds from finger tapping and hand rubbing to walking the floor and kicking the furniture. A generalized, undifferentiated restlessness was viewed by Freud [32] as a prototype of all affective behavior, the discharge of drive tension through the soma.

In between such pointless restlessness and more effective acting to alter, one would probably put energetic application to *work or play* or *physical exercise;* these relieve tension but usually do not change the situation immediately. The functions of work and play have been discussed frequently in our literature; we regard them as the two main forms of constructively used aggressive energy, i.e., destructive drive—harmlessly or usefully directed (and "neutralized").[33] By increasing self-sufficiency, gaining recognition, winning love and success, they make not only for comfort but for strength.

We spoke earlier of boasting and even prevaricating in order to diminish fears. Secret *fantasy formation*—actions taken on the stage of one's "inner world"—can also serve to relieve ego tension. The fantasies may be of carrying out aggressive attacks and even a destructive program; or they may be of compensation, gratification, and indulgence. They give pleasure, but in some curious way they also relieve the excess ego tension, even though they entail some guilt feelings which tend to add to the tension.*

Fantasy formation, if partially conscious, is called "daydreaming." The function of dream work in the diminution of pressure is well known from the elaborate studies of Freud and many succeeding psychoanalysts. Recent studies have demonstrated its vital necessity in the emotional household.[34] A patient of ours, subject to waves of intense anxiety lasting several days, would sometimes lament, "If only I could have another nightmare." He referred to a recurrent dream or type of dream in which he was being overrun by a trampling mob or subject to having the doors of his private chamber forced by a powerful monster. These dreams would awaken him in terror, but they were always followed by several days of relief from his customary daytime "jitters." One of the side effects of some of the ataractic drugs has been an increase in dreaming, or at least of remembered dreams; this may partly account for their effects.

The regulatory, restorative function of *dreams* was recognized by

---

* Dr. Sybille Escalona has called our attention to the fact that this (secret fantasy formation serving to relieve ego tension) has been doubted. "The Lewinian group has attempted some experimentation about it and were led to believe—perhaps on insufficient evidence—that such activities became necessary to the organism when excessive tension is present and under certain kinds of circumstances but that they are signs of the existence of tension rather than effective coping mechanisms and that even lesser degrees of tension will not be drained off unless other dynamic changes occur."

Immanuel Kant [35] a hundred years before Freud's scientific demonstration. In a little-known passage he declared:

> Some persons say that man or animals that have a tapeworm receive it as a sort of compensation to make good some deficiency in their vital organs. Now, just in the same way, I would ask if dreams (from which our sleep is never free, although we rarely remember what we have dreamt) may not be a regulation of nature adapted to ends. For, when all the muscular forces of the body are relaxed, dreams serve the purpose of internally stimulating the vital organs by means of the imagination and the great activity which it exerts—an activity that in this state generally rises to psychophysical agitation. This seems to be why imagination is usually more actively at work in the sleep of those who have gone to bed at night with a loaded stomach, just when this stimulation is most needed. Hence, I would suggest that without this internal stimulating force and fatiguing unrest that makes us complain of our dreams, which in fact, however, are probably curative, sleep even in a sound state of health would amount to a complete extinction of life.

In this list of everyday tension-relieving devices we must mention those inadvertent releases of aggression, in either an actual or a symbolic form, represented by the various *parapraxias*—slips of the tongue and minor accidents or mismanagements. Naturally only those of a harmless type can be included here, since we are not discussing pathological defenses.

At a recent meeting to which psychiatrists from all over the country were called together to advise the American Medical Association in regard to certain actions, the chairman, believed by some to be less than fully sympathetic with some of the purposes, opened the meeting by expressing his hopes that some good would come out of it in spite of the warning that "too many *crooks* spoil the broth." It always seems a little cruel to pick on the flustered individual who has made a slip or had an accident of obvious unconscious intent or made a manifest inadvertent public confession. A distinguished psychoanalyst, now dead, used to blandly excuse himself for forgetting appointments or mixing up people's names by saying smilingly, "You must forgive my unconscious." The implication of this is that we have no control over these things but, of course, that is not quite true. And that is also why they delight others and discomfort (as well as relieve) the individual.

The use of *symbolic substitutions* occurs everywhere in life. It is not surprising therefore to find many common examples—over and beyond those already cited—where a disturbed psychic equilibrium is restored through the ascription of symbolic values to acts or objects having (also) quite other uses and meanings.

The mildly disturbed housewife who goes on a shopping spree obtains not only merchandise but reassurances regarding her power, lovableness, and usefulness. She may at the same time get back at her spouse by disposing of some of his money, or please him by bringing him symbols of her love. In the world of entertainment—the theater, movies, television, circus—symbolism is especially important. Diversion is usually much more than mere distraction from unsolved problems; it may be a substitute gratification, a symbolic soothing, a "feast for the eyes," a vicarious living of a more exciting life. Aristotle called the theater a form of problem-solving. Why is the stupid Punch and Judy show so engaging to children? Someone (else) gets spanked, and various adult offenders get their come-uppances.

Not only the theater but nearly all games and most play from childhood to old age depend upon the achievement of instinctual discharge in modified forms and diverse channels, possible through the use of symbolic representations. These become very complex. In a game of bridge there is far more meaning to the process of bidding than merely the determination of a contract, a leader, and a dummy. Few players realize with what potent and ancient symbols they are dealing when they throw the executioner of Holofernes (the Queen of Hearts) on top of old King David (the King of Spades).

The symbolism of chess is particularly exciting; many psychoanalytic articles have been written about it.[36] In every chess game there are trillions of possible moves and there are almost as many combinations of symbolic gratifications for the players. Some exploit their queen mothers, some corner their flustered fathers, some ride over their brothers on horseback, some have recourse to the power of the church, some take refuge in fantasies of elephantine structure and others in the multiplicity of foot soldiers. In everyday life it is not hard to observe mama's boys and father antagonists and brother-haters, but it is less credible that many of these fantasies can become expressed in a simple, quiet chess game. Play in itself is certainly not a symptom, but compulsive playing, the intensification of any of these elements, a burning necessity to win, overreaction to defeat—these misuses of play represent symptoms.

We are constantly obliged to distinguish between "normal" uses of coping devices in everyday life and the misuse or overuse of them. Many religious conventions provide symbolic devices for the management of tensions. One can go to an extra worship service, pray oftener or longer, meditate more intensely, or sacrifice more often. These are still not symptoms. Religious behavior becomes symptomatic when these practices are carried to a definite degree of imbalance and self-defeating exaggeration. To pray all day and all night or starve oneself can scarcely be described as pure piety.

Giving to charitable causes has many motives—atonement, restitution, humane concern, identification with great purposes or merciful endeavors. But it may also be determined by motives of status-seeking, aggressive competitiveness, indirect bribery, and other less worthy motives.

One of the best illustrations of the way in which the symbol permits the discharge of aggression and the expression of other unconscious intent is in the automobile. Cars no doubt symbolize many things to different people. But their shape, their power, their forward movement, their dangerousness, their appeal to adolescents, all lend a strong sexual coloring to automobile symbolism. This is enhanced by the fact that it is the law and the custom in most places to restrict the driving of cars to people above the age of sixteen, which means that sexual maturity and automobile-driving maturity are concurrent.[37]

In what is called in psychoanalytic theory *reaction formation,* by some curious internal somersault of overcompensation aggressive impulses appear externally in a form exactly opposite to that in which they set out. A man irritated by a troublesome stray cat and bent upon destroying it ends up by feeding, sheltering, and protecting the cat and defending it against indignant neighbors. The *counterphobic mechanism* is similar; instead of being avoided and run away from, danger is eagerly sought and even produced. One sees it in a childish form in the defiance of feared danger, "whistling in the graveyard." This symptom is of particular social importance in adolescents when the temptation to overcome fear by bravado is uncontrolled by mature judgment, with the result that the laws of reality and of the community are apt to be flouted, not so much in contempt of the law as in fear of cowardice. Bernard Shaw's *Arms and the Man* [38] was devoted to this theme. Even in children one sees a form which grows more and more useful as the years advance, namely, the relief of personal "anxiety" by ministering to others. Older children reassure and comfort younger ones, as they will continue to do later as parents, teachers, nurses, doctors, Alcoholics Anonymous workers—and just possibly as psychiatrists! *

One kind of counterphobic mechanism employing symbols consists in

---

* Much argument has been expended on the distinction between reaction formation and sublimation. We here arbitrarily limit reaction formation to those several disguises in which the aggressive drive is still externally operative and apparent, even though modified.

a partial re-enactment of a disturbing experience, in motions or in fantasies and words or in both. This has been variously interpreted as an effort to gain mastery, to achieve a "better" ending, to disprove something. Freud used it as a step in the development of his theory of repetition compulsion.

Finally we must refer briefly to the various *physical and physiological ways* in which tension relief is achieved daily, hourly, perhaps momentarily, from states of tension. Often these are not recognized as having any relation to psychological states. Often they are. Sneezing, coughing, itching and scratching, borborygmus, yawning, the compulsion to get up and walk around, and many other similar measures of relief serve as examples. "Organ language" is a term which has been used to describe the function, expression, and communication which many organs of the body have. It was studied by Darwin * [39] in connection with facial muscles which voluntarily or involuntarily express aggression as well as other feelings and come to have their message recognized by others, so that it is a means of communication. Some organs communicate their message only to the individual himself—palpitation, for example.[40] Some messages are voluntary, such as threatening gestures, and some are involuntary, such as blushing. Familiar somatic devices for relieving excess tension which involve some voluntary nervous-system pathways include such acts as frequent urination and defecation, increased sweating, and increased sexual activity. Just why these phenomena diminish tension derived from conflicts apparently unrelated to them is not always easy to explain, but introspection will probably confirm the clinical observation that, for some people, some of them do, some of the time! Nor is organ language seen only in human beings. Tinbergen,[41] among others, has observed some of the same phenomena in many other animal species.

We shall return to the phenomenon of somatization later as a device for the relief of more severe ego tension.

Recapitulation

Thus far we have been considering what happens when a sufficient and relatively sudden change in the external or internal situation occurs to initiate a minor disturbance of the steady state maintained by the ego. The perceptual "part" of the ego, having become aware both of

---

* But actually Darwin did not emphasize the communication value. This is what he lacked as an explanatory principle.

the external danger and of the increased tension, signals the executive "part" of the ego to use one or more of the coping devices which serve to relieve or regulate the tension increase and restore the balance.

It has been suggested that various "tension-types" of individuals result from different conditioning experiences. Freeman [42] meant by this that "organismic energy systems become so structured by habit [that] their reactions . . . favor a particular form of focal discharge. . . . For example, some people seem to discharge aroused excitation by way of verbal discharge; whether it is an especially appropriate solution or not, they use this as a means to 'blow off steam.' Others use gross skeletal muscular action as the major avenue of discharge; in reacting to problems of increasing difficulty, such persons have been observed to hit the reaction key harder and harder or to engage in nonfocal movements of wiggling. Still others expel nervous excitement with their visceral organs, thereby developing somatic activity, and some discharge primarily on the ideomotor or phantasy level." Freeman suggested the terms Skeletal Discharge type, Vocal Discharge type, Somatic Discharge type, and Ideomotor Discharge type, a classification which might have some usefulness.

A partial list of the normal regulatory devices for the emergencies of everyday life as discussed in this chapter follows:

> Reassurances of touch, rhythm, sound, speech
> Food and food substitutes—smoking, chewing gum
> Alcoholic beverages and other self-medications
> Self-discipline
> Laughing and crying and cursing
> Boasting
> Sleep
> Talking out
> Thinking through, including rationalization
> Working off (physical exercise)
> Acting to alter
> Pointless overactivity
> Fantasy formation and daydreaming
> Dreaming
> Parapraxias
> Symbolism
> Reaction formation
> Counterphobic mechanism
> Physical and physiological processes

The Continuous Process, and the Relativity of Health and Illness

These minor emergency coping devices of everyday life are rarely considered symptoms. They are ordinarily not uncomfortable, they are not ego-alien. They are regarded both by the subject and by those about him as "perfecly normal" or at worst as idiosyncratic characteristics. These are his ways of getting along, his method of coping with life. "This is the way I am."

This emphasizes the usefulness of these devices. They are opportunistic and transitory. When the disintegrative threat disappears, the tension diminishes and the established life style continues virtually uninterrupted. The special coping measures employed are dropped—until the next time. Things go on as before.

But just how *were* things "going on" before? Presumably they went along without causing either the subject or his environment any considerable trouble. Occasional or even frequent minor episodes may have occurred, for these minor emergency coping devices had to be used, briefly. A degree of resiliency and sturdiness * may be engendered by the successful weathering of many such crises.

We must also make the assumption that in some individuals things had not been going so smoothly. An "adjustment" which has perhaps passed for "normal" may actually have been a very tenuous one, with few satisfactions, few outlets for controlled and neutralized aggression, few sublimations, few love objects. This makes for a less flexible, less resourceful personality than we would wish, with less capacity for adaptation to change and to new stresses. The expression "taking something in one's stride" means that one is not obliged to leap or stumble over small obstacles that fall in one's path. But if one's legs are short, or if they are stiff with rheumatism, such obstacles are harder to get over, or be "taken" in stride.

These handicaps and special vulnerabilities may be something congenital, like short-leggedness, or they may reflect some incomplete or improper evolutionary development of the personality, this in turn to be ascribed

---

* Dunbar used the expression of "coefficient of homeostatic elasticity" as an indicator of the person's adaptive capacity, i.e., his ease in recovery when thrown off balance. (Dunbar, Flanders. *Psychiatry in the Medical Specialties.* New York: McGraw-Hill, 1959.)

to the genes, in some instances, and to traumatic experiences in other instances. Events can occur which affect the learning process negatively at certain critical periods, and many of the intensive investigations of psychoanalysis have dealt with the kinds of situations and injuries which thus impede normal development. Incomplete metamorphosis in psychological growth with partial fixations at various points tends to increase the vulnerability of the ego both by diminishing its supports in object love and other gratifications, and by inhibiting the development of impulse-control mechanisms.

And so—whether because of weakness from previous damage or conditioning, or because of the fatigue incident to repeated stressful episodes or cumulative irritations, or because of the occurrence of more severe or sudden traumata—the normal corrective regulatory measures described may fail to effect an equilibrium. External stress, unsuccessfully warded off, is matched by a mounting internal stress ("conflict"). The tension of the ego rises. It rises above the "Plimsoll mark," a nautical expression designating the line placed around the hull of a ship to indicate how heavily it may be safely loaded and retain enough surplus buoyancy to withstand the added stress of storms.

The reader will foresee that we are approaching the topic of "storms." We are about to pass through a zone of indeterminacy separating conditions described as health from conditions described as illness. To define either health or illness is an almost impossible task; the temptation is to define each of them as the absence of the other, and this temptation hides a truth to which we most decidedly hold, namely, that health and illness are words which imply direction and not absolute condition. It would be logically correct to speak only of more health, less health, and still less health, and drop the word illness entirely. But this does too much violence to common usage.

And since common usage is very important and since our book is in part designed to offer some substitutes for some of the errors of common usage, we shall stay with it for the present and seek the patience of the reader in some further thoughts about the state of health and the state of illness.

Many writers have tried to put in words this concept of relativity in regard to health and illness and at the same time preserve the practical implications of the vernacular. In a relatively unknown book written twenty-five years ago an answer to the question was offered by an internist who probably little realized that what he said was more lucidly put than it had been by hundreds of other writers who had tried to say the same thing.

A normal, healthy person may be defined . . . as one who can retain all his organs and tissues in a state of efficient function and physical organization against those external and internal forces that are constantly tending to disturb him. Every function can be stressed beyond the limits of its accepted norm; when this is so, the altered function is called abnormal, and the evidence of it is pathology. In so doing an arbitrary, indefinite line has been created between the two states, which is variably called the "borderline of disease," the "limits of safety," the "limit of tolerance" or the "normal limit," each of which implies that the processes of change have been forced to some point which is intolerable or dangerous.

It is upon the determination of this point that the definition of disease must rest. The term disease implies a state manifestly farther from good health than simple ill-health. The man with a "disease" is looked upon as really sick and no longer just feeling badly and out of sorts; pathology is more than tolerable, functional change.[43]

What William Perkins so ably described applies to psychological and total organismic adjustments and to those adaptive changes which are instituted by the ego to meet special stress. Since both the increased tension and the overworked "stabilizers" are perceived by the ego as unusual and somewhat unpleasant, and because they interfere with satisfactions and production, these adjustment devices begin to be experienced as "ego-alien" and as "symptoms" of something amiss, if not of incipient illness. With an increase in tension there goes an increased utilization of one or several of the "normal" devices described. An individual laughs too loudly, cries too often, swears too much, drinks or smokes excessively.

Although he may concede that he does not feel well, the subject of such symptoms does not consider himself ill. His friends and neighbors would probably not consider him ill. Only in a theoretical sense would we psychiatrists consider him ill. Here we may advantageously quote again from Perkins: [44]

Common experience shows, without resort to scientific evidence, that the organism can suffer from temporary disorders. Everyone knows that there are times when he does not feel right, that he is aware that something about him is not working as well today as it did yesterday. He may feel "bilious," or "liverish"; be irritable and jumpy; suffer from peculiar feelings in the stomach or have palpitations, breathlessness, dizziness, and many other common mild complaints. In many cases there is nothing really wrong with him and these feelings are brought about by nothing more than temporary derangements of mechanisms. These apparent disruptions in many cases are just within the borderland of normal. Although chemical measurements can be applied to them and the microscope may reveal temporary derangements of tissue elements, these changes are within the limits of normal adaptation.

From this one can see how relative and complicated is the distinction between illness and health. If this is true of physical illness, as Perkins demonstrated, it is even more true in that type of illness which is called mental. The uneasy individual may have one view of his affliction; people or the environment may have quite another; and the psychiatrist may have still another. Their views are sometimes widely disparate. But whoever passes judgment or whatever the judgment is, it can be fitted into a concept of the health-illness continuum. This allows for a range from what is considered good adjustment or relative normality or mental healthiness, at one end of the scale, to a zone of abnormality, or maladjustment or mental ill health at the other end of the scale. Between an individual in his most happy, contented, and constructive moment, and that same individual in the extremity of disorganization, there are an infinite number of points representing states-of-being with varying degrees of adjustment from something more than zero per cent to something less than one hundred per cent of satisfactoriness.

We believe it is possible to distinguish certain fairly well-defined steps (up or down) on this continuum in that the manifestations of the increasingly costly efforts made by the ego to maintain order and integrity can be grouped according to certain empirical gross characteristics. These we discuss in the next chapter.

Coda: The Wear and Tear Syndrome

The reader will have deduced that the authors give little weight to the popular notion that mental illness is the product of the stress and strain of *modern* living. The tempo, the complexity, and the insecurity of modern life are no doubt greater than ever before, but the difficulties of adjustment to the stress and strain of contemporary living have been bemoaned and deplored by every generation since long before the Christian era. The theme is perennially revised and not infrequently documented, or at least subscribed to, by prominent physicians. Typical of this is a book written in 1831 by one Dr. James Johnson of London, A Fellow of the Royal College of Physicians and Physician Extraordinary to the King of England. It is entitled *Change of Air or The Pursuit of Health*. Ilza Veith's review [45] conveys the essence of its message and its policy:

. . . it was the wear and tear of early nineteenth-century London life that, according to the author, made a change of surroundings desirable and often mandatory. Dr. Johnson's own impressions upon his departure from the English metropolis in search of better climes present a graphic picture of a "modern" industrial capital. "As the carriage moved slowly up Shooter's Hill, one fine autumnal morning, I turned round to take a parting look at *Modern Babylon*. My eye ranged along the interminable grove of masts that shewed her boundless commerce—the hundred spires that proclaimed her ardent piety—the dense canopy of smoke that spread itself over her countless streets and squares, enveloping a million and a half of human beings in murky vapour."

Inevitably, there follows his nostalgic comparison with his first sight of London thirty years earlier, when it appeared calm and beautiful and promising of a peaceful life. But even then, the "chafing tide of human existence" made him feel annihilated, "lost like a drop of water in the ocean," and he felt certain that there were "few who do not experience this feeling of abasement on first mixing with the crowd in the streets of London." It is this engulfment which, according to Dr. Johnson, first gives rise to ever-mounting tensions resulting in a condition of "body and mind, intermediate between that of sickness and health, but much nearer to the former" which is constantly felt "by tens of thousands in this metropolis, and throughout the empire." Dr. Johnson considered this condition incurable, although he was sure that it added greatly to the practice of the doctors and of the undertakers.

Having established the name of "Wear-and-Tear Complaint," the author suggested that it was a disease peculiar to the English, and he pondered why it should predominate so much more in London than in Paris. The reasons to him were obvious:

"In London, business is almost the only pleasure—in Paris, pleasure is almost the only business. In fact, the same cause which produces the *wear-and-tear* malady, namely, hard work, or rather over-exertion, is that which makes our fields better cultivated, our houses better furnished, our villas more numerous, our cottons and our cutlery better manufactured, our machinery more effective, our merchants more rich, and our taxes more heavy than in France or Italy. If we compare the Boulevards, the 'caffes,' the 'jardins,' the promenades of Paris, with corresponding situations in and around the British Metropolis, we shall be forced to acknowledge that it is nearly 'all work and no play' with *John Bull* during six days of the week, or vice versa with his Gallic neighbours."

His observation had convinced Dr. Johnson that this wear and tear was reflected in the mental and physical constitution of the English. Unlike the fatigue caused by physical labor, the fatigue of the mind could not be dispelled by sleep and rest, for "a chaos of ideas will infest the over-worked brain, and either prevent our slumbers, or render them a series of feverish, tumultuous, or distressing dreams, from which we rise more languid than when we lie down!"

Apart from the general state of tension and malaise that is produced by the wear and tear syndrome, Dr. Johnson saw premature old age as its most devastating effect. He recognized signs of it in the symptoms presented to him by his patients and in their appearance, which was older than warranted by their chronologic age. Indeed, he felt that "This care-worn countenance . . . is a more obvious mark of the *wear and tear* of mind, in modern civilized life, than premature age:—for age is relative, and its anticipated advance can only be appreciated by a knowledge of its real amount, which can seldom be attained."

As contributory to the appearance of aging, Dr. Johnson decried the pallor of the English population. In the laboring classes, this etiolation was the result of unhealthy occupation. Among the fashionable, it was the result of their lack of outdoor exercise, their preference of carriages to walking, and the then current fashion whereby a "mother would as soon see green celery on her table as brown health on the cheek of her daughter."

Although he did not use the expression, Dr. Johnson seemed to consider the wear and tear malady of a psychosomatic rather than a physical nature, and with only a slight reservation he quoted Plato as saying that "all diseases of the body proceed from the mind or soul." This view was not shared by the majority of Johnson's medical colleagues, who were still inclined to think of mind and body as distinctly separate entities, the former surviving the latter in "another and a better world." But Dr. Johnson was convinced that "here below, they are linked in the strictest bonds of reciprocity, and are perpetually influenced, one by the other." In support of this theory, he cited numerous historic and contemporary examples for the "Reciprocities of Mind and Body" where "a sudden gust of passion, a transient sense of fear, an unexpected piece of intelligence—in short, any strong emotion of the mind, will cause the heart to palpitate, the muscles to tremble, the digestive organs to suspend their functions, and the blood to rush in vague and irregular currents through the living machine."

CHAPTER VIII

The First of Five Orders of Dysfunction

SYNOPSIS: *Threatened disorganization evokes tension which may exceed the powers of the habitual "normal" coping devices of the organism. Various special devices are called upon in the emergency to maintain the equilibrium, perhaps at a lower level of total functioning with the best possible façade and with a minimum of discomfort. We identify five levels of such adaptive retreat and describe in this chapter the first of these.*

THE PREVIOUS chapter included a discussion of the borderland between undoubted mental healthiness and beginning mental illness. We referred to it as a discernible degree of disorganization or dyscontrol, a disturbance requiring some special efforts to maintain equilibrium. We tried to show in that chapter how the ego performs its function of regulating minor disturbances so as to maintain an acceptable level of organismic functioning with continued growth and productivity and maximum comfort. We described the recurrence of events tending to disturb the equilibrium of adjustment, both external and internal, but for which the ego usually finds quick remedy by all sorts of accommodations, concessions, and rearrangements. Like the stabilizer on an ocean liner, the ego endeavors to minimize the amplitude of the fluctuations.

But it is also a part of life that events occur and situations arise which more considerably disturb the equilibria and disrupt the patterns of relatively comfortable adaptation to the environment. Satisfactions are diminished; frustration and alarm are experienced; and—most important of all—primitive and aggressive impulses, ordinarily held in check by the ego, become aroused. They threaten to make a dangerous emergence, and the ego becomes alerted to the necessity of more than usual exertion in the function of impulse-control. The minor tension-relieving devices of everyday living become inadequate. Emergency control has to be called upon.

It is as if the instinctual forces were constantly stirring and striving, restless in their restraints and looking for any opportunity for expressive release. One may think of a pack of savage dogs, alerted to the sound of any prowler or passer-by. Once aroused, once released, the excited dogs are not easily quelled. They must be heard, they must be held, and they will do damage if they can—it may be to the prowler, but it may be to others, to "innocent bystanders" or even to the dogs' own keepers.

The aggressive instincts lack discrimination, lack judgment, lack perspective, lack everything but power and a destructive goal. They can be mobilized rapidly, sometimes too rapidly and too powerfully for any control measures to suffice. In the name of self-defense, vengeance, righteous indignation, self-assertion, and all sorts of rationalizations, these impulses rush forth, threatening to elude even the emergency controls. The real need for such bursts of aggression is very rare; the aim is apt to be poor, the weapons inappropriate, the justification questionable, the consequences disastrous.

All this the ego "knows," as it were, and so strives to prevent such direct aggression except in very rare circumstances. As Freud [1] reminded us in *Civilization and Its Discontents*, the opportunities for any of us to settle things by direct aggression have been progressively eliminated by civilization. The violence that once must have constituted an intimate part of the life of every individual in the stages of human development is now theoretically confined to all kinds of institutions, toward which there are conflicting public attitudes.

The energies focused on a "foe" are partly derived from the primary instinctual reservoir. But there are also quantities of aggressive energy which can be withdrawn from their employment against other objects and focused upon the new foe. In addition, aggressive energies can be acquired through a de-fusion of combined aggressive-constructive investment or "sublimation." As explained in Chapter VI, the optimal way to deal with aggressive impulses is to neutralize or sublimate them, i.e., to fuse with them elements of the opposing "erotic" energies and thus transform or modify them in mode or object. Instead of a fist fight, a tennis game; instead of a foray against a person, a crop of weeds vehemently attacked. Such transformations and metamorphoses of the aggressive energies are occurring constantly in everyday life. It is said that Freud did some of his best writing when he was irritated by some of the criticisms of his opponents. And Luther is said to have declared that he never worked better than when inspired by anger. "When I am angry I can write, pray, and preach well; for then my whole temperament is quickened, my understanding sharpened, and all mundane vexations and temptations depart." [2]

We opened this chapter by suggesting that some things could disturb the equilibrium and comfortable adjustment much more than the minor day-to-day events, the coping with which occupied our attention in the previous chapter. We are suggesting that these more serious events operate by setting up or augmenting psychological conflicts and arousing the aggressive impulses. Some external event provokes a departure from the routines of peaceful coexistence, and a surge of aggression arises which requires a surge of special management. This is a much oversimplified description, and we hasten to correct it.

In the first place, the events making for increased conflict and arousing aggressive responses may be direct attacks on the environment or only threats of attack; losses may be feared or actually sustained. Injuries may be suffered. There can be pain, frustration, disappointment, shame, embarrassment, and many varieties of these. There can be temptations! The temptation may appeal to cupidity or to dishonesty or to sexual irregularity.

"Irregularity" is a purposely ambiguous word here; it must have occurred to some readers that we have said nothing so far about the "dangerous" sexual impulse. That means the impulse which seems to the person or the public to be dangerous and is dangerous because of its strange quality or its inappropriateness. Seeming dangerousness is often more inhibiting than actual dangerousness. And sex is never, in its proper channels, aggressive or dangerous; it is only when its expression involves a transgression of mode, of object, of timing, or of purpose that the sexual impulse becomes dangerous, and when such transgression does occur it is because aggressive elements have become mixed with the sexual impulse.

A second correction is needed in the oversimplified description just given. Not all disturbances of internal equilibrium arise from without. We live in the world and cannot escape our environment in some form or other. But previous experiences, wrong learning, painful scars, tender spots, weakened resistances, persistent psychic conflicts—all these make for areas of internal instability which tend to break down. They contribute to a chronic, endogenous state of increased tension within the organism through requiring constant protection. The ego experiences this tension and endeavors to do something about it.

But the ego is constantly threatened by the possibility of a spontaneous, impulsive attempted resolution by outburst, by enactment. A blow is struck, a girl is seized, a watch is lifted, a step is taken; the die is cast. We sometimes figuratively refer to the relief of getting something out of one's system. But the ego's real and lifelong problem in regard to aggression is how to manage without getting out of its system certain things that ought rather to be controlled or to be solved within the system.

Thus, regardless of whether the commotion arises spontaneously or from external stimulation, self-control becomes both the criterion and the objective of good adjustment and good ego management. What we are about to consider are the ways in which self-control becomes more than customarily difficult and requires special regulatory maneuvers.*

Dysorganization and Dyscontrol

We are about to discuss the efforts made by the ego to control disturbances of equilibrium considerably out of the ordinary in degree, devices which differ from those of everyday-life coping in several ways. Perhaps the most important way is that they cost more. They cost extra effort. They cost something, although it may be very little, in efficiency, effectiveness, and level of performance. Finally, they cost some discomfort, ranging from uneasiness and restlessness to much more disturbing sensations.

We propose to examine these efforts as they appear in progressively more strenuous exertion, as it were. We shall gauge these by the extremities to which the ego seems to be put in order to conceal failure. In a sense these represent increasing disorganization, although at the same time they are efforts to *prevent* disorganization, i.e., to prevent *further* disorganization. We recognize a series of levels of control surrender, i.e., impaired management of tension brought about by instinctual pressures resulting from reactions to environmental stress.

It is a problem to find a single word which will pass as a clear and consistent symbol of communication to describe a very complex situation. Aroused instinctual reactions, reactions with the threatened emergence of dangerous impulses, and increasing ego tension require an internal reorganization to meet the emergency. In this sense a *threat* of some, or even

---

* Engel (Engel, George L. *Psychological Development in Health and Disease*. Philadelphia: W. B. Saunders, 1962) offers a good systematic, comprehensive classification of the external injuries which strain the capacities of the organism and provoke stress reactions:

1. Factors which injure by virtue of physical and/or chemical properties.
2. Factors leading to injury when insufficient or unavailable (e.g., oxygen, vitamins, food).
3. Pathogenic organisms (viruses, parasites, bacteria).
4. Psychological stresses, especially loss of love objects, bodily injury, and drive frustration.

much, disorganization exists, against which certain special controls and emergency regulations are instituted. A new kind of internal balance is set up, and a new kind of external balance achieved. There is always some regression, some loss of control, some increased control, some actual *disorganization*, some reorganization.

For this whole process we used for several years the word *dyscontrol*, analogous to *dysfunction* and other *dys-* words that are in common medical use. But *dyscontrol* describes the operation, and we need a corresponding word to describe the state of the organism. For this we coined the parallel word *dysorganization*. We mean by it impaired, expensive, inefficient, perhaps somewhat uncomfortable organization. *Disorganization* goes too far. There *is* organization in these conditions; it has not been lost or destroyed, but only impaired.

The same is true of the word *dyscontrol*; control has not been lost but altered. The dysorganization reflects a concomitant effort to avoid disorganization.

Increasing dysfunction, increasing dyscontrol, increasing dysorganization, can be identified empirically in a series of hierarchical levels, each one reflecting a stage of greater impairment of control and organization. In the text, we use dysorganization, dyscontrol, dysfunction, and disequilibration more or less synonymously to avoid monotonous repetition of any one of them.

The existence of progressive stages of regression, dyscontrol, dysorganization, and the possibility of a relative quantification of them, occurred to me during observations as a member of a commission appointed by the Surgeon-General and my brother, Brigadier-General William C. Menninger,* to study combat exhaustion in World War II. What we observed we wrote down at the time with a vividness which I should like to carry over to these more pedestrian peacetime pages.

> The combat soldier, exposed to internal and external stresses, may suddenly deviate from accepted channels or patterns of behavior in such a way as to render him unfit for duty, so that he becomes a casualty. In trying to present an adequate clinical picture of combat exhaustion it is necessary to begin with the first evidences of an incipient failure in the maintenance of psychological equilibrium.
>
> *Incipient Stage.*—There is almost unanimous agreement among observers that the first symptoms of this failure are increasing *irritability*, and *disturbances of sleep.*

---

* Doctor Will recorded his psychiatric experiences of World War II and related the lessons learned from them to the problems of mental health and illness in postwar life in *Psychiatry in a Troubled World* (New York: Macmillan, 1948).

The irritability is manifested externally by snappishness, over-reaction to minor irritations, angry reactions to innocuous questions or incidents, flare-ups with profanity and even tears at relatively slight frustrations. The degree of these reactions may vary from angry looks or a few sharp words to acts of violence. . . .

The disturbances of sleep, which almost always accompany the symptom of increased irritability, consist mainly in the frustrating experience of not being able to fall asleep even upon those occasions when the military situation would permit. Soldiers have to snatch their rest when they can. They expect a rude and sudden awakening at any time. Opportunities for sleep become very precious and an inability to use them very distressing. Difficulties were experienced also in staying asleep because of sudden involuntary starting or leaping up, or because of terror dreams, battle dreams and nightmares of other kinds. . . .

Stage of Partial Disorganization.—These disabling disturbances in adaptation are shown externally in alterations of behavior or attitude which attract the attention of comrades, officers or medics, and lead to the soldier's being conducted or directed back to the battalion aid station. There seems to have been a considerable variety of these behavior disturbances, occurring in various combinations. The following typical manifestations appear to have been the most common, but not necessarily in this order, either of frequency or of sequence.

(1) General psychomotor retardation, with difficulty and slowness in doing familiar everyday acts, in recollection, in concentration and in responsiveness to order.

(2) A tendency to become seclusive, morose and silent, or the reverse, i.e., to talk excessively, smoke excessively, sometimes, when possible, to drink excessively.

(3) A tendency to discard belongings with the complaint that everything is too heavy, too much to bear, etc. Such men often throw away valuable and much needed personal belongings, military equipment and even food.

(4) An apparent "affective flattening" with a loss of interest in comrades, military activity, even food and letters from home. Food may go uneaten, letters unread.

(5) An increased apprehensiveness and ill-concealed fearfulness.

(6) An increasing dependence upon comrades and others, with unwonted reluctance to accept responsibility or to exert initiative.

(7) A tendency to be confused, even to the point of slight disorientation, with impaired judgment, uncertainty of movement and the like.

(8) Various somatic symptoms such as tremor, vomiting and diarrhea. . . .

Stage of Complete Disorganization.—If such patients are not sent back, the next stage either follows spontaneously or is precipitated by additional stress. Any or all of the above symptoms may suddenly become much worse. The soldier may become unstable, erratic, obviously confused, savagely irritable, quite unreasonable and even defiant and recalcitrant. He may clamber out of his foxhole in the face of danger or freeze to it when danger has passed or when it is safer to go elsewhere. He may run aimlessly about, exposing himself perilously; he may stand mute, staring into space; he may go to his CO pleading that he is not fit to command his detachment. He may break into uncontrollable sobbing or screaming. His speech may become jerky, stammering and incoherent. He may babble like a baby or make smacking or sucking movements of the lips. There is apt to be some tremulousness, especially of the hands and head, physical movements become awkward and incoordinate. Nausea and vomiting are very frequent.

These indications of full-blown demoralization are, of course, practically always sufficient to effect referral to the battalion aid station.

Battalion Aid Station Syndromes.—Patients are seen in battalion aid stations [the first point of medical observation] in all three of the conditions described above as incipient, partial and complete disorganization. It is helpful for the purpose of discussion to divide these patients into two groups, those who come to the battalion surgeon very early in their combat experience and those who come to him after long experience in the combat zone, although these groups are not sharply differentiated by clinical symptomatology.

It was the general consensus that waves of psychiatric casualties came to the battalion aid station after the first baptism of fire. Presumably such initial experiences acted as a screening process which served to precipitate out of the line those of lesser stability or whose greater conflictual tension had brought their adjustment to a marginal level. For others the baptism of fire seemed to act in the direction of preventive inoculation.

The early psychiatric casualty may arrive at the aid station after a day or a week of combat in a moderate degree of disorganization. He is jittery, tremulous, restless, jumpy, obviously frightened or "fright burned." The irritability described as so typical in the field may be diminished with the transfer to the medical station and its relative safety, but sometimes it is increased. One psychiatrist described a typical soldier in this state as "a very weary, dirty and dishevelled man sitting with his head in his hands, trembling and jerking, muttering over and over, 'Shells and tanks, shells and tanks,' or 'It was the 88s, Doc, the 88s all the time,' or 'I can't stop shaking.'" This picture was by far the most common, comprising as we were told from 80 to 90 per cent of the psychiatric cases seen by the battalion surgeon.

A smaller number of patients arrive in the more demoralized state of complete disorganization; they are brought to the battalion aid station, strapped to a litter, fighting, struggling, screaming and yelling. They attempt to dig in the ground or to leap under a bed. They may seem to respond to hallucinations and they may show some degree of disorientation. Still others demonstrate equal demoralization by standing mute, trembling, fumbling, staring into space and making no response to interrogation. A few patients at this stage show classical hysterical (conversion) syndromes with such symptoms as amnesia, aphonia, amaurosis, deafness, paralysis, anesthesia and convulsions.

The experienced soldier may have been hardened and toughened by a succession of combat experiences, so that the terrifying sights and scenes of the battlefield no longer have the fresh impact of novelty. The protective armor of fantasy, rationalizations and philosophy, and above all the self-confidence of experience and the intensified group identification may have strengthened him. But his resistance has been subjected, on the other hand, to assaults from two new quarters. The more powerful of these is undoubtedly the experience of losing comrades. In the opinion of many observers, this is the most destructive influence bearing upon personality integrity in the battle situation. The maintenance of the psychic equilibrium, the defense against yielding to fear and chucking the whole business has its chief emotional anchorage in personal attachments and unit identification. The loss of a comrade, of a respected commanding officer or of a member of the squad which he—the soldier under consideration—has been leading may constitute a wound more painful than that of a bullet through the body. Grief, in short, is, for the veteran, added to fear, fatigue, discouragement and all the pre-existing burdens. In part it is neutralized in some individuals by the incitement of impulses for revenge.

In addition to the grief over lost comrades, however, there is often the added factor of resentment regarding the lack of replacements, or the clumsiness and unpreparedness of particular replacements. Such resentments may be heightened by the interminability of the fighting and the lack of clear objectives or of information about the mission. Anxiety referable to cumulative distrust of command thus contributed to this.

At any rate, grief, accumulated fatigue and resentments (offset to some extent by reinforced fighting motivation) are now added factors which may precipitate a psychiatric disability in the veteran. . . .

Depression is more evident in those patients who relate their chief conscious distress directly to the loss of comrades, or to a line failure in performance or to failing powers of self-mastery. This picture is so common in certain types of older individuals, especially longtime Army noncoms with concern about the loss of soldiers trained by them, that it has been designated in several places "the old sergeant's syndrome." It occurs, of course, in other than sergeants and other than old Army men. . . .

General Discussion of Psychiatric Syndromes Seen at the Battalion Aid Station.—For purposes of clarity in the outline of the clinical picture, we have tried to separate the acute combat cases into groups above described. It should be emphasized, however, that while there are tendencies in the direction of slightly different symptom constellations as mentioned, there is no clear, clinical demarcation so far as we could learn, nor are the patients classified by the battalion aid surgeon on any such basis. In many instances the battalion surgeon probably had no idea and no time to ascertain what length of service his patients had seen. What he saw, in addition to all the surgical cases which poured through his hands, was a number of unwounded men who had been sent back because they couldn't fight any more. Most of them were jittery, tense, sleepless, excited, irritable, sleep-desiring but sleep-deprived, physically weary soldiers. Various battalion aid surgeons interviewed estimated the proportion of psychiatric cases as from one-half to one-fifth of all seen.

It was the conclusion of the Commission, and also of practically all the psychiatrists who were interviewed, that *this picture of psychological disorganization does not correspond either in its moderate or in its extreme form to any recognized or established psychiatric syndrome.* . . .

Metamorphoses of the Syndrome.—Our effort has been to portray the picture of disintegration in a soldier up to the time that he arrives at the battalion aid station. Here several important things take place which have a definite effect upon the subsequent evolution of the syndrome.

In the first place the patient has usually been ordered out of the combat line or taken out of it by some responsible person. This breaks his connection with the unit, but it also removes him from the field of greatest danger.

The breakup in psychic organization is concomitantly a breakup of morale, of self-mastery and of unit membership. The soldier thus affected is in the hands of the battalion aid surgeon to whom he is taken or to whom he goes spontaneously.

In this new situation there is a radical change in the direction of pressures. From being an active, aggressive fighter, he has become a passive, ineffective "patient." He has surrendered membership in a unit of comrades for a lonely, though physically safer, retreat. He is given some food, an opportunity to sleep, a few words of reassurance, sometimes exhortation, by a doctor. He may be impressed by the inflow of seriously wounded comrades with whom he can compare his own disability.

Twenty-four hours later some of these patients, who were jittery, jumpy, jerky, panicky and generally demoralized, are able to shoulder their packs and trudge back to the front lines in a fair degree of composure, ready to reunite themselves with the group, assume their responsibilities and continue on in the same situation of stress and danger as before. It is amazing that some do this; it is still more amazing that so many do. Just how many do it we do not know. We were told by some that 95 per cent of these patients went back to duty within forty-eight hours, and were told by others that less than 3 per cent of them did so. . . .

Clearing Station Stage.—The acute state of complete disorganization seems to tend to change rapidly, at least in many cases. The cases received at clearing stations are less frequently demoralized to the extent described above but are more frequently apathetic, listless, tense, restless, apprehensive, mildly confused, jumping at every sound, sweating excessively, unable to read, write or sleep.

Again, some of these patients improve remarkably after two or three days of rest, sedation, sleep, warm food and sometimes reassurance and counsel by the physician.

Those who do not respond go further back, then, to the Exhaustion Center. By this time—from one to four days out of combat—there begin to be further new clinical features.

Exhaustion Center Stage.—The chief of these is an increasing depression, with self-depreciation and sense of loss and guilt. This is related to reflection upon the separation of the soldier from his unit, his friends, his familiar patterns of behavior and to his feeling of shame for having been unable to "stick it out" and for having achieved a place of safety while his comrades remain in combat. Although usually not talkative, he will often confess his preoccupation with numerous fears—the fear that he is incurable, that he is going crazy, that he is unable to do anything, that he will be blamed for cowardice, etc. He is not relieved by reassurance, even the suggestion that he may be sent home. He may complain of heartburn, diarrhea, polyuria and the feeling that he is about to faint. In the clinical evolution some of the familiar psychiatric "entities" of standard types become distinguishable—crystallize out or split off so to speak—from the main group.

At this stage it is possible to identify a depressed group, a hysterical group, a schizophrenic group, a psychosomatic group, a hypomanic group, a "psychopathic personality" group. But the majority of patients continue to represent a vague, amorphous, anxiety-laden syndrome similar to that seen in the battalion aid station.

Again, at this level, given appropriate treatment of the type to be described elsewhere, a large but variable per cent of the main group recover sufficiently within ten days to be returned to combat or to limited duty. The rest are referred on back.

General Hospital Stage.—Those patients who do not recover within ten days at the exhaustion center reach general hospitals or special psychiatric hospitals, usually within fifteen to twenty days after their withdrawal from combat. . . .

Among patients at the general hospitals there were many who showed a puzzling vagueness in symptomatology. Several whom we saw had headaches, one had a ringing in his ears, one had pains in his legs, one pains in his stomach, several were mildly depressed and all felt incompetent to return to duty. Sometimes we had the impression of the emergence of rather definite "neurasthenic syndromes"—mild depression, slight querulousness, plaintiveness and complaintiveness, obvious discomfort, slight anxiety, and a general lack of zest for life, and so on. As a general rule these patients had been hospitalized for one to two months and had had a good deal of treatment of various kinds; some had developed the invalid attitude and no longer faced the problem of being returned to active duty.[3]

The Five Levels

These clinical pictures of personality dysorganization and reorganization at various levels which appeared so clearly in the war cases can also be seen in the psychiatric phenomena of civilian life, though usually not so telescoped in their course. And in the years that have passed since the war we have had the opportunity to define the levels more carefully. It seems to us empirically that they are five in number.

The *first* level or stage or degree of departure from the normal is that state of external and internal affairs which in common parlance is usually called "nervousness." It is a slight but definite impairment of smooth adaptive control, a slight but definite disturbance of organization, a slight but definite failure in coping.

A *second* level or stage or degree of departure from the normal level to increased disorganization is one which in civilian life rarely results in resignation or hospitalization; it is that group of syndromes which harness individuals with the necessity for expensive compensatory living devices, tension-reducing devices. These are painful symptoms and sometimes pain the environment almost as much as the patient. In the last half-century they have been called "neuroses" and "neurotic syndromes," but these are not good names. The syndromes are thousands of years old.

Our *third* stage of regression or dysorganization or disequilibrium or dyscontrol is characterized by the escape of the dangerous, destructive impulses, the control of which has caused the ego so much trouble. These are the outbursts, the attacks, the assaults, and the social offenses which result from a considerable degree of ego failure.

A *fourth* order of dyscontrol involves still more ego failure. Reality loyalty is abandoned completely or very largely; there is disruption of orderly thought as well as behavior; there are demoralization and confusion. These are the classical pictures of medieval psychiatry, the "lunacies" of our great-grandfathers, the "insanities" of our grandfathers, the "psychoses" of our fathers. We think it is time to abandon all these terms.

A *fifth* and penultimate stage is proposed, an extremity beyond "psychosis" in the obsolescent sense, the abandonment of the will to live.

We shall discuss successively these various levels.*

Dysorganization of a First Order

We are about to consider that slightly greater state of tension, of equilibrium disturbance, which distinguishes what in common parlance we call "nervousness" from the lesser vicissitudes of daily life experience. We must assume that tension has indeed increased; that the ego recognizes a greater than average upsurge of anger, of fear, or of other emotions betraying the arousal of aggressive impulses. Disturbing and arousing incidents can occur in the kitchen as well as in the front-line trenches. Habitual coping devices can be taken off guard anywhere, any time.

The first reaction of the ego to an awareness of such increased tension is automatic, a measure of increased repression. This we know nothing

---

* We learned in the fall of 1962, when Anna Freud spent some weeks at The Menninger Foundation, that she had been working for some time on a schema for the assessment of childhood disturbances in connection with which she had defined certain categorical levels of childhood disturbances arranged in a series with some slight terminological changes. We have tried to indicate the correspondence of her series with our own.

1. Not illness; essentially normality.
2. Mild, transient illness (which corresponds to our First Order)
3. Chronic but moderate degree of disorganization (our Second Order)
4. Classical syndromes (our Third and Fourth Orders)
5. Defect syndromes (included in our Fourth Order)
6. Organic brain reactions (also our Fourth Order)

about. What we are apt to be aware of is the necessity for exerting "will power" for the mastery or concealment of internal reactions. There is a more or less determined effort to not notice, to deny the tension awareness.

This separation, which may become an overworked device, is a conscious effort. Paradoxically, indeed, we speak of the use of self-control only when the much more reliable mechanisms of self-control seem about to fail us. This is true, of course, of the control of many bodily functions. We go on breathing without giving it a thought until we overexert, or until we have a chest X-ray and hear the command to "breathe deeply." We can breathe as fast or as slowly as we like for a short time, but there is an automatic control which takes over when our attention turns aside. This automatic control of breathing sometimes gets out of order (e.g., tetany), and the same thing appears to be true of the control of aggressive impulses. Patterns of self-control are developed by each individual of such a sort that perhaps a hundred times a day minor bursts of aggressive discharge are managed without any awareness of the process on the part of the individual, just as he is unaware of his innumerable moments of oxygen need. But if he turns his attention to it he can often become conscious of irritations or temptations which do slightly disturb him and which may require some conscious effort. In psychoanalytic literature such conscious effort is called "suppression" to distinguish it from "repression," which is the unconscious, automatic inhibition of these impulses.*

Some repression is, of course, always at work; we can scarcely conceive of an individual so sophisticated and so highly developed as to be able to have complete conscious control of all the productions of his instinctual urges. (The practitioners of Yoga attempt to approach the accomplishment of it.) But under the conditions of increased stress which we are assuming, with the appearance of evidence of a slight degree of

---

* We use the word "repression" here to mean both the prevention of certain intentions from coming to awareness and also the blocking of the external expression of these intentions. There is an important difference between these two meanings of the word. In a systematic examination of the concept, Madison has shown that it has numerous different meanings in Freud's writings. Sometimes its essence is that of rejecting something from consciousness, keeping something out of consciousness. Sometimes it seems to mean eliminating something from memory accessibility, i.e., motivated forgetting. Sometimes the concept was used by Freud as almost synonymous with defense in a generic sense; although only one of the dozen ways of achieving ego protection against impulses, it became a blanket word for all of them. Again, "repression" was used by Freud to mean the inhibition of the capacity for emotional experience. (Madison, Peter. "Freud's Repression Concept." *Intern. J. Psycho-anal.*, 37:35–81 [pt. 1], 1956.)

dysfunction, there is probably always an increase of "automatic" repression, *hyperrepression.*

It is characteristic of repression to be somewhat indiscriminate and hence to hold back from consciousness or from expression some things which would do no harm if released, along with those restrained for the good of the organism. This, of course, tends to increase the difficulties of adjustment by a kind of rigidity or blockade which to the outside observer may appear as stiffness, eccentricity, or even total absurdity. A family of my acquaintance was so opposed to the use of profanity that no profane word was allowed in the home under any circumstances. This suppression extended itself to the point that even words that sounded like tabooed words were not used; e.g., the Hoover Dam was never mentioned by name. This is typical of the irrational extension of repression which we designate as hyperrepression.*

Accompanying the hyperrepression, hypersuppression, and tension awareness characterizing the first degree of organismic dysfunction, goes (almost always) an increased alertness and sensitiveness to events and changes in the outside world. In its less marked forms this *hyperalertness* is often aroused by mysterious noises or other strange signals or the appearance of something particularly interesting to the subject. But in the degree now referred to it becomes painfully exaggerated; there is a con-

---

* Bibring and her colleagues have recently prepared a fine set of definitions of various defense mechanisms. Of *repression,* they say, "Repression occupies a central position in the organization of the defensive measures and mechanisms of the ego. In almost every instance of defensive activity, repression plays a part in insuring the effectiveness of the various defenses. Repression is uniquely related to, and predominantly directed against, specific instinctual impulses.

"In the historical evolution of the concept of repression, its special role in warding off unacceptable instinctual manifestations was recognized. In this regard, it is to be distinguished from all other defenses in its singular position in rendering these manifestations unconscious in the dynamic, economic, and structural sense. With the introduction of a systematic ego psychology, the concept of repression gained a new significance with regard to its effect on ego functioning. Much of ego function is in itself unconscious, in particular the operation of the entire defensive organization of the ego. Repression is the paramount mechanism through which this unconscious ego state is maintained, and the activity of the various defenses kept at an unconscious level. As an unanswered theoretical problem, there remains the unique relationship of repression to instinctual drive on the one hand, and its dynamic role with regard to the unconscious ego state on the other hand. As a consequence, the concept of repression is in need of fuller clarification, with special regard to its role in the interrelationship of ego and id, and of drive and ego function. It is our impression on the basis of clinical experience that the instinctual element implicit in defensive activity seems to be more emphatically repressed in the sense of unconsciousness (U cs.) than the ego functional element (U cs. → P cs.)." (Bibring, Grete L., et al. "A Study of the Psychological Processes in Pregnancy and of the Earliest Mother-Child Relationship. II. Methodological Considerations." *Psychoanal. Study of the Child,* 16:69–70, 1961.)

stant listening or peering, or even smelling, without the necessity of specific stimuli. The scanning function of the ego seems to take on increased activity; it looks everywhere for possible dangers. Perceptual functions become exaggerated so that sounds are louder than normal, lights brighter, sensations keener. I remember a patient reacting to battlefront experiences who could hear my watch ticking across the room; the clicking of the door latch caused him to start visibly and shake all over. (One can faintly imagine how he reacted to artillery fire.*)

Another common clinical manifestation of hypervigilance is its effect upon the sleep habits of the individual. Fitful or persistent insomnia seems to say, "I dare not relax even at night; something untoward might happen." Actually what does happen in many instances is a further development of nervous symptoms; in retrospect many patients, or relatives, describe sleep disturbances as the first recognized prelude. It should be mentioned, however, that not a few individuals have less a disturbance of sleep than a disturbance of the sense of having slept. Perhaps it is "normal" to sleep without knowing it. But sometimes we are aware of being asleep at the time we have certain thoughts or sensations, and much more frequently we believe ourselves to be awake while observers are quite convinced that we are asleep.**

Often inseparable clinically from hypervigilance is *hyperemotionalism*. Increased touchiness, tearfulness, irritability, and changeableness are recognized as evidence of a "state of nerves," another common designation for the condition we are talking about. There is a tendency to cry frequently and too easily, to burst into frequent loud, "nervous" laughter,

---

* The only soldier reportedly ever executed in time of war for treason was one who could not bear the noise of the artillery and elected execution by hanging rather than accept an order to expose himself to it. (Huie, William Bradford. *The Execution of Private Slovik*. New York: Duell, Sloan, and Pearce, 1954.)

** George Klein, himself a distinguished psychologist, reported an interesting anecdote. He served once as a subject in research studies linking dreaming with observable fluctuations in electro-encephalographic wave rhythm. The equipment was uncomfortable, the situation a strange one, and it was only with difficulty that he could go to sleep. In the morning he felt that he had barely slept at all, and what sleep he did have was fitful. He was extremely tired.

His expression of regret at having slept so little met with loud laughter, and he was told that few subjects had done *more* sleeping through the experiment than he had. His EEG pattern showed as much as six hours of deep sleep, but there were many "interruptions" when the alpha rhythm indicated a near-arousal pattern.

Apparently these many moments of near wakefulness fused with each other and were experienced as something like a continuum of borderline sleep. This may well be what happens in patients with insomnia who complain that they go for days, weeks or even years with scarcely any sleep; they probably get considerably more sleep than they are aware of.

to repeatedly attempt numerous witticisms that do not come off, to "fly off the handle" in brief temper tantrums or mild rages or to fall into brief spells of moodiness or depression. Of course such depressive reactions should be distinguished from grief related to real loss, but even a grief reaction is sometimes excessive and sometimes merges into the depression and other symptoms just mentioned.

Hyperkinesis is another very common indicator of a mild or First Order level of dyscontrol. The overactivity may be more or less directed, as in the form of attempting to change features in the situation so as to diminish the disturbing external stimuli ("acting to alter" is the classical phrase). But the overactivity is also likely to be impulsive or compulsive, pointless. Restlessness, walking the floor, wringing the hands, biting the fingernails, driving aimlessly about in a car—often too fast—these and similar examples are familiar.* The aggressive component often shows through the thin disguise, and the behavior is annoying or even dangerous.

Along with, or instead of, using his muscles in an effort to obtain relief from increased psychic tension, the individual may make persistent endeavors to think out a solution of one or several of his perceived conflicts or dilemmas. "Worrying" may describe merely anxious concern, but it is more often used in the sense of circular and repetitive thinking, which absorbs psychic energies disproportionately greater than any creative products obtained. The term *hyperintellection* applied to this symptom describes the quantity, not the quality, of intellectual effort. Clinicians use the phrase "obsessive thinking." Combined with small-muscle and thoracic hyperkinesis, it appears as garrulousness.

Some of the evidences of hypertension and dyscontrol belonging to this group of First Order devices go on silently, as it were. Especially common is the multiplication of fantasies which serve to compensate for some of the disappointments or self-deprivations of the day-by-day encounter; recall, for example, "The Secret Life of Walter Mitty." [4] A certain amount of daydreaming is normal, but when it impairs the necessary qualities of reality thinking or of effective acting it must be considered pathological. It is then more than compensation—it is *hypercompensation*.

Another common form of hypercompensation is the overzealous identification with some new cause, some new hero, even some former enemy.

---

* More extreme expressions of floor-walking and hand-wringing, jumping, dancing, hopping, and other forms of great physical activity (to the point of exhaustion) are frequently observed and can be clearly recognized as goal-inhibited or displaced aggressive "attacks." These are properly regarded as more dereistic than the hyperkinetic phenomena here referred to, and hence belong with the Second Order devices.

An impressive expression, "identification with the aggressor," has been coined to describe the sometimes frantic and sometimes merely shrewd maneuver described in the vernacular as "If you can't lick 'em, join 'em!" The opposite form of such hypercompensation is exaggerating one's weaknesses and submissiveness in various forms of "playing the martyr" or "going along for the ride."

The maneuver described in technical language as *denial* seems to the authors to be more serious, more in violation of reality principles, than the other symptoms included in this order. Perhaps we take an overstern view of it; the adjuration to "hear no evil, see no evil, speak no evil" was long regarded as a highly ethical one in the same general areas where it is now regarded as anti-intellectualism, hard-heartedness, know-nothingness, and the like. Perhaps we all "get by" in our daily lives only by means of a certain amount of denial, and in times of stress choose to blind ourselves still further in what may be an ascending scale of obliviousness. Some overstanch partisanships, some elaborate denials of the obvious, some frantic gestures of patriotism, peace, salvation of the race, and the like all belong in the category of pathology. Sometimes denial is a merciful device, as in the temporary relief of grief in one who cannot accept the fact that death has taken a beloved, or in the case of frightful injury and extreme suffering.*

Another group of symptoms of this order depends upon the empirical fact that the body functions and organs can be altered in various ways for the relief of increased ego tension. Some of the devices already mentioned, such as hyperactivity, involve somatic structures other than the brain. But in addition to restlessness there is a galaxy of *somatic discomforts and minor dysfunctions* which serve this role, such as tremor, flushing, palpitation, tachycardia, dysmenorrhea, giddiness, anorexia, nausea, enuresis, diarrhea, belching, hyperacidity, sweating, itching, and many others.** In addition various quantitative and qualitative *impairments of sexual function* occur—diminished potency, inappropriate sexual excitement, premature or retarded orgasm, and many others. These somatic and sexual dysfunctions are usually transitory or of short duration. Prob-

---

* The verbal equivalents of this situation have been neatly phrased by the Hamburgs and deGoza: (1) "I am not in this situation at all but in a better one." (2) "I am hurt, but it is only a minor injury." (3) "I was badly hurt, but I cannot remember it." (4) "I know how seriously hurt I am . . . but I have no feelings about it." (Hamburg, David A., Hamburg, Beatrix, and deGoza, Sydney. "Adaptive Problems and Mechanisms in Severely Burned Patients." *Psychiatry,* 16:1–20, 1953.)
** We discuss the psychological mechanisms of somatic involvements later on (pp. 182 ff).

ably the great majority of them are never seen by doctors. The subject takes an aspirin or a sleeping pill or perhaps a cathartic and expects to feel better shortly—and often does. Others run to doctor after doctor with successive disappointment and dissatisfaction, often coming to dislike the doctors as much as the doctors dislike to see them coming. It would be more accurate to say that this is the way it used to be; doctors today, and the public too, are beginning to understand such conditions better and to treat them differently.

The Meaning of Symptoms

By now it will be apparent to the reader that what we have described as devices employed by the ego to deal with emergencies, disturbed equilibrium and threatened dyscontrol, are what are commonly called *symptoms*. These phenomena *are* symptoms in the sense that they indicate that something is wrong and that help is needed. As such they impel the sufferer to seek relief and constitute a ticket of admission to the doctor's office.

But a symptom has more than merely this distress-signal meaning which expresses the functional and economic aspects of the symptom. We must say something now regarding its symbolic, psychodynamic, and genetic meanings. Charcot and then Freud demonstrated the indisputable fact that symptoms express and gratify wishes. At first this was rejected as utter nonsense; who on earth would *wish* to have a headache? Who would *want* to be paralyzed? Who would crave even the minor discomforts and disabilities that we have been discussing, to say nothing of more serious ones that come later?

To answer and to understand this, in any particular instance, a way had to be found in which to bring repressed and forgotten material to consciousness. Hypnosis and then the more systematic method of free association accomplished this. Buried conflicts could be resolved when their nature could be brought to the surface; until then they were repressed and concealed by symptoms having symbolic meaning. Thus a headache may mean a wish not to think; it may mean a wish to forget; it may mean a nearness to consciousness of an inexpressible hatred or sorrow. The affliction of a hand may be a way of expressing feelings regarding some other organ of the body; sensations about the heart, physically experienced, may mean exactly what those words mean in common sentimental terms. And, because of their highly sensitive and secret nature, the sexual organs acquire many symbolic representations not only in art and language but in fantasy and physiologic function. Correspondingly, anxiety about sexual competence or sexual guilt may be displaced to many different parts and organs of the body, concerning which the subject develops overweening and irrational concern. Much has been made of these symbolic translations of sexual conflict, both in psychoanalytic literature and in general literature, so that the public is not unaware of them. But most people underestimate the extent to which these dynamics permeate clinical symptomatology.

But disguised sexual wishes are not the only thing expressed by symptoms. Freud was able to show that every symptom actually expresses— and at the same time partially gratifies—not *a* wish but a triple wish! One of the wishes *does* have to do regularly with the pleasure-seeking needs of the organism, especially the erotic or libidinous needs.

But a second wish-component of the symptom has to do with aggressive intent. Every symptom both expresses a wish to hurt someone and accomplishes that hurt to some degree, if only in a symbolic way. Sometimes this is completely obvious to everyone, as in the case of an act of a criminal nature. But the same aggressive element is always there, even though it be completely and utterly divorced from any conscious aggressive intent and even though it be concealed from view. It is a part of our civilization to deny any recognition of the aggressive element in a symptom. A sick man is to be pitied, not reproached. But the fact remains that it is unpleasant to be vomited upon; helpless invalidism is a costly burden; putrescent pus is offensive. The actual accomplishment of the aggression is not the point, although it may be minimal or maximal; the important thing is the aggressive *wish*.

That this aggressive wish is present, and partially gratified in the symptom, accounts for the third type of wish expression and wish gratification in any and every symptom. This is the wish to undo the damage, as it were; the self-punishment and atonement wish. This wish may be gratified in physical suffering or psychological suffering in the form of depression, guilt feelings attributed to improper explanations, self-handicap, or outright self-penalization or self-punishment of various kinds. It is usually not difficult to see this aspect of the symptom, though it is sometimes a little hard to believe that it is the gratifying of a wish. But so it is.

We shall come back frequently to illustrations of this complex psychodynamic function of the symptom. From the genetic standpoint, on the other hand, the symptom is believed to be determined in form by childhood experiences which have brought about certain conditioning or special vulnerability. Developmental interference and delays and traumatic impairments of learning and of social adaptation are reflected not only in the kinds of difficulties which appear in later life adjustment but in the kinds of solutions attempted. The symptom always bears some relation to the developmental history.

Without minimizing in the slightest the importance of the psychodynamic, symbolic, and genetic meanings of the symptom, to the understanding of which psychoanalysis has contributed so much, our purpose in this book is to emphasize the economic interpretation, the function of the symptom in the maintenance of organismic equilibrium and integrity. This, we feel, has been neglected and is only recently coming to be fully appreciated. But we shall not cease to remind the reader in pages to come that every symptom has these numerous determinants and these numerous component aspects, even though we do not go into detailed expositions of them.

And, although serving the useful functions mentioned, and gratifying the various unconscious wishes described, symptoms are usually uncomfortable and expensive. Although temporarily helpful in the solution of some problems, of themselves they add to the total difficulties of adjustment. Furthermore, they may become permanent boarders, established as habitual techniques of living. As such they may become more burdensome than the original stresses for the relief of which they were put into effect.

But this is a complication. Ordinarily they have their protective functions to perform and they perform them, even though this is expensive. The ego institutes them as protective necessities, although the sufferer tends to regard himself as their victim rather than as their beneficiary.

Recapitulation and Transition

To recapitulate, we have listed some of the common early indications of mild dyscontrol and threatened disequilibration. We have said that under stressful conditions, which may or may not be known to him or to others, an individual begins to "feel nervous" and to appear so to others. He feels tense, talks too much, laughs too easily, loses his temper frequently, seems restless and erratic in his movements, lies awake at night stewing over problems more or less real, fantasies various ways to correct situations which he regards as unhealthy or unpleasant for him. He may develop any of a long list of physical complaints, yet he does not really regard himself as ill, even though he doesn't feel quite well. He may make sporadic efforts at relief by drinking or smoking too much and taking soporific or ataractic drugs. He may go to a doctor.

These symptoms which we have listed are an expression of a state of partial or threatened disorganization, better denoted *dysorganization.* The equilibrium of relations between the individual and the outside world and the equilibria supporting the internal operations of the organism have suffered impairment. Vital balances have been disturbed and then re-established with the aid of emergency control measures. Although in themselves undesirable, these measures serve a preservative and, hopefully, a restorative function.

The disturbance here described is of mild severity, a First Degree or First Order of dyscontrol. In common parlance it is apt to be referred to only as "nervousness." Psychiatrists sometimes label this degree of dysorganization "anxiety state," "tension state," "mild neuroticism," or "hypochondriasis."

It can be identified by its relative mildness, i.e., there is not a great deal of interference with life activities; there is no detectable regression or dereism, and the devices used are, in the main, merely exaggerations of those common to everyday-life coping methods. We have listed and described the common ones as:

> Hypersuppression (conscious effort at self-control)
> Hyperrepression (inhibition)
> Hypervigilance (exaggerated perception)
> Hyperemotionalism (tearfulness, overgaiety, instability)
> Hyperkinesis (restlessness)
> Hyperintellection (worry)
> Hypercompensation (denial)
> Somatic reactions (minor somatic and sexual dysfunctions)

One swallow does not make a summer. No one would want to say that the presence of one or two of these symptoms was proof positive of illness or even of incipient illness. Indeed the very word "illness" is a convention. Some individuals with many severe symptoms are not regarded as ill, but certainly the utilization of several of the symptoms here described over a period of some days or weeks, let us say, constitutes a definite indication of some wrong. Our book is written in part to discourage name-calling. We are not anxious to prove the appropriateness of the designation "illness." But symptoms of this sort indicate a state of affairs which may get worse.

Usually states of First Order dyscontrol represent a transitional or quickly reversible phase. But some individuals remain "nervous" for long periods of time, never quite able to dispense with some of their symptoms, even when the original stress factors have long disappeared. In the vast majority of cases, when the instance of special need for the emergency device disappears, so does the device. The patient feels "all right" again; his state of indisposition terminates.

But there is a third possibility. Most cases recover; some become chronic. And some, as we shall next try to demonstrate, become worse. The stress situation may not be alterable or at least may not be altered. The burden of First Order emergency symptoms may of themselves aid further progressive disequilibrium. In his account of *physiological* adaptation to stress, Selye [5] describes how the resistance reactions of the body to alarm become exhausted in time; in a similar way the intensification of *psychological* defenses may be described as tending toward exhaustion. Long-continued overvigilance is very tiring indeed; a headache is endurable for a few hours, but if it lasts some days or weeks it is wearing. The same can be said of any symptoms.

As the additional stresses mount, added to the burden of symptoms already present, the threat of further disorganization is perceived by the ego, and internal tension mounts even higher. The ego is not a boiler full of steam or a hive full of bees, but something like steam production or beehive excitement does occur. The ego is aroused to greater activity. First Order devices having not sufficiently or adequately helped to control the aroused aggressive impulses, something further and different must be done. What *can* be done? One might assume from *a priori* reasoning that if two or three First Order devices failed to control the stress satisfactorily, a few more of them would be called upon, or all of them whipped up, as it were, to greater exertion. But this is not the way it works—in most cases. There seems to be a definite limit to the usefulness of the devices of the First Order. This limit relates to the individual experiences and vulnerabilities—perhaps also to constitutional factors. But a limit there certainly is, and at some point the ego begins to institute *qualitatively* different rather than merely quantitatively more strenuous maneuvers.

This leads us to the topic of the next chapter.

CHAPTER IX

A Second Order of Dyscontrol:
the "Neurotic" Syndromes and Personalities

S Y N O P S I S : A second order of dyscontrol and of dysorganization is described, represented by the clinical syndromes formerly called "neurotic," "hysterical," "obsessional," and the like. These are grouped into three acute forms: those in which the discharge of aggressions is blotted from consciousness by dissociation, those in whom the aggressions are reflected back upon the body of the individual himself, and those in whom the aggressions are handled by symbolic and magical transformations.

A fourth, more chronic form is described as a frozen emergency state— variously referred to as "character disorders," "neurotic personalities," and "personality deformities." Typical examples of these are described.

THE ESSENCE of the qualitative changes characteristic of what we call the Second Order of dyscontrol is a slight but definite detachment of the person from his environment, and—simultaneously— from his loyalty to reality. He becomes, as his friends would testify, a little (more) unrealistic.

Several things combine to fill out the picture. Some increment of aggression escapes in various forms less well neutralized than the ego would like. Some of the elements of normal living and normal productivity are sacrificed. There is a distinct lowering of the level of performance and achievement. The ego falls back, as it were, to a second line of defense and takes up the fight to maintain organismic integrity and homeostasis from this new position.

This retreat impairs one of the ego's most cherished tools and talents, the reality-testing function. The ability to correctly identify and evaluate aspects and objects of external reality as the basis of successful existence one would think a first law of life. Thus the partial repudiation of the reality principle is one aspect of a withdrawal; there is a simultaneous withdrawal from the reality objects themselves. Fantasies, false objects, and even portions of the organism itself are substituted for real things and persons with which there was formerly some commerce. Work, play, productivity, and social intercourse are usually to some extent impaired, but this impairment may be covered by a façade. A work level may be maintained which impresses the world as adequate or even superior, but this is achieved at great inner cost.*

This withdrawal from the most effective interaction with reality can be described from the standpoint of organismic theory as a strategic retreat. When the real world is shut out, when the normal sources of energy, nourishment, stimulation, new information, correct bearings, and the like are in any way diminished, there is a partial or threatened closure of the ego system. Autistic processes increase, and, allowed to develop, autism is penultimate death.

One of the most useful of psychoanalytic concepts is that of regression, in which the individual returns to earlier and abandoned techniques or aims of living. There can be regression in all ego functions; one can speak in a more childish way or think in a more childish way or view one's world in a more unsophisticated, primitive, circumscribed way. Some regressive states, such as resting after fatigue, or sleep, are entirely normal and highly useful. The same could be said of many vacations. Sojourns in the desert by Elijah, Jesus, Mohammed, and many others were perhaps regressions in one sense—that of social withdrawal. Most illnesses can be seen as regression of various degrees, in the sense of separation from contemporary modes and contacts of living, and of reducing reality conformity, if not reality loyalty.

Anna Freud reminds us of the necessity to distinguish a restorative withdrawal from a less easily reversible withdrawal which ignores the reality principle to the point of severance. A sleeper may seem to have forgotten the world, but he can be quickly recalled to it when needed—by an alarm clock, the voice of a friend, or some unusual disturbance in the room. The regression incident to illnesses and treatments can sometimes be overcome by sheer will power, duress, or necessity, but not easily. And sometimes it cannot be overcome, even with outside help.

With this dereism go certain other features characteristic, we believe, of Second Order control (or *dyscontrol*, since the necessity of these special emergency measures implies some degree of failure).

---

* One thinks of Florence Nightingale, Dorothea Dix, Charles Darwin, and others.

Clinical Manifestations of the Second Order of Dyscontrol

Prominent in all Second Order devices is the presence of subjective *discomfort*. It may be vague or it may be specific. It may be the uneasiness or "anxiety" described in the previous chapter, a mild depression, a sense of things as not being right or comfortable or pleasant. This is persistent and sometimes almost frightening. More often, however, there is a chronic, gnawing sense of failure, of uselessness, of incompetence, of being a great disappointment to oneself and others. Such feelings may alternate or be tinctured with flashes of envy, jealousy, resentment. Various unpleasant somatic sensations and functional disturbances register themselves, sometimes to the extent of severe pain.

Achievement and work performance may go on after a fashion, sometimes without detectable impairment. But the joy in working is diminished; sometimes it all becomes drudgery. Friends and co-workers seem to be deliberately perverse, indifferent, or provocative. And meantime ghosts and demons harry one—guilty thoughts, absurd fears, ridiculous notions. One keeps doing things one does not want to do and thinking things one does not want to think and failing to do and think what one does want. The perversity of the human spirit, which Saint Paul so vividly described, comes to a clear, naked demonstration in these syndromes of the Second Order: "The good which I would I do not; but the evil which I would not, that I practice."

The word "neurosis" has come to mean too many different things to mean anything. Neurosis once meant a disease of the nervous system; then it came to mean a severe illness, then a mild illness, then a feigned illness. In this book we use the word only in its adjective form to describe a *quality* of the Second Order devices, a quality of painfulness, expensiveness, and inefficiency. As we go on in this section we shall find different ways to characterize or describe the peculiar paradoxical quality implied by the word "neurotic."

Acute emergency devices of the Second Order of dyscontrol are seen clinically in three general groups and may be classified according to the specific way used for handling the conflict.

In the first group this is done by blocking the aggressive and other dangerous impulses out of consciousness by extreme repression and dissociation.

In the second group the aggressive energies are deflected from their target and turned back, not to a substituted external target, but upon the self as a whole, or upon parts of the body.

In the third group the aggressive discharge is altered not so much in aim as in quality; symbolic and magical maneuvers of various kinds carry the aggressive intent, but with a considerable dilution of their original aggressive force and at great expense to the ego.

We now take up each of these groups in some detail, with illustrations.

A. *The Control of Aggression by Dissociation and Disavowal*

This method is the one most closely related to what we have described as normal (or reversible—Anna Freud) regression such as falling asleep. It appears, for example, in the homely phenomenon of *fainting*. In some little understood, automatic way a temporary severance of contact with the outside world is accomplished with a throwing of oneself upon its tender mercies in utter helplessness and oblivion. It is a curious thing that this device is at the same time so familiar and so unfamiliar. Clinically it is rare today, although once it would seem to have been very common in drawing rooms and public places. When it might be most useful—for example, under conditions of torture—it often seems to fail.

Partial but brief obliteration of consciousness occurs more frequently. A friend of mine had the following experience. He had been very worried about his daughter, who was in a hospital awaiting a rather serious surgical operation. He was aware of considerable anxiety about the matter, although he had confidence in the surgeons. There had been some delay in the operation, and a definite date had not been set for it.

One morning he went to his office, worked as usual till noon, and then went out to lunch with a friend. Shortly after returning to his office he realized that he did not know exactly what he had done for some hours. He telephoned the man with whom he had had lunch, who declared that he had noticed nothing unusual at all, and took occasion to say he had been very glad to learn that the man's daughter had been successfully operated upon and was out of danger.

Upon hearing this my friend rushed immediately to a psychiatrist; he still remembered nothing at all about the luncheon, and he knew that the statement he had made to his friend about the daughter was untrue. He had no further attacks.

One patient seen by us for the Air Force was a pilot of excellent record of many years' standing. The divorce of his parents and the death of his brother occurred in fairly close conjunction. He was assigned a confidential mission of considerable importance. On the day before he was to embark he awoke somewhat confused, not quite sure who or where he was, and was uncharacteristically awkward in his movements. His assignment to the mission was naturally suspended. The symptoms continued, however, for a week or more. Subsequently he remembered very little of that period.

The unconscious fantasies which occupy the interval of amnesia and unconsciousness are rarely recovered. But when they can be recovered they demonstrate that dissociative loss of consciousness is actually a device for the control of aggressions and not merely, as is sometimes assumed, a self-anesthetizing device in states of fear. I recall a patient seen many years ago in consultation with a general practitioner. She was a staid schoolteacher whose dreary round of life consisted in early-morning breakfast with her mother, driving some distance to a rural school, a long day teaching, and driving home in the evening. A man to whom she had been engaged came down once a week from a neighboring town and took her to a movie. On Sunday she went to church. The rest of the time she spent caring for her mother, doing her laundry, and sleeping.

A sudden change had come over this young woman. She seemed one morning unable to get out of bed and go to school as she had always done so systematically. Her mother called a doctor, and before he got there the patient seemed to have lapsed into a coma. She continued to doze day and night and could not be fully awakened. A neurological examination to exclude brain tumor was made, and during this examination the patient began to talk in a most astonishing way.

Her conversation was striking for both its content and its style. For she spoke in no refined or schoolteacher diction, but used colloquial, at times vulgar, and occasionally profane language. "What the hell" did she care if it was a school day? The "kids" could teach themselves or "go to the devil." In a drawling, querulous voice she would ask where "the old lady" (her mother) was, how long her mother expected her to "go on with this boring routine of schoolteaching," why her mother "did not die and get out of the way" so that she, the patient, "could marry my boy friend and have a home of my own." Derogatory remarks about the "boy friend" followed. And as for "these stupid doctors pawing over me," what did they really know about her life and her needs, and if they knew, why didn't they do something and give her what she wanted?

These comments and many others were drawled or ejaculated as she lay with her eyes shut as if talking to herself on a desert island. Most of the time she seemed to be in a semi-stupor. Even when she opened her eyes, she gave no evidence of seeing anyone. Naturally her behavior was most shocking to her mother and friends and she was taken to the hospital promptly, partly out of consideration for her mother's feelings. In the hospital she sometimes took her meals, but sometimes had to be spoon-fed and cared for by the nurses as if she were a baby or a complete invalid.

One day about two weeks later she suddenly "came to herself." In a most genteel and well-modulated voice—which we doctors had never heard before—she asked where she was, how it came that she was there, how her mother was being cared for, what arrangements had been made for her pupils, and other appropriate and considerate questions. Her mother was sent for and an endearing scene followed. She was once more a dutiful, cultivated, ladylike schoolteacher who took care of her mother at the expense of postponing her own needs and desires. She never acquired any recollection of what she had said or felt during her illness.

Something like this occurs in the phenomena of *fugue states* and *dual personality formations*, which so intrigued Morton Prince [1] and many since him. Our colleague Henri Ellenberger [2] has written on this topic, recalling the case of Ansel Bourne studied by William James,[3] which is now classical.[4] In Robert Louis Stevenson's famous illustration of Dr. Jekyll and Mr. Hyde the device of dissociation did not suffice to stay a progressive disorganization and severe dyscontrol. When such episodic dissociations permit antisocial or self-directed destruction or show distinct evidence of the repudiation of the ego's commitment to social values, Third Order rather than Second Order phenomena are represented. (See the next chapter.)

Typical of Second Order dissociation phenomena is *sleepwalking*. Ordinarily this can be dismissed as a casual dream enactment of no consequence. But sometimes it becomes a persistent and rather disturbing symptomatic phenomenon. Like all dreams, sleepwalking discharges certain repressed material and intent and, like all symptoms, represents wishes of several kinds. A few years ago I was consulted by an intelligent bookkeeper, a dignified and genteel woman of thirty-five given to no outward manifestations of aggressiveness, who was puzzled and annoyed by her frequently recurrent sleepwalking. At various times in the night she would arise, go to her parents' bedroom and prowl about it, apparently searching for something, which it seemed to her, in the dim conscious recollections she had of the accompanying dream, was something belonging to her that had been hidden, "something which would make me a completely different person." She could easily be awakened and returned to her bed. In the course of psychoanalytic treatment this woman arrived at an understanding of the motives for this symptom which at first she could not accept; it was a campaign of retaliation against her parents, not for their present dependence upon her, but for what she considered to have been an injustice committed by them against her in not equipping her as a boy. She believed that she would find, carefully hidden somewhere in her parents' bedroom, a compensatory corrective for the injury done her.

Less dramatic but far more common than the clinical types of dissociation just discussed are various *formes frustes*. Some of these, like preoccupation, woolgathering, or excessive fantasy formation, rarely come to clinical attention. Actually these usually signify First rather than Second Order dysfunctions (see preceding chapter). But they can reach more advanced degrees which have to be regarded as of clinical concern. We all have selective blindness, selective deafness, and selective amnesia. But when this selectiveness becomes isolation, when Pollyannaism becomes a kind of psychological opiate, when social and human concern is obliterated in the pursuit of some autistic goal, it is possible to consider such isolation or dissociation as symptomatic of Second Order dyscontrol. The clergyman may see this as moral failure, a kind of idol-worship or hardness of heart.[5] It can be that, too!

It may seem strange for us to have left until last a method of dissociation of such great historical and clinical importance as *phobias*. In these reactions strong negative feeling becomes attached to objects or situations, e.g., thunderstorms, high places, snakes, cats, public speaking. Here a secret wish is dissociated and replaced by a fear which seems ostensibly to have no connection at all with the forbidden thought. Something one desires is in a peculiar way "converted" into something so dangerous as to be terrifying and to be avoided. The simple exposure of the wish behind the "neurotic" fear (the spinster afraid to look under the bed) was one of the most convincing steps in the early presentation of psychoanalytic theory. Although Hippocrates described phobias, the term "phobia" in its present use appeared in the psychiatric literature only after the middle of the nineteenth century, and it was fifty to seventy-five years before it came into common usage. Concerning "the morbid condition of Nicanor," Hippocrates [6] observed, "when he used to begin drinking, the girl flute-player would frighten him; as soon as he heard the first note of the flute at a banquet, he would be beset by terror. He used to say he could scarcely contain himself when night fell; but during the day he would hear this instrument without feeling any emotion. This lasted a long time with him. . . .

"Damocles, who was with him, appeared to have dim vision and to be quite slack in body; he could not go near a precipice, or over a bridge, or beside even the shallowest ditch; and yet he could walk in the ditch itself. This came upon him over a period of time."

Phobias may be extended and reversed in an attitude of overcompensation, i.e., pathological boldness and intrepidity. Fenichel [7] first described and Anna Freud [8] further studied this *counterphobic* phenomenon, especially in adolescents, where it is perhaps most conspicuous but apt to be completely misunderstood. A typical form of counterphobic play is the game of "chicken," in which two cars are driven head on toward each other at high speed from opposite directions, and the first driver to become alarmed enough (i.e., sensible enough) to turn aside is regarded as having been defeated and humiliated. Daring one another to play Russian roulette is another form of this self-destructive gambling with absurdly irrational percentages. A "gambling" element is present in much reckless behavior, especially that of adolescents. Most crimes are probably *not* detected; most offenders are not convicted; most convictions are not followed by either punishment or rehabilitation. But the substitution of foolhardiness, bravado, and recklessness for discretion and compliance with the law represents a clear defect in the reality-testing function of the ego. This puts these phenomena definitely in the general category we have been describing, indications of Second Order dyscontrol, even when the pathological nature of the symptoms is obscured by peer-group approval or tolerance.

However widespread such partial dissociation and withdrawal may be, they are—in our present world of culture—clinically important chiefly when uncomfortable enough to lead the sufferer to ask for help. This would indicate that a tolerable equilibrium has not been established by the dissociative device of withdrawal; it has bettered things in one way, but this has proved too expensive for the ego. It has added another burden for which help must be sought—autochthonous help from more devices, or extraneous help from the physician.

B. The Control of Aggressive Impulses by
Displacement to the Body

We are taking it as understood, in all this discussion of Second Order dyscontrol, that some aggression is always being directly and effectively delivered which would not otherwise, i.e., without this disguise, be permitted. A disturbing fly may be swatted, a weed pulled, a marauder repelled, an assailant arrested. But civilization has obliged us to dispense largely with personal aggressiveness against persons. It "isn't done," and, when done, it entails serious consequences. Hence personal vindictiveness and hostility, rational or irrational, have to be suppressed if possible.

But sometimes there may come a time when swallowing one's wrath, or retreating, or sinking back into fantasies of vengeance, or going into a faint, no longer works. One yields to the impulse, regardless of its inexpediency. Let us assume that provocations or conflicts have increased in number or quantity, that tension has increased, that aggressive impulses have been aroused. In the unconscious at least they have been aimed, but for various reasons they have not emerged. Perhaps reason has said that an attack would be too dangerous, that the opponent is too powerful or too sacred or too far away. Or perhaps the superego has raised a finger of caution, or even a counterthreat. We must assume, next, that no substitute object is available for a simple external displacement. What then?

It was an empirical fact of common knowledge long before Freud that many individuals regularly—and all individuals occasionally—take out their rage—and then guilt feelings—upon themselves. To cut off one's nose to spite one's face is by no means a peculiarly human device. It can be observed in many of the lower animals under certain conditions. It is observable in very young children, and many forms of the phenomenon of venting fury upon one's own body have been described in the psychiatric literature. It can be done quietly by abasing oneself, mortifying the spirit and denying oneself pleasures or honors or even the humble satisfactions to which it would seem one is properly entitled. Elsewhere the reader will find reported in detail some clinical descriptions of this curious self-punitive behavior.[9]

Most of these "cases" of self-punishment and self-martyrdom are known to relatives and friends and neighbors but do not come to the attention of psychiatrists. It is a part of the self-punishment mechanism that they deny themselves such help (or defeat the help when it is offered). A more dramatic method of self-punishment which usually does get clinical attention is to be seen in various kinds of self-mutilation. This can be very serious and bizarre, as I and many other psychiatrists have reported in the literature, but now we have in mind minor forms of self-injury usually appearing to be accidental. Perhaps the more characteristic way in which the body is taken as a substitute object for aggression is achieved not through the use of the striated musculature but through internal neurophysiological mechanisms using smooth muscle and glandular tissues. Not the nose, but some other organ or part of the body is "cut off."

We have not agreed upon a word under which to list all these phenomena in which the body seems to bear the brunt of destructive impulses. They may be direct, as in self-mutilations, or indirect, as in accidental injury, or even more diffuse, as in those cases in which physiological processes are used, or misused, as in peptic ulcer. The dynamic mechanisms and the symbolic valence of the symptoms may vary greatly. Thus a swollen hand may be traumatically produced with unconscious intention, or the edema may be "hysterical," i.e., unconsciously effected by vasomotor constriction and dilation, or it may accompany some more general somatic condition. But in all three instances it may have the same unconscious symbolic value, namely, that of an injured and impaired penis. Or it may have exactly the opposite meaning, that of an enlarged and highly sensitive penis. Or it may have little or no symbolic reference to the penis.

Regardless of its symbolic meaning and regardless of its means of physiological accomplishment and regardless of its subjective painfulness, somatization carries with it an unconscious intention to hurt someone which has been partly deflected in its aim so that to some extent the wrong person suffers. Somatization may also be looked upon from the *economic* standpoint as a sacrificial compromise. A part is made to stand for the whole, and this part is proffered or yielded in order to preserve the integrity of the remainder. In ancient religious practice, choice representatives of the flock (and even family!) were offered as a sacrifice in the hope that the gods would relinquish the divine claim upon the remainder of the flock and graciously concede it to the worshipers. When that which is sacrificed is a part of one's own body, the sacrifice is a local or partial self-destruction, even though it may be, ultimately considered, a mode of salvation.

Sacrifices made to reality requirements are usually at least partly conscious, justified as expedient by such proverbs as, "Half a loaf is better than none," and "A bird in the hand is worth two in the bush." But sacrifices made to placate the conscience are often only dimly recognized consciously for what they are, and sometimes not at all. They seem to observers to be quite unrelated to need, reason, or purpose.

The "victim" (subject) of somatization will often cry out to us in pain and distress. He will seek and submit to much, even heroic, treatment. He will often seem to be a martyr to fate, as in the case of those unfortunate individuals whom the newspaper writers often dub "hard-luck champions." Or he may seem to be a martyr to his convictions, as in the numerous forms of pseudo-asceticism; or to surgery, as in the persons who seem to find some need for repeated and often unnecessary surgical operations.

Instead of torturing or mutilating oneself, or offering the sacrifice of an organ in an "accident" or by an unnecessary surgical operation, some persons do themselves in with drugs of various kinds. Alcohol addiction and other compulsive narcotization very clearly illustrate this method of "partial suicide." This is not psychosomatic illness in the ordinary sense, but it does represent self-destruction through an attack on the body purporting to be a relief of pain. The public sometimes sees the self-destructiveness clearly, but it is more apt to be impressed by the social obnoxiousness of drunkenness, the injury to wives and to children and innocent highway casualties, to say nothing of work interruption and other disappointments. What the public almost never sees is the inner suffering which drives the alcoholic to this desperate semi-homicidal, semi-suicidal behavior.

There are other kinds of psychosomatic phenomena and syndromes which are classifiable under Second Order dyscontrol. Instead of actual involvement of an organ in some dysfunction, there may be vivid *fantasies* of somatic affliction, accompanied by real and very considerable suffering. These fantasies often arise in connection with misinterpretation of the sensations from various bodily processes. The "hypochondriac" is unable to dismiss his fantasies and is constantly or recurrently tortured by them and by the fear of permanent invalidism, all aggravated by the ridicule of his friends, who cannot conceal their disbelief. They perceive the increased narcissism and self-concern in a way which the patient cannot. His body has become a love object as well as a hate object. It seems to be the last remaining treasure to which the ego can direct its concern.*

To consciously *simulate* illness or disability is called malingering; this has been discussed earlier (pp. 63 ff.). Much more frequent is the *unconscious* simulation of illness. We continue to call it "conversion hysteria," in spite of the double inaccuracy ** of the designation. In many ways it is the most dramatic and pictorial of all psychiatric pictures and best lends itself to didactic demonstration of psychodynamic principles, such as the mechanism of dissociation, displacement, isolation, introjection and others, the exploitation of bodily structure, and the multiple symbolic values of organs, gestures, and symptoms.

The genetics and psychodynamics of syndromes are important and interesting, but we must not let them draw our attention away from the economic function which they and other "psychopathological" phenomena play. They can be shown to express and partially gratify the three wishes previously mentioned—erotic, aggressive, and punitive. They can be shown to serve both as externally directed and as self-directed aggression. They can all be shown to have connections with deep, long-buried experiences of childhood.

But they can—and must—be seen also as devices used by the ego to forestall further extension of the disintegrative trend. They can be seen as a compromise in the conflict between life and death forces in which life is restricted rather than shortened. Hysterical lesions are a lesser concession to the forces of self-destruction (the process of disintegration) than are structural lesions, i.e., organic disease. The hysterical phenomenon is then a minor sacrificial offering to forestall if possible

---

* Ruth Mack Brunswick first made this point, which was elaborated later by Anna Freud. Doctor Brunswick wrote:

"When watching the behavior of [certain] children toward their bodies we are struck with the similarity of their attitudes to that of the adult hypochondriac, to which perhaps it provides a clue. The child, actually deprived of a mother's care, adopts the mother's role in health matters, thus playing 'mother and child' with his own body. The adult hypochondriac who withdraws cathexis from the object world and places it on his body is in a similar position. It is the overcharging of certain body areas with libido (loving care) which makes the ego of the individual hypersensitive to any changes which occur in them. . . . It would be worth investigating whether the hypochondriacal phase which precedes many psychotic disorders corresponds similarly to a regression to and re-establishment of this earliest stage of the mother-child relationship." (Freud, Anna. "The Role of Bodily Illness in the Mental Life of Children." *Psychoanalytic Study of the Child*, 7:69–81, 1952. See also Szasz, Thomas S. "A Contribution to the Psychology of Bodily Feelings." *Psychoanalytic Quarterly*, 26:1, 1957.)

** Nothing is "converted," and it has no dependence upon the womb (hyster).

the necessity of the greater sacrifice of an organic lesion or illness. Jelliffe repeatedly made the point regarding these hysterical or psychogenic lesions,[10] then called organ neuroses, that "in the neurotic stage of maladjustment the processes are still reversible . . . but after a certain number of years of such faulty adaptation . . . the processes become irreversible. The leaning tower of Pisa has leaned too far and organic disease has begun."

But the organ sacrifice may have to be made. This structuralization of self-destruction illustrates the famous "mysterious leap" * referred to by Freud, from the psychological image to the physical actualization. Actually, there are really three kinds of "leaps" involved. From an unconscious fantasy to its physical reproduction in symbolic form is one familiar "leap"; a patient "punishes" his hand for an offense it (might have) committed, by suddenly losing the use of it.

Then there is a second kind of leap, namely, from the conscious wish to the physical gratification of it in ways not ordinarily controlled by wishing. The best illustration of this is pseudocyesis or false pregnancy. Not all readers may be familiar with this extraordinary and completely baffling phenomenon which occurs not only in women but in some of the lower animals (e.g., dogs). Wishing or believing herself pregnant, the prospective "mother" will cease to menstruate; her abdomen will slowly enlarge in the characteristic way, the pigmentation of the nipples increases, and other phenomena of pregnancy are accurately mimicked.

Can one, by taking thought, add a cubit to his stature? Answer: Yes and no; not a cubit but possibly a few millimeters, and certainly some pounds. Similarly we may ask: Can one, by giving thought to it and acting accordingly, develop a peptic ulcer? Again the answer is: Perhaps; certainly by taking thought some people can *avoid* having an ulcer.

Dynamically it is not the thought but the wish which the thought implies which is effective. Is it then implied that one can acquire not only peptic ulcer but obesity, hypertension, arthritis, and other disagreeable conditions by wishing for them, by unconsciously desiring them? The answer is, again: Yes, one can and many a one does! This is the third type of "leap."

---

* Felix Deutsch and associates believe that there is nothing mysterious about the leap and that we should think of the tendency for some organs to take over the expression of certain wishes as a normal phenomenon, with pathological aspects appearing only in some instances: "Freud's concept of the conversion should be broadened and recognized as a continuous process lasting throughout life . . ." (Deutsch, Felix. *On the Mysterious Leap from the Mind to the Body.* New York: International Universities Press, 1959.)

All this is so well known both in scientific circles and among educated laymen that it is hard to realize how revolutionary such a proposition seemed less than a century ago. What Charcot demonstrated (as some others had done before him) was that suggestion could produce physical symptoms and suggestion could take them away. What Mesmer demonstrated was that an individual would accept suggestions and act upon them without knowing that he was doing so. What Quimby discovered for himself and used to cure many patients, and to inspire one of them to create a religion of it, was merely that some patients are ill in accordance with what they believe. It is more than the suggestion, more than the belief; there is a wish and there is a purpose.

Genetic, constitutional, and psychodynamic factors contribute to determining the particular form and organ of somatic involvement. The head, the feet, the heart, the lungs, the joints, the organs of special sense —any part of the body may be the site of phenomena which fulfill this formula.* The particular ways in which the choice is determined ** and the psychological and physiological mechanisms of its accomplishment are beyond our present concern; we are emphasizing the *economic* role played by such phenomena. They serve as expensive means to an end, but to a very important end—that of preserving the whole through sacrifice of a part. It is a choice of the lesser evil as it seems to the patient. To the doctor, this unconsciously selected sacrifice appears to be an unnecessary one; he believes there are better ways to accomplish the desired end.***

---

* See, for example, the first monumental survey of the subject by Helen Dunbar. (Dunbar, Helen. *Emotion and Bodily Changes.* New York: Columbia University Press, 1954.)

** An able colleague has submitted the very likely proposal that psychogenic somatic symptoms are localized at that part of the body which is felt by the patient to contain his ego and which is therefore most vital to him. For example, patients with psychogenic headaches are more likely to consider their heads to be the most vital parts of their body than are the members of a control group of surgical patients who are not suffering with headaches.[11]

*** The following clipping from a current news journal is not intended to applaud psychiatry but is only to indicate how tenaciously an individual has to cling to whatever self-preservative devices he has elected, until he can be confidently assured of a better device. Until then his symptoms are immune to medication. "A psychiatrist in Columbus, Georgia, last week detailed the amazing case history of a woman who spent seventeen of her twenty-eight years in a psychosomatic marathon. Her ailments included hives, headaches, hacking cough, constant sore throat, nausea, earaches, muscular soreness, and numbness in her right leg. 'The patient was never without some of these symptoms.' She had paid 602 visits to 22 physicians and one chiropractor and was hospitalized five times. She received 33 different kinds of medication, 600 allergy tests, and 1500 injections. Nothing helped. Finally, the last physician advised her that she was 'emotionally ill' and needed psychiatric help.

Doctors assume that there are always better objects than the self for the investment of both aggression and affection. Perhaps in some instances this is not so. But if it is, the condition is theoretically curable. It only remains to find ways to transfer the investment. But this is taking us into the subject of treatment, which is not our present concern.

All that we have said in no wise contradicts the substantial facts of anatomy, physiology, neurology, biochemistry. The "mysterious leap" is not some miracle or metaphysical magic but merely something that we do not fully understand. We do know that physiological reactions are accompanied in all instances by psychological reactions and that psychological reactions to stress are accompanied in all instances by physical reactions. Hans Selye [12] has worked out one logical scheme to describe this process, holding that all stress results in certain psychological reactions (which *he* does not discuss, but which we have been trying to describe) and in certain physiological reactions, which he does describe. The pituitary gland, he believes, stimulates the adrenals (by means of ACTH) and an "alarm reaction" is set up. This corresponds to our First Order ego-tension disturbance. Bodily mechanisms respond to this alarm reaction, Selye believes, by what he calls the general adaptation syndrome. The adrenal elaborates hormone-containing substances which stimulate various and specific reactions of defense.

C. The Attempted Control of Aggression by Magic, Symbol, and Ritual

The third of the principal methods of aggression-control of this order is an executive rather than an administrative one. It consists in a qualitative transformation of the nature of the impulse. At first blush this might seem to be a near-normal or quasi-normal method since, as we assume, aggressive impulses are constantly being transmuted into the energy for useful achievements. This has long been called sublimation, but Heinz Hartmann has proposed and justified the use of the word "neutralization" for this fusion of erotic and aggressive impulses

---

After 32 consultations spread over eight months, 'her symptoms had all but disappeared . . . and she was dismissed.' The patient's total bill: Some $2,700 for medical care, $500 for psychiatry."

in such a way that the original character of both is lost. The outcome is something socially and personally acceptable.

But sometimes neither the fusion nor the neutralization is complete. The aggression is disguised, but its essential quality is not lost. The aggressive impulse emerges; repression and suppression are eluded; the blow is struck. But—*mirabile dictu*—it is not felt! It has been converted into something else, not particularly useful and still undoubtedly aggressive in intent and form, but lacking its destructive effect. This magical conversion differs from neutralization also in that however much it may be eroticized or appreciated for secondary reasons, its essential purpose is to provide a harmless discharge for aggression.

There are many of these magical and symbolic conventions, both private and public * (see pp. 143). Bacchanalian revels of ancient times, Halloween celebrations here, and Guy Fawkes Day pranks in England will come to mind. In an older day the gladiatorial combats, while undisguisedly aggressive, were so to most people only by a process of identification. Essentially the same type of vicarious gratification is supplied today in a thousand coliseums. Some of these are disguised only in respect to the symbolism of the victim; in bullfights the poor bull is a scapegoat for thousands of bad consciences and the vicarious victim of thousands of vendettas. In football, hockey, and basketball games, the aggression is still more attenuated, but is acted out vigorously by a few toward a few others, giving vicarious benefit to many.

Private rather than public rituals are often called upon to assist in the control of aggressions. Some private ceremonials are used by all of us almost every day. These can be described as symptomatic only when they begin to acquire an end-in-itself quality. The ritual then no longer controls the aggression but actually expresses it. One friend of the writers makes such a fetish of cleanliness that he is constantly washing, and with such thoroughness that he keeps his skin inflamed, while acquiring a reputation—not for being clean, but for being tardy everywhere. He is an excellent lawyer but his excessive cleanliness almost prevents his having time to visit with his clients.

Many men and women who regard themselves as mentally healthy put themselves to unbelievable discomfort and inconvenience by calis-

---

* Numerous writers have been impressed with the many symbolic meanings represented by the game of football. For a humorous, but by no means absurd, extravaganza on the theme, see Ferril, Thomas Hornsby. "Freud, Football and the Marching Virgins." In *Readers' Digest*, Nov. 1961, pp. 152–54. Condensed from *The Rocky Mountain Herald* (December 28, 1957), published by Thomas Gibson, 1830 Curtis St., Denver, Colorado.

thenics or dietary rigmaroles which they consider essential to health—daily enemas, prolonged stretching exercises, abdominal massage, etc. Religious practices always appear to non-communicants as aggression-control rituals; take, for example, the daily praying to Mecca of the Moslems (as it appears to Christians), or the regular going to Mass (as it appears to Jews), or the reverential handling of the Torah (as it appears to Mormons), or the reverential handling of snakes (as it appears to Methodists).

Ritualistic control of aggressions depends heavily, of course, upon the use of displacement and symbolism. Symbolism was originally regarded by psychoanalytic theorists as the work of an unconscious, primary-process mechanism. Under the influence of studies by numerous workers [13] the concept has been extended to refer to a conscious or unconscious combining of substitution, condensation, reduction, and displacement. Common sense tells us that many names, gestures, flags, words, and other things of everyday life are symbols; that they are used in order to save time and effort is obvious, but that they may also serve to express aggression is not always so clear. The aggressive element is surely obvious when someone is hanged in effigy, for example.

Symbolic doing and undoing, for example, is a widespread symptomatic maneuver for effecting a blow, and then recalling it and undoing the damage. A mother's envy of her own child's better fortunes or prospects may take the form of harsh restrictions in the name of discipline, or it may take the form of *laissez faire* "permissiveness" in the name of emancipated child-rearing. In both instances the aggressive element is disguised and in both instances there is an automatic undoing and justifying of it. Symbolic doing and undoing fulfill the formula of all neurotic symptoms as given above; they effect (discharge) an aggression under a thin disguise, they gratify an erotic wish, they carry their own built-in punishment, and they achieve their ostensible end imperfectly and at great cost.

The term *compulsion* refers to acts which seem to a rational observer quite unreasonable and unnecessary, but which seem to be irresistible for reasons of which the individual is really unconscious, although sometimes he may try to offer a plausible rationalization. Like all symptoms, compulsions are basically aggressive, although they have some erotic elements and always involve self-punishment. But above all they are functional; they serve an economic function; they exist of a necessity and for a purpose.

To feel that setting a fire to a building is less "wicked" and less dangerous than masturbation seems absurd to anyone whose reality-testing is less impaired, and whose superego is less tyrannical, than in the case of such offenders. To steal quantities of lipsticks or screwdrivers seems silly and superfluous, but it is both more feasible and less dangerous than to attempt to acquire one or more coveted penises (an accomplishment once considered evidence of military prowess in men and still an unconsciously cherished fantasy of some women). Even the looming possibility of detection and arrest may be preferred by some women to the renunciation of all hope for the magical cure for femaleness.

A greedy craving for even more food and other symbols of maternal love or the secret pleasure of heaping up piles of various kinds of filth is present not only in patients who consult psychiatrists but in fellow citizens to whom it never occurs to question the propriety or sanity of their compulsive behavior. Our culture puts a high premium on the acquisition and protection of material possessions. The behavior of certain individuals seen in every psychiatric hospital and prison who filch and hoard trifles of all sorts differs from that of the compulsive hoarders in polite society chiefly in regard to value systems employed. These, of course, depend largely upon circumstances and tradition. The Aztecs, who prized jade, were puzzled by the greed displayed by the Spaniards for gold and their disdain for jade.

Obsessional thinking is another form of handling an oversupply of aggressive drive. Thinking may take the place of action, as Hamlet aptly put it (i.e., instead of merely preparing for or directing action). Shakespeare was right in using the word "sicklied." As the repetitiousness and persistence of the thought patterns increase, both feeling and effective action diminish. But dangerous temptation is avoided, the consequences of direct aggression deferred. Meanwhile there is an appearance of thoughtful and thorough consideration, while indirect aggression is accomplished through reduced productiveness.

Perverse Sexual Modalities

Some of the foregoing material has implied that confused or distorted sexual impulses are frequently involved in compulsive behavior. This is true. Sexual elements are often transparent in fire-setting, kleptomania, addictive gambling, reckless car driving, and various kinds of physical violence. Sometimes, rather than being merely transparently present, the sexual factor is baldly conspicuous.

It is difficult to define sexual perversion in a sufficiently general way to embrace all circumstances and modalities. Everyone knows that there are certain gross and persistent departures in respect to the type of stimulus, to the type of object, to the modality, or to the technique. Freud's comment that no one is completely satisfied with his sexual life can be put another way, that no one's sexual life can be said to be fully normal, i.e., mature. But sexual behavior which overtly violates established modes and customs is always a vehicle for unconscious aggressive impulses. The disguise is operative, of course, only for the eyes of the offender; the raped girl, the seduced boy, the terrified child all perceive the aggressiveness clearly enough. The ardent wooing of Don Juan did not conceal from the perceptive woman his essential contempt for her and her needs.

Bear in mind that the word "sexual" in the narrow sense relates to what is called a partial instinct. It is one form of expression, one aspect, one special direction of the life instinct. There is more to sex (and the instinct which determines it) than reproduction. Sexual desire, sexual pursuit, sexual relations, sexual pleasure, and all the conditions and circumstances surrounding these activities are important; but they are not *all*-important. Although Freud was so bitterly criticized for being pansexual, he was really proposing that sex, while essential and deserving of scientific study instead of hypocritical suppression, is not the main purpose of life. It becomes the primary preoccupation of the adolescent because he is suddenly suffused with so many physiological and social stimuli and is confused over the social regulations and contradictions regarding the expression of his feelings. But with maturity there comes a relegation of sexual feelings and sexual behavior to the roles of marital union and reproduction. Much of the former sexual energy becomes translated into parental concern and family affection.

According to classical psychoanalytic theory, sexual relations are conceived of as predominantly affectionate in character; the erotic factor should completely neutralize the aggressive element—in human beings. In animals there is a great variation about this; in some species the female is graciously courted; in some she is ruthlessly and painfully mistreated. In still other species the male risks and frequently loses his life in the encounter. Human beings are all of the same species, but there is individual variation here too.

Some readers may not know that in some large areas on this planet no one—no man, no woman—expects coitus to be an affectionate act or one giving pleasure to the woman. Avowedly to preclude her having any physical enjoyment from the act, the female child in Arabia is surgically mutilated ("circumcised") routinely, according to information given us by American physicians long resident there. Perhaps this is also true in Yemen and in some parts of Egypt and Africa.*

Ruthlessness and sadism in heterosexual copulation are obviously aggressive and from our standpoint symptomatic. Perversity of object choice or modality is disapproved by the conscience not only because it is disapproved by society, but also because of the conscious or unconscious aggressive component always present in the acts. In spite of this superego disapproval, however, and in spite of reality pressures and inconvenience and danger of arrest and public humiliation and criminal conviction, some individuals become irresistibly addicted, as it were, to these compulsive patterns of behavior. Dreary, dangerous, disreputable episodes, entered into or arranged at enormous effort and psychological expense, seem to them the best possible compromise between strong cravings for gratification and their equally strong fear of normal sexuality.

This strange state of affairs is incomprehensible to the public, which sees such individuals as monsters indulging their vicious whims in lustful dalliance and social ruthlessness. Actually it is usually found that these individuals are relatively lacking in sexual force and in erotic power; they are sexually immature and weak. Their sexual gestures are less erotic than aggressive, and this the public feels and recognizes even when the offender does not.

Of course the same is true to a slightly lesser degree only in the men and women who consider themselves sexually normal or supernormal and who indulge in promiscuity on the assumption that they are expressing their overweening libidinous urges. Philanderers are generally driven less by strength of physical desire than by some secret and perhaps even unconscious sensation of sexual inadequacy—or sometimes, like Don Juan, by the wish to express hostility and contempt toward women.

As in all other psychiatric symptoms, the phenomena of sexual perversion (and promiscuity) arise as a compromise or safety play. The shocking character of some instances gives a hint as to the violence and

---

* "A woman circumciser was operating swiftly on the girls. Each girl sat flat on the ground, braced against the breast and bulwarked by the outstretched legs of her sponsor. No girl screamed, flinched, or wept, for now they were women, rendered respectable and eligible for courtship and marriage. They were now wildly happy, even if it hurt, because no decent man would marry or even lie with uncircumcised girls." (Ruark, Robert. *Something of Value.* Garden City, N.Y.: Doubleday, 1955.)

the hate behind the perversion, a more direct emergence of which the perversions are presumably trying to prevent. These are individuals in whom a normal expression of sexuality is at least partially blocked. But sexual excitement continues. The fusion results in habit patterns involving episodes more apt to be vulgar, lewd, and offensive than outright destructive, but sometimes they are extremely destructive.

Consider for a moment what the psychological state must be in a man, a married man with two children, who drives fifty miles to a small town for the opportunity of exposing his genitals to shock some adolescent girls. To most individuals this seems crude, silly, unpleasant, and quite incomprehensible. "I never had such impulses," thinks the average man. But he probably did. Normally he outgrew them and repressed them. It is the inappropriateness of an infantile act in an adult which strikes us—like wetting one's clothes in a drawing room, or sucking one's thumb at a banquet. These acts, too, were once pleasurable, but most of us have long since given them up.

Or consider the state of mind of a woman who despite a good husband and three children could not resist flirting with and sexually soliciting various acquaintances of her husband or even strangers. She not only could not say "no," as the popular song has it, but she was compulsively impelled to invite overtures and relationships which she did not enjoy. Over and over her husband, whom she loved and who loved her, forgave her and took her back, hoping that she would be able to control this curious and unfortunate compulsion.

One other kind of perversion might be mentioned, not because it is frequent or very important, but because it affords further clarification of the psychodynamic motivation of the sexually perverse act. This is fetishism.

Everyone knows of the attachment of some children for certain cuddly animals, blankets, toys, or even pacifiers. This attachment may be very marked for a time. The object seems to have an enormous importance to the child and is taken to bed with it, petted, loved, and treated as a kind of talisman. Not all children manifest this tendency so clearly, but all children do find some transitional objects between the nursing mother and the final love objects.[14] This is normal.

It has been found by experiment that monkeys deprived of a normal mother and also deprived of adequate transitional objects do not mature sexually. The males are impotent and the females tend not to become pregnant.[15]

With the background of this information—childhood observation and experimental animal observation—one is prepared to understand a kind of sexual perversion in which some object, often a piece of clothing or a slipper or a hairbrush, becomes a necessary trigger to sexual relations. The attachment to this object may become so strong that the coitus becomes quite secondary, and may even be dispensed with altogether. In one of his early articles Freud [16] mentioned that "no other variation of the sexual instinct that borders on the pathological can lay so much claim to our interest as fetishism." He and many other psychoanalysts studied it intently. Why, wondered Freud, do some children tend toward homosexual gratifications as the result of their fears of sexuality, while others avoid it only by the curious device of creating a fetish? (Of course the great majority of people go in neither of these two directions. But that some do is of great importance to all of us.) Freud [17] devoted one of his last, unfinished papers to this subject. This was in 1938. In the succeeding two decades, our colleague Ernst Ticho has pointed out, the stress has been on the disturbances of the early childhood. Greenacre [18] concludes a scientific study of this condition with what she calls "an anonymous contribution to the discussion" which betrays many of its dynamic determinants.

ODE TO THE SHOE

A shoe is a shoe is a shoe—
A shoe and you are two.
A shoe has no teeth—does not bite,
A shoe does not cause any fright.

You can look at a shoe, you can step on a shoe.
You can smell at a shoe and you'll never feel blue.
A shoe keeps silent, a shoe does not speak,
A shoe keeps your secrets, there's never a leak.

A shoe is a father, a shoe is a mother,
Creates only joy and never a bother,
A shoe can be kicked, a shoe can be torn,
And a new one is bought when the old one is worn.

A shoe is a cheap pal, discreet, near and true—
A shoe is a shoe is a shoe.

Homosexuality

Finally a word must be said about the general condition of male *homosexuality*.

One must distinguish an unconscious tendency in a homosexual direction, which may be quite manifest to other people—at least to psychiatrists—and yet unknown to the possessor, from a conscious desire and preference for homosexual contact. One must also distinguish between the preference or propensity and the actual enactment of homosexual acts. And finally, one must distinguish between a few isolated incidents of homosexual contact and homosexuality as a regular and avowed way of life. The latter, homosexuality incorporated in the personality structure as a way of life, represents a syndrome belonging in the final section of this chapter. In our present discussion we have in mind the homosexual act as a symptomatic incident.

It is difficult to make this distinction sharply, because the symptomatic incident tends to become a series of incidents and very quickly the symptom and syndrome become an ego-syntonic part of the personality.

But fortunately this is not always the case, or perhaps even usually the case. When adolescents become aware of this propensity they go through an intense period of suffering. They recognize its essential abnormality and they often recognize and soon discover its selfish and corrupting nature. They struggle against it and often control it fairly successfully, but at great pain. Others find themselves unable to do so.

One of them recently said to me, "Here I am, a married man, a church member, a director in a bank, the father of three children. I am looked up to and revered. Think of it! What if they knew? How can I hold my head up? Something stronger than I am draws me like a chain into the most loathsome combinations under the most dangerous circumstances. If anyone but you knew about this, I would have to commit suicide. But what can I do?"

Of course one thing he could do would be to live continently; there are millions of heterosexually inclined people who are continent for one reason or another, and this should be no more difficult for a homosexually inclined individual.

Another thing he could do would be to get treatment for the condition. Treatment can be efficacious if the afflicted one is not too strongly entrenched in despair or in the rationalizations that there was something wrong with his hereditary genes, that he is condemned to be this way and must make the best of it. The French essayist André Gide took this position and urged his fellow homosexuals to accept themselves and hold their heads up. Conceding that there are homosexual seducers, rapists, and sadists, Gide and his followers insist that these are not characteristic and that physical and erotic and affectionate relations between individuals of the same sex need not express any aggression. This is reasonable, and the Wolfenden Report [19] in England took cognizance of the fact when it recommended that homosexual behavior between consenting adults in private be no longer considered a criminal offense. This does not mean, of course, that it is considered normal behavior.

But the fact remains that as we see homosexuality clinically and officially it nearly always betrays its essentially aggressive nature. What passes for love under such circumstances is largely counterfeit. Inherently there is a process of seduction, seduction accompanied by the degradation of the love object. No amount of euphemism and romanticism can disguise this. The attitude of the public and of the law is harsh, even cruel, and worse, it is in some respects stupid. It was toward the correction of some of these faults that the Wolfenden Committee was appointed through the Welfare Council of the Church of England. But there is no blinking the fact that society recognizes homosexuality's aggressive essence—to be more technical, the lack of a genuine and sufficient neutralization of the basic aggressive drive.

This aggression is often thinly contained. Not only does it overflow in jealous rages or sadistic exploitations, but in backlashes at the despised and despising "normal" environment. Embittered individuals betray these feelings in various subtle or not so subtle ways. Of a recent British motion picture portraying the persecution of homosexual individuals, a discerning critic wrote:

> What seems at first an attack on extortion seems at last a coyly sensational exploitation of homosexuality as a theme and, what's more offensive, an implicit approval of homosexuality as a practice. Almost all the deviates in the film are fine fellows—well dressed, well spoken, sensitive, kind. The only one who acts like an overt invert turns out to be a detective. Everybody in the picture who disapproves of homosexuals proves to be an ass, a dolt or a sadist. Nowhere does the film suggest that homosexuality is a serious (but often curable) neurosis that attacks the biological basis of life itself. "I can't help the way I am," says one of the sodomites in this movie. "Nature played me a dirty trick." And the scriptwriters, whose psychiatric information is clearly coeval with the statute they dispute, accept this sick-silly self-delusion as a medical fact.* [20]

* The same complaint was voiced by a critic in *The New York Times*, November 20, 1961: "Homosexuality is not a forbidden topic. In *The Best Man* it was the dark secret used to destroy a ruthless young politician, and in *Advise and Consent* it was a sympathetically described aberration of a Senator. In both cases it was a facile dramatic device, used without compelling force or overriding need. As long ago as in *The Children's Hour* Lillian Hellman dealt honestly and powerfully with a lesbian theme. There have been a number of works in which problems of homosexuality were probed with directness and integrity. Tennessee Williams' *Cat on a Hot Tin Roof,*

Some colleagues will feel that all and any sexual perversion is prima-facie evidence of gross ego failure and should therefore be assigned to a still higher order of pathology than our Second Order. We disagree. Unless violence and overt destructiveness characterize the perverse sexual expressions, or unless the symptoms have become part of the character structure, they are definitely compromise devices, one of whose purposes is to salvage. If there is overt violence, if the environment suffers notably, the compromise is not working; there has been a partial ego failure or rupture, of which we shall have more to say later. Homosexually inclined men often reach high levels of achievement. Others sneak and sneer and swear and suffer. We cannot, like Gide, extol homosexuality; we do not, like some, condone it. We regard it as a symptom with all the functions of other symptoms—aggression, indulgence, self-punishment, and the effort to forestall something worse.[21]

Old Names for These Syndromes

This concludes a list of what we think can be regarded as the more common acute indications of a Second Order of organismic dyscontrol, of threatened disorganization. These familiar symptoms and syndromes have long gone by such names as "neuroses," "psychoneuroses," "neurasthenia," "hysteria," "psychasthenia," etc. The inappropriateness of these designations for modern use depends upon our radically changed understanding of the nature of these syndromes. They are not due, as was once thought, to a floating uterus, or to an inflammation of the nerves, or to an excess of sexual activity, or to an exhaustion of the mind, or to a myriad of tiny hemorrhages in the brain. The old names are wrong labels and have wrong implications. They have become obsolete and hence dangerous.

Doctors know this; there have been many efforts to correct the dif-

---

Robert Anderson's *Tea and Sympathy* and Peter Shaffer's *Five Finger Exercise* did not dissimulate, and in *A Taste of Honey* a homosexual was portrayed without meanness or snickers.

"Although these are examples of successful plays on delicate themes, there can be no blinking the fact that heterosexual audiences feel uncomfortable in the presence of truth-telling about sexual deviation. And there can be no denying that playwrights interested in such themes continue to attack them tangentially, even disagreeably and sneakily.

"That is why the work of some talented writers seems tainted."

ficulty by announcing a new label, as we have illustrated in the Appendix. In looking back over four decades, I can identify various eras by the popularity and general use by colleagues of various of these designations, which were introduced to correct the error of the earlier ones. A person could almost be "placed" or "dated" as to his professional affiliations by his choice and use of terms. He might refer to a case of "neurasthenia" or "psychasthenia" or use words ending in "-ergasia" or the expression, "defense neurosis," or "tension state."

And nearly a hundred years ago Sir James Paget [22] uttered this plaintive cry: "The name *hysteria* should be abolished. For it is absurdly derived and . . . used as a term of reproach. Hysterical is taken by many people to mean [that a patient] is silly, shamming, or could get well if she pleased. Call them *anything* . . . but hysterical!"

We have proposed an alternative! We call these symptoms the evidences of a Second Order of dyscontrol (or dysorganization), devices employed by the ego when First Order devices prove to be insufficient to control a continued or increased condition of stress and threatened disorganization. Their general characteristics are that they all attempt to reduce an increased state of tension and threatened disequilibration by effecting a compromise between the dangerous impulses which seek discharge and the sense of expediency and wisdom of the ego—or perhaps it is fear—with reference to permitting them to be discharged. They effect a discharge, which is more or less disguised; the disguise involves a partial erotization of the impulse and an associated factor of penalization. These are the psychodynamic qualities of all symptoms. The economic value of the Second Order devices relates to their success in preventing a more serious consequence, perhaps the uncontrolled emergence of the aggression, or perhaps the more serious disintegration of the organism.

Second Order symptoms may suffice to tide over the emergency and may then subside. After doing their job they may disappear. Statistics would seem to show that this happens to the great majority of cases in time, although the disappearance may not be permanent. Many patients, however, prefer the help of treatment in the hope of dispensing with the symptoms sooner.

On the other hand, Second Order symptoms may not be sufficient. The stress and tension may continue to mount and the threat of disintegration increase. Then symptoms of a Third or Fourth or Fifth Order of dyscontrol may put in their appearance. These we discuss in the next chapter. But before doing so, we must speak of one other contingency.

D. *Frozen Emergency Reactions: Personality Deformities*

We have not yet mentioned what is probably the most common "solution." Sometimes the situation does not get worse, but neither does it get any better. The acute emergency situation which gave rise to the First and Second Order devices may become a "chronic emergency," or it may, in fact, disappear, leaving no change in symptoms. The devices instituted for the management of the original tension increase may become accepted and slowly established as permanent ways of living.

This tendency to "accept" an emergency measure and to adopt it as a permanent feature of the personality was described in connection with the discussion of First Order devices on page 173. We explained there that these went to make up the personal idiosyncrasies and peculiarities characteristic of a particular individual. At a card table one player hesitates and deliberates and oscillates over every bid and sometimes every play. Another throws each card upon the table as if in a rage. Still another talks continuously while playing, and if no one listens he talks to himself. We glean hints from this about how these same individuals handle other situations in their lives at which we are not present. But such personality characteristics, which are merely exaggerations of everyday-life coping devices, are not symptomatic of illness; they are not clinical.

Institutionalization or incorporation of the Second Order devices as permanent features of the character structure is a much more serious matter. The Second Order devices represent the reaction to an emergency; they are expensive, they are always slightly dereistic. Hence their *permanent* employment by the ego is a heavy liability. It is as if a fire-extinguisher, picked up by a janitor in the excitement of a threatened blaze, were to be continuously carried about by him thereafter, perhaps supplying him with water for scrubbing floors. A better figure might be that of a man who had broken his leg and had a cast applied, and who then continued to wear the cast or to use a crutch or both indefinitely afterward, even though the bones had healed.

Many of us, no doubt, retain some of these scars of earlier battles; sometimes we know about them and try to conceal them, and sometimes we cannot conceal them. They may, like the pearl formed by an oyster, be something highly prized by the outside world—more so, indeed, than by the oyster, to which it represents only a silent, peacable dealing with an intruding irritant. This is particularly transparent in certain exhibitionistic talents and was vividly illustrated in Andreyev's play of the clown who amused the crowd by submitting himself to slapping.[23] More commonly, perhaps, the maladjustment residuum may be highly prized by the individual but thoroughly despised by the outside world. The ego seems to become oblivious or indifferent to the distressing consequences *to others* which result from this cherished, or at least condoned, peculiarity. Like evil, the symptom may be

> . . . a monster of so frightful mien,
> As to be hated needs but to be seen;
> Yet seen too oft, familiar with her face,
> We first endure, then pity, then embrace.[24]

All sorts of eccentricities, perversities, private rituals, irregular pleasures, secret phobias, and unlovable traits may thus be accumulated in various patterns of crystallized chronicity of maladjustment. We may say of someone that he is a miser, a braggart, a bully, a "sissy," a worrier, a "fussbudget," a liar, or other designation based on one of his "accepted" symptoms. This name-calling is actually a kind of psychiatric diagnosis. But this kind of diagnosis almost never implies "illness," because the acceptance of the traits (symptoms) by the subject is taken for granted. This, of course, is not necessarily true; many of these individuals are well aware of their afflictions but think that nothing can be done about them, that they must "learn to live with it," bear their cross bravely.

As we know from earlier discussions, these devices always express directly some thinly veiled aggression and some distorted sexuality. Personal charm, wealth, power, and other factors may guarantee considerable social tolerance. There was not much the Roman populace could do about the pathological behavior of Nero and his infamous predecessors and successors. As Alexander [25] clearly expressed it, if one has sufficient money he can indulge in behavior with impunity which would land an impecunious man in jail as a criminal. And going back to Janet's classification,[26] in between the rich "eccentric" and the poor "criminal" —both guilty of the same persistently aggressive behavior—there is a middle zone. Is the prominent lawyer's wife who repeatedly lifts stockings from department stores criminal or eccentric? Is the teen-ager who is a persistent speeder and car-wrecker, and whose father is neither a millionaire nor a slum denizen, "sick" with something? Is the businessman who furtively exposes himself defective or merely delinquent? What is the corporation vice president afflicted with who officiates in church on Sunday, and on Monday conspires with the officers of other companies to defraud the government?

Actually such questions as these rarely arise, because the public has stereotyped ways of thinking about misbehavior which depend largely upon the social class of the offender. If a poor man steals he does so in order to acquire something he did not want to work for, but if a rich man steals, it could not possibly be for that motive. And what other motive is conceivable in a healthy-minded person? Since the man was successful he certainly was healthy-minded—not a born "crook" like those other fellows—and if he has now done something reprehensible, without any motive, surely he is not himself; he is sick. He should see a physician.

For present purposes we do not have to decide the sick or not-sick issue; all that concerns us is that such behavior departs from the standards of the community and of the individual himself. It is a form of coping which is expensive, unpleasant, offensive, always more or less unrealistic and always handicapping. It is, therefore, definitely psychopathological, and, although incorporated as an ego-syntonic aspect of the personality, these devices embarrass the ego's elasticity in its efforts to react to further emergencies.

To use another figure (taken literally from the diagnostic manual of the American Psychiatric Association), the psychopathology of these individuals is such as to leave them little room to maneuver under conditions of stress except into "actual psychosis." By this latter phrase the authors refer to conditions we shall describe as Third, Fourth, and Fifth Order dyscontrol.

Personality deformity characterized by psychopathological traits may become ego syntonic. This simply means that the individual accepts them not only as necessary but as desirable. He "embraces" them. Alexander [27] proposed that we call these "neurotic personalities," emphasizing their alloplastic offensiveness as contrasted with the autoplastic symptomatology of the classical "neurotic" patient. If put into simpler English, the point is that these individuals usually do not think of themselves as patients and even deny that they are suffering; it is those about them who suffer. But this distinction is untenable, for many of these individuals do indeed suffer, both from internal stress and from the rebuffs and rebukes received from the environment because of their ineptness. All of these personality disorders permit the release of aggressiveness in various ways, but self-injury is also always present and usually self-recognized.

Psychiatrists speak of immature personalities, rigid personalities, inadequate personalities, inhibited personalities, schizoid personalities, hysterical personalities, cyclothymic personalities, paranoid personalities, compulsive personalities, sexually deviant personalities. Their general nature can be inferred from their names.

This is not true of certain designations in common use, of which I take cognizance only to condemn. "Psychopathic personality" and "sociopathic personality" have become too vague and too pejorative for any scientific use. "Emotionally unstable personality" is a meaningless expression; everyone is emotionally unstable or else hopelessly rigid. "Passive-aggressive personality" is perhaps the most frequently used designation at the present time and the most completely absurd one. To confess the whole truth of the matter, the "passive-aggressive personality" is frequently further described as being "of the aggressive type" or "of the passive-aggressive type." I blush for the inanity of an *official* designation such as "Passive-aggressive Personality of the passive-aggressive type," but it exists.

What all these names mean is simply what we declared in Chapter II. The old names and concepts no longer fit. There are all sorts of queer pictures in the patterns of human behavior. If these patterns become consistent and stylized, as it were, we can sometimes identify them by names referring to conspicuous features.

The reader might get a better picture of what we are talking about from a few thumbnail sketches of various so-called character malformations.

For example, individuals who can be described as possessing *inadequate personalities* may, like all the others, erect a fairly deceptive façade. The inadequacy may never become common knowledge. In general, such individuals, although awkward, gauche, inept, and generally disappointing, may find their niche and carry on in a bungling way until projected into the limelight of medical attention by some acute stress.

The *infantile personality* is likewise apt to escape notice if he—or more frequently she—can arrange a proper social camouflage. Many a girl in certain circles and areas is reared to believe that a façade of fragile helplessness is calculated to get her the kind of economic security and social status that she wants. And, alas, some men's concept of women reaches out to meet just this distorted notion. The baby-doll type, the social butterfly, the beautiful-but-useless house decoration—these are well known. There are recurrent instances in psychiatric practice of little girls in the dress and stature of adult women, but totally unprepared to live the part.

I think of a woman who has been seen by at least twenty psychiatrists. Although her husband is a competent and respected lawyer, she manages to humiliate him in public to the point of frantic exasperation by flirtation, drinking, temper tantrums, and social indiscretions for which she is forgiven because of her childlike innocent smile, her tearful penitence (and her husband's decency). She behaves like a little spoiled girl who can do anything she wants anywhere and any time and expect to be forgiven. Solemn apologies, wistful pleading, a few tears, and then a sunny smile, and everything is all right again; why is everybody making so much of it?

Schizoid personalities are a little more difficult to understand. The wounds of childhood deprivation or trauma make for a certain strangeness and tenuousness in their human attachments. There are chronic skepticism, coolness, even fearfulness toward other people, and an over-development of consolatory or compensatory fantasies. Unlike the infantile personality, the schizoid individual is never really accepted, never popular, never socially comfortable. He may be admired for achievement or respected for his intelligence, but not loved or capable of deep loving.

The *cyclothymic personality*, so called, often makes its possessor very popular because of his friendliness, generosity, emotional responsiveness, sympathy, energy, and enthusiasm. But this tends to fluctuate, to change with too slight provocation into the opposite mood. It has been said that this is only an exaggeration of normal human temperament, and perhaps it is. Clinically some individuals seem to be typified by an excess of emotional liability and are "too human," as it were.

The *narcissistic personality* is a familiar one in supercilious, selfish, vain —sometimes artistic or otherwise gifted—individuals. The dynamics are very obvious: the self has become the chief love object. Usually this is a kind of consolatory compromise, but sometimes it seems to be an enthusiastic preference from the very beginning.

Closely related to narcissistic personalities are *negativistic personalities*. I do not know to whom to give credit for a story about President Jefferson and a group of companions, riding horseback cross-country, who were obliged to ford a swollen stream. A wayfarer waited until several of the party had crossed and then hailed President Jefferson and asked to be ferried. The President took him up on the back of his horse and later set him down on the opposite bank. "Tell me," asked one of the men, "why did you select the President to ask this favor of?" The man answered, "I didn't know he was the President. All I know is that on some faces is written the answer 'No' and on some the answer 'Yes.' His face was one of the latter."

There are some individuals who first say "no" to almost everything proposed to them. Psychiatrists are familiar with troubled patients who have always been proud of being "no" men. They have made no unsound loans. They have made no unwise investments. They have wasted no money. They have sponsored no extravagances. They have "never voted for a liberal cause." They have never endorsed any "hare-brained schemes." But they can become increasingly overcautious and rigid, chronically unhappy individuals, bitter, insecure, and often suicidal.

I see a good many patients who have reached middle age, proud of the heaps of possessions they have accumulated, but utterly unhappy—and partially disintegrated. They cannot permit themselves to break their lifelong habit of always driving a sound bargain. They really never took seriously the comment that "you can't take it with you," and never realized that, skillful as they were at acquiring, they had no capacity whatsoever for skillful dispensing.

In every community there are individuals of this type who cannot permit themselves the pleasure of giving. Many of them have no idea in the world what to do with their money, but to give any of it away is unthinkable. Sometimes they compose fantastic schemes for dumping burdens of wealth upon their defenseless children, concealing this cruel blow by rationalizations about "providing security for the family." As one who has also treated a great many of the ill-blessed children of these families, who were given much "security" but no love and no example of generous living, I may be permitted to speak with fervor. King Midas, who turned everything that he touched into gold, is almost too stylized a figure for us to feel very sorry for him, but there is no doubting the suffering, the inner coldness and desolation of some King Midases who excite so much envy and seem so little to need pity. That they come to a psychiatrist at all is never from a discovery that they are so pathologically stingy, for they never connect this symptom with the thing that hurts them.*

---

* There is an unfulfilled implication here; readers will want to know what such patients ever *do* come to a psychiatrist for. Of the last few I have seen, I recall these presenting symptoms: Mr. A., aged 33, sleeplessness and excessive worry over details of the business; Mr. B., aged 55, a sudden inexplicable, clumsy attempt at suicide which frightened the patient almost as much as it frightened everyone else; Mr. C., aged 40, a messy, complicated affair with three women; Mr. D., aged 42, a messy affair with

Dishonesty and Fraudulence

Much as we would like to do so, we cannot assume that telling the truth is the normal human reaction. Concealment and escape by dissimulation seem to be almost universal among living creatures. Civilization, on the other hand, requires by mutual agreement that the almost instinctive method of self-defense be abandoned and replaced with an adherence to literal truth, the slightest departure from which is regarded in the scientific world, the legal world, and the financial world as highly reprehensible.

There are certain circumstances and conventions in which lies and deception are permissible to avoid causing pain or unpleasant situations. In some games, such as poker, there is a complicated tradition about deception. The one who can best deceive other players in regard to his actual holdings is apt to be regarded as the most skillful. But this deception must be done strictly according to certain rules. One can bluff, one can lie, one can pretend all sorts of things just as long as he does not take for himself an advantage which the others have forsworn with him. One instance of "cheating" and he is out of the game permanently. "Play" which reverts to undisguised aggression is unacceptable.

Ibsen portrayed the universality of deception in his play *The Wild Duck*. One of the characters there says, "Take from the average man his 'life lie' and you bereave him of any happiness." This play goes on to illustrate how the destruction of the "life lie" brings catastrophic consequences to a whole family. In the Russian "purge" trials it seemed to Westerners as if scores of men preferred execution rather than surrender their "lie." A Swiss psychoanalyst [28] has collected a series of cases in which destruction of the "life lie" resulted in acute, severe mental illness.

one boy; Mr. E., aged 49, brooding suspicions that he was being plotted against by associates and subordinates.

All of these men were immensely wealthy; none of them had made the slightest investment of himself in anything but making money. All were regarded as tycoons, thoroughly feared and thoroughly hated by many. I suggested to one of them that he put a library in honor of his mother in one hundred small towns in her section of the country, which had no libraries. (He had made his money manufacturing books.) This total contribution would have used up no more than a tiny fraction of his immense wealth. The idea fascinated him! End of the story.

I suggested to another one that he establish playgrounds and equip them for children in the county seats of the state in which he was reared. Because of certain tax advantages this would probably not have cost him *anything*, but it was an outlay, and so he asked, "It sounds wonderful but would it be a good investment?"

O'Neill's *The Iceman Cometh* proposes that every man must have his pipe dream.

This preamble regarding deception is to introduce the incorporating in the character structure of a compulsion to deceive, as a broad streak of fraudulency. We hear it said sometimes that a certain person would rather tell a lie than the truth, even when the latter would be easier. But for some people with this *fraudulent personality*, the lie in different forms becomes a habitual way of life.

The use of the lie aggressively rather than in mere self-defense is most dramatically seen in those cases of mythomania in which an accusatory fantasy is announced as a reality, and announced with such persistence and conviction as to obtain some degree of credence. Hitler actually persuaded many Germans to believe his accusations of the Jews.

There are no doubt some innocent people in prison at the present time because of the "success" of some unrecognized, accusative mythomania. I recall a young unemployed woman who had always been a social misfit, who went to the office of a seventy-year-old vice president of an advertising company to receive a prize for having won a contest. She had never seen him before. She was in his office less than an hour. She subsequently charged that he had assaulted her sexually "dozens of times" there and thereafter. It is almost certain that, beyond the possibility of an awkward attempt at a kiss, the man was completely innocent; nevertheless, he spent the next ten years in a penitentiary. The girl became a complete recluse; she never recanted her testimony. This is an extreme instance of deception, illustrating both the aggressive and the self-comforting functions of the lie.

The accusatory lie may be self-directed. The frequency with which unsolicited false confessions of crime are made to police departments is little recognized by the public. Many motives enter into this, sometimes sensationalism, more often the wish to propitiate an unconscious and pathological sense of guilt. The most surprising thing is the utter conviction of some false confessors that it is really they who are guilty of the specific crime they confess.*

There are other forms of compulsive aggressive deception. That one must not claim to have money in the bank that isn't there, or sign somebody else's name to a promise, is perfectly well known to the people addicted to this type of fraudulency. But they can't resist doing it, given the slightest financial pressure. Of course our present penal methods of

---

* See the dramatic account of one such case in *The New Yorker*, May 2, 1953, pp. 37–49.

handling this propensity are utterly ridiculous and futile. As one warden remarked to me, "We go through the motions of keeping these folks in here awhile, and they behave perfectly well and we even get to liking them, and we send them home with a pat on the back and a stern warning not to come back. But they will forge a check at the bus station to get a bus ride home."

Some will wonder if we are logical in seeking to include such things as check-forging and shoplifting in this category of character deformity or neurotic character rather than in the category of behavior characterized by direct aggressions, which we consider in the next chapter. The reason we have done so is that we consider most theft and certain kleptomania-like stealing, check-forging, swindling, and other such behavior far more self-injurious than socially injurious. Some of our lawyer friends will not agree with this, but that is because they see the social injury and hear all about it; they rarely hear or have the opportunity to observe either the inner disorganization which brings about the aggression, or the consequences of the aggressive pattern. But in any case it is true that this is a borderline area. Perhaps these patients *do* belong in the next chapter.

There is another type of personality deformity which is so ancient and classical, so commonly assumed to be prevalent, and yet so rare, that we must list it out of sheer curiosity. It is the compulsive deception represented by the feigning of disease. Curiously enough, the individual who does this, the malingerer, does not himself believe that he is ill, but tries to persuade others that he is, and *they* discover, they think, that he is *not* ill. But the sum of all this, in the opinion of myself and my perverse-minded colleagues, is precisely that he *is* ill, in spite of what others think. No healthy person, no healthy-*minded* person, would go to such extremes and take such devious and painful routes for minor gains that the invalid status brings to the malingerer.

The average person imagines that people feign illness for obvious and, in a way, sensible reasons, to avoid military service, to escape from jail, or to get out of work. Once this was so, no doubt. One of the most horrible aspects of slavery was the fact that ignorant owners and overseers commonly assumed that any symptoms of weakness, pain, or physical disability on the part of slaves was malingering, and malingering for an obvious purpose. The result was that the already suffering wretches were given the added misery of kicks and lashes. Hundreds of books and articles on malingering are listed in the catalogue of the library of the Surgeon-General's office. Even Galen, in the second century, composed a treatise on "How to Detect Malingerers." [29] Later, it seems, Galen himself was guilty of malingering, with great success. But today we know too much about illness for malingering to be very easily accomplished. When it does occur today, one of the most puzzling things about it is that the motives are so obscure.

The simulation of illness is particularly irritating to doctors. Although it involves some self-injury and suffering, malingering is extremely aggressive. It misleads people and wins for the "victim" pity, attention, and even money. From the physician it elicits first solicitousness, then treatment, then chagrin, and finally anger and even vindictiveness. He feels deceived, teased, challenged, ridiculed, "taken in." I recall a patient who kept neurologists and surgeons sitting up most of three nights because of bleeding from her ear, suggesting skull fracture; we finally discovered that she was surreptitiously pricking her ear with a pin! [30] Of such a patient, who "had our medical department in an uproar off and on for forty days and forty nights," Dr. William Bean [31] has described in clever verse the amazing repertoire of symptoms and suggested the designation "Munchausen syndrome."

Addictive Characters

Living as we do at a time when there are five million fellow Americans disabled by reason of alcohol addiction, and a much smaller but significant number addicted to other drugs—not counting nicotine—we cannot pass over the obvious fact that some people live their lives by means of a partial, discontinuous narcotization. This makes the syndrome of addiction, the character deformity in which narcotization is incorporated as a necessity, the most widespread single psychiatric affliction in the United States. If five million Americans were suddenly disabled with some distressing skin disease, Congress would call a special session, if necessary, to appropriate enormous sums for its study and eradication. The affliction would be visible to everyone, and the pain of its victims would arouse unusual pity. But alcohol addiction, which is also painful and disabling, can be hidden, at least for a time. The suffering it causes is not so evident; we are more than apt to laugh at its victims. And if it gets unpleasant we can always stay away from "those people," especially since we have the suspicion that it is a gluttonous indulgence, a chosen vice of a few ill-bred individuals. In the case of special friends and relatives, we are willing to say that it is more than a vice, it is a "disease."

The commonly associated traits and tendencies of people who become alcohol addicts have been the subject of many studies, including some by ourselves,[32] so we shall not go into further detail about them here. Addictions to morphine and other drugs, including marijuana—which is an increasing problem in the rising new continent of Africa—are problems in which much more psychiatric research is needed. What we can be certain of is that these artificial regressions, these chemically induced escapes from reality, usually start out to be brief vacations but become substituted for the things from which they were to enable escape. They clearly represent a partial ego failure.

At first the overuse of alcohol is usually a First Order device. Then it *becomes* a definite Second Order device. When, later, it is incorporated into the character structure so that we have an irresistible addiction, it must be recognized as a Third Order syndrome which may go further. Alcoholic debauches and excitements belong in the Third Order of dyscontrol; delirium tremens, hallucinosis, and Korsakoff's disease belong to the Fourth Order.

Coda (for Doctors Only)

It is an open season for the renaming of syndromes, and the reader may suspect that any new designations would be better than some of our traditional psychiatric jawbreakers. Most of these labels were determined empirically and have been used by certain groups as a kind of local jargon, which sometimes spreads to a larger psychiatric community. A few years ago some witty caricatures of personality-typing along ornithological lines appeared, which candor compels us to say are often more easily recognized than are our more pedestrian technical designations. Recently this idea was continued in a young and irreverent magazine for resident physicians, interns, and senior medical students published by Medical Economics, Inc. The following familiar medical personality types were listed and illustrated:

Quailing Lab-Warmer: Usually found in a nook or cranny of a big medical center, nursing his characteristic unimportant little project. Has completed ten years of assorted residencies but still peeks over the edge of his warm nest, afraid to fly. Only bird with an umbilical cord.

Brooksbrothered Backslapper: Having just molted his white feathers, this newest attending appears in magnificent plumage (though his grade-school children are still being fed on free samples of baby food). Flits from M.D. to M.D., shaking hands and passing out business cards. Operative flights range all the way from circumcisions to hemorrhoidectomies.

Starchy Whistler: Old as the dodo, but far from extinct, this female has been chief nurse on the service since the attendings were in diapers. Her song consists of a monotonous blowing of the whistle on each step of any young doctor she considers out of line.

Self-billed Olympian: Hatched with his own pedestal, this chief medical bird early surrounds his head with a nimbus. Even a young Olympian knows he's congenitally smarter than birds of surgical, obstetrical, or any other species.

Nerve-Racker: This old bird, notable for his fixed, piercing eyes, hovers in the front ranks on grand rounds. When the resident describes some heroic therapeutic struggles of the night before, the nerve-racker points a claw and cackles through his sharp beak: "You did WHAT?" [33]

Recapitulation

The commonly observed clinical syndromes representative of Second Order dyscontrol as described in the preceding pages may be summarized here in outline as follows:

A. Aggressive discharge blocked from consciousness by dissociative withdrawal:
    1. Fainting
    2. Brief dissociation
    3. Sleepwalking
    4. Phobias and counterphobic states
B. Aggressive discharge displaced to the body:
    1. Self-imposed restriction and abasement (asceticism)
    2. Self-mutilation
    3. Somatization (in fantasy, function, and structural impairment)
    4. Intoxication and narcotization
C. Aggressive discharge effected through symbolic and magical modifications:
    1. Rituals, public and private
    2. Symbolic doing and undoing
    3. Compulsions
    4. Kleptomania, pyromania, etc.
    5. Obsessional thinking
    6. Perverse sexual modalities
D. Frozen emergency reactions—personality deformities:
    1. Inadequate personalities
    2. Infantile personalities
    3. Schizoid personalities

4. Cyclothymic personalities
5. Narcissistic personalities
6. Negativistic personalities
7. Fraudulent personalities
    a. Lying
    b. Check-forging
    c. Malingering
8. Addictive personalities

CHAPTER X

A Third Order of Dyscontrol:
Naked Aggression

SYNOPSIS: Continuing the theme of the preceding chapter, a third stage of dysorganization is described. This one is characterized by the escape of more or less directed undisguised aggression.

The chapter is introduced by a general discussion of aggressive behavior, including some forms which are still socially condoned. This is followed by a clinical description of the premonitory evidences of dangerously high ego tension and the devices of displacement and projection and paranoid attitudes.

The occurrence of ego rupture is manifested by two general syndromes —the chronic, repetitious occurrence of relatively milder although still serious aggressions, and the sudden, explosive outburst of very serious aggressions.

WE HAVE called the devices used for the control of increased tension, described in the preceding chapters, *emergency* measures. They represent the ego's endeavor to maintain the integrity and survival of the organism in spite of disruptive threats. Some "discharge" of the dangerous destructive drives which are responsible for the tension increase occurs, but this discharge is accomplished in as disguised and controlled a way as possible, and much of its net aggressive effect falls back upon the individual himself. It is he who bears most of the pain and disability, although his symptoms may cause the environment some pain, loss, or embarrassment.

When the aggressive drive is expressed directly upon the environment, we have to assume either that the ego was unsuccessful in its efforts to restrain, divert, or neutralize the dangerous impulses, or else that the ego "came to the conclusion," as it were, that efforts to control an aggressive act should be suspended in the interests of self-preservation or the total good. Such justifications for the expression of violence—"self-defense," "a blow for righteousness," "the destruction of evil"—are often formulated only after the act and are apt to smack of self-deceptive rationalization. Self-defense has been used as a justification for nearly every war that has ever been fought between nations, and individuals employ the same logic as diplomats.

But for many acts of violence there is no such attempt at logical explanation or justification. The individual considers his act a private matter, an affair of vengeance, sometimes merely a "human" yielding to greedy or envious or lustful temptation. He may offer no explanation whatsoever. When asked why he did it, the only truthful answer that an offender can make may be, "I don't know," which, as Alexander [1] commented in his study of "The Criminal, His Judge and the Public," is the one which most infuriates everyone.

Do you mean to imply, asks a reader, that all aggressive behavior connotes a degree of personality disorganization? Is the violent act—except in rare instances of emergency—*prima facie* evidence of ego failure? Socrates, Jesus, Gandhi, and a few others thought so. Should they be considered paragons of mental healthiness? Some would find no difficulty in accepting this, and the general trend of our culture might seem to be in that direction. Overt aggression, once a hallmark of manliness and courage, has largely gone out of fashion. Most people today eschew direct aggressiveness, try to contain it with regard to themselves and vigorously condemn it in others. Our civilization has become so organized that there seem to be relatively few occasions when direct aggression is indicated. This is reflected in the disappearance of dueling, the public whipping post, public abuse of animals. It is reflected in the gradual disappearance of corporal punishment in hospitals, public schools, prisons, and homes. It has become a matter of common knowledge that it is really possible and perhaps preferable to rear children by means of love and example rather than by means of pain and fear.

There are, to be sure, a few amenities, a few special permits for direct aggression, concerning which there is sharp difference of opinion. A small minority of adolescents and adult males continues to find the pursuit of and violent destruction of wild animals peculiarly thrilling. They are vigorously encouraged in this, of course, by numerous business interests which seek to rationalize it as the exemplification of virility, the appreciation of natural beauty, the return to the freedom of primitive life, the reduction of "varmints" or overstocked species, the escape from debilitating effects of city life, and so on. All these rationalizations cannot disguise the fact that hunting exploits the pleasure of causing fear, suffering, and death in other living creatures, who have as much right to live as we unless their death furthers human welfare in some respect other than amusement. However, to call such individuals sadistic, uncivilized, and psychopathic is just as untenable as to call their opponents idealistic, fanatic, and sentimental.

If direct, overt aggression can be denatured, as it were, both of the hostile feelings which originally aroused it and the guilt feelings which it tends to arouse; if, in short, it can be delivered in the name of sport or courage or discipline, it can be indulged in with a zest that seems almost obscene to those not in accord with its philosophy. And yet I know certain generous, intelligent, decent fellows who live eleven months of the year in happy anticipation of November, when they can go and hunt. What I am writing here will seem totally incomprehensible to them. There is simply no meeting of the minds.

But reflect on the psychology of the hearty, friendly, exuberant fellow who can write with such pride the following account. The reader will bear in mind that euphemisms like "solid thump," "hitting home," "smacking against ribs," and the like refer to gouging and tissue avulsions causing pain of the sort that in a human being would evoke screams or choking moans. But, says this gleeful fellow:

> I hiked further up stream, watching the ridges on both sides. I had crossed a small clearing, and was heading along the side of a steep ridge, when I heard two quick shots across the stream. I stopped and waited to see what was up. The shooting was fairly close by and I figured somebody may have jumped a buck in the thick popple over there. I wasn't long in waiting. A little up stream from me, I heard the brush move and a deer broke cover. It was coming down stream on the other side and it did have a rack, but not a large one. My heart started to pound. This was the buck I was sitting for. I raised the old 38-55, and when the deer was broadside I let go my first shot. It proved good. He dropped to his knees, but was up in an instant and was on his way. As I hurriedly pumped in another cartridge the buck jumped into the stream and was bounding through the icy shallows to my side. I let my second shot go when he was about midstream, and heard the solid thump of the 255 grain bullet as it hit home, but the animal didn't even waver. He kept right on coming and when he hit the bank on my side, he started up the ridge straight for me. I heard my third shot smack against his ribs, but no use. That deer was intent on going somewhere, and there was no stopping him. About fifteen yards from me, he turned slightly, and went by me only about ten yards away. I let him have another slug when he was broadside. It slowed him somewhat, but it didn't stop him. A short distance up the ridge I let my fifth and last shot go. He reared back on his hind legs and turned around, trotting back in my direction. About ten paces away, his legs slipped from under him, and he rolled against a rotten log and lay still. . . . He had enough holes in him as all five of my slugs hit home, but I don't believe the last four would have been necessary. My first shot had done the work. It hit low in the front quarters, passing through and shattering the heart. That accounted for the crazed action of the deer.[2]

Some will hold, as did the early American colonists, that animals (like Indians) have no souls and are here for the pleasure and benefit of man, however he may seek to find that pleasure and benefit. For over two hundred years it was considered perfectly all right in places to have a little fun in the dull days of winter by hunting down Indians and their wives and children and shooting them on the run or on their knees.*

But children, we all concede, have souls. How, then, shall we regard outright aggression directed against them? Why, as a feature of discipline and child guidance, of course. The Reverend John S. C. Abbott, in *The Mother at Home, or Principles of Maternal Duty*, gives a vivid account of up-to-date child care in the 1830s:

> I have known many such contests, severe and protracted, which were exceedingly painful to a parent's feelings. But when once entered upon, they must be continued until the child is subdued. It is not safe *on any account*, for the parents to give up and retire vanquished.
>
> The following instance of such a contest occurred a few years since. A gentleman, sitting by his fireside one evening, with his family around him, took the spelling book and called upon one of his little sons to come and read. John was about four years old. He knew all the letters of the alphabet perfectly, but happened at that moment to be in rather a sullen humor . . . when his father pointed with his knife to the first letter of the alphabet and said "What letter is that?" he could get no answer. . . .
>
> "My son," said the father pleasantly, "you know the letter A."
>
> "I cannot say A," said John.
>
> "You must," said the father in a serious and decided tone. "What letter is that?"

The upshot was that the father dragged John out of the room and "flogged him severely." Nothing doing. John was adamant. Father dragged him out again. The Rev. Mr. Abbott goes on:

> Again the father inflicted punishment as severely as he dared to do it, and still the child, with his whole frame in agitation, refused to yield. The father was suffering from the most intense solicitude.
>
> The mother sat by, suffering, of course, most acutely, but perfectly satisfied that it was their duty to subdue the child, and that in such a trying hour a mother's feelings must not interfere. With a heavy heart the father again took the hand of his son to lead him out of the room

---

* For a documentation of this favorite sport of the whites in northern Canada (among other places), take a look at the article in *Maclean's* for October 10, 1959. The unarmed quarry was routed out of tents in the dead of winter before they could get dressed, and driven naked out on frozen lakes, where they were easier to see. Men, women, and little children were shot down like jackrabbits or coyotes. This popular amusement went on for over two centuries, and no white man was ever prosecuted for it. But a whole nation of handsome, proud, and peaceful Indians (the Beothucks) was extinguished.

for further punishment. But to his inconceivable joy, the child shrunk from enduring any more suffering and cried, "Father, I'll tell the letter!"

The Rev. Mr. Abbott then smugly describes how Father and John went back to where they had started from, until John had answered "A" to everyone's satisfaction. Then he adds, "And John learnt a lesson which he never forgot—that his father had an arm too strong for him . . . but perhaps someone says it was cruel to punish the child so severely. Cruel! It was mercy and love!"

If this seems a bit old-fashioned, don't laugh. There are plenty of present-day counterparts both of this philosophy and of this treatment. Usually they are kept under cover. Sometimes an "accident" occurs. It may make the headlines:

FATHER ON TRIAL IN FATAL BELT BEATING OF SIX-YEAR-OLD SON

Erie, Pa., Sept. 15 (AP)—A young father being tried on a murder charge in the death of his 6-year-old son, told a criminal court jury that he beat the boy with a belt for refusing to tell where he had hidden a toy hammer.

"I told Jackie a father sometimes has to do things to their children they do not like," Ralph J. Hoge, 26, of Harbor Creek, Pa., said Tuesday.

Dr. James E. Wallace, pathologist at Hamot hospital, previously testified the boy died last May 30 as a result of repeated blows, "probably 100." There were at least 93 abrasions on the child's body, he said.

District Attorney Damian McLaughlin has indicated he would seek a second-degree murder verdict with a maximum penalty of ten to 20 years in prison.

Hoge testified that after the beating he put his son to bed and massaged his wounds with vaseline.

"Jackie told me, 'I still love you, daddy,' " Hoge said. "Those were the last words my son said to me." [3]

Life magazine has several times exposed public spectacles of zestful sadism; for example, in one issue six hundred smiling boys, women, and men are shown gathered about, beating small foxes to death with clubs. In another issue a proud huntress poses in front of the stuffed carcasses of the many elephants and lions she has slaughtered.

One other type of glorified violence which, while condemned by many, is still condoned and exploited is prize fighting.* Recently there has been some public agitation to abolish this remnant of barbarism; neurologists and other physicians [4] who observe the permanent brain-tissue damage inflicted for this amusement for the masses have been joined by officials and

---

* "As operated today, prize fighting is a cruel, crooked, senseless racket that serves only to batter and cheat hapless young fighters and enrich their mobster bosses." (Stewart-Gordon, James. "Abolish Professional Boxing." *Reader's Digest*, April 1960.)

former aficionados.* One is reminded that only a little over a century ago in this country human beings were kidnaped, chained, trained as fighting animals for public exhibition, and bought or sold on the basis of their performance.[5] This slave practice and its present-day counterpart,

---

* "*Priest Sees Boxing as 'Indirect Suicide.'* Boston (RNS)—Prize fighting was condemned as 'indirect suicide' by a Roman Catholic priest here who is the founder of Rescue, Inc., an organization that has prevented hundreds of suicides. Commenting on the death of boxer Benny (Kid) Paret from injuries received in a New York bout March 24, Father Kenneth B. Murphy declared: 'Professional boxing, as it exists today, can be suicide for many a participant.' There is sufficient evidence to warrant condemning it on both moral and medical grounds, he asserted.

"Citing statistics, Father Murphy said studies show that 60 per cent of all boxers develop neurological and psychic changes in a brief span of years.

" 'Prize fighting is morally evil,' said the priest, 'and will remain so until the second "foul" line is declared at the chin to diminish all danger of head injuries and scrambled brains.'

"Father Murphy observed that of 'all forms of so-called sport in which man is pitted against man, boxing alone had as its prime and direct object the physical injury of the contestants.'

"If boxing is to continue as in the past, Father Murphy maintained, then a pension plan for fighters should be instituted because of the short span of their earning capacity." (*The New York Times*, May 5, 1962.)

"The primary responsibility lies with the people who pay to see a man hurt. The referee who stops a fight too soon from the crowd's viewpoint can expect to be booed. The crowd wants the knockout; it wants to see a man stretched out on the canvas. This is the supreme moment in boxing. It is nonsense to talk about prize fighting as a test of boxing skills. No crowd was ever brought to its feet screaming and cheering at the sight of two men beautifully dodging and weaving out of each other's jabs. The time the crowd comes alive is when a man is hit hard over the heart or the head, when his mouthpiece flies out, when blood squirts out of his nose or eyes, when he wobbles under the attack and his pursuer continues to smash at him with pole-axe impact." (*Saturday Review*, May 5, 1962, p. 14.)

"Let's go to the prize fight, buddy,
Where the punches whistle and sing;
Let's sit where it's smelly and bloody,
Close up, with our knees on the ring.
Maybe we'll see a jaw shattered,
Or a pug lose the sight of an eye,
Or an amateur brutally battered—
Maybe we'll see a boy die.

"Get a load of the houseful of patrons,
Ogling the boy on the stool,
Gamblers and students and matrons,
Expectant, avid and cruel.
Smell the good smells of the fight pit,
The smoke and the hatred, the fear
Of the untutored tyro who might quit.
Chum, aren't you glad that you're here?

"There's music in gloves that are soggy
In face bones that shatter and crunch,

What a thrill when you see a boy groggy,
Then starched with a powerful punch.
There's delight in a referee calling
The count to a kid on his back.
How jolly to see a kid falling
Unconscious, uncaring and slack.

"What if he ends with the mumbles?
What if he walks in a fog?
A white cane will help if he stumbles,
And there's always a Seeing-Eye dog.

"We're off to the blood-letting, pally,
Let's sit where we won't miss a thing,
Knockdown and knockout and rally—
It's a spectacle fit for a king.
Boos for the purist and crackpot
Who thinks fighting a sport to decry;
Tonight we may hit the jackpot,
Tonight we may see a boy die!"

(The Tribune Publishing Co., Oakland, Calif., 1962)

illustrated in the movie *Requiem for a Heavyweight*,[6] answer the question as to whether observing the exhibition of violence diminishes the need for the personal expression of it.

We cannot close our chamber of horrors without mention of the epitome of aggression in a civilized society, the imposition of capital punishment, mercifully unseen by the public or by those who order it. While the main argument for the retention of capital punishment is its deterrent effect, it is ironic that it is almost impossible for anyone to be admitted to an execution in order to experience its deterrent effect at close range. This argument would logically demand that executions be open to the public, or at least be broadcast on radio and television like other spectacles. Instead, they are carried out in almost complete secrecy, usually in the middle of the night. This furtiveness suggests some awareness that the social climate has shifted to such a degree that the community at large would not tolerate capital punishment if it could actually see its official representatives taking the lives of inadequate and often obviously disorganized individuals.

But some will say, "We agree with your position regarding brutality, sadism, and violence, even in those forms which some portions of the community condone. We concede that most aggression * and most fighting are not only foolish but even 'psychopathic' or psychopathological. But don't you go too far? Are there not occasions where a man *must* fight? Indeed, is it not indicative of psychopathology of some kind if an individual fails to stand up for what he believes? Must he not align himself with the forces of righteousness, even to the giving of his life, in defense of his home, his loved ones, his country, his principles?"

Certainly. There is no question about this. Negative aggression, the failure to defend oneself or one's home or one's principles is indeed a symptom, and sometimes a fatal symptom. There are evils in the world which have to be destroyed, there are dragons to be slain, there are enemies of society to be sought out and dealt with. Dangers constantly arise which threaten our existence. We are daily obliged to make decisions and choices, some of which involve at least a *show* of force. But in actuality the occasions for a real exertion of destructive force become more and

---

* The essence of aggression is the infliction of injury or at least pain. Our use of the word corresponds with the definition in Webster's dictionary. Aggression does not mean assertiveness, liveliness, or energetic pushing; it means the naked use of fang and claw. It means acts intended to injure or hurt some feature of the environment, usually intentionally, often, but not always, with premeditation and malice aforethought, and usually, but not always, with conscious feelings of anger, hate, or fear.

more rare. There is positively no resemblance whatsoever between real-life situations and the sluggings, punchings, clubbings, eviscerations, slaughter, and destruction daily exhibited in television shows. These are fantasy, remnants of what was once a way of life for a few people, but a comforting fantasy for the weak child or even the weak adult who was or who felt that he was at the mercy of powerful parents or masters.

For the child this power is highly personalized in the parents; later it becomes "the government" or "they" or "the labor unions" or "management." In reality the threats to our existence are usually far more impersonal. Something unexpected happens every minute. Accidents occur. The explosions and mistakes of other individuals set off chains of events which excite violence, and sometimes counterviolence seems the only possible way of managing the situation. Victor Hugo [7] portrayed this vividly in his famous account of a gun carriage on wheels which becomes unleashed during a storm at sea and hurtles about on the deck, crushing sailors like a juggernaut. A leopard recently escaped from the local zoo. It was a prized animal and the keepers made strenuous efforts to recapture it without harming it. It remained nearby but would not return to the enclosure, and the calculated risk of leaving it at large was too great; destruction became necessary.

Thus we repeat our concession: There are indeed occasions when aggression seems to be necessary and hence normal. A part of the reality-testing task of the ego is to determine as well as it can in the light of its past experience and the temper of the prevailing culture what constitutes common or individual danger requiring defensive aggression. Only then can it without penalty permit the release of pent-up destructive energy. Only then can the requirements of social conventions and cultural patterns be transcended.

As we have become more and more civilized, the situations in which personal violence is expected or considered appropriate or even tolerated have become increasingly few, and except in the rarest of situations it is no longer possible to justify morally acts of personal violence. This shift in the moral climate has been such that one can now say that the appearance of direct aggression is always prima-facie evidence of some failure or injury or impairment in ego functioning.*

---

* The legal term prima-facie precisely describes the situation; it means that the burden of proof has shifted to the one who wishes to rebut the proposition. In other words, while we acknowledge that there may be times that aggression is necessary, these occasions are now so few that the burden of proof of demonstrating that the aggression is necessary, that is, realistic and therefore not a sign of disorganization, now falls to the aggressor.

Failure may be that of judgment, but it may also appear as a failure of effort to comply with the judgment. Obviously this kind of dyscontrol is more serious than those forms in which there is at least some disguise of the aggressive impulses. Thus aggressive outbursts represent a wider divergence from reality adherence than occurs in states of disorganization characterized by Second Order devices. In more customary parlance, these aggressive-act phenomena indicate a greater degree of personality disorganization than do those formerly described as "neurotic," but less than those for which the designations "psychotic," "committable," "schizophrenic," and the like have been applied.

Whether or not individuals exhibiting Third Order dyscontrol are called "sick" is entirely a matter of custom and common knowledge. Time was when no patients exhibiting psychological symptoms were regarded as sick. Later the more extreme cases in which disorganization was inescapably visible ceased to be regarded as bewitched and were considered brain-damaged and hence sick. "Neurotic" symptoms, on the other hand, were not regarded as worthy of medical attention, while phenomena of the type represented by Third Order dyscontrol were (and still are, for the most part) clearly evidences of perversity and wickedness.

When an individual begins to strike out at his wife, his child, his acquaintances, or even complete strangers, we may well suspect on an *a priori* basis that a gross failure in ego functioning has occurred. Its restraining control has been eluded. The façade of social conformity has been demolished, and the hateful murderousness which the ego had been trying to control is partially exposed *in action*. What might be called the last-minute efforts of the ego to restrain or deflect the aggressive outburst may be perceptible; the wrong target is often hit; the recoil (internal and external consequences) is seriously injurious to the aggressor. The parent may speak the truth when he says that a whipping hurts him—and the rest of the world—worse than the child. It is a grim but true fact that most murderers *suffer* more than the ones murdered.

There is much evidence that public attitudes are rapidly changing. It is neither necessary nor, in our opinion, desirable to force the issue of whether or not this is correctly called a sickness. There is no question about its being a state of dysorganization. And it is our proposal that it represents a third line of defense, as it were, against further disintegration. We do not mean to evade the technical question of why we speak of Third Order emergency control devices when the aggression is no longer controllable, or at least no longer controlled. The point is right there; it is our proposal that direct aggressive discharges are in all cases somewhat controlled, somewhat modified, somewhat restrained. They are never as direct or as complete or as devastating as they might be. In theory at least they are held to the minimum; they are the smallest possible package, as it were, the releasing of which will enable the ego to reorganize and reharness its system. The rupture may be catastrophic, but usually it can be held. Of this we shall say more presently.

The Appearance of Overt Aggression; Premonitory Signs

We are always surprised when someone—a friend, a patient, an unknown offender described in the newspaper headlines—wreaks an act of aggression upon us or upon others. It always seems to come out of a clear sky. It is "news."

And yet actually it is never entirely surprising to everyone. Some people have known, as a rule, that a certain individual was close to the breaking point and that he had propensities of overt destructiveness. Unpredicted the act may have been but not necessarily unpredictable. Evidences of accumulating tension which tax the ability or even Second Order coping devices usually contain some warning of the possibility if not the imminence of a break. Hence, before discussing the clinical forms of impulsive, aggressive behavior, we should give some attention to the premonitory signs of those appearances.

First, at the risk of sounding pedantic, we are going to remind the reader that the ego is presumed to have at its command, for the management of aggressive impulses, quite a number of different tools or programs. It can suppress such impulses, fully recognizing them but blocking their expression. It can repress them without ever permitting them to come to consciousness. It can neutralize them, employing the modified energies harmlessly or even constructively. It can reflect some of them back upon the self as a whole, or upon parts of the body. It can deflect them to targets better able to endure them than the intended target.

This deflection of a blow to a substitute target goes beyond being merely poor aim or physical awkwardness. It involves a self-deception such that the false target seems to be the right one, the one toward which retaliation or defensive attack is properly directed. The convictions of its dangerousness or undesirability, the feelings of fear or hatred, and the impulses to hurt and destroy become united in their displacement from a real and provocative object often miles or years away to an object which is more available, perhaps more vulnerable, perhaps less likely to retaliate. The new object must be a plausible one, it must be accepted, so to speak, just as the moving scarf of the bullfighter must catch the attention of the bull. But it is an illusion.

Although rediscovered by Freud and elaborated in his systematic studies, the mechanism of projection, i.e., displacing hate or love to substituted objects, is as old as the human race. It is as old as playing with dolls, kneeling to idols, offering sacrifices, releasing scapegoats, or burning in effigy. It is scarcely possible to conjecture how far this mechanism pervades cultural practices. The motion picture *Twelve Angry Men* [8] shows with brilliant simplicity how much the most apparently objective and impersonal decisions depend upon the arousal of emotions related to similar but different situations, bringing about displacements which utterly corrupt the ostensible "objectivity." Most popular elections probably depend more upon displacement than upon reason—both in votes *for* certain candidates and in those *against* certain candidates. What indeed are all prejudices, extreme aversions, and fanatical attitudes, pro as well as con, but the substitution of someone or some group of ones for certain other objects less available for receiving the fear, the hate, or the love? [9]

One often reads with dismay of ruthless vandalism in a beautiful library, or of the unprovoked beating up of innocent individuals, the knocking over of tombstones, the defacement of schools and synagogues. Sometimes these despicable acts will have the presumptive meaning: "We don't like you. But we are too insignificant to have our protest otherwise noticed and we are ashamed to take the known responsibility for our acts." At other times they may mean: "You have bullied and humiliated us; now we get back at you."

When, as is occasionally the case, one can make a thorough clinical investigation of such acts, it is usually discovered that the substitution of object was made without the understanding of the actor himself. He may clearly admit that he has no idea who it is he hated enough to do so much damage. Or he may name the Jews or the Negroes or the Democrats or the Catholics or the Capitalists or the Communists. These ascriptions rarely make sense except in terms of the private phobias and secret delusions of the hater. The bitterness of marital disappointment, of sexual incompetence, of business inadequacy, of social ineptitude, and of a hundred other reality situations can be forgotten if one finds an opportunity for the discharge of what would otherwise be self-reproach in what appears to be a high-minded and wholly legitimate cause, by finding a group of fellow dissenters and joining the hue and cry against a highly magnified, if not imaginary, foe. One can transmute personal misery and insignificance into what gives the illusion of being chivalrous, noble, and patriotic.

An editor recently showed me a letter from a friend we both share, containing a vitriolic attack on the editor, declaring that he was a Communist and a traitor and should be hounded out of town. Although I had known the writer for thirty years, I had no suspicion that he was inwardly so disturbed, or that his disturbance was likely to appear in this way.

Neither employers nor fellow employees were prepared to understand the case of a man of thirty-four who in the eight years since his graduation from Harvard held fourteen important jobs. Each one of them was well handled and he gave complete satisfaction in his work. But each time he resigned because of the increasing conviction that he was not appreciated, that he was about to be fired, that he was picked upon and discriminated against. Most remarkable of all was the fact that this man himself knew, with a part of his mind at least, that his fears and suspicions were untrue. But he could not live without them.

One day he went to a senior officer in the company with which he was temporarily associated and laid before him a list of seven reasons why he should commit suicide. His astonished employer said that he himself had a dozen reasons, but didn't intend to do it, and thought this should settle the matter. It only convinced the employee that this man was the ringleader of his enemies. He resolved that instead of himself it should be this man who died. At the same time he felt relieved and comforted that he had pinpointed his foe. Fortunately, he was not permitted to resolve his dilemma by violence.

Displacement is apt to go beyond mere clumsiness of aim and the transposing of aggression from a forgotten object to a contemporary one. It has been found empirically that the suspicions or accusations directed toward the false object are apt to be an inversion of hostile, destructive wishes. "It is not I who hates and wants to hurt this fellow; it is he who hates and wants to hurt me. Hence I have to defend myself." This is the logical extension of displacement, and it illustrates the real psychopathological nature of projection.

Displacement and projection become clinical and earn the name of "paranoid" when their intensity is such as to seriously disturb either the individual who is using them or those about him. This occurs when the misapprehensions continue, uncorrected by the continuous reality-testing of daily life. The rationalizations organized to justify a contemplated attack ordinarily become dissolved by the stubborn persistence of contrary fact. Suspiciousness, hypersensitiveness, over-reaction to minor incidents or clumsy remarks, querulousness about details—these are the indications familiar to all of us that such devices are being used to a greater or lesser degree, used and then abandoned in the light of better judgment. We all use displacement and projection every day, and yet to speak of projection of a normal amount is like speaking of poison in non-toxic doses. By definition projection is a departure from reality. If the departure is slight, if it is recognized for what it is and corrected, the device may yield some temporary benefit.

But projection, like alcohol, tends to get out of hand. Its "as if" nature is too easily forgotten; its conclusions become the justification of aggressive action. This is why psychiatrists look with such concern upon the appearance of definite and persistent projective (paranoid) ideas and attitudes. They are in many cases the precursors of direct outbursts. Every American president who has been assassinated has been the victim of a man with accumulating pressures. Hitler could never correct his delusion that the Jews were enemies of Germany; he had to persist in it once he had acted so violently on the assumption. Shakespeare's Coriolanus was a man whose inability to control attacks of rage led to his ultimate destruction. "Ostensibly his anger [was] directed against the plebeians and the foes of Rome, but evidence in the play supports the conclusion that his rage [was] displaced to them from its real object, his mother" who continually drove him, taunted him, harassed and threatened him.[10]

Overuse of the psychological mechanism of projection may lead to becoming fixed or frozen in the way described in the previous chapter. Projection becomes incorporated as a chronic paranoid armor against the world. Behind a sour, skeptical, suspicious, cynical, bitter, grouchy, misanthropic, hostile front, a precarious balance is maintained with the aid of self-justifying fantasies. This attitude tends to appear in every response to social approach—in words, acts, and facial expression. A certain kind of formal relationship is maintained with the outside world and a further internal disintegration is halted, but halted at the cost of a deformed personality.

Paranoid trends may, on the other hand, disappear completely even after having reached extensive development. This happens less frequently than we might wish. Many psychiatrists might be inclined to doubt it. But I remember several occasions when I was obliged to alter a gloomy prognostic estimate I had made. One young engineer, after making steady advancement in his organization for perhaps ten years, began to suspect nearly all of his co-workers of being involved in a plot to get rid of him.

He interpreted many trivial occurrences as supporting his theory; for example, he was sure that the ties certain of his associates wore on certain days had special meanings regarding movements for the day in fulfillment of the conspiracy. He consulted a lawyer who fortunately recognized the psychopathology and counseled patience; this advice only convinced the young engineer that the lawyer was himself in the plot. In one way, perhaps, this was true. The lawyer felt very uneasy about having his client continue to work with a group of unsuspecting associates, and yet constrained by his professional ethics not to say anything about it to them. He did, however, cautiously question the company physician, who told him that his client's queer behavior had already caused them some concern and that he, the physician, had intended to look into it. He asked the young engineer to stop in at the medical department for a check-up, which threw the poor fellow into a panic and he refused. Matters remained in this stage for a matter of two or three years, with everyone afraid to take any definite action. But then, as insidiously and inexplicably as it began, the syndrome melted away. Time passed, and everyone seemed to forget about it. The actual technical work of the man improved to the point that he was given a highly important assignment in one of the company's South American plants. He returned from that to be made director of one of its California divisions, where he remains to the present day, highly regarded and apparently well adjusted and comfortable. It has been nearly twenty years since that very worried lawyer came to see me.

Ego Rupture

Sometimes paranoid mechanisms grow progressively more extreme until relieved by an explosion. Gathering resentments breed suspicion; the suspicions become delusions; the delusions determine action. Nonexisting plots, entanglements, insults, and injuries are discovered, collected, and nursed. Finally the unsuspecting offenders are accused or even attacked; they in turn often react defensively, and thus the circle is rounded. This extreme state of boiling delusional, paranoid preoccupation represents so marked a degree of reality severance that such syndromes probably belong in a Fourth Order of disorganization, presented in the next chapter.

For the present we are considering the prodromal evidences of imminent ego rupture, and these are by no means limited to paranoid rumblings. First, and especially Second, Order devices of many sorts have usually been employed increasingly. Sometimes there is much warning, with few symptoms and little self-deception.

It is an unforgettable experience to sit vis-à-vis an individual who is acutely aware of an impending ego rupture. Often he is quite inarticulate, but speaks clearly with posture and facial expression. I recall vividly one patient who was given an emergency appointment because of the obvious urgency of his symptoms. He was a large, handsome, healthy-appearing man of forty who sat tensely on the edge of his chair, gripping his hands, occasionally clenching his teeth so that the contraction of the facial muscles was clearly visible. In a low voice, obviously controlled with great effort, he appealed for help thus: "I have no pain: I have no symptoms. I am not what most people consider sick. But I am scared to death! It's not the ordinary sort of fear; I am not a coward, but I don't know how long I can keep from exploding." In humility rather than in boastfulness, he described the contrast between his role in the community and his state of mind as he saw it. President of the Rotary Club, a member of the school board, father of three children, the owner of one of the largest businesses in his town, he was a man apparently in full command of himself and others. "And yet, day and night it takes all the energy I have to keep myself from violence. No one knows the agony of realizing how destructive and murderous he is while all the people about him regard him as a benevolent angel and protector. If you won't lock me up, which I am begging you to do immediately, I am afraid that I will kill someone. I am not even sure who it will be or how many it will be, I don't even know why, but there is murder in my heart and I don't believe I can control it much longer." *

---

* Distinctions must be made between the individual thus aware of an impending ego rupture, perhaps for the first time, and an individual who is familiar with the experience and has a history of great ruptures, but is, or had been until recently, in relative equilibrium at the time he is seen. In the latter case, the dramatic picture before described is rarely seen; the man is more apt to concede more or less calmly that he knows his past history and his tendency and has some concern about it. These individuals are often seen just after an outburst—a decompression, so to speak—and anything they say about having lost control of themselves (similar to the foregoing) is apt to be taken as an attempt at exculpation. Some individuals, feeling an ego rupture to be pending, may ask for help. But since they do not always present a dramatic picture, they are too often ignored or laughed at.

The son of the governor of one of our states, while attending a university in the East, three times asked to see a psychiatrist. His parents discouraged him; his dean discouraged him; a very competent medical colleague discouraged him, or at least discouraged the relatives from taking his request seriously. When the explosion came, everyone was embarrassed, everyone was apologetic. The psychiatrist was as-

Such a vivid description of the subjective feelings of inner tension helps to visualize the model we have in mind when we speak of the ego as being on the point of bursting or rupturing. It is a figure of speech, of course, and one which may seem to violate our earlier definition of the ego as a group of functions. "One falls only too easily into the mental habit of assuming substance behind the substantive," wrote Breuer [11] in an early classic. But we have many precedents for doing so, none more striking than Freud's own vivid metaphor: [12] "It is always possible for the ego to avoid the rupture in any of its relations by deforming itself, by submitting to forfeit something of its amity or, in the long run, even to be gashed and rent."

These are subjective feelings which we have all had, no doubt, even when we were considerably removed from the degree of tension now being considered. People do seem at times to suddenly lose control of themselves, after going to great lengths to avoid doing so. Let us grant that "ego rupture" is a figure of speech, and an imperfect model, but let us use it as far as it will go without violence to the facts.

What we try to express by the figure of a rupture of the ego is a disruption of the ego functions of instinct-control. There is an emergence of more or less naked aggression after subjective or objective evidences of a mounting pressure, which is clearly diminished after the aggressive discharge has occurred. These Third Order devices are distinguished from First and Second Order devices by the following criteria:

1. The aggressive impulses seem to elude or discard as unnecessary any disguise or concealment of their purpose or character.

2. They tend to show a dereistic disregard for customs, social regulations, laws, and other strictures of reality, and are usually accompanied by little or no disturbance of conscience.

3. Immediately preceding, accompanying, and following the actual physical enactment of the aggression, impairments of perception, judgment, and consciousness often occur.

4. Following the aggressive act there is usually a detectable reduction in tension, as just stated, and this is reflected in the disappearance or lessening of First and Second Order symptoms which may have been in evidence before the explosion.

5. The discharges may be relatively minor but frequent, or relatively major in scope and infrequent. Repetitive major explosions are rare, per-

---

sured by the various friends that they had not meant any reflection on psychiatry by their counsel. But they "just wondered" about the stigmatization; they "just thought" the man was being a bit sorry for himself and needed to "buck up."

haps because the ego becomes too disorganized; single minor episodes would not be sufficient to constitute the syndrome.

What we believe happens is that after the ego pressure has been temporarily lessened by the explosion, the internal forces are usually rearranged or reorganized at a tolerable level, pending the reaccumulation of unmanageable stresses. Ego rupture permitting some aggressive energy to be discharged has the economic value of affording sufficient temporary relief from internal pressure for the healing-over of the ego's ruptured wall to occur. The internal pressures having been lessened by the explosion, the internal forces and balances can be rearranged so as to bring about a tolerable degree of tension and an acceptable level of performance pending the reaccumulation of otherwise unmanageable pressures. In this way these sudden phenomena serve the same purpose as other symptoms: they are a choice of the lesser evil made to avert the greater disaster.

Twenty years ago the late Robert Lindner [13] put it brilliantly thus:

It has been brought home to me ever more forcibly that the aggression, the hostility, the rejection of authority, the migratory tendencies, the impulsiveness, the destructive and blind lashing-out of the psychopath—all of these are homeostatic adjustments operating to restore a dynamic equilibrium within the personality. As I see it, the personality of the psychopath is the battlefield whereon a titanic struggle between . . . drives or needs and social or superego prohibitions is being waged. The tension produced by such a conflict accumulates to a point beyond tolerance, to where the organism is threatened with disintegration and destruction. Exactly at this point, in order to restore the disturbed balance and achieve a relative quiescence, the aggression (personal or social) is released with explosive force. Whether the emergent behavior involves what seems to be an impulsive killing, an aggressive burglary, or an attack against a superior, it serves an homeostatic end. It represents the best adjustment the personality can make under its peculiar circumstances.*

This is our present view of it, precisely and eloquently stated.

---

* Elsewhere Lindner puts it thus: "[Treatment] becomes a matter of aiding the personality in obtaining the sought-after dynamic equilibrium by ways more highly regarded socially. We must train ourselves to regard the behavior we see as a mechanical adjustment, a process of striving for satisfying quiescence, for balance so that life can continue in what the individual organism regards as a health state. Upon the establishment of motivating factors, treatment should substitute adjustment modes of a higher order, should aim to instill new ways of response to unbearable inner tensions and conflicts. Viewing apparently maladjustive behavior not as an end-result but as an automatic striving for the recovery of balance, as homeostatically initiated and sustained, our job is to make acceptable behavior serve the same purpose." (Lindner, Robert: "Psychopathic Personality and the Concept of Homeostasis." *J. Crim. Psychopath.* 6:150–156, 1945.)

Allchin, more recently, develops the economic functions of the aggressive symptom

Open Aggression

Aggressive behavior can be classified in many ways. Textbooks on criminology have many different categories of "bad" behavior based on types of offense. More abstractly, all such phenomena could be arranged in an order of progressive severity, based on the extent of destruction accomplished. Or they might all be grouped according to techniques of the attack: verbal, manual, genital, instrumental, conspiratory, and so on.

Another way in which to classify them would depend on the state of consciousness during the acts. Some individuals are clearly conscious and aware, some appear to be in a daze or "trance," and still others are definitely unconscious and later amnesic for the episode. Such classifications have more legal than scientific definiteness. Other classifications could be based on the degree to which the behavior is rationalized or on the degree to which it is accurately aimed, or on the social interpretation of the explosion, e.g., wife-beating, child-clubbing, fire-setting, check-forging, car-stealing, shoplifting, bank-robbing, and sexual attacks.

Many other classifications have been offered and many explanations and many descriptions given.[14] * I have even taken a hand in this myself. But after many years of experience I have concluded that these classifi-

---

in a way very sympathetic to our own concept. Among the positive aspects of delinquent behavior he lists its function as a form of communication, its function in establishing a feeling of identity, its function in calling the attention of the physician or others to the existence of need, its function as an appeal for help to the more general environment—"Somebody help me lest I go crazy"—and its function in denying a feeling of being controlled by its replacement with a feeling of being able to control something. (Allchin, W. H. "Some Positive Aspects of Delinquent Behavior." *Brit. J. Criminology*, 3:38–46, 1962.)

* The systematic scientific study of offenders long urged by Ben Karpman and attempted in some measure by him, by the Gluecks, by William Healy, ourselves, and a few others, is still something for the future of psychiatric research. Until then we cannot seriously offer any valid nosological subdivisions of sociopathy. Nor do we believe that there is any useful differentiation between "sociopathy" and what has been persistently called, in spite of its vagueness and many definitions, "psychopathy." There have been many attempts at this, as the exhaustive reviews of the literature by Sydney Maughs and others show. Karpman made a distinction between those in whom psychogenic factors can be found and those in whom they cannot be, the latter possibly depending upon an organic brain defect or damage. Frosch and Wortis have made a useful proposal to expand Fenichel's notion of "impulse neurosis" into a category of syndromes to include most of the perversions and "monomanias" (episodic phenomena) *and* "psychopathic personalities" of various kinds. While details of the classification differ from ours, the essential idea is the same, i.e., that there is an irresistible episodic discharge of an original impulse with minimal distortion which manages to acquire some degree of ego approval.

cations are intellectual exercises and not useful differentiations. In what is to follow we offer the common patterns of aggressive discharge characteristic of Third Order dyscontrol. First we describe the persistent, repetitive, aggressive patterns which seem to indicate a kind of chronic permeability of the ego. Then we present various types of sudden eruptive violence which seem to represent gross but usually reversible ego rupture.

A. Chronic, Repetitive, Aggressive Behavior

In a motion picture The Wild Ones (based on actual occurrence) some black-jacketed Nazi-imitating motorcyclists are terrorizing a small town in California. A frightened waitress addresses one of the bullying terrorists: "You fellows call yourselves 'black rebels.' What are you rebelling against?" One of them shrugs and replies, "Name it; we're against it. What have you got?" This characterizes the overtly hostile, hateful, embittered revolt of this syndrome. These individuals are the rebels in search of never-found causes. They are only too familiar to all police, judges, social agencies, and psychoanalysts.

The aggressions of the individuals with this syndrome are often poorly aimed but usually succeed both in damaging and in inflaming the environment. Hence, in spite of the high degree of selfishness and lack of human cathexis, their behavior is usually conspicuously self-injurious. The outbursts tend to recur, as if the subject were unable to learn from the past or to acquire any better coping devices. But the time and sometimes the circumstances of recurrence are highly unpredictable; it is rarely at regular intervals and, indeed, sometimes does not occur at all! This is a highly relevant and significant admission to make, because the matter of recidivism, repeating the offense or the offensiveness, constantly arises when these patients come into the courtroom or are about to leave the hospital.

This is a characteristic cycle: Persistent hooliganism of one kind or another results in expulsion of a boy, whom we will call George, from school; at great trouble and expense the parents get him admitted to another school, where he does well for a time and leads his family to have some hopes that for once he has found a milieu in which he is happy. They have no sooner permitted themselves this encouragement than they get word that he has assaulted a teacher, cheated in an examination, or gotten himself arrested for some prank which to the community was not funny. Again, the family makes strenuous efforts and perhaps finds a job for him by importuning a business friend or relative; he does well in this job for a time, only to be discharged for alcoholism and absenteeism. He disappears, and a stream of no-fund checks flows back to his (father's) bank. He is finally located, driving a stolen car, and is arraigned for trial. The family by this time is so wrought up with a mixture of anger, alarm, shame, pity, and worry that everything they are doing and planning is impeded. The daughter's wedding is postponed, a business project of the father's has to be abandoned. The other children in the family become self-conscious socially; all family efforts have to be concentrated on doing something about George. A lawyer and perhaps a psychiatrist are employed, and a plea is made to the court. George is examined. The psychiatrist (if he is of our persuasion) points to the clear record of defective impulse control, the impaired sense of identity and also of reality, the pliable or corruptible ego, and hence the need for thoroughgoing rehabilitation and personality reorganization. To obtain this the judge may give him a bench parole, or George may go to prison for a time and after a few years be paroled from there. He tells people that he wants to make a man of himself; he may even say that he realizes that he needs treatment.

Treatment may even be arranged for and begun, although this is not typical. A few weeks before his parole period has expired, George will find some absurd excuse to cross the state line, or get into a public brawl, or write a no-fund check at an all-night poker party, or exhibit some other piece of social, parental, or legal defiance which brings him back as a parole violator into the prison he so much detested.

Most of these cases are too poor, too proud, too rebellious, and too provocative to obtain psychiatric care, but some of them have a peculiar penchant for getting themselves seen by a psychiatrist, even when the parents and others think it is absurd or useless. This sometimes encourages psychiatrists to believe that they are dealing with an exception, a man who "really wants" help, and sometimes they are. Unfortunately, most of these people manage to defeat treatment efforts just as they have defeated themselves in everything else.*

There are often clear indications of why this is so. Imagine the state of mind of an adopted child whose parents informed him that he was adopted only after he had been teased about it at school at the age of

---

* But as we were writing these lines a letter came from one of these lads, who was brought to treatment by three deputy sheriffs about eight years ago. It was a most unprepossessing prospect, very similar to the model just cited. But the envelope received today contained an invitation to the exercises for his graduation from a leading law school!

nine. To "justify" having kept this information from him for so long the parents—in one instance of our knowledge—made the additional mistake of assuring him that his own parents were no good and they did not want him to find out about them because he would be so ashamed. They had to further confess to him, they said, that his behavior in school, his poor grades, his tendency to get into fights, his temper tantrums, and his pilferings had led them to suspect that bad heredity was making its appearance.

He reacted badly to what he regarded as his foster parents' perfidy and condescension. He coupled this with great envy and jealousy of their real son, who was a little younger than he and whom they strongly favored. Then this real son was killed in an automobile accident, and although our patient had nothing to do with it, he felt that he was in some vague way blamed. He assumed an attitude of frozen indifference, and this angered the parents further, so that he was sent away to a boarding school. There he showed poor attention, poor grades, irresponsibility, immaturity, lying, and grandiose bragging. After about a year he ran away from this school and came home, where he fell in love with a neighbor girl and seemed to be settling down at a job, when he impulsively joined the Marines and was shipped off. In the Marines he had a series of homosexual affairs and then went AWOL "in a panic." He was recaptured and put in the guardhouse, where he made a suicidal attempt, which led to his being discharged from the Marines "without honor." He was next picked up by the police for car theft, sent to prison, paroled, arrested for parole violation (he thought the parole officer "wouldn't catch him"), returned to prison, served his sentence, and was released to take a job which had been obtained for him with great difficulty through his father's influence. He stayed on the job about three months and was arrested for attempted rape.

The reader will recognize how similar these case histories are, and the data of the psychological examinations are also very similar. But something which is not conveyed by the record is a subtle, intangible appeal these patients have. One faces them at first with a certain perplexity at their perverseness, almost a sense of annoyance; they seem to have been so unnecessarily troublemaking, so determined to thwart any help. They seem to be so unaware of the trail of tears and curses they leave behind them; one even suspects they rejoice in it. They are experts at coarseness; they pick their teeth and noses as they wait to be interviewed; they sneer and sniffle and smoke cigarettes with an insolent disregard for the furniture.

There are a lot of such desperate, immature, hostile, lonely individuals, and when they get together a gang is born.[15] And when a gang is born, juvenile delinquency is apt to follow. By this time it is very difficult indeed to reach individuals, difficult but not impossible.

As a matter of fact, there is a strongly paradoxical professional attitude toward them. On the one hand they have, to use a slang expression, kicked everyone in the teeth. They have made themselves public enemies. But their defiance is somehow pitiful in its inappropriateness, like a little child making fists and crying when angry. Unattractive as their records may sound, they are often artists at subtle importunity, combining wistfulness and penitence in a kind of Prodigal Son appeal. Some of them verbally disdain all help; others plead for it, without being clear as to what they want. "I just want to get out of here and be given one chance." "One of the fellows got some psychotherapy and it helped him." "I want someone to talk to." "All I need is a job so I can show you what I can do." There are a hundred varieties of such appeals.

One has to be very much of a cynic not to believe that there is some body to this line of good intentions. But it is very easy to become cynical when one has heard it many times. However, our cynicism only reflects our ignorance. The psychological study of these individuals is always hampered by the emotions they arouse in the examiner. An unhealing rupture or defect in the ego which permits the very behavior which the rest of us have struggled to avoid is an ugly thing to see—like looking at a gaping abdominal wound. If we can approach it, however, in a surgical manner, as we would approach a surgical necessity, we can often do something. In many instances one can discover with considerable presumptive accuracy the reasons for this ego weakness: hypocritical or ambivalent parents, unbearable rivalry with a brother or sister, strong identification with the mother and uncertain sexual identity—these and many others. On the basis of a sufficiently penetrating diagnostic study and a sufficiently skillful and prolonged treatment, there can be a retraining and repair of the ego in some instances. But it is first necessary to see clearly how the disorders of these patients resemble, as well as how they differ from, personality disorganizations of lesser and greater degree.

The variety of aggressive behavior of which human beings are capable is exceedingly great, even though it can all be summed up as injuries inflicted upon people, animals, or things. If one bears in mind that the object back of it is to hurt someone—and usually not the person actually hurt—one can begin to get a different viewpoint about the whole business of crime and criminality. Take stealing, for example (and stealing represents the essence of three-fourths of all delinquent behavior). Stealing is the taking of something belonging to another, but it is almost never done for the purpose of acquiring the thing taken. More frequently, perhaps, stealing is a symbolic method of attempting to obtain the love which one feels—often correctly—that he has been deprived of. At the same time, as George Gardner [16] pointed out many years ago, stealing is essentially a destructive act; taking unto ourselves and for our own use that which was once a belonging or a part of some other person is destructive in a double sense: it adds to one's self the object taken, and at the same time symbolically robs, strips, mutilates, or destroys a part of another person. Stealing "symbolizes unconsciously the *destructive* taking of [a part of someone], a wrenching it away. . . . All other 'causes' of stealing . . . (poor training, deprivation, rejection, symbolic fetishistic stealing, demonstration of physical prowess, etc.) . . . have their full meaning and relative significance for us only in the light of this concept."

Diagnostic characteristics of the "anti-social character" do not depend upon age except for the nature of the work and play activities. Typical features of this syndrome in pre-adolescent children are the mistrustful, defiant, aggressive, but always superficial, relationships to those about them, the lack of emotional respect or concern, deceitfulness and evasiveness, pilfering, wandering, running away, bed-wetting, fire-setting.[17]

From the technical standpoint, all aggressive behavior *is* dereistic, as Karpman [18] also persistently reminded us, all his life, in that it ignores the practical consequences of the social disapproval it arouses, and in that it pays incredibly high prices for minuscule material gains. This is the very essence of "irrationality." The individuals manifesting these syndomes are more aggressive, more lacking in common sense, more unrealistic, more detached from a sense of the past, and more lacking in a reasonable vision of the future and more disinclined to seek or accept help than are individuals commonly described as "neurotic." But at the same time the former are less disorganized and less out of contact with reality than are the patients sometimes described as "borderline" or "psychotic." *

---

* Makkay and Schwaab feel that it is important for proper treatment to differentiate the various syndromes of dyscontrol, even those which occur in childhood.

Both the borderline and the antisocial character-disordered children exhibited more consistently hyperactive, aggressive, and destructive behavior in the clinic than did the neurotic child. However, the borderline child's aggressive, destructive

Not all of the behavior of this group is explosive, but outbursts of undisguised and seemingly uncontrolled aggression are characteristic of it and hence justify the inclusion of this syndrome in our category of Third Order dyscontrol.

B. Episodic Impulsive Violence

The preceding pages might have been more convincing had we postponed reference to *chronic* repetitive minor explosions until we had first submitted the more spectacular, once-in-a-lifetime (or at least very infrequent) outbursts. The very violence of the latter makes their pathology the more obvious and also—if it does not lead to capital punishment—leads to vigorous corrective measures.

A morning newspaper reported the terrible beating given by a road machine operator to his seven-year-old crippled son. Having read this with feelings of revulsion, I had some strong feelings of reluctance when I was asked to see this man in consultation with state officials.

He turned out to be a small, wizened, gnarled laborer who operated the largest earth-moving machine of a highway-paving company. "I had to show them that just because I was short and light didn't mean I couldn't go along with the best of them," he said. "It wears me out but I can do it. The fellows all kid me for taking such a tough job; they call me 'Shorty' and 'the Runt' and it makes me mad so I drink a little; then I don't mind it so bad."

But drinking made complications at home. Especially it hindered him

---

behavior was rarely observed to be expressed toward human objects in an organized, direct fashion, but seemed to represent a more diffuse explosive type of motor discharge (Rank & Macnaughton, 1950). On the other hand, the antisocial child's aggression was always largely directed toward people and objects in response to frustration and with the aim of control and manipulation. In relation to persons, the implicit demand of these children seemed to be either *to give* or *to give in*. In conferences with school personnel, we learned to give considerable diagnostic weight to the reactions and feelings of counterhostility which school personnel had developed toward the antisocial child. Although the severely disturbed borderline children created anxiety, concern, and aggravation for their teachers because they presented many management problems to school personnel, hostility toward these children was generally much tempered by an awareness that they were "sick" or severely handicapped children emotionally. Not so with our antisocial children. Here the object-directed aggression and demands for narcissistic gratification on the part of the child tended to arouse intense counterhostility (the image of the "bad" child, the "bad seed") to a far greater degree. (Makkay, Elizabeth S., and Schwaab, Edleff H. "Some Problems in the Differential Diagnosis of Antisocial Disorders in Early Latency." *Journ. Amer. Acad. Child Psychiatry*, 1:414–430, 1962.)

in helping his seven-year-old crippled son with his homework. "You see my wife doesn't like the boy. She won't help him. And he isn't very good in school work.

"But then that lady came from the school and told my wife the boy was feeble-minded and we would have to take him out of the school. That made me awful mad. My wife laughed and I wanted to kill her. I quit drinking and I helped that boy with his lessons every night when I got home from work. I know he isn't feeble-minded.

"But the day they are talking about, the day I did that awful thing, I came home from work and I was never so tired. But I wouldn't take a drink. My wife had a little supper for us and then I sat down to help the boy. They said he couldn't count up to twenty and I was bound he could, so we kept at it. He would get as high as thirteen and then he would get mixed up and couldn't go any further.

"Just then the old lady came by and gave me an 'I-told-you-so' look and I went to pieces. The boy kept saying, 'Thirteen, twelve, twelve, twelve.' 'Go on, I said. Go on, go on.' But he couldn't. I don't remember anything else but I know what I did was terrible. I just blew up. I grabbed him by the hair and I hit him. I beat him. It was awful, I know. The next thing I remember was the neighbors screaming."

He related the circumstances without sparing himself, but showed an affection for his son and a troubled concern for his future, fully realizing that the consequences of his rage had brought complications which only made bad matters worse.*

Of course the more dramatic instances of this syndrome relate to murder.** It is not the usual product of episodic dyscontrol, but if murder

---

* This uneducated but highly motivated man proved to be an excellent subject for psychotherapeutic help; he reported to the clinic faithfully, continued to work, continued to eschew alcohol, and continued to nurture his son with kindliness and real affection.

** In 1827 Esquirol introduced his concept of periodic homicidal monomania, arising suddenly in an individual with or without delusional ideas. This concept provoked a storm of indignation among contemporary judges and lawyers. French forensic psychiatrists such as Marc, Morel, and others continued to fight for a century before this concept was recognized. In the United States, the celebrated case of Mary Harris, diagnosed as periodic homicidal mania, was reported in 1860 by Dr. Charles Henry Nichols, first superintendent of St. Elizabeth's Hospital. Mrs. Harris had three subsequent admissions to the hospital and was finally discharged in 1881 as "recovered." (See Lebensohn, Zigmond M. "Contributions of St. Elizabeth's to a Century of Medical-Legal Progress." *Medical Annals of the District of Columbia*, 24:469–477, 1955.)

Wertham has suggested the name *catathymic crisis* for some of these cases. (Wertham, Frederic. *The Show of Violence.* New York: Doubleday, 1949.) The term "catathymic" was suggested by Hans Maier of Switzerland to designate delusions, hallucinations, or "morbid actions" originating from a central representation with high *does* result, the offender is apt to be arrested, detained, and sometimes carefully examined. Such examinations often reveal an understanding of the murderous act which is far different from that gained by casual—or even a judicial—reading of the "facts."

One particularly tragic murder occurred in the case of a petty officer who had an excellent Navy record. In spite of the fact that he had upon one occasion "gone berserk" in a bar, smashing it up and assaulting numerous other individuals, the general feeling about him was one of confidence. He had attained the rank of chief petty officer, taught a class in the base Sunday school, took classes in the night school, adopted two foreign orphans, and was regarded as living, for the most part, a sober, respectable married life.

On an afternoon in November 1953, while going home late from the hospital where he was in charge, he met the daughter of one of the high-ranking officers of the station; she dismounted from her bicycle to walk along with him, laughing and joking. Without (known) provocation he suddenly seized her, choked her to death, and threw her body into a nearby irrigation ditch.

He was so highly regarded by everyone on the post that it was quite natural that he should be among those who made a vigorous search for the assassin. But after a week or so, although no one had suspected him, he went to the authorities and made a full confession. He could offer no adequate explanation for what he had done. The death sentence was pronounced, and he expressed himself as considering it appropriate. A careful investigation of the history showed that this man had once been employed by a civilian hospital, from which he was discharged for having struck at a patient and for having possibly killed another patient. In addition to this, he had made impulsive, aggressive attacks upon several other occasions, which were so out of keeping with his character, as most people saw it, that no charges were preferred and, indeed, doubt was thrown upon the stories tendered by the accusers.

Several other cases in this category of episodic dyscontrol which were examined by us may be briefly abstracted: [19]

A twenty-four-year-old corporal looking for a prostitute near a French town was approached by a thirteen-year-old boy who persistently asked him to change Army scrip into French currency; when refused, the boy

---

emotional load. As an instance of catathymic murder, Maier gives the assassination of the Austrian Empress Elizabeth (1898) by an Italian anarchist who wanted to avenge himself for the injustices he had suffered. (Cf. Maier, Hans W. "Uber katathyme Wahnbildung und Paranoia." *Zeitschrift fur die gesamte Neurologie und Psychiatrie*, 13:555–610, 1912.)

seemed to mock or make fun of him, whereupon he struck the boy. The corporal insisted he had no intention of killing the victim and did not recall the actual killing. When he "found out" what he was doing, the victim's body had been severely mutilated.

A twenty-year-old laborer and truck-driver, frightened and angry following an argument with a friend, picked up a fourteen-year-old boy to whom he suggested homosexual relations. The boy refused and kept "nagging" the driver to take him back home. He struck the boy, and began choking him. He said he didn't intend to kill the boy, but "found" the victim was dead.

A forty-three-year-old married Negro soldier lapsed into a dreamlike dissociative state under the taunting and mocking of a prostitute who was attempting to seduce him and get his money. He struck her with a tire jack, discovered that he had killed her, and then mutilated and dismembered her body.

These were bizarre, apparently senseless, spur-of-the-moment murders. In each instance our opinion was requested because someone connected with the case was dissatisfied with previous psychiatric examinations and explanations. "How," they asked, "could a person as sane as this man had seemed, and *now* seems, commit an act as crazy as the one he was convicted of?"

In each instance, the murderers themselves were puzzled as to why they had killed their victims, and all attempts to reconstruct a rational motive were unsuccessful. In no case was there any gain to the murderer; in no case were there any accompanying or complicating crimes. In all four cases the victims were relatively unknown to the murderers, and the method of murder was haphazard and impromptu. Not one of the murderers used a conventional weapon, but killed with bare hands or whatever weapon could be pressed into use. And in all four instances the murder was unnecessarily violent.

Bear in mind that we are emphasizing here the *economic* rather than the dynamic elements of the act. Dynamically there were some explanations to be offered which are mentioned in the original article. The second case, for example, seems to have been close to suicide, the victim representing his own hated self-image. The first one may have been ridding himself of a dead sister with whom he had had incestuous relations.

But these dynamics do not explain the extremity of the act, the violence or the apparent meaninglessness of the act. Our theory is that these explosions do have a certain general meaning or use; they represent an effort to forestall something worse. But what, one might ask, is worse than murder? The ego in distress often "thinks" in primitive language, in primary-process terms. According to this, the ego would rather kill than be killed, or, what amounts to the same thing, suffer a completely disruptive disintegration. Thus, murder is frequently committed, according to our theory, to preserve sanity (as well as in other instances to preserve life).[20] Some colleagues [21] have proposed that murder and suicide may both serve as defenses against "psychosis." Certainly this would sometime seem to be the ego's "intention." And it usually works. Such "temporary insanities" rarely become long-term "insanities" and indeed, it is just this fact that so perplexes juries in attempting to fix a degree of "blame" on an offender whose "insanity" seems to them to have been too brief to have been real.

This concept lawyers and judges find very baffling. But it is no more obscure in principle than flooding an area to relieve an overtaxed dam, or inoculating with cowpox to prevent smallpox, or incising an abscess to prevent it from bursting. From the standpoint of society, the explosion of murder is disastrous, but from the standpoint of the individual himself it may be the way to survival, the only solution which, at the moment of decision, the crippled ego could find.

We have been using murder as a dramatic exemplification of ego rupture and episodic dyscontrol. It is probably much the least frequent result. Suicide is probably more frequent, but after a suicide there is no one left to study. Most suicides, we believe, belong in another category, which we shall discuss later, but there is an impulsive gesture of suicide in which the fatality is probably quite unintended. Circumstantial evidence often suggests that these individuals neither wanted nor intended to die. They expected (i.e., hoped) to be rescued.[22]

Other Types of Episodic Dyscontrol

Another clinical type of episodic dyscontrol is represented by the states of demoralization which occur under the stress of battle conditions. Symptoms of various kinds may have for some time preceded the break, but often a soldier never showed any evidences of his mounting internal stress until more or less suddenly he would "go to pieces." Some soldiers would freeze to the spot in a kind of panic paralysis. Others would be seized by uncontrollable trembling and weakness. Others would begin to scream and dash wildly about in apparent disregard of all danger. Still others would laugh incessantly or sob or babble. These pictures have been described by many observers of the military scene and have been called all sorts of names—shell shock, combat exhaustion, ten-day schizophrenias, amentia.*

In civilian life somewhat similar pictures of dereistic trancelike states or delirious excitement are not infrequently seen, and are also called by all sorts of names. A blanket description applied to many of them was "situational psychoses," since they seemed to depend so directly and obviously upon the immediate stress situation.

A "travel syndrome" is quite familiar in Air Force hospitals.** Characteristically a recruit or dependent has been traveling alone for several days on a bus, train, or plane, with irregular eating, minimal fluid intake, and occasionally some alcohol. Insomnia may be the immediate premonitory symptom leading to an explosive outburst of delusions, illusions, and ideas of reference occurring after a few days of continuous travel.

One of the classical forms of these episodic disorganizations and re-organizations was long called "prison psychosis," the derivation of which is obvious. For many individuals, squalid confinement is more disintegrative than danger situations. A major element of stress in prisons is the rigid repressive atmosphere, with the consequent lack of opportunity to discharge aggressive energy. Prisons contain a high proportion of individuals whose psychic equilibrium demands action, and it is almost impossible for some of these action-oriented individuals to maintain their equilibrium under situations which are totally repressive. Neher, of our staff, observed and followed a number of cases of young men who could not control their behavior and who were, therefore, sent from reformatories to progressively "tougher" prisons, finally ending up in Alcatraz. There, under conditions of almost total repression, they became disorganized and had to be sent to the Medical Center for Federal Prisoners in Springfield, Missouri, for psychiatric treatment.

There have also been many reports of episodic psychological disorganization in the isolation experiments in which an individual is deprived as much as possible of all perceptual stimuli. Something similar to this happens in patients who, following cataract operations, have had

---

* There is a strong suspicion that many of these patients were left with some impairment of ego functioning and predisposition to the recurrence of episodic dyscontrol. See for example "Gross Stress Reaction in Combat—a 15-Year Follow-up" by Herbert C. Archibald, Dorothy M. Long, Christine Miller, and Read D. Tuddenham (*Am. J. Psychiatry*, October 1962, pp. 317–322).
** Twenty-two cases were seen in one Air Force hospital over a three-year period. (Flinn, D. E.; Gaarder, K. R.; and Smith, D. C. *U.S. Armed Forces Med. J.* 10:524, 1959.)

both eyes bandaged,[23] also in poliomyelitis cases who are treated in a tank type of respirator, and in numerous other medical and surgical conditions as recently surveyed by Leiderman and others.[24] It is also seen in prisoners who have been placed in solitary confinement without light or contact with guards. Characteristic of this group of syndromes is the fact that a severe degree of disorganization appears and rather promptly disappears. Perhaps the phenomena are related to the demoralization of experimental rats (and other animals) produced, for example, by placing them in situations of insoluble conflict.[25] The remarkable objective similarity of these acute disorganizations to epileptic attacks in human beings has been remarked.[26] The contribution of indigenous factors—which is always present—is for practical purposes ignored.

In some individuals, however, certain internal "sets" may predispose them to episodes of transient disorganization in which the external factors are apt to be lost sight of because of the conspicuousness of the *internal* factors. Typical of this is the syndrome long designated hypomania—a sort of runaway acceleration of the psychological process. Hyperalertness, hyperintellection, hyperactivity, and an elevated mood combine to give the impression of a human engine which has temporarily lost its governor. Such individuals talk too much, go too fast, sleep too little, appear to be tireless in their incessant reactions to everything, to the point of being highly annoying or merely amusingly troublesome. Their impaired judgment is usually quite obvious to everyone, including in most instances the patient himself. But in contrast to the case in the more healthy-minded individual, this insight is not able to exert sufficient deterrence in the hypomanic patient. As in the other cases which we are describing as phenomena of episodic dyscontrol, the type just described generally runs a brief course and recovers. This fact has been known to medical science for hundreds if not thousands of years. These patients cause an enormous amount of alarm and inconvenience before they get well, but generally they do get well, and often manifest superior talents.

As these pages were being written, I was interrupted by a visit from a former patient now living in another city. Thirty years ago he had had an episode of excitement followed by a depression of some months. He came now to tell me that he had just sustained a second attack of something similar. His previous illness was no secret, but he had in the meantime built up a successful insurance business in one city and an even more successful mercantile establishment in a town not far away.

He had become convinced that his town needed a building-and-loan association. He persuaded several of his friends to join him in organizing and developing one. He was working exceedingly hard on this when it became apparent that reality severance had occurred and that he had definitely lost control of himself.

"My wife said I was on Cloud Seven all the time. First I was worried half sick, and then everything was just rosy, better and bigger and finer, except I wouldn't stop for a minute to eat or sleep. My wife said maybe I wasn't crazy, but I was driving all the rest of them crazy."

The patient laughed at his little joke and went on: "I have been in the hospital a few weeks now. I think your doctors are going to let me go home in a couple more. It is ridiculous for me to blow up like this again after thirty years, but I guess it is the only way I know how to get myself a little rest. Sorry I worried so many people—I know they called you up in the middle of the night, and some other people too."

These "manic" attacks, as they have been ungrammatically called, serve as defense measures, i.e., they protect the individual from a more serious disintegration, perhaps severe depression or impulsive abandonment of a familiar way of life, and they do so, let it be clearly understood, by the release of aggression. The manic attack is sometimes obviously and seriously aggressive, but even when it is disguised by humor, conversation, puckish behavior, or other devices, it is basically aggressive. Many psychoanalytic studies, following Abraham,[27] have shown clearly the intense cannibalistic oral aggression accompanying the hypomania and sometimes clearly perceptible in the voracious and insatiable approach of the manic patient to various aspects of his environment. He devours people, as it were. Moreover, this syndrome is usually accompanied by a high degree of hypersensitiveness, if not frankly paranoid fantasy-formation. Bateman and others [28] point out that manic attacks serve the secondary purpose of protecting the patient from external interference while he is attempting to regain "psychic equilibrium."

Davidson [29] tacitly supports our position by describing the attack of manic-depressive illness as "the result of failure of the hierarchical organization of the total personality" under the effect of acute or continuous stress. "The system of defense of the total personality will break down, particularly the mechanism of repression, and compensation and overcompensation will seek to save the person's self-esteem." *

* The author endeavors to correlate this point of view with the biological research of Humphrey and of Hebb. (Humphrey, George: *Thinking: An Introduction to Experi-*

In Lewin's book, *The Psychoanalysis of Elation*,[30] he quotes Freud as saying:

> Denial disclaims the external world, then, as repression disclaims the instincts. . . . Just as there are negations, contradictions, and delusions to offset the intellectual contents [of the pathogenic conflict] so there may be odd moods, depressions, elations, perplexities, confusions, states of dim awareness, even stupor, which insistently pervade the affective apparatus of the mind (the thymopsyche) and leave no place for anxiety.
>
> Like an instinct, an event (or stimulus) in the external world may be taken as having two aspects: its intellectual representation or idea, and its emotional bearing or impact. Hence, denial may operate like repression in a dual capacity. It may oppose the intellectual recognition of an external fact, say a death, and state that it did not occur, and this may lead to a negative or positive delusion. Or it may oppose the affective impact of the external facts; although admitting that a death did occur, the ego's point of view would be that it did not matter. In the elations we shall find that it is chiefly this aspect of denial—the denial of the emotional impact of reality—which influences the clinical picture. . . . The effect of denial is to rupture the intellectual rapport or emotional attuning of the ego with its environment.

In some instances, of course, manic and melancholic attacks become florid and resemble the textbook illustrations of "mania" or "melancholia," which are not Third Order conditions but Fourth Order syndromes.

C. Disorganized Episodic Violence

In contrast to somewhat focused and directed aggression of the syndromes just described are the equally violent but completely unfocused discharges of energy in the *grand mal* convulsion. It has been suggested many times that this sudden release of disorganized violence is like an enormous, clumsy temper tantrum. The loss of consciousness which accompanies it is usually so complete that the convulsion has been described as a "little death." The tendency of patients with this diathesis to injure themselves during the attack is well known.

What is less well known is that most of these patients feel better for a while after the attack. An unlettered prison guard of long experience was conducting me, many years ago, through the dreary "snake-pit" wards of a state prison in which the "insane and epileptic" prisoners were

mental Psychology. New York: Wiley, 1951. Hebb, D. O.: *Organization of Behavior.* New York: Wiley, 1949.)

kept. "We always breathe a sigh of relief," he said, "after them as has fits comes around with one of their spells and has it over with. Then they don't give us no trouble for a while. Seems like they store up a charge of meanness that just has to come out that way. When we have trouble down here it is likely to be just before several of them epileptics is due." (This was in the days before any effective anticonvulsant drugs were in use, at least in prisons.) Janet [31] noted this clinical phenomenon and suggested that if we could just find a way to produce convulsions, we could probably cure many nonconvulsive psychiatric patients. This shrewd observation anticipated the accidental discovery of convulsive shock therapy.

Note that we are speaking here particularly of the function of the symptom, not its provocation or its psychological mechanisms or the psychodynamics or the anatomical structures involved. Convulsions may, of course, occur under many circumstances and conditions from glioma to uremia and from drunkenness to *lupus erythematosus disseminata*, but the psychological function performed, i.e., release of unbearable tension, is conceivably always the same, regardless of the crucial precipitating cortical stimulus, or the predisposing cortical structure. The effect upon the environment is vastly different, of course—convulsions arousing our dismay and pity, intentional aggression arousing our anger.

Numerous workers today are concerned with other bonds of linkage between these phenomena, the diffuse discharge represented by a convulsion, and the focused discharge represented by aggressive acts.[32] One of our former associates was among the first to note the high frequency of pathologic electroencephalographic findings in "psychotic" federal prisoners.[33]

Russell Monroe, who was himself one of the contributors to research along these lines, was convinced of the validity of such a correlation. Commenting on our theory, he says, "It seems to us that there is accumulating more and more evidence that paroxysmal activity in the second system of the rhinencephalon could very well lead to severely disordered behavior with the adaptive failure so great that such patients are generally considered psychotic." [34]

A closely related syndrome associated with abnormal discharge patterns in electroencephalogram brain tracings has been differentiated sharply by some investigators from epileptic disorders. The behavior of children and adolescents with the "6- and 14-per-second positive spiking" pattern often includes fire-setting, aggressive sexuality, murder, and other acts of violence.[35]

Woods [36] is careful to point out, however, that this disorder is one of psychological disturbance, not simply a neurological disease.

It is my hypothesis that the dysrhythmia does not itself induce violence, but rather that it serves as a biologically determined stress on an already impoverished ego. In the resultant regressed ego state, there is the emergence of primitive nonneutralized aggression, with the violent acting-out of conflict previously held in check by the defensive system of the ego. This is contrasted to epilepsy, where the presence of a seizure discharge provides a "short-circuiting mechanism" with considerable relief of tension.

From the economic standpoint, it is unnecessary to demonstrate or even to assume that these widely differing clinical syndromes have an organic injury or defect in common. The possible inference is that a pattern of explosive discharge is related to the damming-up of strong, poorly controlled aggressive impulses. Several psychoanalytic studies strongly support this.[37]

Woods [38] emphasizes the interrelatedness of structural defects and psychological dysfunction not only in his own cases but in the descriptions of such cases by other investigators.

Ego function cannot be separated from the organic matrix through which it operates, and the ability of the ego defenses to contain psychic conflict is in part determined by the continued integrity of this organic matrix. As an example, regression to primitive levels of ego functioning, with the explosive acting-out of conflict, may be seen under the toxic influence of alcohol or drugs. In the case of epilepsy, Gottschalk has stressed the fact that both psychological factors and disturbed cerebral function are necessary for the production of seizures. Fenichel regarded the epileptic seizure as a kind of special affect attack, occurring in organically predisposed personalities, with the attack serving as a short-circuiting of mental impulses. Freud, in his remarks on Dostoevski's epilepsy, saw the seizure as an expression of inhibited rage and an outlet for inhibited incestuous sexual drives. Sperling and Riemann viewed the attacks as having genesis in overwhelming aggressive impulses; while Greenson was impressed with the role of inhibited sexual desire.

Epstein and Ervin [39] hold that "mounting insoluble psychological tensions . . . are one of the factors determining the onset of a given seizure," and that "seizures have an adaptive value representing miscarried attempts to dispel mounting psychological tension not immediately soluble in reality." Barker [40] proposed that the *petit mal* attack "abolished consciousness when unconscious emotional responses and their demand for action seriously endanger the patient's consciously acceptable patterns of behavior." Some patients with convulsive tendencies certainly show clinical evidence of a "build-up" of tension prior to a seizure, with a period of relaxation for some time after the seizure.

It is not easy to demonstrate this. One of us made a special study of these cases before and after the seizure and was unable to find any psychological-test evidence of either the pre-seizure build-up of tension or the post-seizure reduction of tension.[41] Rather he found an increased disequilibrium after the attack. This was also noted by Kurt Goldstein [42] in his description of "catastrophic breakdown." However, said Goldstein, these are "the only means by which existence for these individuals can be maintained."

It is increasingly accepted that recurrent convulsions are never "purely" neurological, but always possess strong psychological determinants. Frequently the best approach, or at least a necessary cooperative approach, to therapeutic control is psychological.*

Numerous other clinical syndromes may belong in this category, such as certain fugue states,[43] some menacing attacks of psychomotor "equivalents" of "epilepsy," some brain-damage syndromes, and some chronic encephalitic behavior. All of these, while less frequent than those mentioned, are still too frequent for our peace of mind. They are peculiarly resistant to treatment.

In some of them, as clinical readers will know, the history of healthy well-behaved childhood was followed by the noted occurrence of a not particularly severe attack of influenza. Some weeks or months or sometimes even years afterward neurological symptoms would appear, then disturbances of sleep, restlessness, increasing unmanageableness, disobedience, fighting, delinquencies of many kinds. The rapid "moral disintegration" of these patients is particularly heartbreaking to parents, who blame themselves quite unjustifiably.

A typical example of this is a child who for several years had compulsively beaten himself on the head unless his arms were restrained by an attendant. His stomach, he said, was very cruel and told him two million things, all bad; told him to knock his eyes out, to hit and kick and spit and die, said that nobody was keeping him from it. In addition to mistreating himself, he pinched, scratched, kicked and spat on playmates, threw water on the adults, smeared saliva over his food, and otherwise made himself highly offensive as well as pitiable.[44]

---

* Only 20 percent of the known epileptics in the United States are receiving adequate treatment, according to Robin White. Four national agencies may be consulted: United Epilepsy Association, Inc., 111 West 57th St., New York 19, N.Y.; The Epilepsy Foundation, 1729 F Street N.W., Washington 6, D.C.; National Epilepsy League, 203 North Wabash Ave., Chicago 1, Ill.; and the American Epilepsy Federation, 73 Tremont Street, Boston 8, Mass. ("The Epileptic's Battle for Understanding." *Saturday Evening Post*, June 8, 1963.)

No case should be considered hopeless; the very presence of these symptoms is, according to our own theory, a basis for some hope. One of the most disturbed brain-damaged cases in our files was a boy of sixteen considered by all consultants to have no chance of improvement, after a catastrophic car-wreck injury. But after six years he was not only improved but almost completely recovered.

Even in individuals in whom great disorganization has already occurred, in so-called "dementia" patients who may seem to be "vegetating" only, sudden eruptions of anger, excitement, fear, and destructiveness may appear. This suggests that even in conditions of extensive disorganization there is still a tendency to attempt to preserve whatever integration may be salvaged.[45] Obviously, however, such fluctuations in the course of regressed states do not belong in the present clinical category, although they illustrate the same mechanism.

Recapitulation

We have proposed in this chapter that the exhibition of direct aggression, except in certain conventionalized forms, is a manifestation of acute or chronic ego failure. We have suggested that the resulting dyscontrol is usually an explosive, destructive act or series of acts always accompanied by other evidences of internal disorganization, and sometimes by loss or disturbance of consciousness. We hold it to be a more serious clinical indication than the symptoms of Second Order dyscontrol in the sense that it indicates more ego weakness, or at least less success in the ego's efforts to restrain and control dangerous impulses. It represents more reality denial, more impairment of achievement, and more actual injuriousness to subject as well as environment.

The functional episodic dyscontrol, acute or chronic, is presumed to be the averting of greater failure, a more catastrophic disintegration. It is this economic principle which we have been emphasizing and according to which we have arranged our clinical syndromes.

The syndromes cited in this chapter illustrating Third Order dyscontrol were as follows:

A. Chronic, repetitive, aggressive behavior
B. Episodic, impulsive violence
   1. Homicidal assaultiveness
   2. Demoralization syndromes

CHAPTER XI

Dysfunction of a Fourth and a Fifth Order

S Y N O P S I S : Organismic dysfunction of a Fourth Order is represented by those extreme states of dysorganization, regression, and reality repudiation which constitute the classical picture of severe mental illness —so-called psychoses. Many names have been given to different forms which emerge from behind various façades of quasi-normality. They represent a penultimate effort to avoid something worse, viz., Fifth Order dysorganization—malignant anxiety and depression eventuating in death, often by suicide.

WE COME finally to the consideration of those extreme states of personality dysorganization, regression, and reality repudiation which constitute the classical notion of mental illness. These are the "psychoses," the "insanities," the "lunacies" of an earlier day. They are the extremes of personality dysorganization.

The phenomena recorded in such variety in the many preceding pages are for the most part only recently envisaged as mental illnesses. In the minds of some it will seem as if we had traversed a long corridor of minor exhibits leading at last into the central core of psychiatric reality.

But it is not a long corridor in which we have been walking, nor is it tangential or peripheral to our material. Psychiatry is no longer a small circumscribed collection of curiosities and monstrosities; it is a great, wide community, for which we have suggested some hierarchical zones. One is reminded of the experience of the uninitiated visitor to London who learns with surprise, after a long ride through varied metropolitan scenery, that he has only now arrived at "the City" of London—a small area within the great metropolis.

And just as the importance of the old City of London is now primarily historical and symbolic, so it is today in psychiatry: the conditions of extreme disorganization which formerly occupied the attention of psychiatrists and constituted the body of mental disease are no longer the central focus of our attention.

Inspection of the many taxonomic lists of "the insanities" collected in the Appendix will lend eloquent confirmation to this statement. The phenomena studied and classified by our professional ancestors were chiefly these conditions of severe disorganization, "true madness." As a rule no connection was seen between these phenomena and the lesser degrees of disorganization, controlled by less radical devices, but in accord with the same basic principles, which were apt to be dismissed as eccentricity, perversity, or viciousness. Such persons were not likely to be taken to a physician or to go voluntarily.

Our well-meaning ancestors little realized that they were permitting or encouraging or even forcing the development of these "end states," the extremities of madness. We have tried to emphasize the relatedness of these to the milder phenomena of lesser disorganization and to show how progressively more energetic efforts are attempted by the ego to avoid being swept into the vortex of the maelstrom of disintegration. But sometimes the ego cannot stay it, unaided, and former treatment programs often offered little help.

At the risk of tiring the reader, we venture to repeat the formula: Stresses accumulate beyond the powers of the habitual coping devices of the individual to manage smoothly, and devices characteristic of a First Order of dyscontrol are employed to handle the emergency. In the vast majority of instances these succeed and no more is heard of the matter. In a certain percentage of instances these emergency devices threaten to fail or do fail and a Second Order of dyscontrol develops with a somewhat different quality of emergency management. Again the devices may suffice, and they may be continued indefinitely; they usually disappear. But they may fail. Then evidences of a still more severe dyscontrol appear; the ego sustains—perhaps permits—a rupture in order to manage the rapidly increasing tension. This we have called a Third Order of dyscontrol. The devices used to control it always involve some external damage for which restitution of some kind has to be made, and always some internal suffering.

These explosions characterizing Third Order dyscontrol are more severe, more destructive, more alarming than the minor blow-ups that characterize phenomena in everyday life—temper tantrums, blowing one's top, going on a spree and the like—but resemble them in serving to afford the ego some respite. The ego soon recaptures its authority and resumes its ministrations, so far as is possible in view of the environmental reactions which have been provoked by the outburst. The ego's tasks of adaptation were already presumably great and may now become greater. Life is more difficult. This is one of the reasons that Third

Order phenomena, once instituted, tend to recur.* The explosion may have occurred many times and thus periodically afforded some relief and prevented further disintegration. Or, on the other hand, it may never have occurred at all.

In schematizing this process we have introduced an element of oversimplification. It should be remembered that this regressive course may seem to encompass only a few months or a few years, but actually covers much of the life of an individual. A person who seems suddenly to develop symptoms of Third Order dyscontrol or Fourth Order disintegration will, on careful examination, show that there was a time, perhaps even in his childhood, when an attempt was made to hold the line with Second and First Order devices. One may have to search carefully and far for the indications of the ego's vulnerability which may "suddenly" become overt in the eruption of a mental illness.

Thus there may not even have been any considerable number of Second Order devices in use. The ego may have been so weakened over the years as to lack the power to employ the emergency devices that would stem progressive dissolution and demoralization. External help may be—for many reasons—unobtainable or not forthcoming, and a process of progressive decay and mounting tension may be going on beneath a completely deceptive external façade.

Façade

This is the place to describe a coping device which belongs to all orders. Perhaps it should not be called a coping device at all. It has to do with the way we present ourselves to the world. A child early learns that he is obliged to be different things to different people, and what he is to each and to all of them may be quite different from what he is to himself. One presents himself as different from what he feels not only for self-protection but for the protection of the public. Thus a façade is of the greatest social usefulness. It permits the social amenities and a public peace of mind; it represents consideration for the feelings of

---

* Pictorially minded readers may think of some membranous tissue like an eardrum or an automobile tire which has sustained a rupture and been patched either by man or by nature. There is a feeling that a weakness remains and that another blowout may occur more easily. This is one way of looking at it. The other way of looking at it is to discard the membranous model of an ego boundary and think rather that the consequences of the explosion have irritated or inflamed the environment so that restrictions and threats which did not exist before now exist.

others. At the same time, by very virtue of its external uses, a façade can bolster self-esteem. By concealing unpleasantness and deficiencies, it spares embarrassment and a feeling of exposure, and in these many ways helps the maintenance of ego control. A façade is, therefore, more than merely putting a good face on things, or sweeping the dust under the rug, as it were—valuable as these measures may be at times. It is definitely a coping device, a way of living. A façade is a necessary part of the personality; the very word "personality" comes from a Latin word meaning "mask," and woe to him who has not learned to wear his mask(s), as one of Pirandello's characters says.

But this same façade may be a liability as well as an asset. It may so completely conceal the sufferings (i.e., the internal instability) of some individuals as to preclude either help or appropriate consideration. The façade may enable individuals whose internal state of disorganization is very considerable to go long unobserved by the outside world, especially if all internal complaint can be squelched.

The use of the word "façade" is a little misleading to the degree that it implies fraudulency. In a certain sense, to be sure, all fronts are fraudulent in that they do not represent the whole self. But they do represent one aspect of the self, and they do have a function. The front may be an unpleasant one, a truculent or contemptuous one, or haughty, concealing a great secret fear of rejection. Or a façade may be one of serenity and an avowed wish to please, quite contrary to some of the internal impulses. The façade may serve to conceal suffering and incompetence from the world as well as aggression and bitterness. To call it hypocritical, insincere, dishonest, phony, fraudulent, is only to say that we are aware of a discrepancy and one which troubles us— us outsiders. We do not know why it is necessary. But to clinicians, this discrepancy is itself a very significant clinical indication.

When one's internal world is crumbling, or when one is withdrawing from what has been one's world to live in another, so to speak, the façade becomes a concession made to the conventional world of reality in order that one may be permitted existence in his own world of unreality. The façade exists, so to speak, to hide the ego's shame; from another point of view one might say it conceals the ego's secret joy. In either case it is the configuration of behavior upon which we have to judge the outer semblance of reintegration and equilibrium-restoration. Recovery, as it is seen externally, is often a matter of the restoration of a familiar façade, characteristic of the individual as he had been known to his associates. This façade may be thick or thin, strong or fragile. What it presents of the patient's purposes, comprehensions, attitudes, emotional responses, serenity, good will, and so forth, these are important; but what it conceals is also important.

This façade may crack. Repeated explosions may not sufficiently relieve the tension. Second Order devices may mushroom and hypertrophy. Everything, in short, may fail and the ever-imminent catastrophe ensue.

Fourth Order Dyscontrol

What is this great catastrophe, this awesome disaster which the ego so dreads?

What the ego fears most is a collapse, a general loss of all control and of all identity. A seemingly complete demoralization and disorganization is never a complete disintegration—even though it may appear so—for there is another stage beyond, an extremity of failure and reality separation which we shall discuss later.

In the type of dysorganization which we are now to discuss, a façade is no longer maintained. Actually this is not true; even the most disturbed patients often attempt, pathetically, to conceal some of their symptoms. But the self-control is so impaired that aggressive impulses emerge into consciousness and in various abortive ways into action, as if the ego were paralyzed. Loyalty to reality is repudiated to varying degrees. Perceptual processes distort the picture of the outside world.

The cognitive processes become snarled, confused, and poisoned. Emotional reactions are inappropriate and exaggerated. Behavior becomes unpredictable. Productivity falls to near zero. Linkages with the outside world are severed. There is a retreat into a self-created "autistic" world which has been called by various sensitive writers "the outward room," "the closed door," "the forbidden path," and "the world next door."

It is no wonder our ancestors believed that such patients were scarcely human, that they were unaware of cold and heat or of hunger and thirst. It is faintly understandable how some could believe that if the right kind of pain could be inflicted, if a sufficient surprise or fright or discomfort could be induced, the patient might return to us, so to speak, readapt to our world of reality and pursue our methods of self-expression and self-comfort. For, externally regarded, such patients do often present a strange appearance. Read some classical descriptions by a master clinician.[1]

I will first place before you a farmer, aged fifty-nine, who was admitted to the hospital a year ago. The patient looks much older than he really is, principally owing to the loss of the teeth from his upper jaw. He not only understands our questions without any difficulty, but answers them relevantly and correctly; can tell where he is, and how long he has been here; knows the doctors, and can give the date and the day of the week. His expression is dejected. The corners of his mouth are rather drawn down, and his eyebrows drawn together. He usually stares in front of him, but he glances up when he is spoken to. On being questioned about his illness, he breaks into lamentations, saying that he did not tell the whole truth on his admission, but concealed the fact that he had fallen into sin in his youth and practised uncleanness with himself; everything he did was wrong. "I am so apprehensive, so wretched; I cannot lie still for anxiety. O God, if I had only not transgressed so grievously!" He has been ill for over a year, has had giddiness and headaches. It began with stomach-aches and head trouble, and he could not work any longer. "There was no impulse left." He can get no rest now, and fancies silly things, as if someone were in the room. Once it seemed to him that he had seen the Evil One: perhaps he would be carried off. So things seemed to him.

As a boy, he had taken apples and nuts. "Conscience has said that that is not right; conscience has only awakened just now in my illness." He had also played with a cow, and by himself. "I reproach myself for that now." It seemed to him that he had fallen away from God, and was now as free as a bird. His appetite is bad, and he has no stools. He cannot sleep. "If the mind does not sleep, all sorts of thoughts come." He has done silly things too. He fastened his neckerchief to strangle himself, but he was not really in earnest. Three sisters and a brother were ill too. The sisters were not so bad; they soon recovered. "A brother has made away with himself through apprehension."

The patient tells us this in broken sentences, interrupted by wailing and groaning. In all other respects, he behaves naturally, does whatever he is told, and only begs us not to let him be dragged away—"There is dreadful apprehension in my heart." Except for a little trembling of the outspread fingers and slightly arhythmic action of the heart, we find no striking disturbances at the physical examination.

The [next] patient has almost to be carried into the room, as he walks in a straddling fashion on the outside of his feet. On coming in, he throws off his slippers, sings a hymn loudly, and then cries twice (in English), "My father, my real father!" He is eighteen years old, a senior in high school, tall, and rather strongly built, but with a pale complexion, on which there is very often a transient flush. The patient sits with his eyes shut, and pays no attention to his surroundings. He does not look up even when he is spoken to, but he answers, beginning in a low voice, and gradually screaming louder and louder. When asked where he is, he says, "You want to know that too; I tell you who is being measured and shall be measured. I know all that, and could tell you, but I do not want to." When asked his name, he screams, "What is your name? What does he shut? He shuts his eyes. What does he hear? He does not understand; he understands not. How? Who? Where? When? What does he mean? When I tell him to look, he does not look properly. You there, just look! What is it? What is the matter? Attend; he attends not. I say, what is it, then? Why do you give me no answer? Are you getting impudent again? How can you be so impudent? I'm coming! I'll show you! You don't turn whore for me. You mustn't be smart either; you're an impudent, lousy fellow, an impudent, lousy fellow, as stupid as a hog. Such an impudent, shameless, miserable, lousy fellow I've never met with. Is he beginning again? You understand nothing at all—nothing at all; nothing at all does he understand. If you follow now, he won't follow, will not follow. Are you getting still more impudent? Are you getting impudent still more? How they attend, they do attend," and so on. At the end he scolds in quite inarticulate sounds.

The patient understands perfectly, and has introduced many phrases he has heard before into his speech, without once looking up. He speaks in an affected way, now babbling like a child, now lisping and stammering, sings suddenly in the middle of what he is saying, and grimaces. He carries out orders in an extraordinary fashion, gives his hand with the fist clenched, goes to the blackboard when he is asked, but, instead of writing his name, suddenly knocks down a lamp, and throws the chalk among the audience. He makes all kinds of senseless movements, pushes the table away, crosses his arms, and turns round on his axis, chair and all, or sits balancing, with his legs crossed and his hands on his head. Catalepsy can also be made out. When he is to go away, he will not get up, has to be pushed, and calls out loudly, "Good-morning, gentlemen; it has not pleased me." The only physical disturbance worth noticing is a considerable acceleration of the pulse to 160 beats.

The factory-girl, aged thirty-two, who now comes into the room with an awkward and very deep curtsey, presents an entirely different aspect from the last patient. She declines to sit down to talk to us, thanks us for the "honour," goes up and down with affected, waddling steps, and begins to declaim and recite verses, and to interpolate witty remarks in our discussion of her condition. Her name is what the parson christened her, and she is as old as her little finger. She knows her position, the date, where she is, and the people around her, and can give the most exact information about her past experiences. She does not consider herself insane. She often interweaves her disconnected talk with scraps of bad French and senselessly altered quotations, such as, "Ingratitude is the world's praise," "Many hands, many minds." She rides single phrases to death in uninterrupted repetition—"Devil's dung on the soul's foot, the soul's foot in devil's dung." She often uses very strange and almost incomprehensible compound words and phrases.

Her mood is silly, cheerful, sometimes erotic, and then again irritable. She takes pleasure in the most indecent sexual allusions, and occasionally in outbursts of the wildest abuse. She does not obey orders, and refuses to give her hand on the ground that they are *her* hands. She will not write, and pertly refuses to do anything she is asked. She chatters continually, and will not let anyone get in a word. Her speech is extremely laboured. She cuts the separate syllables sharply asunder, accentuates the final syllables sharply, pronounces g like *k*, and *d* like *t*, talks like a child, in imperfectly formed sentences, distorts words, inserts senseless expletives and strangely-formed words, and constantly changes the subject. All her movements and gestures are clumsy, angular, and stiff, and are very lavishly employed, but monotonous; she hops about, bends down, claps her hands, and makes faces. She has ornamented her clothes in an extraordinary way with embroidery and crochet-work of startlingly bright wool. From her talk it appears that she looks on herself as the mistress of the house; she pays the nurses and appoints them, and will hire herself better doctors. Moreover, she complains of being exposed to sexual assaults, and says that her lungs, heart, and liver have been taken out. She says she is engaged to a doctor in the asylum where she was before. She tells her name with the prefix "von." She also seems to have heard voices, but will only make evasive statements about them.

Her talk was at that time much more irrelevant and incomprehensible than it is now. She offered the doctor a piece of bread, and added, "Here you have the oxen. I am an ox, am an ox; take it, I am an ox." In this there appears still more distinctly than in what she has said today the inclination to senseless repetitions of the same expression, which we have so frequently remarked in katatonia. Another time she exclaimed, "I have not winked, I have not wished, I have not stolen. I fare as I have never done at home. Baking ovens are not persons." Together with the forced phraseology, one notices a senseless forming of new words, which is a very familiar accompanying phenomenon of confusion of speech.

The patient was indifferent to, or irritated by, the visits of her husband. She devoured the eatables he had brought with him in a very greedy and disgusting way. Hallucinations also apparently existed—at all events, transitorily—although no further detailed information was to be learnt about them from the patient. But she spoke of a smell of death in the food, saw her brother go out, and thought it was said that she would redeem every soul. Finally, one was struck by the great slowing of the pulse.

This is the way patients in this state of organismic dyscontrol appear to the outside observer—bizarre, chaotic, incomprehensible. And yet, as Carl Jung first convinced us, there is a discoverable meaning in the most senseless babble and the most preposterous behavior. A patient listener and observer can often piece together threads and fragments and establish by deduction and reconstruction the relation of these fantasies to the needs and past experiences of the patient. Working with less disorganized patients, Freud discovered many of the principles of such alien levels of psychological organization and was able to construct a systematic theory and description of their relation to "normal" personality development.

This "natural history" of the evolution and growth of personality has been quite generally accepted in psychiatry and is probably well known to most readers. It assumes the continuous adaptation of growing and changing needs of the infant, the child, the young adult to the world about him. This represents a gradual exchange of complete passive dependency for increasing active interchange and give-and-take for mutual benefit with the world about him. In the course of this evolution an internal regulator of sanctions replaces the external compulsion for complete dependency. This structure itself has a natural history; all sorts of contracts are entered into between the superego and the ego, some of them based on archaic and repressed interpretations of rightness and wrongness and others based upon later acquired ideals and concepts of "the good." Sometimes the burdens imposed by the superego are too heavy. Sometimes its culpability is only too evident. But in all cases the ego faces the various threats of actual and fantasied world destruction, internal demolition and disorganization. These threats relate in part, perhaps, to existential anxiety and the fear of death, but perhaps even more to the fear of being unloved or unlovable. This helps us to understand such bizarre symptoms as that of a patient frantically hugging and kissing himself, and less obvious and often subtly misleading symptoms of other kinds. In the past few decades psychiatrists have—through patient listening—learned some of the content and trends of thought in these states of severe disorganization. It has been shown that just this process of gaining an understanding of the patient's hopelessness and terror can assist him in a recovery.

The essence of these inner feelings is nothing so strange. It appears in less desperate form in the life of every man, in the vicissitudes of every person's life experiences. Consider the familiar story of Robinson Crusoe and think of it as Robert Koff [2] suggests, not as a mere fanciful tale of adventure, but as the portrayal of the psychological aspects of a progressive disintegration and ultimate recovery.

A young man—that is to say, a beginner in adult life—breaks with his father and leaves home against his father's wishes. Punishment inevitably follows; he nearly drowns in a storm and is captured by pirates who make him a slave for two years. Then he turns the tables and himself becomes the owner of slaves as a prosperous planter in South America, where he is for the moment, in conventional terms, "successful and normal."

But then he tempts fate again; he goes to sea to obtain more slaves for his plantation. A terrible storm destroys his ship. He alone is washed ashore, cast out of the water on his birthday! This is a typical rebirth fantasy.[3] Total destruction of ship and crew occurs, which is symbolic of his own inner disorganization.

The story's continuation concerns his reconstruction of (his) world. He makes for himself a small-scale model of the civilized world which he had left behind him. But, he reflects, "Here I am cast upon a horrible desolate island, void of all hope of recovery. I am singled out and separated, as it were, from all the world to be miserable. I am divided from mankind, a solitaire, one banished from human society. I have not clothes to cover me. I am without any defense or means to resist any violence of man or beast. I have no soul to speak to, or relieve me."

These are precisely the inner feelings of some patients with severe mental illness—not the earliest feelings, but the later ones, which impel the effort toward a reconstruction (cf. the story of the Prodigal Son). Crusoe attempts to explore his island and to construct a boat in which to sail back to the mainland (the outside world), once more there to enjoy the pleasures of human companionship and normal life. He is frightened by the dangers of navigation in the open sea, and particularly with one experience he has with a whirlpool. He is on the point of resigning himself to a permanently solitary, withdrawn life when he discovers the human footprint not made by himself. This frightens him again, as he fantasies being devoured by cannibals.

He finds a cave into which he can creep on all fours through a long tunnel and be housed in a "most delightful cavity—though perfectly dark" (intra-uterine fantasy). He again becomes preoccupied with fantasies of escaping to the mainland with the help of some of the cannibals, whom he hopes to capture and enslave and force to help him escape. Ultimately he comes to see Friday as a human instrument to help him escape from his isolation back to the mainland of human life. Whether the portrayal of Friday properly describes the role of the psychiatrist, we shall consider in the final chapter.

Syndromes Characteristic of the Fourth Order of Dyscontrol

In the older psychiatric literature much space was given to elaborate differential diagnoses of the different clinical pictures presented by patients seen at various times and places in various cultures. The subspecies and varieties, the regroupings and the altered designations of these clinical pictures had great usefulness at one time; their delineation led to careful clinical study of individuals whom laymen and scientists alike tended to ignore as incomprehensible or ignorable. As we have seen in Chapter II, and as is illustrated more fully in the Appendix, there have been a vast number of names for these pictures.

Empirically there are, to be sure, various recognizable groups of symptoms which can be observed in association more or less frequently. These syndromes vary from time to time, from place to place, and from person to person.* And to assign names to some of these syndromes has a certain

---

* "A psychosis is generally a complicated structure which may manifest itself in very different ways, not only from one patient to another, but in the same patient at different times. The manifestations were formerly taken for the diseases themselves, and even yet it is of practical value to emphasize them as pictures of morbid states and as syndromes. . . ." (Bleuler, E. Paul, tr. A. A. Brill. *Textbook of Psychiatry.* New York: Macmillan, 1924, p. 161.)

pragmatic usefulness. It is helpful in the general provisions for treatment and in the making of administrative or legal decisions, and also in professional communications, to be able to refer to a depressive, a paranoid, or a phobic syndrome. The danger to be avoided is the assumption or inference that these terms describe specific "diseases." They are not diseases. They are various forms of the penultimate stage of organismic disequilibration and disorganization, with minor variations in the forms of reconstitution, compensatory effort, fusion, and defusion. Differences in appearance must not mask their essential identity in degree of disequilibration.*

In our opinion all these conditions represent one and the same "illness" and the same stage of that illness, despite their differing forms. We *must* free ourselves from the misleading implications that have become attached historically to the various disease labels.

Some of the generally recognized, variably designated syndromes of a Fourth Order of dysorganization are as follows:

1. Pervasive feelings of sadness, guilt, despondency and hopelessness, with convictions of inadequacy, incompetence, unworthiness or wickedness—or several of these. Psychomotor retardation is usually present, sometimes stupor or restless activity, even agitation. Delusions or delusional trends appropriate to feelings of guilt, defection, unworthiness, and self-disparagement are common—such as fantasied offenses or fantasied punishment to come.

   (This picture has been called *melancholia, depression, thymergasia, affective disorder,* and other names.)

2. More or less continuous erratic, disorganized excitement, accompanied by a corresponding excess of verbal and motor production and emotional heightening, elation, excitement, irascibility, etc. In this syndrome over-activity, volubility, and impulsivity may be at times self-injuring, at times bizarre, meddlesome, exhibitionistic, and socially annoying. The characteristic feature is the great and continuing overflow of poorly controlled energy.

   (These pictures have been called *mania, hypomania, delirium,*

---

* "The different clinical pictures [of psychosis] [are] in part determined by [different] defenses the ego is able to apply *instead of* neutralization of aggression. . . . Depending perhaps on quantitative factors, the defense against the aggression is dealt with by withdrawal, projection and varying grades of regression of the ego to the point of its undifferentiated phase." (Bak, Robert C. "The Schizophrenic Defense Against Aggression." *Int. J. Psychoan.*, 35:129–133, 1954.)

furor, frenzy, recurrent mania, hyperthymergasia, moria, dysergasia, catatonic schizophrenia, status epilepticus, and many other names.)

3. Autistic regression and self-absorption, silliness, mannerisms of speech and behavior, bizarre delusional ideation, irrelevancy and incoherence of speech, posturing and gross (apparent) indifference to social expectations. Inertness, or automaton-like behavior, often mutism or hallucinations, apparent indifference to the external world, but occasional sudden "impulsive" outbursts of speech or action are also typical.

(These pictures have been called *hebephrenia, parergasias, amentia, autism, chronic delirium, dementia simplex, catatonia, chronic deterioration, regressed states, nuclear schizophrenia,* and many other names.)

4. Delusional preoccupation with one or several themes, usually persecutory in trend, and usually accompanied by defensiveness, resentment, suspiciousness, grandiosity, condescension, irascibility, etc. A façade of dignity and sensibleness may partially or occasionally obscure the underlying picture.

(These pictures have classically gone under many compound names containing the noun *paranoia* or the adjective *paranoid*.)

5. Confused, delirious states with disorientation, bewilderment, amnesia, confabulation, and sometimes hallucinations and hyperactivity. These are commonly seen with severe injury, intoxication or inflammation of the brain, hence with encephalitis, arteriosclerosis, alcoholic and other poisonings, Huntington's disease, Alzheimer's disease, and so forth.

(These pictures have been called many things, chiefly *dementia* and *delirium*.)

These are the five classical syndromes of conventional nineteenth-century psychiatry, i.e., the typical pictures of severe dysorganization. They are essentially the pictures originally recognized by Hippocrates twenty-five hundred years ago. The dissection and elaboration, subdividing and regrouping that have been given them by thousands of colleagues over the years has not changed their basic forms. They are not separate diseases, but varieties of one disease, one illness, in its principal variations of extreme development. They are the extremities to which the ego can be pushed and still be able to re-establish itself.

For, catastrophic as these states seem to be, and indeed are, they are not the end. The ego has sacrificed much but not everything. The versatility and tenacity of its regulatory function are the more conclusively demonstrated by the empirical fact that all these syndromes are reversible (with the exception, perhaps, of some of the brain-injury reactions). They are states of disorganization which represent extreme phases of a usually reversible process.

These cases are well advanced, but all tend to recover. The demoralization may recede, the forces favoring reintegration may once again gain the ascendancy, and the evidences of extreme crisis and disorganization may be left behind.

The Fifth Order

A moment ago we spoke optimistically. This is a much needed mood in the field of mental illness, which has been too much permeated by pessimism. Most of the patients we have been describing do recover, or could do so under favorable circumstances. The circumstances not being favorable, many of them do not recover nor do they die; they continue on a plateau of chronic maladjustment or, rather, adjustment at a very low level. In large part this is the consequence of our neglect or our ignorance.

But it is not true of all cases. It cannot be denied that in our present knowledge some patients cannot be helped. In spite of our efforts a few remain disabled. Some get continuously worse until they die. This is a small percentage and it should be still smaller.

But our insistence is that such a termination is not inevitable. Mental illness is not an invasion, but a defensive reaction. Hence it has no natural predetermined course of development, no typical evolution. We repeat: The vast majority of cases improve or recover, even from such serious states of demoralization and disorganization as we have just described. But a small number of them neither get better nor get worse, and a still smaller number will proceed to a still more serious phase, a complete disorganization.

The reader may well ask, what could be worse than what has been described? The desperate stages of illness just considered can scarcely be surpassed. Can personality disintegration reach any further point?

The answer is simple: Yes.

From the biological standpoint death is worse than any kind of life. It is a stage beyond the feeblest and most ineffective survival effort and organization attempt. But is there, short of death, a stage of complete disintegration, representing complete and irreversible ego failure? Can the ego be completely demolished or dethroned or disabled and the organism still survive at a vegetative level?

The answer to this would depend somewhat on how the functioning of the ego is defined. If it is assumed to have any relation to the regulation of physiological functioning, the answer would have to be no. But if the ego is thought of as responsible chiefly for psychological functioning, one could certainly testify that states of bare, insensate existence are to be seen—the individual seems to have little that can be called consciousness, but continues to breathe, to digest, and to excrete incontinently. The condition has been denoted *aphanisis*.

One also sees occasionally the failure of any such plateau, with a progressive diminution of one psychological function after another and then of physiological functions, too, until death supervenes.

Sometimes there is simply a progressive worsening of some of the pictures of illness described previously. Continuous wild excitement with struggling, screaming, pounding, kicking, and fighting develops which is difficult to control with any drug therapy. Death usually follows from exhaustion.

A clinical picture, about which anthropologists know more than psychiatrists, is commonly but awkwardly designated *psychogenic death*. According to the literature this may come about as a result of suggestion, based upon strongly held beliefs, or it can be spontaneous and autonomous. There can be no question that some people can be "scared to death." A kinsman and colleague, Menninger von Lerchenthal [4] of Vienna, has collected instances of this in the literature since 1900. Numerous case reports have also been collected by Simon et al. [5] An early and extraordinarily interesting case history of death from fear was reported by Antonio Benivieni (1443–1502). [6] Our colleague and fellow author Ellenberger, [7] in a paper summarizing the literature, felt he could distinguish three types of acute psychogenic deaths. In central Africa (Congo, Uganda) psychogenic death occurs as a consequence of the infringement of an important taboo. Death occurs rapidly, sometimes in a few hours. In Polynesia psychogenic deaths also occur after the infringement of a taboo, but more slowly. From Australia and Melanesia come numerous accounts of psychogenic deaths occurring rapidly as a result of a curse solemnly performed by a magician. In the African and in the Australian-Melanesian cases, death occurs more rapidly, but can be averted by the intervention of a medicine man, whereas Western medicine is generally ineffective. In the Polynesian type, death seems to be inescapable. A physiological interpretation of acute psychogenic death based on Australian-Melanesian accounts was published by Cannon.[8] Such anthropological instances of psychogenic deaths should be compared with clinical cases from military psychiatry.[9] However, the concept of voodoo death has been vigorously attacked as based upon unreliable reports.[10] *

Mira [11] described an epidemic of "malignant anxiety" in Spain, in which 97 out of 100 persons succumbed to progressive fear:

> They showed anguish, and perplexity rather than fear or excitement; they remained sitting or lying without any spontaneous activity, barely answered questions, except with "Yes" or "No," could scarcely concentrate, but were not very confused; the pulse rate was permanently above 120, and the respirations were 40 or more (in two cases . . . 75 per minute). At first sight they looked like overstrained dogs. The tendon reflexes were much increased; the cutaneous reflexes were exaggerated but were more variable. No focal symptoms were observed. The urine was concentrated and extremely acid, with a peculiar smell.
>
> At the end of the first week, sometimes even earlier, the temperature rose very quickly and the general state became worse. The tongue became ulcerated and blackish; the skin was slightly jaundiced, the abdomen tympanitic. The mental state changed; although the anguish remained, the patient became restless and exhibited an increasing number of automatic movements; carphologia appeared; subsultus tendinum and facial spasms, specially roused by touch, were observed. In almost all cases signs of hypocalcemia were observed. Death occurred after three or four days . . . there was no delirium . . . the cerebrospinal fluid was normal except that the pressure was always increased and no focal symptoms were observed. In some, post-mortem examination showed swelling of the brain and even haemorrhages.

Meerloo [12] tells of death from "sudden panic," which he explains as asphyxiation due to sudden cataleptic rigidity of the muscles of breathing:

> . . . in the spring of 1943 a London shelter was overcrowded, there was a bomb explosion nearby; the electric power failed, lights went out and somebody stumbled on the stairs. There was a sudden upheaval of tremendous fear in the pitch dark; no yelling or crying were heard. When first aid arrived nearly 200 of the 600 people were dead. Post mortems revealed no significant anatomical changes in the victims.

Self-Destruction

The pictures of the terminal phase of progressive and irreversible disorganization just described have in common, presumably, the uncon-

---

* Lambo describes this symptom as widespread in connection with criminal conduct in Africa. (Lambo, T. A.: "Malignant Anxiety." *J. Ment. Sci.* 108:256–264, 1962.)

scious determination to die. Such cases might be said to represent illustrations of a rapid ascendancy of the death instinct. In this sense the Fifth Order of dyscontrol is merely the phase of terminal collapse. There is another way of looking at it. We may think of the Fifth Order level as the greatest extremity to which the ego can be pushed, not in respect to actual death and dissolution, of which the ego can probably not even conceive, but rather in respect to something the ego does perceive as "the farthest out."

What then *is* the most extreme perversion of the life instinct, the most antithetical, the most extreme affliction, as it were, which the ego could exhibit? We submit that this can only be the repudiation of life, the conscious resolution to end it, to effect total self-destruction. When the virtually unquenchable spark of life flickers out in despair, when all hope, need, and effort give way to futility, when the only relief seems to be the ending of all further struggle, then a Fifth Order of disintegration has been reached and death by one's own hand often follows.

Suicide is one of the great paradoxes of human existence. It apparently denies all biological principles; at least, it refutes the most basic one. Until Freud initiated his studies in depth psychology and proposed some hypotheses regarding its motivation, suicide was virtually inexplicable.[18]

Goethe said something to the effect that philosophy was an examination of an attitude toward the phenomenon of death. On this basis suicide, or even the wish to destroy oneself, is almost in itself a terminal reductionistic philosophy. When to the ego the only appropriate behavior seems to be the initiation of a series of events expected to end in self-extermination, the ego has already virtually died.

We should note, however, that actual or attempted suicide is by no means necessarily an indication that dyscontrol has reached the Fifth Order level. To the outside observer suicide plainly demonstrates complete destruction, but to the one attempting suicide the contemplation of suicide may represent other and quite varied things.

The suicidal process (and it *is* a process, a series of acts) is almost always tinctured with elements of the integrative efforts of the ego, and indeed with love and the wish to live and be loved. One can perceive these clearly in the poem just quoted. Perhaps no suicide is ever completely wholehearted, and certainly many of them are less than halfhearted. There can be no doubt that many attempts at self-destruction occur for the purpose of testing a loved one and are accompanied by the fantasy of being rescued as the climax of a grand and noble act.

Everyone who has seen or read about the indecisively inhibited, suicidally inclined individuals who linger upon the edges of roofs [14] or in open windows must have reflected upon the meaning of the extraordinary efforts that are undertaken toward saving such individuals. Perhaps at no other time in their lives have people seemed so interested in them, so concerned, so energetic in their determinations to rescue one who only a few minutes before may have felt utterly unloved and unnoticed.

Although suicide as a gesture must be distinguished from suicidal attempts which are unsuccessful,[15] the great excess of unsuccessful suicidal attempts over "successful" attempts suggests that many of the latter are actually bungled attempts. The wish to *die*, the wish to *kill*, and the wish to *be killed* all enter into suicidal motivation in different proportions, as I have pointed out elsewhere.[16] But none of these is an undisguised representation of the "death instinct."

Meerloo [17] modified and elaborated my proposals [18] regarding the unconscious motivations of suicide into a number of categories based on the inferred meaning of the final act. He subdivides it into suicide as being killed, suicide as killing, suicide as communicating, suicide as getting revenge, suicide as escape, and suicide as magic reversal or transformation.

The subdivisions of some of his categories are especially interesting. Thus suicide as a way of being killed magically is sometimes a self-offering to the gods, sometimes a death sentence after the transgression of a taboo, sometimes a negative magic gesture: "See, they killed me!" As a communication it sometimes says, "I must do as they have done" (especially in the case of familial suicide); or "See how I have suffered"; or "Please, won't you help me, rescue me?"

Suicide is often revenge, i.e., an aggression or partial killing, on those who remain. The survivors all feel to some extent guilty, as no doubt the victim expected. "Now you will be sorry that you were not kinder to me. Remorse will follow you to the grave. The dead exert great power and my death will haunt you." No doubt some such psychology as this entered into the stylized ritual of hara-kiri.

Suicide may be even more aggressive, even an actual murder, as in the famous last act of Samson (more recently repeated by some individuals who take bombs into airplanes and blow themselves and others to pieces). In fantasy, suicide is probably always a psychological murder, a killing of the world or some important person in it—an unfaithful lover, a resented parent, an internalized tormenter, which may be the conscience.

Suicide may be a flight from pain, incurable disease, the threat of helpless senility, or violent death on the gallows. It may be a flight from anticipated rejection or result from a fear of becoming dependent. Or it may be a flight from self-depreciation, feelings of sexual or general inadequacy, humiliation, unknown danger.

We are indebted to Dr. William Simpson of our staff for the following poem written by a fourteen-year-old girl who suffered intensely from depression and despair. She made numerous suicidal attempts, one of which was successful about a year after this poem was written:

> I wandered the streets,
> I was lonely; I was cold.
> Weird music filled the air.
> It grew louder and louder.
> There was no other sound—
> Only weird, terrible music.
>
> I began to run as though I was being chased.
> Too terrified to look back,
> I ran on into the darkness.
> A light was shining very brightly, far away.
>
> I must get to it.
> When I reached the light,
> I saw myself,
> I was lying, on the ground.
> My skin was very white.
> I was dead.

And just as suicide can be a fantasied end, it can also be a fantasied beginning, a magic revival. The death-and-rebirth fantasy represented by suicide has already been mentioned; this may involve joining a dead leader or parent. Thus some suicides are prompted less by despair than by hope. They are poorly chosen techniques for endeavoring to live in spite of the apparent inevitability of death in the ordinary sense, or death in some terrible and fearful representation. These considerations will place this type of suicide in the range of Third Order devices—impulsive, aggressive outbursts—rather than in the Fifth.

But we propose now that there is in the suicidal determination an exposition of that deepest and most incomprehensible yet inevitable characteristic of man, his self-destructiveness. Freud repeatedly emphasized that the manifestations of the self-destructive instinct were never nakedly visible. In the first place, the self-destructive instincts get turned in an outward direction by the very process of life, and in the second place, they get neutralized in the very process of living. Self-destruction in the operational sense is a result of a return, as it were, of the self-destructive tendencies to the original object. It is not *quite* the original object as a rule, because the object of redirected aggression, aggression reflected back upon the self, is usually the body. And since a part of the body may be offered up as a substitute for the whole, this partial suicide, as we have called it, is a way of averting total suicide. But if that part of the body is a vital part, the partial suicide becomes actual suicide. The fantasies involved in the modification described by Meerloo are there, but they are not determinant.

This is not to say anything new. Just as every symptom contains by hypothesis an aggressive element, so one may say that every clinical entity contains a self-destructive element. One authority of such experience, Friedman,[19] goes so far as to say that "there exists no clinical entity in which suicidal *ideas* and *impulses* are absent" (italics ours). For these depend upon vicissitudes of the aggressive instinct. With intuitive understanding of the unconscious, even before Freud had pointed it out, Wilhelm Stekel said in 1910: "No one kills himself who did not want to kill another or, at least, wish death to another." Seven years later Freud commented, "It is this sadism (aggression), and only this, that solves the riddle of the tendency to suicide which makes melancholia so interesting —and so dangerous . . . It is true we have long known that no neurotic harbours thoughts of suicide which are not murderous impulses against others re-directed upon himself, but we have never been able to explain what interplay of forces could carry such a purpose through to execution." [20]

Early in the professional career of the senior author he was impressed with the central position in all psychiatry held by the phenomenon of suicide. It is considered irrational in most cultures; in some societies it is unknown; it is strangely overprevalent in certain very civilized countries. It increases with prosperity. Rationalized as it may be by intellectuals, its occurrence is always somewhat uncanny, incredible, inexplicable. It is a little difficult for survivors to conceive of anyone having been *quite* so hopeless, *quite* so heartless, *quite* so unrealistic. It is, indeed, a last act, an irreparable, irreversible, final blow. Its dreadfulness, its aggressive impact, is felt by relatives and friends and physicians, which, of course was partly its victim's intent.

There are different kinds of suicide—we speak now not of the method used but of the motivation. There are accidental suicides, there are suicides which are substitutes for murder, there are suicides which are a cry for help and suicides which are miscarriages of an attempt to get oneself rescued. But some suicides are also expressions of total despair and ruthlessly directed at one's own self-annihilation. The essence of this ultimate form of suicide is the disintegration of the ego and the overwhelming of the organism with self-directed destructiveness. It is the final and ultimate catastrophe of the organism. It expresses a suffering so terrible, a hopelessness so great, that only one resolution pervades the mind. Dissolution seems the greatest desideratum. It is as if the end were already here, as Emily Dickinson [21] described it:

> I felt a Funeral, in my brain,
> And mourners to and fro
> Kept treading—treading till it seemed
> That sense was breaking through—
>
> And when they all were seated,
> A service, like a drum—
> Kept beating-beating—till I thought
> My mind was going numb—
>
> And then I heard them lift a box
> And creak across my soul
> With those same boots of lead, again,
> Then space—began to toll,
>
> As all the heavens were a bell,
> And Being, but an ear,
> And I, and Silence, some strange race
> Wrecked, solitary, here—
>
> And then a plank in reason broke,
> And I dropped down, and down—
> And hit a World, at every plunge,
> And finished knowing—then—

Recapitulation

This chapter has continued a description of the pictures of dyscontrol begun in a previous chapter. In spite of strenuous efforts to deal with situational stress beyond the powers of its ordinary coping equipment, the ego may not be able to avert a worsening of the situation. A rupture of the ego may occur which permits direct aggressive outlet. This affords the ego temporary relief from pressure, but the external damage done may greatly complicate the situation and add to the ego's burdens. Thus "ruptures"—explosive discharges—may recur over and over.

Rupture does not always occur, and, occurring, it does not always avert further disintegration. The graver states of more severe disorganization have been attention-arresting since the beginning of history because of their striking departure from ordinary behavior patterns. They have gone by a thousand names, but their basic forms or clinical pictures are not many. And, as we have tried to emphasize throughout, they are all variant appearances of one stage of one process, a process continuous with the phenomenon of ordinary everyday human living in a constantly changing world.

CHAPTER XII

Determinants of the Course of Illness

S Y N O P S I S : Patients not only get worse, as has been described; they —usually—get better, sooner or later. Getting better involves a progressive reintegration with the environment, a diminution in internal tension, a disappearance of symptoms and a resumption of adequate self-regulation. There are always forces working for and against this recovery, both internal and external forces, and the changing net balance of their effort determines the course of the illness, i.e., the trend and rate of change. Some of these positive and negative factors are here listed.

FOR CENTURIES, as has been pointed out previously, it was the accepted belief that mental illness led regularly to mental disintegration. To "lose one's mind" implied an irretrievable loss. A living extinction in oblivion was considered the terminus of the "natural history" of nearly all forms of mental illness.

Today we know how absurd this is. The great majority of instances of mental illness reveal themselves as episodes and disappear—some in a matter of days, others after some weeks or even months. True, even with the most intensive treatment, some patients remain ill for years, for a lifetime, but these constitute a very small percentage.

The point implied here by these generalities is that no established "natural course" of mental illness exists. Every instance of mental illness runs a course, to be sure, but this course does not have, in Sydenham's sense, a characteristic predetermined form based on its category.* The progressively more severe pictures described in our chapters on the hierarchy of emergency control measures were intended to describe not a natural history of mental illness, but rather its range and variety.

Some colleagues in refutation will point to the characteristic recurrence, in some individuals, of waves of depression or excitement. But a tendency to recurrence and oscillation does not establish a definitive course of illness. Some cyclothymic patients have severe depressions once in a decade but may have one or two attacks and then not again for

---

* Some physical diseases comply with Sydenham's model, such as measles and cancer; many do not, such as arthritis and diabetes.

thirty years. It is true that some cases show an apparent regularity of recurrence, but even this does not describe any typical or predictable natural history of the syndromes in general.

Process

Here it would almost seem as if we were only saying something which everyone knows. When *The New York Times* [1] reported a recent study [2] showing that 80 per cent of a sample of citizens were aware of some degree of mental illness, it used a small headline. No one is surprised at this amazing statement any more. It has come to be common knowledge. It is no longer a question of, Has he a mental illness? but How much illness has he and what is its trend?

Trend and process have been the chief emphasis of this book. The various orders of dyscontrol which we have described and illustrated are not pigeonholes into which people may be fitted; they are only still photographs of a moving picture of human life. In every individual are potentialities for destructiveness and self-destructiveness, and in every individual there are potentialities for salvage, concern, growth, and creativity. The ceaseless struggle between these opposing trends occupies all the energies of our lives. One could say there were all degrees of failure, but one could also see these as all degrees of success. It is an act of faith which will win. There is no question where our hopes lie, and hence our sympathies and our responsibility.

If the phenomena of human life are looked at in this way, psychiatry passes from being a science of classifying and name-calling into a discipline of counsel for the maximizing of the potentialities of the individual and the improvement of social happiness.

Mental illness, being an aspect and phase of the course of a human life, fluctuates and varies with the ebb and flow of living. Sometimes the disruptive process rushes on breathlessly, frighteningly; sometimes it vanishes into thin air; again, it seems to grind to a stalemate stop, to cease moving entirely in a state of chronic dissatisfaction. Now rest is not the natural state of affairs in the universe. Atoms, molecules, planets, and suns keep moving; so do the processes of life, *and* of mental illness, even when they appear motionless. And while we cannot always predict the ultimate direction and degree of movement, as we can with planets, we have learned to detect the *trend* of an illness process *toward* recovery or —temporarily—*away* from it.

"Recovery" is an ambiguous word. It is sometimes used to describe a continuing trend toward improvement; this is the recovery process. The end state of that process is also called recovery, the condition of a person *after* having been sick, and now sick no more.

When illness is essentially the reaction to invasion by a noxious foreign body, the elimination of this invasion initiates a trend toward recovery and resumption of the "normal" state of affairs, save for the permanent damage done to the structures. The normal processes held in abeyance by the illness are once more activated in full flow. The patient begins to walk and to work; he feels first "better" and then "all right" again, and after a confirmatory period of observation we say that he has "recovered."

But if the disease is not an invasion or wound so much as an accumulation of mismanagements and emergency compromises, recovery appears somewhat differently. We assume that a *relatively* * effective and comfortable pattern of adjustment has been surrendered or compromised by various emergency arrangements, some of them very expensive, to insure survival. The illness is in the nature of a strategic retreat, hence the first "step" in the recovery process is in precisely the opposite direction from "recovery." Thereafter, we expect the course of illness to fluctuate, sometimes appearing to recede and sometimes to proceed. Reintegration and reconstitution of the organism tend to occur *pari passu* with the compromises and regressions necessary in making the best of a bad situation. Thus it is more accurate to speak of an "illness-recovery process" to indicate our recognition of the fact that *recovery is still illness and illness is, from the start, recovery.*

Many years ago the philosopher Schelling expressed this concept of conflict-in-balance in these eloquent words: "In every single body attracting and repelling forces are necessarily in balance. But this necessity is only felt in contrast with the possibility that this balance will be disturbed. . . . If the secret of nature lies in its ability to maintain opposite forces in balance and in a continuous never-decided battle, then these same forces, as soon as one of them achieves a continuous gain, must destroy the very condition which they produced in an earlier phase." [3]

In describing the extraordinary care with which a disastrous airplane accident was investigated, Morton Hunt [4] cites the director of the Bureau of Safety of the Civil Aeronautics Bureau as saying: "In most cases of

---

* Of course our whole thesis is that few people are completely effective and comfortable *all* the time, and that many are far from it. We shall discuss this "starting point" versus "end point" later. But for schematic presentation we must postulate a *relatively* high starting level.

pilot error, we've found that it has taken six, seven, or even more unfavorable circumstances, all working together, to cause the accident. If any single one of them had not been working against the pilot, he would have recognized and corrected his situation in time—which, I suspect, is just what happens all the time in normal flights, *and in our daily lives*" (italics ours).

He was speaking of airplane accidents. He might well have been speaking of mental illness. In most instances there is a dominance of self-righting factors, and the patient *does* recover. Sometimes there is concatenation of "unfavorable circumstances" and a plane goes down.

Detection of Change

A clinical illustration will assist the reader to visualize this dynamic concept of recovery. Let him picture in his mind a severely ill patient—a man, let us say, who had been hale and hearty but who had progressively declined in efficiency, productivity, and sense of well-being. As he became more and more erratic and uncomfortable, he made strange remarks and seemed to be increasingly withdrawn and inaccessible. He was taken to a hospital, where his confusion and helplessness at first deepened. With help he could be gotten to dress himself in the morning, but he would then sit about his room vacantly or go walking with the nurse silently like an automaton.

Let us assume that some weeks have passed during which energetic treatment efforts have been pursued with little perceptible effect. Then, one day, a slight difference is observed. When the nurse approaches him in simple greeting or in food service, or merely in passing, the patient nods. Perhaps he even smiles faintly or whispers, "Thank you."

Next it may be noticed that his face seems more relaxed and less vacuous. There is less stiffness in his posture. He looks about him inquiringly.

In the days to follow, if the upward trend continues steadily, he is progressively brighter and more alert. He seems to notice more things and to take a slight interest in some of them. He smiles frequently now and speaks words of response to greetings instead of returning silent stares. He moves about more, and with less aimlessness. He listens to other patients and occasionally even addresses questions to them.

He begins to express wishes to do certain things or to go certain places. Sometimes it is necessary to refuse these requests, and the disappointment may be followed by a recession lasting some days, or even longer.

His physician may be obliged to be out of town briefly, and his substitute is not welcomed by the patient, who retreats further. He may express considerable peevish or even bitter resentment.

But this mood passes and again there begins a slow but definite turning toward a reacceptance of reality. This is usually a halting, wistful approach rather than a vigorous striking out, although the latter may occur, even literally. However, even a blow is sometimes a frantic effort to recapture or re-establish a relationship with the real world.*

Along with these efforts to find us and to communicate with us and to interact with us—"us" of the world about them—patients progressively relinquish various of the peculiarities symptomatic of their illness. They begin to eat and sleep better, to converse, to be more alert to changes in the environment, and to be able to turn their attention to things without distraction or confusion. Emotional reactions become increasingly appropriate and hence more flexible, so that demeanor and behavior conform more and more to general social standards.

These successive replacements of emergency regulatory devices with less and less costly ones are not all there is to recovery. It is also necessary for the patient to "climb back up" to the levels of functioning and productivity which were surrendered with the development of his illness. As his interest in the world about him increased, the patient we have been describing found increasing pleasure in being with people (instead of the reverse) and then in *doing* with them. He showed an increasing desire to express his energy usefully or in ways approved by his peers, by his friends, and by his doctor, to exercise his skill—or perhaps even his awkwardness—to paint something or make something or grow something or learn something.

The recovering patient thus extends more and more tentacles into new sources or possible sources of satisfaction. In doing so he expresses both his commonality with the fellow human beings about him and his uniqueness. He wants to do some of the things others do. He wants to play with them, and in playing he wants, sometimes, to win. He wants to work with them, and he wants to do some things better than they. He finds increasing pleasure both in the giving of pleasure to others and in the

---

* Dr. Bruno Bettelheim has described an immobile, emaciated, and dehydrated child of seven, who after she had been in his school a few days "began to eat bits of food. Then she began to respond to an unplanned game. Her counselor, while putting raisins into the child's mouth, dropped some on the bedspread. The child picked them up and ate them; it was the first time in four years she had fed herself. The game continued until the child resented being fed, and fought anyone who tried it. Her therapists rejoiced." (*The New York Times*, May 8, 1960.)

receiving of deserved approval. He can even give approval to others, and to himself.

Thus he begins to give and take, earn and spend, work and play, live and let live—all with a favorable trade balance and an increasing *joie de vivre*. He "feels better," life seems more "worth living." There is a prevalent mood of optimistic expectation about the future which we can perhaps call hope. This sketches in descriptive terms the course of illness of a hypothetical patient with emphasis upon the recovery phase.

It is difficult to describe the course of any illness precisely, partly because we are handicapped by a lack of terms and our expressions of "much" improvement and "little" improvement sound vague and inexact to scientists who desire more precision. Terms commonly used in clinical reports such as "movement," "structural shift," "reconstitution," "coming along," and "working through," imply various models and employ various metaphors which may or may not convey definite information to one who is not in communicational tune, as it were, with the writer or speaker. With the aid of this jargon, the therapist is trying to tell us something that he feels about his patient, something that he thinks he perceives in respect to the changes occurring in his patient. But it is easy to be misled by one's own hopes, and even easier to be betrayed by one's own inarticulateness at the very moment one thinks one is being precise.*

The oversimplicity of the sample case given partially obscures the value and the need of precision of language in describing the course of illness and the levels reached in the recovery process. It is an "ideal" case; it represents a *frequent* course of recovery, but by no means the only one or perhaps the most frequent. There usually occur many ups and downs, many falterings, slight or greater recessions, fast or slow movements in one direction or another with arrival at various temporary "resting places" along the way.

Compare this with an interesting analysis of the "process of becoming

* One of the achievements of our Psychotherapy Research Project at The Menninger Foundation is a development of certain definite clinical criteria in place of these vague phrases. (The Psychotherapy Research Project of The Menninger Foundation. "Rationale, Method, and Sample Use: First Report." *Bull. Menninger Clin.*, 20:221–278, 1956. Article IV. "Concepts." Robert S. Wallerstein and Lewis L. Robbins, pp. 239–262. The Psychotherapy Research Project of The Menninger Foundation. "Second Report." *Bull. Menninger Clin.* 22:115–116, 1958. Article II. "Treatment Variables." Lester Luborsky, Michalina Fabian, Bernard H. Hall, Ernst Ticho, Gertrude R. Ticho, pp. 126–147. Article III. "Situational Variables." Helen D. Sargent, Herbert C. Modlin, Mildred T. Faris, Harold M. Voth, pp. 148–166. Wallerstein, Robert S. "The Problem of the Assessment of Change in Psychotherapy." *Int. J. Psa.* 44:31–44, 1963.

chronic" made by two colleagues.[5] They start out with the individual who becomes ill. His symptoms may or may not be noticed by his family and friends. If unnoticed, the symptoms may eventually disappear; if they are noticed, something is apt to be done about them. Indeed, two things can be done. The behavior can be "accepted" by the family and friends and allowed to get worse or get better of its own accord or on the basis of the patient's own action. Or the symptoms of illness may be handled in the logical scientific way and the patient brought to the attention of a doctor (or perhaps the police).

Then *three* things can happen: (a) He can begin a treatment relationship with a doctor, remaining an outpatient and presumably trying to work. (b) He can enter a hospital for total treatment. (c) He can reject all treatment and stay (or run) away from medical help.

Let us assume that he enters the hospital. Again, he may receive treatment, improve, be discharged, and go home, or he may receive treatment but show minimal improvement and remain hospitalized.

In other words, just as in the Army cases, some patients seem to make a turnabout after various levels of regression have been reached and a certain low point touched. The illness trend sometimes remains at any of several plateaus, then heads downward, sometimes upward. The physician looks hopefully for changes in the direction of trend, especially those toward improvement. But, from the technical standpoint, he is just as interested in the turning points preceding a worsening.

The recovery process is an aspect of the illness process, and of as much interest to the physician as the development phase. Recovery is something we expect, and we take it into account in our diagnostic appraisal. We assess the potential for recovery, and the forces favoring or obstructing it. To do this, we need to have a feel for the essence of the recovery process, whether we call it "resilience" or the "synthetic function of the life instinct" or the "self-regulating equilibrations of an organism geared biologically to optimal survival." Something happens, we do not always know what; the trend of the process changes its direction.

The Turning Point

In the revised edition of our *Manual of Psychiatric Case Study* [6] we have shown how graphs could be drawn describing the course of any particular psychiatric illness and its quantitative changes over measured periods of time. Such graphs bring out vividly those critical moments in the course of an illness when there is a definitive change in the direction or in the speed of change of the process. All physicians and many laymen are familiar with the dramatic, climactic course of lobar pneumonia.

It is always a temptation to ascribe a change in the direction of an illness process to some event conspicuously contiguous in time or space. This or that preceding event is so easily the "explanation." But it is the perennial duty of the scientist to be slow in accepting the "truth" of the obvious. We speak of the "precipitating events" related to an illness with a tacit recognition that this implies a readiness of the organism for the sudden appearance of an imminent, if previously invisible, adventitious phenomenon. Similarly, when an illness improves, what we describe as the effective "curative" factor is usually only one of many which brought about the favorable shift.

The deceptive conclusion of *post hoc ergo propter hoc* is the more baffling because it is not always wrong. The "*straw* that breaks the camel's back" may actually weigh a ton. A cup of water may start a process of recovery not through correcting dehydration, but because the giving of a cup of water may have a powerful symbolic effect.* The element of magic is always present and it is powerful. "Our medicines," wrote Father Joseph LeMercier, who was present in an epidemic among the Huron Indians in 1637, "produced effects which dazzled the whole country, and yet I leave you to imagine what sort of medicines they were! A little bag of senna served over 50 persons; and they asked us for it on every side. . . ." [7]

All of us have seen seemingly intractable conditions in patients over whom we have labored long and hard yield promptly to the casual attention of a new group of doctors. Over the years I can recall numerous patients who were given the very best treatment we could give them, and after the relatives had become completely discouraged, and resigned to the probability that their loved one would never get well, they removed the patient to another—often much less comfortable or energetic—hospital, where he promptly recovered!

Such cases have frequently been reported in the literature. Schwartz [8] described three severely ill patients who were given much treatment without benefit and then more or less neglected for a period of time; thereupon they improved and even recovered. This author suggests that some patients resent the efforts of other people to make them well and may

---

* Cf. the scene at the well in Lew Wallace's novel *Ben Hur* (New York: Harper, 1922).

be rebelling against this coercion. Hence, when abandoned to hopelessness, such patients become aware of the necessity for self-help and if motivation for recovery is powerful enough, the ego seems to find the needed strength.

The daughter of a friend of mine was treated in our hospital for several years, and it was very sad to have to tell him month after month that she was no better. The physicians became very discouraged with her lack of progress and finally told the father that she was hopeless and should be removed to a custodial institution. He came in some distress to see me about this verdict. I told him that I did not quite agree with the opinion of my colleagues and certainly did not approve of their using the word "hopeless." I said I could not deny the fact, however, that his daughter was showing no positive response to anything that we did and was actually getting worse. Reluctantly he removed her to a small, adequate private sanitarium where good care but no particular treatment would be given. It was expected by all that she would remain there the rest of her life.

Less than a year later I had occasion to be visiting in the city where her father lived and expected to be met at the railroad station by him. Imagine my astonishment when, instead of him, the patient herself turned up, driving the car that was to convey me to their home. She laughed heartily at my amazement and assured me that she was well now —and was a good driver. She thanked me for having helped to accomplish this by moving her to a place where she had had "no one but myself to depend upon." The implication that she would not be *made* to recover against her "will," as it were, is a disturbing one to most physicians, although some have emphasized that every patient has a "right to remain ill." [9]

Such cases make us keenly aware of the necessity for appraising as accurately as we can all the factors which enter into the resultant change, and, of course, all the factors which oppose it. Let us cite another illustration,[10] one which occurred on a rather large scale and upon which some systematic research was done.*

In June 1940, during the German invasion of France, a psychiatric hospital (La Charité-sur-Loire) was in the direct line of the German advance. Preparations were made for evacuating this institution. A special commission of psychiatrists screened all the patients, and all those who

---

* We are indebted to our colleague and former associate Henri Ellenberger for this vignette.

were only moderately ill were sent back to their families. The severe and supposedly incurable cases were retained in the hospital. At the last moment, when everything was ready for the evacuation of this final group to the south of France, news came that all bridges had been destroyed. Panic ensued. Nurses, aides, and patients fled.

After several days order was re-established, but 153 "incurables" were missing. A few of them were later recaptured; but four or five years later a special commission was appointed by the French government to find out just what had happened to the others. *Thirty-seven per cent of them had re-established themselves in various communities—presumably "recovered."*

Paradoxical Cure

External events may have a paradoxical effect upon the course of illness. The most favorable circumstances, the most assiduous treatment, the most felicitous environment, and the most persistent efforts may all prove unavailing. On the other hand, a most unlikely move or event sometimes presages a recovery.

Intercurrent illness sometimes has a beneficial effect upon the course of another illness, for example, malaria upon paresis, foreign protein reactions on arthritis, hyperinsulinism upon various psychiatric conditions. Such observations date back to Hippocrates and his immediate successors, who held long discussions on such matters as the healing effect of hemorrhoids.[11] Other writers have reported the beneficial effects on various illnesses, especially mental illness, of many different affections. During the influenza epidemic of 1918–1920 (and in many previous epidemics) psychiatric patients with mental illness were frequently observed to improve mentally during and after their attacks of influenza. My personal experience with some of these cases was unforgettably impressive.[12] *

---

* For example, a child of four was seen at a school for mental deficiency. She had been studied by a competent staff (and seen, after her remarkable change, by many visiting colleagues). Her American-born, college-bred parents had brought her to this school because, although her physical development corresponded with her age (four years), her mental development was then estimated to correspond with that of an infant of ten months. Details of her birth history and early infancy are recorded elsewhere (Menninger, Karl A. "Influenza and Hypophrenia." *J.A.M.A.*, 75:1044–1051 [October 16] 1920) and, together with psychiatric and psychological examination details, will be passed over here. She was observed and cared for in this institution for a year without significant change.

Fourteen months after admission she was severely ill with influenza, plus broncho-

These paradoxical cures by the worse-added-to-worse method make us somewhat uncomfortable—supporting, as they might seem to do, the various cruel, startling, and unpleasant methods of treating the mentally ill in ages past. They are the very antithesis of the (to us) more logical procedure of tempering the wind to the shorn lamb, of nursing, soothing, supporting, and encouraging the afflicted. They point up the complexity of the illness process, in which we are never able to identify all of the determining factors. We cannot be sure in advance how effective an interposed measure, a well-reasoned intervention, may be. The influence of influenza is more apt to be deleterious than helpful, but the reverse can happen; the influence of a sympathetic friend or a book or an operation is apt to be good, but it may be the reverse.

This digression regarding the paradoxical cure was introduced to emphasize the risk of attributing a cure to a certain supposedly beneficent effort or event bearing a close chronological relationship to the shift in the course of illness. We like to believe that, in most cases, treatment efforts made by the physician assist in determining a turning point. But many times the turning point occurs after most unpropitious and even inexplicably related events. Some patients get well for reasons that are extremely obscure, and some patients remain ill for reasons equally obscure.

But it is not all obscurity. We do understand, *in part*, the process of favorable change and propose now to submit some reflections about its determination.

Which Miracle?

If illness be viewed as an alteration in regulation produced by dynamic factors, recovery will be seen as a further alteration in the regulation of the same factors, brought about by some change in the constellation, internal and external. New sources of energy become available, fearsome threats disappear or lose their power, forces in conflict come unblocked,

---

pneumonia and empyema. A long convalescence followed. During this convalescence from the infection she began to show marked evidences of mental awakening! Her automatic purposeless movements disappeared, she took an interest in things about her, became tidy for the first time, learned to dress and feed herself, and participated in kindergarten activities. In six months her intelligence quotient went from 27 to 40; a year later it was 52, two years later it was 68. Her mental age, in other words, increased more rapidly than her chronological age. At eight years of age (1922) she had reached a mental age of nearly six, was doing first-grade work, and was removed from the state school to a public school.

aggressive energies find harmless and even constructive outlets, latent resources are tapped and exploited, the emergency devices cease to be necessary.

But why does this not happen to every sick patient? Is recovery or chronicity the norm? Is change or inertia the more fundamental? Do we not generally assume that health is normal? Why should there ever be an unnecessary persistence of symptoms and illness in this fine world? When the storm passes, the sun comes out; why need symptoms remain when the illness-producing stress has disappeared?

The opposite paradox is equally impressive. Why should the organism exchange a safe position of retreat for a dangerous position of advance? Is not the bird in the hand worth two in the bush? Is it not possible that by giving up the safety of regression, expensive as it is, one may loose powerful and uncontrollable forces so disintegrative that all the king's horses and all the king's men would never get Humpty-Dumpty together, again? Our colleagues of a generation ago considered recovery from mental illness exceptional, a minor miracle. Why *should* one recover?

An economic-dynamic theory can explain how and why emergency measures come into being, and how and why they are—in some cases—gradually abandoned in favor of more efficient and stable steady states. Can it also explain why they are sometimes not abandoned, why the illness persists despite favorable circumstances and therapeutic efforts?

We think it can. We see illness and the maintenance of symptoms as a phase of life, a way of living in the presence of many opposing difficulties. It is an extremity to which the organism is pushed and must await release by overbalancing pressures in the other direction.

In our studies of reactions to combat stress in World War II [13] previously referred to, we were very much impressed with the way in which a set of forces began a phase of great stress and simultaneously aroused certain opposing forces which helped to maintain a balance. Then came more stress and more defense. Gradually the stresses seemed to become greater than the defenses, so that there occurred a lowering of achievement level, a partial retreat, the employment of emergency regulatory devices, evidences of threatened disorganization, and then, usually recourse to medical aid.

With sedation and a few hours of rest many of these individuals were able to resume their former efficiency and return to the battle. Heroic and admirable as it was, this was not too difficult to explain. But other individuals had the same treatment and were not able to return to the front lines. Their symptoms persisted. This too we could understand:

more time was required, more rest, more recuperation, further removal from the imminence of renewed combat stress.

But now comes the enigma. Many of these patients were sent back to the base hospital for care, nursing, protection, rest, and treatment. We saw some of them there, later. Many had improved or were improving; some had returned to duty (but usually not to combat duty). What impressed us most was that some of them were not better; they were under treatment of sorts, but they were worse. There was, for them, no more battle stress, no more physical exertion and deprival, no more threat of death. There was not even any considerable probability of further duty assignment. Bright, or at least safe and comfortable, situations lay ahead for them. Why did not the symptoms disappear?

In analyzing the nature of the stress they had undergone, we began to realize this was different from what would appear on the surface. In the beginning these men had experienced fear, fatigue, resentment, hunger, cold, and other things. But they were sustained, there, by many things, too: self-respect, pride-idealism, courage, devotion to duty, training, and habituation to routine. Moreover, there was a strong support from relations with comrades and officers and units. The sudden increment of stress which precipitated the symptoms was frequently the loss of one of these human supports by death or transfer. In other instances cumulative fatigue seemed to be the most important factor.

For these men, then, who did not respond to battalion-aid-station treatment, the nature of the stress had changed; but it did not diminish quantitatively as the casual observer might have assumed. The threat of danger was gone, true, but so were the excitement and the routine activity. The weariness was gone, true, but so was the companionship of fellow soldiers. The unpleasant physical conditions were corrected, but in their place was the guilt feeling of abandoning one's comrades and the fear of accusation of cowardice. Painfully disturbing was the dilemma that if one mastered his distress he would be sent back to duty, but if one admitted it he would be retired. A retirement could be cleared of all tincture of suspected cowardice only if it took the form of something called sickness. Efficient warfare and humane medical science are antithetical, and sooner or later the antithesis shows up in the individual.

This balance of pros and cons is present in every illness. Forces which favor a restitution of the ego's best control and the organism's highest efficiency are opposed by forces which oppose this restoration. Let us consider some of these antithetical pressures in general terms, beginning with some of the pro-illness factors.

Internal Forces Working against Recovery

Alien wishes to remain ill, to handicap and cripple oneself, to exult secretly in suffering, and to avoid measures leading to recovery are detectable in every illness. The assumption prevails that what we call health, that relatively comfortable, relatively effective, and socially tolerable way of existence, is "just naturally" what everyone wants. If someone does not want it he is unnatural ("neurotic," "masochistic," "perverse," "psychopathic," and so forth).* Freud coined a special word for the opposition erected by every patient against the work of his physician; he called it "resistance." Something within the patient resists change for the better. This resistance is supplemented and supported by many and diverse secondary gains, which may overrule the importance of suffering. Perhaps resistance represents the psychological equivalent of the physical concept of inertia. The many ways in which it is manifested constitute much of the content of any systematic description of psychotherapy.

The phenomenon of resistance is one of the central topics of psychoanalytic theory and psychoanalytic practice. I have written at some length about this in another book, from which I should like to quote now; [14] that book was designed for students of psychoanalysis, and this technical point should, in our opinion, be more widely and generally known about.

> . . . When we say that Freud "discovered" resistance we mean that he brought to the attention of physicians that in psychological medicine resistance is a factor which cannot be ignored and which can be dealt with in certain ways. Experienced clinicians have known for thousands of years that something in patients under treatment seems to impel them to work

---

* Even in a progressive, therapeutic hospital, the very process of being considered a patient is charged with conflictual meanings and expectancies: the patient is expected to want treatment, and he is also considered to be unable to want this, on account of his failures to maintain adequate reality contact. When within the hospital the patient's aberrant behavior is politely accepted without retaliation or scorn, he becomes alarmed that he might not be considered seriously ill, and must therefore show proof that he *is* sick! He carries with him an image of the outside world which requires him to justify his seeking help within by demonstrating that he needs it, i.e., displaying certain manifestations of what the public calls "illness." When he shows "normal" behavior as a part of recovery processes, he feels that he is losing his right to patienthood from the point of view of the public. In K. T. Erikson's words: "He is left in the exposed position of one who has to *look* incompetent even while learning to become the exact opposite." (Erikson, K. T. "Patient Role and Social Uncertainty—a Dilemma of the Mentally Ill." *Psychiatry*, 20:263–274, 1957.) The social role of the "mental patients" is exceedingly unstable and conflict-laden, and in the search for greater structure and stability of that role the patient must often give in to his illness and perpetuate his unhealthiness.

against the efforts of the physician to cure them. But the traditional attitude of medicine throughout the centuries has been to ignore this opposition, to treat it with equanimity, as Osler said in his classical essay. The dentist does not lose patience with a man whose tooth has stopped aching after an emergency appointment has been arranged. The (good) surgeon does not get angry with a screaming child who dreads the lance. But the reluctance of such patients to accept treatment is ascribed to fear, in the hands of which they are considered helpless. But Freud showed us that resistance is more than fear, that it is a force related perhaps to the inertia discovered by Newton to reside in all matter, a reluctance to change position. The suffering patient submitting himself to our profession at no mean expense in time, pain, and money seems to be demonstrating how much he wants to get well. But there are always indications that he is a man divided against himself and that he does not *wholly* want to get well! He also wants to stay sick! Freud's genius was reflected in his discovery that this paradox has deep meaning, that the conflict is of the essence and not a mere complicating nuisance, and that the intelligence is our best weapon against it. . . .

In [a famous essay] Freud [15] listed five types of resistance. The first of them he called *repression resistance*, which comes from the persistent, automatic, normative tendency of the ego to try to control dangerous tendencies by blocking them off. The ego has the habit, so to speak, of solving its problems in this way as far as possible, and it resists the process of "free thought" and ventilation of preconscious memories lest the change upset the homeostatic balance and permit the emergence of *dangerous* tendencies. It is the ego's lifelong "business" (in part) to hold back certain things from expression, and this is automatically extended to the analytic situation, especially when the expression of previously repressed impulses (as distinguished from *suppressed* material) becomes likely to occur.

The second of the types of resistance listed by Freud is *transference resistance*. I should prefer to call it *frustration resistance* or *revenge resistance*. It expresses the patient's resentment at not getting from the analyst (as a representation of an earlier figure) the expected response; it bespeaks the mounting frustration and anger of this disappointment. It is as if such a patient were sulking or, to put it more urbanely, as if he had become less eager to try to please the analyst, and almost too angry to want to tell him anything.

Third, there is the *epinosic gain resistance*, which has to do with the reluctance of the ego to give up the advantages that have accrued to the patient as a whole as a result of an illness. These secondary gain resistances are related to the repression resistance just mentioned, but are more superficial; they are more recently acquired devices rather than lifelong habits of action and lie predominantly in the conscious and preconscious.

The fourth variety of resistance listed by Freud emanates, he believed, from the Id; he called it *repetition compulsion resistance*. It was the last to be discovered. As Freud put it, "We find that even after the ego has decided to relinquish its resistances, it still has difficulty in undoing the repressions," despite the rewards and advantages we have (by inference) promised the ego if *it* will give up *its* resistances (the three types just listed). This period of strenuous effort which the ego makes following its decision to relinquish them is called *working-through*. This is carried on against the resistance of the repetition compulsion, "the attraction exerted by the unconscious prototypes upon the repressed instinctual process." This form of resistance is related to the self-destructive principle which operates behind the ego, as Freud put it in *Beyond the Pleasure Principle*.

Fifth, there is the resistance which emanates *from the superego*, deriving from a need for punishment. This may be a socialized form of the preceding type, but one which is very characteristic of human beings in our culture and era. "I do not deserve to get well; it is fitting that I should suffer [*some*]." This is the inexpedient but partially effective way in which guilt feelings are atoned for and kept in a kind of spurious balance which resists change.

To summarize, Freud suggested that there is resistance derived from unconscious fear (repression resistance); there is resistance derived from disappointed expectations in the analysis (transference resistance); there is resistance derived from inertia, false prudence, and short-sighted opportunism (secondary gain resistance); there is resistance derived from self-directed aggression on the basis of a deep biological pattern (repetition compulsion resistance); and there is resistance derived from the feeling that one should suffer (superego resistance).

Another type of resistance is seen in the "acting out" aspects of forgotten episodes of earlier life without being able to remember them. One remembers not in words but in behavior. "He repeats it without of course knowing that he is repeating it." [16] This we described in the clinical section of the present book, where we said that symptoms instituted as emergency devices to insure survival may become incorporated into the character structure. They are treasured for obscure reasons after the original need for them has disappeared and become the "ego-tolerated" traits. Then they tend to continue their own necessity, as it were, as in the case of alcohol addiction.

Another form of resistance derives from secondary narcissism, i.e., self-pity and preoccupation, which begins as a protective ointment on the wounds of frustration and loss and injured pride, but may become a coat of insulation about the individual, thus interfering with the establishment of effective therapeutic relationships as well as social and love-object attachments.

Thus there are many ways to fight off help and all sorts of rationalizations for it. We are too proud, we are too strong, we are going to be all right in a few weeks, we do not want to give in. We have very important things to do, we do not want to hurt someone's feelings, we do not want to become dependent upon the help.

As I write these words, I have before me the morning paper reporting that a fifty-seven-year-old man, a man of some importance, committed suicide yesterday because he had been depressed recently and "feared that he might be obliged to enter an institution for treatment." What did this mean? Certainly not what it says. This man knew hospitals are not that bad. He need have had no fear of disgrace, for his friends knew that he was subject to severe depressions and would have respected him for getting proper treatment for them. Prisoners we examine often declare that they would rather be executed than "called nuts" and spared on the basis of mental incompetence and subjected to psychiatric treatment. Think of the paradox: thousands of people in queues and on waiting lists seeking psychiatric treatment, while others, who need it no less, prefer some form of violent death to the undertaking of treatment aimed at their betterment.

Seen in this way, resistance as an internal force working against recovery is *de facto* self-destructive. It would be a mistake, however, to dismiss all resistance as arising directly from the "death instinct," i.e., from deep instinctual self-destructive trends. These trends undergo many vicissitudes before they finally appear in the self-destructive direction of resistance.

Some resistance, including some of the examples just cited, can be seen as the realistic consequences of ignorance or of unrealistic fear. The typical example of this can be seen in the way a child jerks his hand away from a mother who is endeavoring to remove a splinter from his finger. Misinterpretations of reality may be based on ignorance, upon misinformation, or upon an adverse conditioning dependent upon early childhood experiences. The effect of the latter may persist throughout a lifetime unless some kind of re-education or "de-conditioning" occurs. The child reared by a devout Christian Science mother can easily come to have an attitude toward all physicians which is just as pathological as that of the child whose mother died despite the efforts of a good physician, leaving an orphan who attributed death to something the physician did to her mother. In both instances the child will probably never feel "right" toward doctors nor see objectively the benefits of medical science. These early experiences deflect the course of a patient's life in a way similar to what might happen to a ship near whose compass someone had placed or unwittingly dropped a magnet. The "unwittingly" element in the illustration will reflect the fact that in many instances the individual guilty of consistent misjudgment in regard to certain matters has completely forgotten the events which gave rise to his bias. Chronic difficulties with authority, with responsibility, with married life, with social obligations, and, indeed, with all kinds of life roles, tend to arise upon the basis of just such long-hidden misdirections.

The consequence of such misdirection has to be distinguished from more direct expressions of aggressive or reflected aggressive intent. That there is a latent capacity in all of us to extend a measure of hospitality to these deep self-destructive trends can scarcely be doubted. It is an unpleasant thing to face and we like to shut our eyes to it, as Freud did in his earlier years of theory-construction. Later he faced it and described and defined it. It is there for anyone to see or, rather, to clearly infer. Self-destructive trends rarely appear in the nude, as it were; they are apt to be disguised, or at least thinly clad, and to some extent denatured. But they ride freely on the backs of many tolerated practices—alcoholism, gambling, asceticism, martyrdom, fanaticism, speeding, sexual perversions and excesses, and a great many forms of physical affliction.

In such forms as those mentioned the self-destructive pattern is obvious, especially if attention is directed to it, and its opposition to recovery and to efforts made toward achieving recovery is always considerable. But in addition to the obvious, one must accustom one's eyes to looking for fluctuating, evanescent, disguised manifestations of the same thing, sometimes acute, sometimes chronic. Especially is this important in the appraisal of illness. In seeking to identify the internal forces working against recovery one must ever be on the lookout for these traitorous elements in the personality.

External Factors Working against Recovery

The emphasis of the preceding pages has been on the *internal* forces which work against recovery. In bringing these forward we have not meant to minimize the external burdens and bruises of life,

> The slings and arrows of outrageous fortune . . .
> The heartache and the thousand natural shocks
> That flesh is heir to . . .
> . . . the whips and scorns of time,
> The oppressor's wrong, the proud man's contumely
> The pangs of despis'd love, the law's delay,
> The insolence of office and the spurns
> That patient merit of the unworthy takes. . . .

Shakespeare was true to life, as always, when he had Hamlet list not only big things, but little things which add up. Undoubtedly the great majority of external difficulties are adequately coped with *most* of the time by most people. But hope deferred maketh the heart sick, and naggings and goadings and minor wounds and chronic irritations can have a cumulative effect.

In the early days of psychiatry it was a presumption that a specific mental illness could be ascribed to specific causes. These causes were usually painful pressures of some kind—the loss of a friend, a great fright, anxiety of impending bankruptcy. Sometimes the cause was not an event or experience, but rather a kind of behavior, which today we would regard as symptomatic rather than etiologic. Examples of this taken from actual hospital records are: "overwork," "excessive dieting," "intense love affair," "masturbation," "sleeplessness." These are good examples to indicate how difficult it is to distinguish the pressures which are most responsible for increasing the tension and the pressures which are most sharply felt or which the outside observers think ought to be or probably are more strongly felt. It is important to realize that the disturbances of equilibrium do not always come from the tragic and painful blows which have been referred to. Unexpected bonanzas, sudden success, attractive temptation, inappropriate reward—these may be equally devastating. In other words, what appears to be good luck may, from the standpoint of its effects, be very bad luck indeed.

A lawyer of my acquaintance had established a good practice and was well known not only for his professional abilities but for his wide interests in social and cultural affairs of the community. He carried on a lifelong feud with one of his wife's relatives upon whom he actually had no claim whatsoever and whom he rarely saw. When this relative died she left a large bequest to the patient's wife, which was equivalent to giving it to the patient. He immediately went into a decline. He began worrying as to whether or not the title to the property was really clear, whether all the inheritance taxes had been properly paid, whom he should lease it to. At the same time he began complaining to his wife of weakness and shortness of breath. He stopped going to his office and walked restlessly about the house, depressed and occupied with obsessive thoughts which were in no conscious way related to the bad feelings he had always had toward his benefactor.

Another instance: A younger man, the son of a stern, ultra-conservative banker, joined the Army, partly perhaps to get away from his not too happy home. He did well in military life but was offered a good business opportunity and resigned to accept it. He bought a subsidiary plant which rapidly increased in value, and this he sold for a large profit. Almost immediately he began to have anxiety attacks which increased in severity until he was completely incapacitated and hospitalized.

Sometimes happy occasions, such as a marriage or a family reunion or a trip to Europe, will precipitate a mental illness in what seems to be a most paradoxical way. But it is not paradoxical if we remember that all change is difficult and changes involving considerable shifts in the pattern of interpersonal relationships are particularly taxing. And, as we pointed out in an earlier section of the book, the margin of safety, the degree of elasticity and resilience of the ego, varies greatly in different individuals. What we can always be sure of is that the precipitating event is not the whole story, indeed, not half the story. Increments of responsibility, pain, reaction to loss, frustration, physical illness, disappointment, accident— all these things add up, mostly in secret, to burdens for the ego. When these have been reacted to by what we call illness, by the special adaptive devices that we have described, the pain does not necessarily disappear nor is the loss necessarily recaptured (although it may be in a hallucinatory way). These forces then continue to operate in some degree against recovery.

One of the external forces of great moment is the attitude of the environment. When mental illness was regarded as *prima-facie* evidence of wickedness * the environment only added its cruel blows to those already suffered by the patient. Sometimes, paradoxically, this does relieve the patient. His sense of guilt no longer requires his own self-punishment.

---

* "Heinroth (1773–1843) set out with the artificial distinction of a good and an evil principle, which he assumed as specific, independent, and constant entities. Life becomes teleologic, and represents continually the result of the conflict between these two principles. The pestilential doctrine that man is by nature inclined to evil was the cornerstone of Heinroth's system. However, 'Purity and integrity in human nature, while by no means unattainable, are attainable only by the religious point of view, and we know no other true religious standpoint than that of the redeeming faith which Christ brought into the world and the apostles spread abroad.'

"Here we have a clear statement of scholastic dogma which constitutes the foundation of Heinroth's psychiatry. Page after page of his textbook, published in 1818 while he was associate professor at Leipzig, we pore over, fancying that we are in the depths of some medieval treatise on theology. His psychology he draws from the Gospels, much as others have attempted to reconstruct geology from Genesis. The life of mental health is the life of piety. The etiology of madness is sin. Repentance and a return to faith are the means of cure.

"'Whatever one may say,' exclaims Heinroth, 'there is no mental disease, except where there is complete defection from God. Where God is, there is strength, light, love and life; where Satan is, weakness, darkness, hatred and destruction everywhere. An evil spirit abides, therefore, in the mentally deranged; *they are the truly possessed.*' Anticipating the charge that this is an absurd opinion, he neatly justifies it by saying that it is no more absurd to hold that the insane are children of the Devil than that the righteous are the children of God. 'In short,' he concludes, 'we find the essence of mental disease in the partnership of the human soul with the evil principle—and not merely in partnership, but rather in its entire subjection to the latter. This is the complete explanation of the lack of freedom or unreason in which all the mentally disturbed are involved.'" (Farrar, Clarence B. "Some Origins of Psychiatry: Part VIII." *Am. J. Insanity*, 66:277–294, 1909.)

But this is no sensible justification for a hostile attitude toward the mentally ill. What is far more common is an attitude of indifference, condescension, or even contempt. The social stigma which still attaches to psychiatric illness, and especially to hospitalization, remains a painful and regrettable deterrent to recovery or even to acceptance of proper help.

An individual's adjustment always means his reaction to a reaction to a reaction to a reaction, etc. And when an individual has fallen or wavered, his struggle back to the line of march is often handicapped by the attitudes which have been created in the environment by the development of his illness. Even when recovery has clearly occurred, often as a result of the hospitalization, an attitude on the part of relatives, friends, employers, and others will have developed tending to force the victim back into his illness.[17] Another example is the difficulty former prisoners find in obtaining employment. Suspicion of their possible defection denies them the economic opportunity to make the defection less necessary. Nathaniel Hawthorne in *The House of Seven Gables* said well what we psychiatrists know well: "The sick in mind . . . are rendered more darkly and hopelessly so by the manifold reflection of their disease, mirrored back from all quarters in the deportment of those about them; they are compelled to inhale the poison of their own breath, in infinite repetition."

There is nothing more expressive of a barbarous and stupid lack of culture than the half-unconscious attitude so many of us slip into, of taking for granted, when we see weak, neurotic, helpless, drifting, unhappy people, that it is by reason of some special merit in us or by reason of some especial favour towards us that the gods have given us an advantage over such persons. The more deeply sophisticated our culture is the more fully are we aware that these lamentable differences in good and bad fortune spring entirely from luck.

It is luck: luck in our heredity, luck in our environment, that makes the difference; and moreover at any moment fortune's erratic wheel may turn completely round and we ourselves may be hit by some totally unforeseen catastrophe. It is luck, too, springing from some fortunate encounter, some incredible love affair, some fragment of oracular wisdom in word or writing that has come our way, that launched us on the secret road of health and on the stubborn resolution to be happy under all upshots and issues, which has been so vast a resource to us in fortifying our embattled spirit. At any moment we are liable, the toughest and strongest among us, to be sent howling to a suicidal collapse. It is all a matter of luck; and the more culture we have the more deeply do we resolve that in our relations with all the human failures and abject and ne'er-do-wells of our world, we shall feel nothing but plain, simple, humble reverence before the mystery of misfortune.[18]

The eloquence of this famous passage does something to pierce the presumptuousness and indifference of the unthinking; it presents vividly the imminence of the overwhelming blow, attributed to what Powys calls luck, which we could translate into something like the unpredictable exigencies of living. Charles Peirce attempted to develop a theory that all life could be conceived of as operating upon laws of pure chance, which may be true in a highly mathematical sense but not in a clinical sense. Clinically it would be absurd to deny the occurrence of chance, but much which is called "luck" has to be attributed, upon closer examination, to the plans, conscious and unconscious, of the individual. Thomas Mann felt that the greatest contribution of Sigmund Freud was his proposal that we think not in terms of "look what fate has done to this individual," but rather "look what this individual has done with his fate." Look to what extent he has helped to build his fate. Look, we might add, at what we may possibly do to assist him to change what would otherwise seem to be his fate.

In addition to the social forces there are, of course, impersonal factors of time and space which may act against recovery. There is no question about the greater elasticity and adaptability of youth as a general thing. We all keep growing older and as a rule less flexible, less adaptable, less resilient to shock and change and frustration. There are protective compensations for this diminished flexibility; wisdom is supposed to accumulate, and experience has increased caution and discovered danger points. But with age and wisdom come the successive loss of friends and the tendency for increasing withdrawal. These forces undoubtedly work against recovery, but as a rule their weight has been overestimated. It has been a most agreeable surprise to discover in the increasing attention given to geriatrics that many of the conditions which were formerly called "senile dementia" and looked upon as terminal states, sometimes painfully protracted, are often transitory and reversible conditions. The tolerance of the elderly is often greatly diminished. But so are their needs. And these needs must be correctly interpreted.

This section of our chapter is a thin and shallow one; the forces working against recovery are only those concatenations of circumstances which occasionally overwhelm the ego. Most of them tend to disappear and some can be removed or alleviated. The forces which the ego has most reason to fear are the forces operating against recovery from within.

Internal Facts and Forces Working toward Recovery

For while many factors are opposing recovery, many others are exerting pressure in the opposite direction, i.e., toward health. And, as before, some of these forces appear to come from without, while some appear to arise—or at least to operate—within the organism.

Consider the internal pressures toward recovery first. Among these *pain* [19] is of course pre-eminent. Pain is man's friend, in its curious, paradoxical way.[20] It may announce a wound or it may reflect the organism's reactions to wounds. A bee's sting hurts, and the swelling it excites also hurts. A third type of pain derives from readjustments incident to the illness reaction—the losses, the renunciations, the costs of retaliation.

The first waves of pain after an injury—humiliation, rage, fear, jealousy, sorrow, or whatever—may lead to retreat, perhaps counterattack, perhaps effort at altering the situation by manipulation. In any case, the pain will not disappear immediately, and new pains will be added as readjustment is attempted. First Order devices will diminish but not quell the pain, and soon the pains of remorse, guilt feelings, self-distrust, and discouragement will ensue.

The persistence of this suffering is important in the pursuit of a better solution. One external hope held out for every sufferer is the physician and all he stands for. But long before he consults a physician every sufferer has done something on his own, as it were, to find a more comfortable position. Various regulatory devices are called upon to cope with the mounting internal tension. Alcoholic inebriation, resolute denial, and various kinds of distraction efforts may be tried. These rarely vanquish all the pain, which remains as a nagging incentive toward finding a better solution. Many people simply learn to bear pain stoically and get along with it, so to speak, or even to make of it a kind of unpleasant "old friend." [21]

The most poignant pain in many individuals derives from the loss of satisfactions and opportunities, the failures in productivity and achievement. A sense of unworthiness and uselessness augments this, as does the painful memory of plan and promise.

But both the perception of pain and the capacity to endure it seem to vary a great deal in different people.[22] This was amply demonstrated in the various reactions to torture, an official medieval pastime which became popular again under the Nazis and then under the Communists.[23] There is actually such a thing as congenital indifference to physical pain, although probably quite rare.[24] Insofar as psychological pain is concerned, however, an acquired indifference to it actually constitutes one of the commonest secondary symptoms. It is common observation that many people—whether or not they be patients—*seem* (we cannot always be sure) to suffer very little from a sense of guilt for their social aggressions or from painful regret at their failure to develop their potentialities. Some even make a virtue of their vices, as it were, and pride themselves on their niggardliness or their callousness or their stupidity. In many instances some of us often wish that the pain were sharper and more insistent and more general.

The public reads eagerly of new drugs to bring about a temporary serenity; some of us would be more interested in drugs that would evoke aspirations or spur a desire for learning or increase displeasures in wastefulness and self-preoccupation. We cannot be enthusiastic about chemical methods to produce a state of *sans souci*; what the world needs and what more human beings need, for their own mental health and that of their universe, is not to care less but to care more. For this we have no chemicals. There are no drugs "to keep the soul alert with noble discontent."

Drugs cannot inspire or encourage or comfort. Only a person can heal a person, said Schilling two centuries ago. Perhaps this is only partially right, but it was a word spoken against mechanistic drug therapy long before ataractics were heard of. This is not to decry the use of drugs to relieve anxiety, but only to point out that just as relieving a sharp pain in the abdomen with morphine may mask the development of an appendicitis, so the taking of sedative drugs often masks the development of dangerous pressure and retards steps toward its proper correction. Chronic psychological pain, the so-called pervading sense of inadequacy or inferiority, is less likely to be relieved by drugs, but unfortunately this type of "pain" is also less likely to stimulate self-corrective efforts. The feelings of inferiority are accepted as a correct self-judgment and an alibi against improvement or even normal achievement.

The establishment or re-establishment of relationships with fellow human beings is the basic architecture of normal life; hence it is not only the index of recovery but one of the methods of recovery, one of the forces making for recovery. To live, we say, is to love, and vice versa. If a patient is not frozen in his primary narcissim, or drowned in the secondary narcissism which developed from his previous failures in attempting to establish and maintain love objects, he will continuously strive to find and touch persons and things about him. He will keep reaching out first a receiving and then a giving hand, making acquaintances and then friends, and finding more and more satisfactions and identifications. This is not to imply that love consists in an endless mutual hand-holding or that life is a pure culture of love. But predominantly positive relationships are ultimately productive, as well as satisfying. The production of a baby is both an example and a symbol of this, but there are other kinds of re-production in the world. All of them require goal-seeking efforts; all of them which are really creative require the investment of love.

Love in its modifying function determines those essential ways of life which we call work and play. There seems to be a great variation in the capacity people have for doing and enjoying *work*, not only to harness aggressive energies, but to further the productiveness just referred to. *Play*, likewise, seems to be very easy and rewarding for some, very difficult for others. These variations are important, since much of our treatment program depends upon their exploitation and development. More important than either play itself or work itself is the balance (an ever-recurring word in this book) which is established between the two. All play and no work has just as bad an effect on Jack as the oft-cited reverse situation.

Similarly, the individual's appreciation of time, space, and other realities, his reactions to authority, power, and responsibility, and his philosophical, social, and religious concepts can be viewed as the products of what in the broad sense of the word can be called his *education*. If this education has been a good one—and there is surely no need to explain here what we mean by good—the lessons learned in these areas will all help in times of emergency, bearing strongly toward re-establishment. It is easier to see how a defect in one of these areas has the opposite effect—a hypersensitiveness to authority, a refusal to take responsibility, a feverish lust for power, a poisonous prejudice against some social groups, or a vacuum in religious convictions.

In the history of medicine there have been periods in which a basic force toward recovery, namely the *vis medicatrix naturae*, was assured, with the physicians functioning as its ally. This important idea referred in an inclusive sense to all the internal factors favoring recovery. This concept will be reviewed in a subsequent chapter.

External Factors Favoring Recovery

The external factors favoring recovery are far better known than the internal factors which we have just been discussing. In a general way they include all those events and persons and things and opportunities in the environment which tend to fulfill critical needs of the harassed patient. These needs are those of all human beings, but sometimes in greater amounts or in greater emphasis or in easier availability. They include whatever will give the patient the sense of relief from anxiety, assurance of security, knowledge of possibilities remaining, encouragement to proceed, assurance of affection. Other patients will most need opportunities to make restitution or atonement or to mourn or to meditate undisturbed. Still others will require new forms of sublimation, new objects of interest, new friends to replace old.

It is almost axiomatic to say that new or more strongly invested love objects are factors in the furtherance of recovery. It has been said in a dozen ways that love is the touchstone of method in the modern psychiatric hospital. Elizabeth Barrett Browning [25] wrote:

> How sick we must be, ere we make men just;
> I think it frets the saints in heaven to see
> How many desolate creatures on the earth
> Have learnt the simple dues of fellowship
> And social comfort, in a hospital.

Many a man, like the Flying Dutchman, is saved from self-destruction by his wife, and others by the love of their children or their pets. In the hospital we deliberately make use of what we call "transitional love objects." We encourage the warm friendship which develops between the patient and his aide, or his nurse, or his physician. Professional people are trained in the skillful management of such attachments and in the moral wrongness of exploiting them.

But other patients do their part, often a very considerable part. Transitional love relationships sometimes become permanent relationships, either as lifelong friendships or even as marriage compacts. And contrary to what one might assume, these marriages often turn out well. I can remember several times when we were much concerned because two very unstable patients "ran away from" treatment, and got married. Such a marriage certainly is not the ideal prospect, but I must record that several of these turned out very well. Love for each other accomplished more than the treatment could; but perhaps it would be fair to give some credit to the treatment for making the marriage possible.

A word should be said here, too, about those invaluable twentieth-century inventions of psychiatric hospital operation, *volunteers*. It is not quite accurate to imagine that they are entirely a modern invention; in the Middle Ages the only food and care that many hospital patients got was that which was brought in by charitable minded citizens. But today the well-organized volunteer services in public hospitals do a great deal, not only to make patients more comfortable but to develop or retain for them a feeling of personal relationship with non-professional, non-paid, non-technical individuals—just fellow citizens like themselves who happen not to be sick but who happen to care about those who are.

And, since we are attempting to be somewhat encyclopedic, we must not omit the obvious fact that hundreds of impersonal things contribute to recovery—everything, in short, which belongs to a healthy way of living. This means the opportunity and the encouragement to work, to play, to create, to communicate, to enjoy beauty. Sometimes in the retreat from a painful aspect of the life situation into the protected milieu of the hospital there is a tendency to relinquish the very activities which the patient needs more, not less. Hence the modern hospital program tends to be increasingly an educational one, a training in practice living, with the guidance of teachers who used to be called recreational therapists and occupational therapists. And while, as with all other staff members and, indeed, all teachers, their personalities and examples are important, their special skills regarding the use of certain techniques of living are their special advantage.

And just as there are tragic accidents and incidents which bring about the collapse of self-regulation and the development of an illness process, so there are accidents and incidents quite unplanned and unexpected which may have a most beneficent effect that sometimes turns the scales. These may or may not have been precipitated by the occasion of the illness, but sometimes the emergency removal to a new environment seems to change everything. Or the visit of an old acquaintance starts a new train of thought. Such events are like the (usually legendary) experience of receiving a legacy from a deceased second cousin. And sometimes the external forces favoring the recovery are not only unexpected but quite paradoxical, as illustrated earlier in this chapter.

These forces are not always so clearly positive or negative as they have been presented. Some of them fluctuate—now strong, now weak—

and some change sides, working at times for recovery, at times against it. It is certainly not our conception that the whole process of mental illness can be described with mathematical precision, but we think it can be more accurately described if we think of it as being a highly fluid, dynamic process determined by many factors—strong ones and weak, internal and external, positive and negative. Some of these forces we can identify and perhaps even measure. Some of them we can infer or hypothesize, and some, no doubt, we know nothing about at all. But we can look for the turning points, the changes of direction, changes in the rate of change, and, comparing these with our total supply of information, we should be able to make fair presumptions about the reasons that some of them occur. Such presumptions will be tested by experience and sometimes by experiment. Gradually we acquire a few facts and a little knowledge, and by this the physician is guided.

The Physician as a Force in Recovery

Finally, one of the external factors working in the direction of recovery, or so we believe, is the physician.

Thus we come at last to what must have seemed all along a most conspicuous omission. It may have seemed that we were describing an automatic process, a process *in vitro et vacuo*. A complex machine, temporarily overcome by the unpredictable exigencies of fate and circumstance, runs up and down the gamut of illness and recovery, observed, studied, but uninfluenced by us who are credited if the outcome is favorable and forgiven if it is not.

The discoveries of Albert Einstein and Sigmund Freud taught us all that no observer can remain outside the process he observes. Hence we cannot take seriously reports of spontaneous recovery, since we know that if recovery was reported it might have been observed, and if it was observed it was not "spontaneous." And we must deal now more seriously with the role of the observer, which is always more than observation. We must consider in what way he becomes one of the forces which influence the course of illness and in what way he can mobilize or alter other forces so as to change the balance in the direction he seeks. Most physicians assume that at least some of the time they can do something. Some overrate their powers and knowledge, while others distrust both; still, few can relinquish the conviction that they can and do influence the course of illness in many instances.

This conviction is an act of faith. Its assumptions are often disputed. It is constantly being doubted. Honest research has refuted the usefulness of a thousand methods and ten thousand drugs. And every day of his life the observing physician is reminded that his ministrations alone are not what effects the cure. Indeed, sometimes he seems to do nothing at all except stand by in sorrowful helplessness; in spite of all he can do, his patient gets worse. Yet the faith persists—in the doctor, and in his patients. And this mutual trust requires that art continue, even where science fails.

We shall try to go beyond or beneath the faith and the art and endeavor to see if we can identify some of the specific functions or roles, which the physician plays in the recovery process, especially in the case of the psychiatric patient. This we shall undertake in our next chapter. We shall expect to find the physician to be one of the many vectors of force converging upon the patient and his situation.

CHAPTER XIII

The Role of the Physician in the
Illness-Recovery Process

PART I: DIAGNOSIS AND TREATMENT

SYNOPSIS: *The physician's role as healer in mental illness is beset by temptations, traditions, beliefs, fads, and various conscious and unconscious motives. These must be constantly checked by self-criticism and controlled by scientific principles and methods. In psychiatry, this control is effected in part by systematic psychiatric case study, the main features of which are outlined in this chapter, with particular reference to the determination of the factors which impede recovery and those which favor recovery.*

THE INFLUENCE of the physician upon the course of illness was referred to in the previous chapter and deferred for a fuller consideration. It is a matter lying at the very heart of scientific medicine, and we propose to devote the final chapters of this book to it, with particular reference to the responsibilities of the psychiatrist.

No more moot and debated point exists than that of the contribution of the doctor to the illness-recovery process. On the one hand, he professes to be ready and able to attempt help; on the other hand, suffering drives patients to seek help. Mutual need and social custom thus bring them together; help is asked, help is tendered, and help is accepted.

But with what demonstrable results? Patient and physician both have James's will to believe; both want the same thing and both want to believe that it can be accomplished. Both may be gratified; but one or both of them may be disappointed and react to that disappointment with bitterness and withdrawal.* Disparagement and distrust of medical

---

* Since the especially intense relation of doctor to patient imposes responsibility on the physician, he naturally cherishes the freedom of action which he thinks necessary to meet that responsibility. He develops a strong need to be untrammeled, and this need is sometimes frustrated in the hospital environment, where many individuals are restricted in their rights and duties in the interest of orderly coordination. Communication between the doctor and patient is unbalanced; although the patient must recite

science in the patient are paralleled by a therapeutic nihilism and cynicism in the physician. Rather than these extremes, an attitude of cautious expectancy is perhaps more common. The point of it all is that neither patient nor physician can possibly be fully objective in an appraisal of the specific contribution made by the doctor.

Motives of Medical Men

That the doctor is on the side of recovery is presumptive; that he is not always successful, that the effect of his efforts cannot always be detected or proved, that some patients even get worse under his ministrations—these do not affect the principle. It is his avowed wish to relieve and restore his patient; this he professes, this he intends. And his motivation is powerful and complicated.

Who was the first physician? Was it a mother so skillful in her ministrations to her own family that she was called upon by the rest of the tribe to share her powers and herbs? Was it a wise elder, a chieftain or a prophet who turned from the active pursuits of war and hunting and agriculture to the observation of the stars, the seasons, and the forces of nature and tried to relate them to man's life by naming them and describing their influence? Was it a priest assaying to dispense divine power and blessings? Was it, as Celsus declared, a philosopher seeking self-cure?

---

his symptoms and history, it is the physician who speaks in tones of knowledge and authority. The doctor is expected to dominate this situation. Yet his hospital duties increasingly involve him in cooperative relationships in which the accent of authority must be modulated toward the orchestration of a total treatment effort.

"If clinical diagnosis and creative surgery confirm the impression of medicine as an art, the battery of techniques and mass of verified knowledge also characterize medicine as a science. This complicated art-science holds much genuine pleasure for the practitioner. The artist's joy in discovery, the scientist's thrill in research, the man of action's deep satisfaction with concrete practical accomplishments—all these are potential rewards for the doctor. Medicine, however, has such stature as a field that the public harries it with overexpectations. Patients expect their problems to be solved, and doctors themselves, in expressing the fundamentally American belief that answers ought to be available, may sometimes foster too high a level of anticipation. Therefore a feeling of intense disappointment may accompany any ineffective medical work regardless of the realistic factors in the situation. The job is laden with possibilities of psychic strain; defense against an overinvolved sympathy with patients often takes the form of a protective callousness or cynicism, which may be misinterpreted by the layman as a sign that the doctor 'doesn't care' when in fact it may be a defense against caring too much." (Burling, Temple; Lentz, Edith M.; and Wilson, Robert N. *The Give and Take in Hospitals.* New York: Putnam, 1956.)

Or was it perhaps a former sick man, resolved to turn his experience to good account? *

May it not have been a captive of war, a slave, forced to tend those unfortunate sick who seemed fated to die, to care for those whom others shunned in fear of contamination?

Certainly these elements are all to be found in the make-up of the physician: the maternal ** concern to allay suffering and to comfort, the desire to master the secrets of nature and to control the fate of man, the compulsion to maintain a lonely and often dangerous and disagreeable vigil, the feeling that one is permanently set apart from normal pursuits in the company of a lost remnant of people who, if they live, may not remember or be grateful. There may be some less worthy motives—to inflict pain,*** to command deference, to deal condescendingly with the helpless, or to acquire wealth.

Driven by whatever constellation of conscious and unconscious motives,[1] the doctor has remained throughout centuries a man set apart, belonging to a special class ****—as are also those who take the step of approaching him for help. The latter, dubbed "patients," are both pitied and envied, as their doctors are revered and dreaded. Patients become isolated in sick chambers, and doctors in laboratories and offices. Their fears and doubts, their sustaining faith, their responsibility for the life and death of their fellow men they share with one another. Toward the

---

* In his account of Babylonian customs Herodotus wrote: "I come now to the next wisest of their customs: having no use for physicians, they carry the sick into the market-place; then those who have been afflicted themselves by the same ill as the sick man's or seen others in like case, come near and advise him about his disease and comfort him, telling him by what means they have themselves recovered of it or seen others recover. None may pass by the sick man without speaking and asking what is his sickness." (Herodotus: *History*.)

** If such traits are commonly ascribed to feminine weakness, it may be only because we have a curious anthropocentric misconception of the nature of strength and an artificially inverted hierarchical order of the sexes. (The *Hymenoptera* are under no such illusion!) The maternal identification of physicians is often very conspicuous, sometimes well disguised. It might be expected to be most obvious in pediatricians, but a survey of our colleagues will discover maternal qualities in all specialists and in general practitioners. It is significant that in Russia, where prodigious effort has been made to eliminate sentimentalism and tradition, a majority of the medical students have been women.

*** "As a medical student, Freud wrote wittily to a school friend: 'I have enrolled in another laboratory. Here I am preparing myself for my real profession to torture animals or to torment people. I come to favor more and more the first term of this alternative.'" (Glauber, I. Peter. "A Deterrent in the Study and Practice of Medicine." *The Psychoanalytic Quarterly*, 22: 381–412, 1953.)

**** "All idiots, priests, Jews, actors, monks, barbers and old women think they are physicians." (Medieval Latin proverb.)

public they turn faces of calmness, wisdom, and serenity, but secretly they hold fast to one another's hands.

There are many sufferers in the world, and there are many who seek to afford them relief. Among the latter there are those who follow intuition and inspiration and there are those who adhere to a convention of checks and balances which we call the scientific method. For the former, healing is more important than truth; for the latter, truth more important than healing.

In the performance of healing acts, the scales are weighted heavily against scientific truths. Patients long to be deceived. Driven by pain, desperate with fear, they are ready to seize at straws of hope. They prostrate themselves before the doctor; they queue up in weary, straggling lines, awaiting the opportunity to submit themselves to humiliations and new sufferings, or even to hear but a few words of reassurance.

"There is nothing men will not do," declared Oliver Wendell Holmes,[2] "there is nothing they have not done, to recover their health and save their lives. They have submitted to be half drowned in water, and half choked with gases, to be buried up to their chins in earth, to be seared with hot irons like galley slaves, to be crimped with knives, like codfish, to have needles thrust into their flesh, and bonfires kindled on their skin, to swallow all sorts of abominations, and to pay for all this, as if blisters were a blessing and leeches were a luxury. What more can be asked to prove their honesty and sincerity?"

Besieged by multitudes of such petitioners, often with gifts in their hands, the doctor—knowing his limitations—must try to be patient, kind, merciful, and honest. But simultaneously he must try to be "objective," to be influenced in his acts and words only by "scientific facts." The desire to bring comfort, the need to earn one's living, the suppressed longing for prestige and popularity, the honest conviction of the efficacy of a pill or a program, sympathy for the pleading sufferer— all these throw themselves upon the scales in the moment of decision. Thus every physician in the world has heard the devil whispering, "Command that these stones become bread. . . . All these things I will give thee if thou wilt fall down and worship me." And sometimes he falls down. He commits the sin of presumptuousness, *hubris*.

The legend has it that Aesculapius so far pursued his medical studies and achieved such skill in the healing art that he essayed to reverse the hand of death and restore the dead to life. For this he was removed by the jealous Zeus. He had abandoned a first principle of medical art and medical science—humility.

The doctor must ". . . beware the pitfall which awaits all physicians, when and if they lose their sense of humility. . . . Our patients often assume that we have knowledge or skill or power which we do not have . . . that we are the *only* ones who can help them. . . . Sometimes for a few moments we may dare to think we are as good as they think we are!" [3]

My brother here touches upon the well-known fact that for his efforts to do something a doctor frequently receives more credit than he deserves. True, he usually receives money too, but sometimes neither money nor gratitude. The *unconscious* needs and conscious hopes of those who appeal to the doctor for help can easily strike a responsive chord in secret fantasies of the healer or the helper, particularly when some effort of his is blessed by success. Wrote Bunyan:

> Christ Jesus, as you may perceive, has put himself under the term of a physician, a doctor for curing of diseases; and you know that applause and fame are things that physicians much desire. That is it that helps them to patients, and that also that will help their patients to commit themselves to their skill for cure with the more confidence and repose of spirit. And the best way for a doctor or physician to get themselves a name is, in the first place, to take in hand and cure some such as all others have given up for lost and dead. Physicians get neither name nor fame by pricking of wheals, or picking out of thistles, or by laying of plaisters to the scratch of a pin: every old woman can do this. But if they would have a name and fame—if they will have it quickly, they must, as I said, do some great and desperate cures. Let them fetch one to life that was dead; let them recover one to his wits that was mad; let them make one that was born blind to see; or let them give ripe wits to a fool; these are notable cures; and he that can do thus, and if he doth thus first, he shall have the name and fame he desires; he may lie abed till noon.[4]

This is the reason that doctors must share with teachers and ministers the necessity for constant self-searching, conscientiously rejecting deification and the appeals of "Lord, Lord." Doctors, like clergymen, are called in at times when the need for them is strongly felt. They have certain jobs to do which seem forced upon them. But they have prepared themselves to accept the responsibility; they have been trained to do this very thing. More than that, they feel a compulsion, an obligation, to do it. This feeling is enhanced by many factors, as we have seen—sympathy, curiosity, cupidity, pride, challenge, and others. It imbues doctors with a sense of necessity, sometimes a heavy fever of determination to change the patient's condition, whether he wants it changed or not.

"Indeed," writes Hayward, an English colleague,

> one of the most important problems in psychiatry is the problem of the doctor who feels he must cure his patients. We must teach our doctors that

their approach in psychiatry must be an understanding of the patient's situation, and that treatment may or may not come out of this understanding as a side issue. . . .

This need to cure is seldom, if ever, a sublimation; it is nearly always a reaction-formation against underlying destructive needs and wishes, and this is why the need to cure is so dangerous within psychiatry. It does not matter in surgery; but in a mental hospital the patient may never react to what is on top in the doctor, but to what is underneath. Many of our patients will not be in touch with the reaction-formation of the doctor's need to cure him, but only in touch with the underlying destructive impulses. From this spring many of the patient's fears. We need, therefore, doctors who, besides accepting their traditional role, are able to accept and be at ease with their own omnipotent fantasies; to take over ill patients in a supportive and expectant way, content to provide them with simple things; and to help them to find a solution to their illness in whatever way they are able to go. We must have doctors who can allow patients to be ill.[5]

Besought by the multitudes to relieve suffering, correct disability, predict outcome, and forestall death, physicians feel obliged to respond, to act. Yet life is short and the art long; experiment perilous, decision difficult, delay dangerous.

What shall one do? He may bleed, he may physic, he may poultice, he may trepan. He may prescribe goat gallstones (bezoars) or powdered unicorn horn * or the ancient elixir of theriac, of marvelous renown. Mattioli, too, is powerful; it contains 230 ingredients. Or usnea, listed in our official pharmacopoeia until the nineteenth century and carried in all apothecary shops. It consisted of moss scraped from the skull of a hanged criminal. Or crocodile feces or the powdered lungs of a fox.

These are the medicines which Shakespeare knew. These are the remedies our forefathers were given. Benjamin Franklin and Isaac Newton would not have laughed at these *materia medica*, nor Galileo, Miles Standish, Cotton Mather, or J. S. Buck. And there were many other treatments besides drugs. The point is that the sick want to be treated and doctors have always wanted to treat them.

---

* "Unicorn's horn was another highly prized remedy of the medieval period and Renaissance. Unicorn's horn was sold for an enormous price; a specimen in Dresden was estimated in the sixteenth century to be worth $75,000. . . . Paré tried unsuccessfully to abolish the custom prevailing in the French court of dipping a piece of unicorn's horn in the king's cup before he drank, as a precaution against poisoning. Instead of abolishing the custom Paré precipitated an attack against himself for his skepticism, on the ground that the king had refused to part with his horn for a hundred thousand crowns, and that fact in itself was proof that the horn must be useful. In England the belief in unicorn's horn as an antidote for poison lasted until the reign of Charles II, when the Royal Society was requested to investigate the properties of a cup made from rhinoceros horn. The society reported that the cup was useless as an antidote. . . ." (Haggard, H. W. *Devils, Drugs and Doctors*. New York: Harper's, 1929.)

No better illustration of the *furor therapeuticus* need be sought than the record of Benjamin Rush. Here was an energetic, animated, intelligent man who was into everything in a lively fashion. He was a signer of the Declaration of Independence; he was a founder of the American Psychiatric Association; he was an active humanitarian, highly esteemed by most of his compatriots. Oliver Wendell Holmes [6] wrote of him in 1860:

> If I wished the student to understand the tendencies of the American mind, its sanguine enterprise, its self-confidence, its audacious handling of nature, its impatience with her old-fashioned ways of taking time to get a sick man well, I would make him read the life and writings of Benjamin Rush. . . . His own mind was in a perpetual state of exaltation produced by the stirring scenes in which he had taken a part, and the quickened life of the time in which he lived. . . . He taught thousands of American students, he gave a direction to the medical mind of the country more than any other one man; perhaps he typifies it better than any other. It has clearly tended to extravagance in remedies and trust in remedies, as in everything else.

Benjamin Rush, for all his virtues, almost certainly brought about the premature death of many patients by the senseless, painful, depleting procedure of bleeding. Justifying his treatment, he developed a theory

> that all diseases were due to essentially one cause; i.e., vascular tension, and that the universal remedy was to attempt to decrease tension by removing blood in great quantity. Included in his regimen was the administration of ten grains of calomel and fifteen grains of jalap along with the removal of as much as four-fifths of the estimated total amount of blood in an effort to deplete the patient and remove the tension. Unfortunately for some of his patients, in Rush's day the amount of blood was thought to be almost twice what we now consider it, and it is readily seen that removal of an estimated quantity based on that erroneous figure might have amounted to almost complete exsanguination. Despite strong opposition from many of the medical practitioners of Philadelphia, Rush waded through the great yellow fever epidemic of 1793 in Philadelphia in a bath of his patients' blood. His opponents called him a murderer, and public concern was greatly aroused; but Rush pushed on with his theory and his bloodletting and may well have been responsible for some part of the large mortality which the epidemic carried, for Rush's practice was very extensive, and his belief and enthusiasm never faltered.
>
> Although the violent measures advocated by Rush declined in popularity, bleeding continued to be a general practice over the world. In 1833 it was still in full swing. Broussais and Bouillard were its chief exponents. By the mid-nineteenth century mention of bleeding as a therapeutic measure became more and more infrequent in the text-books of the time, largely because of the doctrine and influence of Marshall Hall of England who at one time had been an enthusiastic bleeder but recanted his earlier views most emphatically.[7]

Read the full description of "total push" treatment in the seventeenth century as applied to King Charles II of England:

Some idea of the nature and number of the drug substances used in the medicine of the past may be obtained from the records of the treatment given King Charles II at the time of his death. These records are extant in the writings of a Doctor Scarburgh, one of the twelve or fourteen physicians called in to treat the king. At eight o'clock on Monday morning of February 2, 1685, King Charles was being shaved in his bedroom. With a sudden cry he fell backward and had a violent convulsion. He became unconscious, rallied once or twice, and after a few days died.

Seventeenth-century autopsy records are far from complete, but one could hazard a guess that the king suffered with an embolism—that is, a floating blood clot which had plugged up an artery and deprived some portion of his brain of blood—or else his kidneys were diseased.

As the first step in treatment the king was bled to the extent of a pint from a vein in his right arm. Next his shoulder was cut into and the incised area "cupped" to suck out an additional eight ounces of blood. After this homicidal onslaught the drugging began. An emetic and purgative were administered, and soon after a second purgative. This was followed by an enema containing antimony, sacred bitters, rock salt, mallow leaves, violets, beet roots, camomile flowers, fennel seed, linseed, cinnamon, cardamon seed, saphron, cochineal, and aloes. The enema was repeated in two hours and a purgative given.

The king's head was shaved and a blister raised on his scalp. A sneezing powder of hellebore root was administered, and also a powder of cowslip flowers "to strengthen his brain." The cathartics were repeated at frequent intervals and interspersed with a soothing drink composed of barley water, licorice and sweet almond. Likewise white wine, absinthe and anise were given, as also were extracts of thistle leaves, mint, rue, and angelica. For external treatment a plaster of Burgundy pitch and pigeon dung was applied to the king's feet. The bleeding and purging continued, and to the medicaments were added melon seeds, manna, slippery elm, black cherry water, an extract of flowers of lime, lily-of-the-valley, peony, lavender and dissolved pearls. Later came gentian root, nutmeg, quinine, and cloves.

The king's condition did not improve, indeed it grew worse, and in the emergency forty drops of extract of human skull were administered to allay convulsions. A rallying dose of Raleigh's antidote was forced down the king's throat; this antidote contained an enormous number of herbs and animal extracts. Finally bezoar stone was given. Then says Scarburgh: "Alas! after an ill-fated night his serene majesty's strength seemed exhausted to such a degree that the whole assembly of physicians lost all hope and became despondent: still so as not to appear to fail in doing their duty in any detail, they brought into play the most active cordial." As a sort of grand summary to this pharmaceutical debauch, a mixture of Raleigh's antidote, pearl julep, and ammonia was forced down the throat of the dying king.

King Charles was helpless before the drugging of his physicians, who wished "to leave no stones unturned in his treatment." [8]

And if this sounds too medieval or old-fashioned, consider this illustration noted down by one of us while in attendance at a seminar in one of the leading medical centers of the United States on April 20, 1948. A case was presented whose clinical chart contained *sixty-three pages* of "doctors' order sheets." Professor B. himself counted them and exclaimed about this to us. It seems that in spite of much treatment the patient had grown progressively worse and was about to die. All treatment orders consequently had been suspended, whereupon the patient immediately began to improve! (She was ultimately discharged, cured, with a diagnosis of Simmonds' Disease, a pituitary gland disorder, supposedly incurable.)

These were the efforts of honest physicians, experienced and no doubt competent. It is difficult to see how they did anything to help their patients recover. Sometimes they did, but not so often as they thought they did. They believed they were curing patients, and they got the credit.

It is important to emphasize that all these doctors—1685, 1793, 1948—were sincere, earnest, assiduous. They believed they were benefiting their patients.

So did Dr. Elisha Perkins. He is almost unknown today, but 150 years ago he was one of the great healers of the age. In 1796 he "discovered" that two metal rods, each three inches long, made of specially compounded metals, could be placed on an area of the body of a sufferer from pain or disease of some kind, and when they were drawn out along the body and to one of the extremities, the illness left the body and followed them. Americans rushed to buy these "tractors," as they came to be known. Apparently no price was too large. George Washington bought tractors for his entire family.

> There seems to have been no doubt that Perkins was sincere. When the great yellow fever epidemic paralyzed New York City, Perkins rushed to the scene and personally attended the stricken. Observing the tortured victims of the infection, he decided his tractors alone were not enough and he advocated oral administration of vinegar in various combinations with the magical tractors.
> Confidently, fearlessly, he applied his cure. Three weeks later Dr. Elisha Perkins was dead of yellow fever. . . . [His] finest hour [had been] his ultimate discovery—vinegar to cure yellow fever. . . .[9]

Compare the record of this great, sincere, evangelical quack, and his conviction that imbibing vinegar would cure disease, with this fact: in 1962 one of the nation's best-selling books (over 500,000 copies to date) offered relief from headaches, arthritis, diabetes, and other scourges by imbibing—yes, you guessed it—vinegar (mixed with honey)! As Deutsch exclaims, "Shades of Elisha Perkins!"

The bleeding to which Dr. Rush was addicted and the application of tractors which Perkins advocated were both *physical* measures of therapy; but Perkins, it will be noted, reverted in the extremity of the epidemic to the philosophy that medical relief must come through a *chemical* alteration of the organism, the older medical concept.

Back in Chapter IV we tried to demonstrate that through the ages what doctors do depends upon what they believe about disease and diseased organisms. Their reasons for particular acts are not questioned by their patients, who want only results. But some rationale is demanded by the physician himself, *for* himself. This is partly for the purpose of improving his practice, by logical extensions or corrections of theory; partly for both self-comfort and self-discipline; and partly because it is of the charter and dogma of a scientific profession. Saint Paul counseled the early Christians to be ready always to give a reason for the faith within them—despite the contradiction of terms. There is actually *something* of the same contradiction in the rationalizations for therapeutic procedure, but it is of the *essence of science* that we continuously strive to reduce our "irrationalities" by logical demonstrations that appeal to or survive the objective judgment of our friendly and hostile colleagues.

Hence it is not sufficient for the genuine doctor to have "cured" a patient, or to have seen one get well; he must attempt to explain to himself the recovery, and his own involvement in it, as best he can. Only then can he feel justified in repeating what seemed *this one time* to be beneficial when similar needs for it again present themselves. Even then he may conclude "wrongly," under the influence of his strong *wish* to be helpful, and his melioristic philosophy. Therapy—"like any other helping procedure—presupposes belief in the possibility of changing conditions for the better, an optimistic attitude in spite of insight into the enormous difficulties, or even doubt as to the results of the effort. That alone can help the therapist to bear his own sacrifice—the inability to do a better job—without being too much disturbed in his own self-realization."

Even when this knowledge was mistaken in fact, it was orderly in theory. Hence from the days of Hippocrates to the present time it has been a keystone of medical science that treatment follows, depends upon, and is determined by diagnosis. We must try to understand the nature of what we are taking steps to alter, else we are charlatans or magicians. Having made a diagnosis and administered the treatment thereby indicated, the doctor—likewise the patient—awaits the expected results.

Examinations having determined the strategy, the battle is joined. Help has come. The beleaguering forces of evil are to be attacked; the resisting garrison of health is to be supported. Soon now the pain will cease, the old strength return, and the shadow of death fade away. The patient may fear the physician, he may distrust the treatment, he may dread the costs in money and in pain. But his desire for relief outweighs all deterrents, and his hopes have found a foothold.

The doctor, especially, must now guard himself against easy conclusions and false interpretation, particularly if they reflect credit upon him and his treatment. Over and over he must ask himself probing questions: Was the change in this patient directly attributable to something I did, and did deliberately? Did the improvement come about consequently, incidentally, accidentally, or "naturally"? Was my intervention logically planned or blindly empirical? Beyond my presence, my reassurance, my intentions and hopes, was I actually a factor determining the changed course of my patient's illness? The difference between the charlatan and the scientist lies in the internal attitude regarding these questions; we cannot always answer them, but we should always *ask* them of ourselves.*

Not only must the doctor question the meaning of his "results," but he must submit his data and conclusions to his colleagues. And dare he do this? Can his pride, his self-esteem, endure it? Indeed, dare he scrutinize himself too closely? Dare he distrust his therapeutic potency? May it not be too devastating for doctors to discover what a minor role they have played in recoveries for which they have been given so much credit? Can they face the certainty that some of their former patients were afterward the worse for their "treatment," and that some whom they believe to be well and happy are now dead, or in the hands of other physicians? Does the humility dictated by science and intellectual honesty impair clinical effectiveness?

---

* In our own Psychotherapy Research Project at The Menninger Foundation we are concerned with just such questions—not only of what changes occur during the course of psychiatric treatment, but how those changes have come about. It is too easy to assume that changes occurring during treatment are necessarily consequences of treatment. Our research investigates the interaction of three major sets of factors in relation to treatment course and outcome—factors in the patient, in his personality organization, and in the nature of his illness, factors in the treatment, in the therapist, and in the nature of the therapist-patient interaction; and factors in the altering life-situation of the patient. We hope in this way to disentangle the varying roles of the patient, the treatment, the therapist, and the life-situation in the change which comes about.

The answer to these questions must be sometimes yes and sometimes no. Certainly a self-confident and cheerful charlatan will bring more comfort to some individuals than a grumpy, pessimistic, but scientific physician. Science is neither optimistic nor pessimistic. Optimism, nevertheless, has a therapeutic function; it implies a faith in change, not necessarily in one's own abilities but in the latent forces for "good" in the universe. The strictly objective scientist cannot acquire the healing art, however much he may know of medical science. The therapist, on the other hand, may not abandon his loyalty to scientific principles, for all the optimism and faith in the world will not permanently cloak charlatanry, fraudulence, and self-deception.

Psychiatric Examination and Diagnosis

It has become an accepted axiom, which commends itself both to common sense and to scientific principle, that diagnosis must depend upon the acquisition of certain general and certain specific knowledge by the physician. He must know about disease in general, and he must know the details about the particular patient's condition. This requires an examination. The meaning of the physical examination has become well known to the general public, but to this day there is little understanding of just what the psychiatric examination entails.

Read, for example, the following press report of a psychiatric interview in which the attitude of the psychiatrists was obvious. The purpose may have been a little less obvious; it will be explained later. But this is one kind of psychiatric diagnosis.

> Two physicians sat at a bare green table in a bare green room, facing an unshaven man in a rumpled sports shirt. They were preparing to answer this question: "Is he insane?" The examination lasted just two minutes!
> "Who brought you here?" asked Dr. F.
> "My wife," said the man, James R.
> "Now, why did she do that?"
> "That's what I'd like to know."
> "Don't lie to me—you think she's trying to poison you?"
> James R. shook his head, rubbed his forehead. Obviously it was a question he had heard before. He said:
> "I don't believe so, I didn't say that, I . . ."
> Dr. F. interrupted. "You wouldn't eat what she cooked?"
> "No sir, I won't. It's slop."
> Dr. F. began writing, in pencil, on a form labeled "Report of Commission," and said:

"Why did she say you think she's trying to poison you? You think she's persecuting you?"

"I don't know."

"What do you think?"

"I don't think nothing."

The doctor looked up from his writing. "You don't think?"

The man, sensing now that he was caught, hung his head and muttered: "I don't think nothing. I don't know."

One more question, this one from Dr. I.: "What kind of a place is this —do you know?"

"Sure, I know. It's the nuthouse."

He was not correct—not quite. For him, a mental institution was still one day away. But he'd get there. He would get there—committed by order of Cook County Mental Health Court—without having a chance to confront his wife, to challenge her story, or to call witnesses in his behalf. James R. was a patient in Cook County Hospital's Mental Health Clinic, aboard a beltline to a state institution. His diagnosis—schizoid reactions, paranoid type—was determined by two court-appointed physicians, Drs. F. and I., in a two-minute hearing.

To assist them, the doctors had at their disposal—a "Case History" compiled by a social worker after an interview with just one person, [the man's] wife, who frankly said she wanted him committed; and a five-line report by a psychiatrist who saw James for less than thirty minutes, and found him to be "in contact and oriented, but hostile." [10]

These examiners were employing a traditional method of psychiatric examination. They were endeavoring to establish the presence of "reality severance" in this frightened, threatened, confused, and doubtless *ill* individual. This was not for the purpose of affecting the disease process; it was a legal "gimmick" intended to *enable* treatment (and a further examination) to be given. It used to be a primary function of psychiatric diagnosis to determine the presence or absence of dereism, i.e., departure from or repudiation of the interpretations of reality common to the culture and the community. The upshot of inquiry was to determine whether the patient was experiencing hallucinations, entertaining delusions, or withdrawing his orientation to the world about him. If one could say that the patient was hearing voices, had delusions, or was disoriented, one could certify him as having "a" mental illness requiring involuntary hospitalization.

All this is a relic of the Middle Ages, when mental illness—"insanity" —was almost *prima facie* evidence of an evil nature come to light: sin, wickedness, immorality, vice. Commitment was essentially a sentence to life imprisonment, and the psychiatric examination was a modified and somewhat softened criminal trial. Attached to it were all kinds of social complications—stigmatization, suspension of voting privileges, separation from family, prejudice regarding civil and legal rights. A guardian might have to be appointed, and a guardian's ideas about investing or spending a patient's money might be quite different from those of the patient. Hence the patient stood to profit little or none by being committed—but it protected others from retaliation by the patient, who might later think he had been wronged. It had to be gone through with in order to justify the state in expending monies for the treatment of the indigent, to enforce treatment upon the fearful and unwilling, and to control the violent and unruly without risk of legal charges. Today with patients knocking on the doors of all psychiatric hospitals, psychiatrists have little heart for forcing any patient to accept treatment. The commitment device is an awkward and antiquated one and should be replaced.

It *is* necessary to know *early* in the handling of a new or prospective patient how disturbed—how *dysorganized*, in our sense—he is, how much he is aware of a need for treatment, and how consistently he can cooperate with those who can provide it for him.

In common speech we frequently hear someone exclaim, "Why, that man is crazy!" A friend may comment, "But he has always been so. Didn't you know it?" And the reply might be, again, "But now I mean he is *really* crazy."

What the speaker has in mind is the same thing that the alienist of old had in mind; someone's repudiation of reality has escaped all concealment, compromise, façade. He has renounced what we all struggle to maintain—and perhaps he too had struggled. But he has crossed the line into perdition; he has betrayed the presence of "it." This "it" is that peculiar, mysterious essence of alienation, of uncanny, other-worldly, far-offness. Actually, it is only a greater degree of something present in all of us all the time, but this is hard to accept. And the sleuthing search for the damning proof of irrationality often leads to the reinforcement of a façade, to evasion and escape; or to vigorous counteractions.

The approach to and the outcome of the interview just cited might have been different if the examiners had not been determined to find this "it," but had sought rather to learn how this man was ill, if at all; and if so, how ill he was, and why, and whether he might be helped.

Let's try it over again. The reader will have to imagine the inflection to be sympathetic and inquiring; he will have to imagine us speaking slowly and quietly, and he will have to imagine a facial expression of friendliness and concern. The interview, then, might have gone something like this:

"Good morning, Mr. R. My name is Dr. F., and my associate here is Dr. I."

The patient may have muttered an answering "Good morning," or he may have remained silent. It was still the doctor's move.

"We are doctors, Mr. R. Someone wanted us to talk with you, to see if we could help you. Was that your wish? Did you want to see a doctor?"

"No, I don't see any sense in it."

"Well, you are here in a hospital, and I'm a doctor. Did you ask to see a doctor?"

"No. My wife brought me here."

"Did she want you to have some treatment, maybe?"

"I don't *want* any treatment. I don't *need* any treatment, and I wish my wife would let me alone! She nags me all the time to have my mind examined."

"Perhaps your wife thought we could help you."

"No, she didn't! She just wants to get me locked up so she can get my money. She don't love me."

"But perhaps she thinks you are sick and wants you to have treatment."

"No, she doesn't! She doesn't want any good for me. She has been trying to get rid of me for a long time. She's got me so discouraged and mixed up I don't care any more. She just goes on pestering me and lying to me and tricking me and I think she wants to get rid of me and I guess she will. She even tried to poison me once."

"Well, would you be willing to stay here awhile and let your wife go home and stay there? You can tell us the whole story, and we'll give you your own room, with no molesting. Then we'll talk with your wife. Maybe we can help her to understand things better after we get the whole picture of it."

"She wouldn't come back; she wants to get rid of me."

"Will you stay here and let us look into this?"

"Well, I might."

It might have gone something like that—and the "alienists" would know just as much as they learned from the actual interview. They knew he needed treatment; they suspected that he was delusional; they despaired of getting his cooperation and assumed forcible treatment provision to be necessary, as it *may*, indeed, have been. But the patient *might* have agreed, by word or gesture, to cooperate. A compact must be set up between doctor and patient such that the illness process and its investigation becomes a common problem. Only then can the psychiatrist really make an accurate assessment of the difficulties and of the resources available. The psychiatric examination has begun.

Establishing this relationship is an art, one never perfected, but capable of being improved throughout one's professional life. The greatest agility is required to adapt oneself to the particular situation and the particular façade, and the tempo of approach must be carefully regulated, with an infinite respect for sore spots, reticences, pride, and dignity. No surgeon any longer operates without the merciful aid of anesthesia. No psychiatrist should torture or shame any patient with too personal inquiries or bewilder him with jargon.

Here, then, is surely one important function of the physician. With—but preferably without—the legal stipulations, he can advise whether or not hospitalization is indicated for a patient, and assist the patient or the relatives to accept this unpleasant move.

In or out of the hospital, even before the physician has said or done a single thing, even before he arrives at the patient's bedside, or before the patient arrives in the doctor's office, powerful psychological pressures have been set in motion working toward recovery. Scientific medicine does not deny this psychological factor, nor does it rely heavily upon it. It is a consistent feature of medical practice to constitute an orderly program of objective case study, a prosaic diagnostic appraisal based on prescribed steps of investigation. The doctor listens. He observes. He inquires. He palpates. He tests. He reflects. He begins a process of putting together observed and reported facts and correlating these with memories of experience—his own and that of others.

Making this contact is a far more important matter in psychiatric cases than in medical cases. Except in the case of a child or an unconscious victim of accident or disease, physicians do not usually offer their help until it is requested; and when they do, they expect cooperation. Psychiatrists are prepared for the opposite state of affairs and proceed upon quite a different principle. They often take the first step and persist in their efforts even when ignored by the patient or vigorously rebuffed. They know that such fronts often cover feelings of almost extinguished hope of obtaining helpful notice or real concern. Some mutuality is essential, and it is the psychiatrist's duty to try to establish it.

Guttentag [11] describes three stages in the development of a patient-physician relationship. There is a state of compassion, the basic, subjective stage dedicated to alert listening and careful history-taking. Presently the physician can detach himself a bit, entering the stage of estrangement. He is more objective, scientific; he begins to compare the data of the patient's affliction with established data and known facts. Finally there is the stage of personal communication and action.*

The effect of establishing a contact is to start certain processes of interaction and of internal change. The patient begins to orient himself toward the inquiries of the physician. The physician begins to study, appraise, and evaluate the patient's suffering, his complaints, and his symptoms in the light of the situation in which he lives. This, of course, is diagnosis.

As the physician becomes better acquainted with the patient, the patient becomes better acquainted with the physician. The illness is no longer the private property of the patient; it becomes also the doctor's illness, his problem. He, with the patient, must seek a better arrangement of things, contriving and working together toward a more acceptable solution.

The doctor and the patient thus enter into a compact, while continuing their separate relationships with their common environment and with their own particular sub-environments. The two-party affair between the patient and his environment now becomes a three-party arrangement: environment, patient, and the physician, who is part of the environment but also becomes an internalized part of the patient. The environment is related to this new corporate compact in the three ways suggested: the doctor has his own environment with its norms and expectations and restrictions; the patient has his own special environment into which the doctor will inquire and perhaps bring some change; finally, the two of them have a common environment of which they have common knowledge and over which they very likely have common control.

The Psychiatric Case Study

The first object of the establishment of a relationship is the diagnostic case study. This is a basic function of the psychiatrist. It is done not

---

* Guttentag ascribes these three steps in the nature and structure of patient-physician relationship to von Gebsattel. (Von Gebsattel, V. E.: *Prolegomena einer medizinischen Anthropologie.* Berlin: Springer, 1954.)

with the aim of detecting weaknesses alone but with the aim of assessing a human being in the midst of a complex life task. We must know his strengths as well as his handicaps, his uniqueness and his special vulnerabilities, if we are to understand his failure and his despair.*

The method of procedure is not like that of a traveler going from one landmark to another, but rather like a scientific explorer following an untutored native guide who presents the various sights and scenes in his own order of importance and with his accustomed routes and circumlocutions. As the native senses the explorer's authority and friendliness, he relaxes his guard and seeks to impart more information where the explorer shows sympathy and interest. So they go on together day after day, until they venture into remote and dangerous wilderness places which are taboo to strangers. All the time, the explorer goes on making notes, revising his map, filling in details, correcting his observations, until the whole is recorded and the dangers, real or imaginary, are exposed and confronted.

Perhaps this is an unfortunate simile. The patient is not as much the native of a strange and distant land as he may feel himself to be. Yet an uncharted exploration of his "life space" *is* required. What is the patient trying to do, or say, or avoid? What life problem is he trying to solve? What appropriate and inappropriate assumptions is he making about his problem and what solutions can he see among those realistically open to him? What does it cost him in disturbed functioning to persist in trying to solve his problems in the way he does?

Assisted, in ideal circumstances, by members of the diagnostic team skilled in doing so, the psychiatrist initiates an examination of the environment from which the patient comes and to which he belongs, simultaneously with the examination being made of the patient. Appraisal of the environment calls for a definitive statement about four general areas:

1. The general features of the man's life—geographic, climatic, national, linguistic, economic, and social.

2. The more immediate features of the environment, such as family, neighborhood, work, school, church, union.

3. Particular and significant sources of support and help to the patient

---

* The authors have written a practical guide for physicians entering the field of psychiatry. It supplies a plan of procedure for the study of psychiatric patients and for recording clinical data in a way that can lead to useful conclusions and recommendations. (*A Manual for Psychiatric Case Study*. New York: Grune & Stratton, 1962.)

and the reverse, i.e., special burdens, injuries, harassments and over-stimulation. (In this we bear in mind that appearances are nearly always deceiving and the obvious rarely the real.)

4. Injuries and hardships inflicted upon the environment by the patient. (These are often ignored in cases coming to the psychiatrist via medical routes, and exaggerated in cases coming via legal routes.)

While the appraisal of the environment is proceeding, an appraisal of the patient is also being made. To obtain this information there must have been systematic investigations of the past and present, the "history-taking" aspect of the case study. Psychiatric social workers are highly skilled at this, interviewing as they do many different people connected with a single case. But historical data will also be collected by the physician in the course of and as a part of the psychological examination as of here and now. This collection is made by the psychiatrist, the psychologist, and the internist or neurologist, i.e., the rest of the diagnostic team. They examine the patient with all the refinements of modern techniques. We want to know his assets and liabilities, both physical and psychological.

The general meaning of physical assets and liabilities requires no explanation here because physical health and the impairment of social and psychological functioning which physical handicap or physical illness brings about is something easily grasped by the layman.

But it will not be so obvious what is meant by specifying psychological assets. In the older procedure of psychiatric examination no mention was made as a rule of a patient's healthy psychological functioning. But it is important from the standpoint of planning treatment to know something about his potentialities, his talents, his psychological equipment. How intelligent is he? How well educated? How flexible? How ingenious? How amiable? How courageous? What kind of front does he endeavor to present to the public eye?

This front may be a truculent or a contemptuous one, beneath which exists a great fear of rejection. On the other hand, it may be a façade of social conformity, internal serenity, and an avowed wish to please. Such a façade may well be considered an asset for the patient. In some cultures it is highly esteemed, and it may save much social unpleasantness. We tend to call it hypocritical and insincere and dishonest and phony. All these things it well may be, but it is also an effort on the part of the patient to conceal his suffering and his incompetence from the world.

Looking beneath this façade, we may discover evidences of impairment and malfunctioning of long standing, chronic personality deformities or defects, for some forms of which we have empirical designations. There are the organically handicapped, the hypophrenic, the immature, the schizoid, the antisocial personalities. These are not the names of diseases; these are the partial descriptions of certain lifetime compromises of familiar conformation. We take note of them; we record a reference to them in the diagnostic conclusion, bearing in mind that these designations are at best only crude approximations of the individual character structure.

The Psychological Examination

Psychological examination (formerly called "mental status determination") has long outgrown the old-fashioned format which emphasized the identification of disorientation, amnesia, delusions, and hallucinations. The areas to be explored are now greatly expanded to include all accessible phases of the patient's psychology. We systematically investigate the patient's processes and styles of perception, i.e., how he sees the world, how clearly and accurately. We inquire into how he deals with what he perceives internally. We examine his memory, his store of knowledge, his ability to recall. We examine, too, his ways of thinking, his trends of thought, their coherence and relevance. His intellectual flexibility, his capacity for abstraction, his abilities in communication are noted.

Our preoccupation with the patient's cognitive processes never excludes attention to his emotional reactions, their intensity, their appropriateness, their persistency, their blunting or perversion. What does he feel strongly about and how does he show it? And do his emotions correspond to his ideas, on the one hand, and to his behavior on the other hand? Does he "emote" without action or act without feeling, or think without acting or feeling?

Behavior is the final resultant of psychological processes—not the only resultant, because the sensations related to affect are also a product. The fact that actions speak louder than words does not mean that we do not consider the words or the feelings accompanying them. The action patterns are examined in a systematic way from the standpoint of energy level, vigor, adroitness, directness, and effectiveness. We must assume that they express the resultant of all the conflicts of impulse—the pros and the cons—and we are just as interested in what the patient does not do as in what he does do. It is not enough to say that the patient dresses neatly, plays with his children tenderly, and forges checks; we must also know what he fails to accomplish.

Behavior is then examined from another standpoint; namely, the degree to which it expresses self-destructiveness. This is particularly clear in what is called symptomatic behavior; in fact, it can almost be said to characterize symptomatic behavior. This point has already been discussed at length in the text; here is where the matter belongs insofar as systematic psychological appraisal goes.

But this is only a beginning. Having obtained information regarding these part-processes of psychological functioning, the psychiatrist can look for evidence *in the patient* of what the history and the environmental investigations have suggested regarding his integrative and adaptive successes. In his relationships to people he has established various patterns, with prevailing techniques of social encounter. There will be major attachments and minor attachments; there will be best friends and worst enemies. The quality, depth, consistency, and satisfaction of the linkages will be studied, the patterns of relationship, the "kinds" of ambivalence betrayed, the dependencies, active and passive.

Besides people there are concrete things—animate and inanimate—which become a part of the personality through established relationship. What a patient does with his money, his car, his lands, his books, his clothes, his dogs and cats—all these come under scrutiny and one investigates particularly the extent to which they replace human love objects and to what extent they serve as narcissistic extensions of the self.

Two of the most important patterns of social integration are the way in which he works and the way in which he plays. Add to this the purely quantitative estimates of too much or too little play, too much or too little work, and a gross imbalance between these modalities of living. Each man must find satisfactions in his life efforts; food, warmth, and sexual relations are primitively important. But they do not suffice civilized man. He may think, he may even say that these are what he works for. But this is never the whole truth. Actually there are always some satisfactions in the work itself as well as satisfactions in escape from it and satisfactions in doing other things or in doing nothing at all. The complete psychiatric case study of any individual must deal sooner or later with many intangibles such as his philosophy of life, his religious life, his concerns, his ideals and aspirations, his attitude toward authority and responsibility, his prejudices and predilections, his self-image and self-confidence.

All this leads to and includes, inevitably, the patient's view of his present difficulties—his illness. Its sources, contributing factors, evolution, and present manifestations will be recited. His version will be compared with the versions of the relatives, friends, employer, or police. And certainly all these will be compared with the examiner's own observations—supplemented by those of other members of the diagnostic team, particularly the psychologist. The latter may also interview the patient, observe him, listen to him, or record and study his reactions to standardized problems and stimuli. He will correlate his findings with those of the psychiatrist.

The well-trained clinical psychologist is quite capable of making a comprehensive psychological examination and an appraisal of psychological functioning. In practice he usually does not do so, partly from tradition, partly because of the special skills in psychological testing which many clinical psychologists have acquired, and partly because of the advantage possessed by the psychiatrist in being a physician and hence one to whom a sufferer looks for help and in whom he confides secret or embarrassing information.

But the psychologist is nevertheless an indispensable member of the diagnostic team, his precise functioning varying with the particular case, with the clinic, and with the psychologist. The trend, however, is for him to spend a larger and larger portion of his time as a therapist, i.e., as a member of the *therapeutic* team, partially replacing the psychiatrist there, and permitting the latter to give more attention to diagnostic functions. Of this we shall have more to say later.

The historical and examinational data collected by the psychiatrist—or by the members of the diagnostic team—have to be organized, combed, correlated, and integrated. Otherwise they remain a meaningless mass of facts. We have to arrange those facts so as to get a picture of the individual, or as much of one as is relevant to the understanding and correction of the troubles for which he came to examination.

The individual who is now our patient was once the patient of an obstetrician, who "handed him over" in time to a pediatrician. The nucleus of the personality present at birth, that combination of hereditary and congenital items which suddenly appeared, was acted upon and interacted with many changing features of the new world. First there was a little world of mother and brother and rattle and bottle. The larger world beyond them—a room, rooms, grass, trees, sky, people—gradually took shape. This growing personality, with the aid of parents and peers and teachers, ultimately discovered and explored more of the various environments about him—some intimate, some proximate, and some more remote. He established relationships with parts of these environments, and to some extent changed them. By this he himself was changed, and his change again affected the environment. Each continually made new requirements of the other, but certain habits and balances and expectations became established. If these were occasionally upset by unexpected events, they were shortly re-established in the main, and "life went on."

Most contacts between environment and individual are pleasant or at least tolerable; some of them are necessarily painful and intolerable. The environment of the particular individual under study may have seriously injured or crippled him, intentionally or otherwise; he, in turn, may have seriously damaged or inflamed parts of his environment. Some situations are easy to overcome, some are mastered with difficulty, some are overwhelming. Accidents and fortuitous events keep occurring which rupture patterns of adjustment so that compensations and rerouting have to be made.

Diagnostic Formulations

We used to say that to diagnose an illness we should endeavor to discover what evidences of psychopathology a patient under examination revealed (or concealed). Was he correctly oriented, or perhaps somewhat disoriented? Was his memory within average standards of effectiveness?

Was he hallucinated, or delusional? If so, we might be able to identify the several symptoms observed as characteristic of an established, recognized syndrome. We might—we often did—make, then, a definite diagnostic conclusion, for example: "This patient has dementia praecox, hebephrenic type. He is committable as insane." Such a diagnostic statement is preferable to the older statements to the effect that "the patient is out of her mind; she is a lunatic; she is bewitched."

It was another step forward to recognize that these pictures actually represent not different diseases but different forms of one disease. Emil Kraepelin, dismayed by the vast number of variously labeled syndromes, attempted to bring order out of the chaos by a shrewd and arbitrary grouping of symptoms, considering their evolution over long periods of observation. This was useful in reducing psychiatric designations from thousands to a few score, and Kraepelin's exquisite designations and convincing delineations gave his taxonomy great popularity and influence.

Adolf Meyer, who introduced Kraepelinian psychiatry in America, later did his best to reject and extrude it. He tried to supplant it with the concept of mental illness as an undesirable reaction to environmental stress, capable of being described in terms of inept energy expenditure of different kinds. As a result of his efforts and those of William Alanson White, American psychiatrists began to ask, not "What is the name of this affliction?" but rather, "How is this man reacting and to what?" This led, of course, to the third logical question of a triad, "What does he have to react with?" This, in turn, led to the formula described, "With what, to what, and how?" But gradually this had to be amended. For instance, just what is implied by the question: "What does one have to react with?" Almost simultaneously in a dozen places psychologists (and a few psychiatrists) began to be concerned with a systematic and consistent theory of personality. At the time Freud began his work and, indeed, until a few decades ago, there were few books about personality *theory* and, indeed, few systematic theories.

But suddenly * treatises on personology began to appear—Lewin's in 1935, Allport's in 1937, Murray's in 1938, and after that Goldstein's, Angyal's, Sheldon's, Cattell's, Collard's, Sears', and Gardner Murphy's.**

Case-study method had to be enlarged not only in respect to the reaction capacities of individuals, i.e., according to some theory of personology, but in regard to the reactions produced or observed. More and more careful psychological and physiological and anatomical examinations began to be made. Just as progress has been made since the days in which a physical examination consisted in taking the pulse and temperature, so, similarly, great progress has been made in the techniques and scope of the psychological examination since the days when our chief preoccupation was to discover whether or not the patient was "oriented" or professed hallucinatory experiences.

Finally, the *to what* element of the diagnostic triad has undergone

---

* Gardner Murphy has reminded the writers that the psychology of personality, or personology, did not come into existence so suddenly. From the 1880s forward there were Ribot on *Diseases of Personality*, Binet on *Alterations of Personality*, William Stern on *Psychology from a Personalistic Standpoint*, and considerable French, German, and Italian work; Rorschach, for example, drew upon it.

** These and other theories have been analyzed competently by Calvin S. Hall and Gardner Lindzey in their *Theories of Personality* (New York: Wiley, 1957.)

much change. Freud's discoveries demolished for all times the easy assumption that human reactions are ever to *one particular more-or-less obvious thing*. Reactions are always to more than the one person or event. True, the event may be overwhelming, such as a blow on the head, but even such events are never entirely disconnected from the other events and persons in the universe or from the memories and the previous experiences and conditionings of the patient. The older state hospital legal forms used to require that "the cause" be identified in the case of each patient admitted. It is amusing to find in these records long lists of such things as "alcohol," "masturbation," "meanness," "deserted by husband," "loss of virginity," "financial difficulties," "business failure." It may be taken as axiomatic that psychiatric illness always represents multiple and complex reactions to multiple factors—factors in the body, in the environment, in the memory, even in the imagination. Established equilibria are disturbed, self-regulation is impaired, and disorganization of the internal government is threatened.

There is, in short, some degree of *dysorganization,* as we have defined it in this book. And the appearance, meaning, and trend of this dysorganization must be stated, as well as the degree. How "sick" is the patient, and *how* is he sick?

First of all, to what degree has dysorganization proceeded? Is it, in the language of our earlier chapters, dyscontrol of the First Order? of the Second Order? of the Third or Fourth or Fifth Order? Are the emergency-coping and tension-relieving devices called upon characteristic of what we defined as First Order dyscontrol or of more severe distress?

In practice we often use simpler and less specific terms than the mention of these five Orders. The average physician and the average judge would find them recondite and obscure. We prefer to say simply that the dysorganization manifested by the patient was of mild or slight degree, of moderate or more severe degree, or of very severe degree. "Mild," "moderate," and "marked" (or "severe") are relative terms which allow for the relativity and variability in the syndrome. And they are universally understood adjectives, but for diagnostic purposes must be given more precise definition.

It is not sufficient to mention the degree simply. Something should be said about the timing and rhythm of the illness, i.e., whether the symptoms have appeared acutely with rapid development, or insidiously with slow development. We should know whether the illness phenomenon is episodic and irregularly recurring, chronic and stationary, or highly variable.

If possible one should carry this further by saying whether the dysorganization appears to be increasing at the time of examination or whether it is now decreasing, and whether this change is occurring rapidly or only slowly.

We come finally to the matter of syndrome designation. The unitary concept of mental illness does not mean that no differences can be distinguished between the various pictures of mental illness. Groupings of symptoms in certain constellations have long been recognized. There is no need to discard useful adjectival references to classical syndromes. If a patient is depressed or hypomanic or pyromanic—in the well-understood meanings of these terms—his condition may be so described. Carefully worded definitions of agreed-upon reaction patterns are listed in the official nosology of the American Psychiatric Association—"depressive reaction" (or syndrome), "schizophrenic reaction" (or syndrome), and so forth. But in every instance the syndrome should be followed or expressed by a listing of the symptoms which comprise the picture in *this* patient and which are essential for accurate and explicit description.

When we have completed an appraisal of the environmental situation and of the patient who is having difficulty in and with it, we have almost completed a diagnostic description. We are prepared to say now that Patient X is a man of Y years who was born and reared in environment A (dominated perhaps by a certain mother or brother or racial situation) but now lives in environment B (which may be important because of a wife, an employer, or a job failure). Because of certain predispositions from the period of environment A and certain stresses arising in environment B, Patient X has become uncomfortable, perhaps even desperate. He manifests symptoms M, N, O, P, and Q, which we recognize to be indicative of a certain degree or level (I, II, III, IV, or V) of *dysorganization*.

All these facts and conclusions we can list. We can coin phrases; we can, if the temptation is irresistible, name some names. But what of it all? *What can be done for the man?* What shall we do for those contiguous to him? In order to answer these questions and institute treatment based on a certain rationale, it is necessary for us to offer some explanation, not so much as to *how* the patient is ill as to *why* he is ill and what his illness represents. We must attempt to explain how the observed maladjustment came about and what the meaning of this sudden eccentricity or desperate or aggressive outburst is. What is behind the symptom?

No man steals a watch for the sole purpose of obtaining a timepiece.

No man cuts his throat merely in order to die. No man interrupts a successful career from the sheer wish to loaf. Human motivation is not that simple. There are easier ways to attain the objectives of these examples than to buy them at such a great price. What do stealing or throat-cutting or loafing mean to these individuals in the totality of their experience and life and personality and environment? Why had they become so highly prized? Why were they so necessary?

It is this complexity which we try to grasp and partially simplify in our diagnostic conception. We try to discover and describe the nature of the mounting pressures and how certain events touched special vulnerabilities and made for special stresses. We try to see why a man of such-and-such endowment with such-and-such training and opportunity now exhibits such-and-such signals of distress, betraying internal and external imbalances. All this goes to make up a total picture of the personality and his illness—a slanted picture, to be sure, an oversimplified picture, an imperfect picture, but a picture by means of which we can convey to others our view of the dynamic nature of the problem for which we have to find a "therapeutic" solution.

In the course of the past few decades all sorts of names have been applied to this: "the dynamic analysis of a case," "the dynamic synthesis," "the case formulation," "the explanatory hypothesis," and others. Anna Freud [12] refers to it as a "comprehensive metapsychological picture." * Its name is not important, but its function very much is.

For example, to say of Abraham Lincoln that he had melancholia tells very little indeed. One may say, on the other hand, that, reared under conditions of insecurity and privation, inspired by a loving mother whom he lost too early, Lincoln lived under a lifelong shadow of loneliness, irreparable loss, and a compulsion to be to others what he felt someone had not been (or too early ceased to be) to him. Usually this appeared as concern and compassion; sometimes it took the form of depression and despair.

---

* She was speaking of a child under study, but this term could also apply to adult cases. Her idea of such a metapsychological picture is one based on dynamic, structural, economic, genetic, and adaptive data. She considers successively: the child's (i.e., the patient's) developmental history, the degree of regression, dynamic and structural assessments on the basis of examination and history, the assessments of general characteristics such as frustration tolerance, sublimation potential, and over-all attitude to anxiety.

She suggests that the conflicts be classified into the external and the internalized, and, depending on the nature of the conflict, an estimate be offered as to the level of maturity, the severity of the disturbance caused by the conflict, and the intensity of the therapeutic efforts probably needed for alleviation or cure.

The reader may think such an explanation offers little clue for treatment. But this is not so. However, we shall postpone relating the conclusions of these explanations to specific treatment programs.

Of another "case," recently studied, we might say that his disorganization is of moderate degree, now slowly recovering, manifested by mild depression, diminished efficiency, ruminative doubt, with vague delusions of persecution. But this state of affairs becomes more intelligible if we explain that this Blackfoot Indian grew up on a Montana reservation, hungry most of his early life. He lost his mother when he was ten and was reared by relatives who had a variable but predominantly negative attitude toward him. Convinced finally that even the much feared and suspected white man might have something better to offer than the sparse opportunities of his village and the surrounding farm community, he accepted the government's offer of industrial placement in Chicago. Here he was given a rent-free apartment for three months and a job in one of the meat-packing houses on the West Side. He worked daily in the packing house and knew no recreation or distractions for Saturdays and Sundays except walking about the streets or lounging in a beer hall. He met a few other members of his tribe but felt distinctly isolated from the whites and the blacks who worked in the factory with him, and became increasingly lonely. Criticism by his foreman was taken by him as a rebuke and an insult; he quit his job and sat about in a beer hall most of the time, dreading to apply for work. He had a gradually elaborated theory that he was the object of persecution, and tried to assuage his alarms with increasing alcohol ingestion.

Or take another example, a lonely only child of austere parents, who found his principal pleasure in scholastic activities. His precocious development in boarding school and college discovered for him few friends or pleasures. A political job, threatened by an approaching election, served to revive childhood feelings of anxiety, insecurity, and incompetence.

Prognosis

All three of the examples given lack a specification of the asssets, internal and external, upon which treatment and prognosis so much depend. This is an important difference between the old type of case study and the new. So long as psychiatrists were concentrated upon the identification of psychopathology and psychopathological syndromes the tendency was to emphasize the pathological, ignoring the healthy aspects of the personality. This is in keeping with medical practice; the physical-examination report on a healthy man given in complete detail makes very dull reading. It is like a superficial book of anatomy. The practical physician ascertains an acceptable level of cardiac, pulmonary, and renal functioning and, hearing no adventitious sounds and finding no evidences of pathology, he proceeds on his search to other parts of the body. Healthy physiological functions are usually silent, and therefore silence is usually taken to be health. But in psychiatry we make less use of terms like "healthy" and speak rather in qualitative terms. One man may be intelligent, another very intelligent, and still another extremely intelligent. All of them are healthy, all of them are normal. One obviously has a greater asset in this area than the other. Intelligence is not the only personality asset; we look as well for such things as:

1. Ease of social interaction
2. Capacity for pursuit of realistic goals
3. Fulfillment of biological needs, such as childbearing and rearing
4. Satisfying sense of social belonging: sensitivity to the needs of others
5. Feeling of adequacy in social roles (particularly sexual)
6. Optimal balance between independency-dependency, rigidity-plasticity needs
7. Capacity for utilization of essential creativity
8. Capacity to accept deprivations and individual differences
9. Conservative handling of hostilities and aggressions
10. Identification with ethical and moral values
11. Adaptability to stress (homeostasis)
12. Healthy acceptance of self (e.g., body image and ego image) * [13]

In addition, as we explained in an earlier chapter, we look for the forces working toward reintegration and recovery as well as the forces working against it. For example (as we suggested in our *Manual for Psychiatric Case Study*),[14] considering first those forces or circumstances which seem to work *against* improvement, we ask ourselves such questions as these:

(a) Are this patient's prospects for improvement pre-limited by un-alterable factors such as organic defect, developmental lag, advanced age, progressive physical disease?

(b) Are the patient's prospects for improvement impaired by conditions unlikely to be altered, such as irreparable loss, psychological rigidity, various physical diseases, actual guilt, or realistic economic and other fears, legal entanglements?

---

* Lists of positive qualities like this always sound banal and added together seem to characterize some kind of boring paragon. One is reminded of Dante's magnificent description of a "normal man" in *Inferno* (tr. Sinclair, New York: Oxford, 1961).

(c) Does the patient's life history indicate that his aggressive impulses are extremely difficult to deflect, modify, or placate?

(d) Is the patient's narcissism so extreme as to preclude object attachments? (This often handicaps therapeutic relationships.)

(e) Are the indirect satisfactions from the illness enough to impair motivation for being treated?

(f) Is there conscious acceptance of self-destructive intent?

(g) Is the "ultimate" environment to which the patient returns a frustrating, corrupting, overwhelming, or otherwise harmful one?

Concerning the forces and factors which seem to be on the side of recovery, working *toward* improvement or capable of being exploited in therapy, one asks oneself such questions as these:

(a) How much does the patient's pain (anxiety, apprehensiveness, depression, guilt feelings, excitement, shame) motivate him to seek a more favorable compromise? Cf. item (e) above.

(b) Opposed to the positive pain referred to in the preceding question, how much does he sense painfully the loss of satisfaction?

(c) A large factor in treatment depends on the patient's intelligence; how well endowed is he in this respect? How accessible to reason, re-education, counsel is he?

(d) Does he show some propensity for acquiring and using transitional love objects—other patients, aides, nurses, physicians, others?

(e) Are there latent capacities for recreation, and if so, are they likely to be for narcissistic, libidinous, or aggressive expressions?

(f) If self-punition is a marked feature in his symptomatology, is it susceptible to the substitution of symbolic forms of penance or realistic restitution?

(g) Is there evidence of undeveloped potentialities for creativity and healthy living?

(Items c, d, e, f, and g imply the presence of intact areas of functioning which might be extended by and through treatment.)

(h) Is the home situation or other "ultimate" environment to which the patient returns attractive to him?

(i) Is the patient's temperament essentially optimistic or pessimistic?

We have discussed in detail how we think a psychiatrist should proceed in obtaining this information and in organizing it. We shall only summarize it here by citing our outline for summarizing the psychiatric case study, taken from our *Manual*,[15] omitting or condensing parts irrelevant to our present discussions.

The Outline for a Summary of
Psychiatric Case Study Findings

I. Administrative Data (the patient's file number, age, sex, nationality, ethnic group, marital status, occupation, religious affiliation, place of normal residence, referring physician, and so forth)

II. Clinical Data

    A. Historical data

    B. Examinational data

    C. Observational data

III. Diagnostic Conclusions

    A. Appraisal of the patient's environment

        1. General features, such as geographic, climatic, national, linguistic, economic, and social

        2. Immediate features, such as family, neighborhood, work, school, church, union

        3. Particular and significant sources of support and help to the patient, and special burdens, injuries, harassments, and over-stimulation

        4. Injuries and hardships inflicted upon the environment by the patient

    B. Appraisal of the patient

        1. Somatic structure, functions, and reactions

            a. Special assets (physical, psychological, neurological)

            b. Impairments (use standard nomenclature and give date)

        2. Psychological structure, functions, and reactions

            a. Assets and potentialities (sublimations, talents, intelligence)

            b. Impairments and liabilities

                (1) Pre-clinical (predisposition, personality disorder)

                (2) Present dysorganization

                      (a) Degree (mild, moderate, severe)

                      (b) Type (acute, chronic, episodic, recurrent)

                      (c) Trend (increasing, decreasing; slow, fast)

       (d) Syndrome (most nearly appropriate
            APA designations)

       (e) Symptoms and signs

  C. Explanatory formulation of the case—including the illness—
     on a genetic, developmental, or dynamic basis

IV. Prognostic Conclusions

  A. Probabilities regarding the further trend of the dysorganization
     with and without therapeutic intervention (listing, if helpful,
     the determining forces pro and con)

  B. Accessibility of the patient to treatment (motivation, coopera-
     tion, economics, geography, etc.)

  C. Possibilities of changing the environment in a favorable direc-
     tion

Quod Erat Demonstrandum

The outline just submitted puts in a condensed, practical form the essence of our proposals. We submit that it is a primary function of the psychiatrist, with the aid of colleagues who together compose the diagnostic team, to arrive at an understanding of a patient, his environment, and his illness such that rational treatment may be planned and a logical prognosis offered. This understanding must be articulated and recorded in a form which communicates information to other people concerned in the behavior of this patient.

We have outlined the principles of organization and organismic functioning and self-regulation and disturbances of regulation. These make it possible to describe an individual as being in a state of mild or greater distress and dysorganization. Assuming that it is a temporary and constantly fluctuating state which is a function of interacting factors in the environment and the individual, we believe that its manifestations and mechanics and meanings can be described, the process analyzed, and some of the determining factors identified and even traced to their earliest appearance and effects.

On the basis of such an explanation and such an understanding of the affliction, the physician can decide what might be done to change the balance of forces in the desired direction, and say how probable and how prompt such a change would be. This is the information desired by the public; this is what the patient wants to know, as well as his friends, his employer, his lawyer. It depends upon the art of pursuing a diagnostic process, or arriving at a diagnosis which is a true understanding of what the patient's illness means, and on putting oneself in a position to recommend treatment, and recommending that treatment in language comprehensible to all those who are concerned with its administration, its execution, its cost, and its benefits. The language used by a psychiatrist has every reason to be understood by any physician, lawyer, judge, social worker, or intelligent layman, and such witch-hunting designations as "schizophrenia," "neurosis," "insanity," "psychopathic personality" are not really understood by these people or—for that matter—by anyone else. Their use only disguises essential ignorance or incompleteness of knowledge.

To insist on a comprehensive diagnostic description of the type we have offered, refusing to employ jargon as a matter of principle, runs the risk of exciting ridicule. "We have got to call it something," someone jeers. "Are you going to resort to sign language?" ask others. "Do you mean to say," thunders a judge, "that with all your purported psychiatric knowledge and experience you don't know what disease this man has? Do you mean to say you don't know what name to call it? *Is* it or is it *not* schizophrenia (or psychosis or insanity)?"

Many colleagues cannot endure the humiliation of such pontifical browbeating; others are for peace at any price. Even a controversial term, they say, is better than none; even though it implies a definiteness that we do not possess, it allays the anxiety of the ignorant. Even though we don't agree on what it means or whether it exists, we can use it in public and argue about it in private.

At the risk of sounding prudish or fanatical or afflicted with scrupulosity, we adhere to our position that to create a false sense of security, to assign class membership and employ designations of tainting and corrupting significance, is to wrong the patient and mislead those who await our opinion, even when they think they know what we think we mean. This kind of dishonesty is precisely what the holistic concept of mental illness eschews, and it is because of this that we affirm the necessity of cutting the Gordian knot and *using no names at all* for these conditions of mental illness.

On the other hand, we offer a medium of discourse which is useful at the same time to those who must deal with behavior in terms of the law, those who must deal with it in terms of religion, morals, and education, and those who deal with it as physicians. There is no copyright on simple, descriptive English words. But the trouble is not just with the words. It is where the words are placed and how they are used. We have offered not only a change in phraseology and designation; we have offered a model of psychiatric illness which, if understood and agreed upon, will permit the psychiatrist to offer a description of the illness which is comprehensible to his colleagues and to the relatives and to the judge. It is a description which aims at the central question, which is: How can something be done toward betterment?

A Second Basic Function Performed by the Psychiatrist

What has just been said implies, correctly, that the planning of treatment is another basic function performed by the physician. But one cannot call it secondary except in the sense of timing. All patients prefer treatment to diagnosis. Treatment depends upon diagnosis, and even the matter of timing is often misunderstood. One does not complete a diagnosis and then begin treatment; the diagnostic process is also the start of treatment. Diagnostic assessment *is* treatment; it also enables further and more specific treatment.

Psychiatric treatment is too big a subject to be dealt with in a book whose primary emphasis is on diagnosis. We have said all along, however, that our understanding of diagnosis implicitly and explicitly moves toward a plan of treatment. Treatment must be designed, it must be directed, it must be administered. More and more these three aspects of treatment are being separated and redefined.

We began this chapter with a highly abstract physician, starting with an ancient model and coming up to more recent ones. But, as the discussion has proceeded, the reader will have perceived the tendency for us to speak less and less of the individual psychiatrist and more and more of the psychiatric team, diagnostic or therapeutic. This shift of language describes something which has actually occurred in psychiatry. The classical practice of one doctor treating one patient (at a time), usually in his office but perhaps on a hospital bed, is today still an actual occurrence in psychiatry, indeed, a widespread and increasing occurrence. Fifty years ago there was no such thing. Today thousands of individual psychiatrists are seeing patients in their offices, making diagnoses, and administering various kinds of treatment. Given time enough and given access to sufficient borrowed professional help (laboratory examinations, X-rays, psychological tests) a psychiatrist can make a diagnosis without the assistance of a team. But the temptation is to make an incomplete examination, sometimes omitting one or more of the essential examinations, and hence to that extent guessing at a diagnostic approximation rather than arriving at it by the scientific method.

Most of the time of the individual psychiatrist is apt to be taken up with treatment. The patients for whom the preferred treatment is something that can be done in an office—psychoanalysis, psychotherapy, perhaps electro-shock—are usually patients of Second or Third Order levels of dyscontrol, in our terms, for whom part-time treatment, a few hours of treatment a week with a therapist, are all that is necessary. However, the change effected by part-time treatment is apt to be relatively slow and spread over a longer time than in the case of the full-time treatment of hospitalization. This is why outpatients often seem to the outsider to require so much more treatment than the more severely ill. It is not a matter of more so much as a matter of less intensive and more gradual.*

In spite of the rapid progress that has been made in methods of treating outpatients, both by individual physicians and by teams of various kinds, and despite the tardiness of many hospitals to introduce modern treatment programs, the fact remains that the great majority of patients in the United States receiving psychiatric treatment at the present time are being treated in hospitals. It is wishful thinking indeed, as R. E. Reinert has recently put it with great cogency, to think that more provisions for outpatient treatment will dispense with the need for inpatient treatment. "I know of no state hospital that has reported a decreased admission rate because of the increase in outpatient facilities; quite the contrary; even in those communities that have more than the usual number of outpatient clinics and community services . . . the admission rates to the hospitals have gone up measurably." [16]

Said *Time* recently: "If all the 15,000 [psychiatrists] in the United States, plus all the psychiatric social workers and all the psychologists trained as therapists spent all their working hours with individual patients, they would still only be able to treat one in ten of the patients who need help for emotional ills." [17] This is why forms of therapy such as milieu therapy, group therapy (industrial and recreational), and group psychotherapy hold so much promise for meeting the broad practical problem of many patients and few therapists. Of these methods, group psychotherapy is recently the most popular.

In short, therapies are multiple and require increasingly multiple and

---

* In addition to these patients who come regularly, one or several hours per week, every psychiatrist has one or more patients who come at relatively long intervals, but regularly, for reassurance, comfort, encouragement. Their psychiatrist is their friend, their counselor, their monitor. But patients of this sort take relatively little time.

preferably a cooperative approach. Diagnosis, on the other hand, is unitary
—or should be. This is our thesis. The paradox is that the unitary diagnosis may, and perhaps is, ideally arrived at by a polydisciplinary staff.
Many patients require more than one physician. Many physicians now
treat more than one patient at a time. And many a patient has numerous
people treating him, some of whom are not physicians but who work with
a doctor in a therapeutic team. Just as the trained nurse is less and less
involved with the bedside nursing of patients, where her profession began,
and more and more occupied with the direction and supervision of others
in performing clinical duties, so the psychiatrist is more and more dependent upon many therapeutic assistants.

Professional Teams

The therapeutic team may be identical in constitution with the diagnostic team, each member assuming new functions. The social worker,
who is in touch with relatives, friends, employers, and others connected
with the patient, assists them in making such changes in the environment
as are indicated as desirable or necessary for the mutual benefit of patient
and surroundings. The psychologist will assist in the continuing observation of psychological change and reactions, checking the course of the
illness. He may also personally assist the patient to make corrections in
his perceptions, associations, attitudes, and behavior; in short, he may
undertake, vis-à-vis, some form of re-education or psychotherapy with the
patient.

The internist or the neurologist—in fact all the workers—may continue
to see the patient helpfully, and of course the psychiatrist may continue
treatment in the form of counseling at shorter or longer intervals. Any
of these functions the psychiatrist *could* perform, and sometimes does.
But the virtue of the team idea is not so much the distribution of labor
as the development of special skills, *plus* the value of exchange and comparison of observations and opinions in conference.

And there are usually many other members of the therapeutic team.
If the care of the patient has been completely taken over for a time, i.e.,
in hospitalization or boarding-school care, the nurse, the nursing aide, the
dietitian and her assistants, the housekeeper and her assistants, the chap-
lain, and the clinical teachers of the various prescribed activities * all par-

---

* The designations "music therapist," "recreational therapist," "industrial therapist,"
"occupational therapist" arose during the developmental period of modern psychiatric

ticipate in the treatment. These are really subspecialties of patient-care contributing to total psychiatric treatment. In one sense the individuals are all part of the therapeutic team. But in a stricter sense—since their very numbers would defeat the purposes of conference planning—the individual workers are adjunctive members of the team and are usually represented on the team by their leader or someone else; they carry out parts of the prescribed treatment, delegated to them by the psychiatrist.

For the psychiatrist is the leader of the therapeutic team. He is responsible for its effective orchestration. Contrary to the general knowledge of the people and contrary to the concepts of some of the older physicians, the great bulk of psychiatric therapy is not carried out by the psychiatrist but by other members of the therapeutic team. His responsibility is the prescription of that treatment, its direction, its supervision, its modification, and its discontinuance at the right time.

The mere existence of a patient as a target is not sufficient to maintain group unity and clearly focused attitude and action. The psychiatrist must be a leader, a leader who plans and directs, but who does so in such a way as to hold group solidarity.

SAYING 17

A leader is best
When people barely know that he exists,
Not so good when people obey and acclaim him,
Worst when they despise him.
"Fail to honor people,
They fail to honor you";
But of a good leader, who talks little,
When his work is done, his aim fulfilled,
They will all say, "We did this ourselves." [18]

The metamorphosis of the roles played by the psychiatrist is a topic which right now commands the attention of all thoughtful persons in our field.[19] One can no longer answer the question, "What do psychiatrists do?" with a simple statement. Diagnosis and the prescribing of treatment, certainly; but these are general topics, as we have shown, accomplished in a process which has usually involved many other people. The psychiatrist often does more than direct a team of experts seeking a diagnosis or carrying out a treatment program. He may participate in

---

treatment. We prefer the honored name of "teacher" for all these fine and useful people, who teach the art of living to persons who may never have quite learned it or, if so, have lost it for a time.

the treatment, not only as supervisor of a program, but as an active therapist—a counselor, an admonisher, a comforter, a teacher.

These and other person-to-person therapeutic efforts are generally called "psychotherapy," a concept of treatment which has finally achieved respectability. At one time it meant "fooling" the patient with placebos, spectacular maneuvers, and gadgets, or "mesmerism." Even now it is difficult to define scientific psychotherapy—and even the most chauvinistic psychotherapists do not deny the large component of art in admixture with the science.

Psychoanalysis as a treatment method is regarded by many as the most scientific form of psychotherapy—and yet it is the only one for which some *years* of intensive training are required before it may be practiced. Hence, while perhaps as many as ten thousand patients are being treated in the United States today with psychoanalysis, it is probable that over a hundred thousand patients are being treated with other forms of psychotherapy, many of which depend ultimately upon the scientific principles for furthering recovery through psychological means established by Sigmund Freud.

This is the more remarkable when one considers that psychoanalytic treatment is actually *not* a "treatment" as much as it is a prolonged, detailed diagnostic study, stressing the patient's participation in events in which he had regarded himself as passively victimized. This ultimately leads not only to discovering and hence better controlling dangerous tendencies, but to discovering talents and potentials not previously recognized.

Most patients do not require so long and exact a diagnostic study as psychoanalysis. There are simpler and shorter and less expensive ways to discover the difficulty and assist or stimulate the recovery process. Indeed, many psychiatric patients do not even require the complete case study outlined in this chapter. The art of medicine consists in part in knowing how to make shortcuts, and when it is wise, and permissible, to do so.

Every medical teacher hesitates to say what I have just written, because he knows the temptations of the overworked, harried practitioner to neglect thoroughness, to make quick guesses and "do something"— prescribe an ataractic, order shock treatment, offer some opinionated advice, or give some hasty comfort or easy dismissal. At times these may be quite adequate and sufficient treatments, but in other cases they may be pitifully inadequate. The dilemma of the psychiatrist is that it takes a relatively long time to make a case appraisal, and a quick appraisal is so apt to be incorrect or seem careless and lead to improper treatment. Yet the pressures continue. There are so many troubled people pleading for assistance. And many of them will have to be studied and their condition diagnosed by a man working alone, unassisted by a team, and in a relatively short period of time. Naturally the more experienced he is—the more cases he has studied—the more accurate he is likely to be in this effort to reduce the time required by diagnostic study. At best this is bound to be more art than science at the present time. But the art must be based on the science, and on the knowledge derived by scientific procedure.

In the next chapter we try to illustrate the processes and procedures of diagnosis and treatment as they cccurred in an actual case. This will bring out some of the points made in the present chapter.

CHAPTER XIV

The Role of the Physician
(CONTINUED)

THE CASE OF MARY SMITH

SYNOPSIS: To further illustrate the many functions served by the physician in his work with the patient, this chapter presents the case history of a patient who after a long, chronic illness seemed to respond particularly to a relatively brief contact with a doctor and members of his therapeutic team.

The functions served by the physician in this case are examined, particularly that of listening, from which a digression is made into the matter of psychotherapy. Involuntary roles played by the psychiatrist by reason of the phenomenon of transference are also examined.

WHAT WE have spelled out in the previous chapter regarding the diagnostic and therapeutic functions of the psychiatrist can be seen in a better perspective if presented in connection with a particular case.

But what case? We would have to submit a hundred case histories to give an adequate picture. If we cite only one, should it be a case in which the physician fails, one in which his efforts are unavailing? This would not be very convincing of anything. Or shall we cite a case in which he succeeds? Would it not inevitably appear to be weighted or slanted? And a case in which the doctor sometimes failed and sometimes succeeded might become very boring, for such cases are indeed long and wearisome and vex the spirit.

And since no illustrative case is going to be just the right one, we shall do the best we can and draw such conclusions as we may from one at hand. The case history we have selected has certain dramatic qualities; if these make it more intriguing for the reader, so much the better. But drama is not of the essence. Nor is recovery, although this woman did—ultimately—recover.

We shall give an account of this case—a reading account, not a technical history. We shall disguise the name and identity of the patient. We shall give the diagnosis arrived at and the treatments given and the course of illness up to the present day. Then we shall go back and trace some of the functions performed by the doctors, noting their influence on the course of the illness. And we shall hope to demonstrate that the concept of illness and the method of case study and the formulations of diagnosis proposed in this book were useful in determining an effective treatment.

On November 22, 1936, at the age of sixty-three, a patient whom we shall call Mary Smith was admitted to the Blank State Hospital. She declared that she lived in fear of her husband, that he had once driven her from their home with a shotgun, with which he had also threatened the neighbors. Apparently on the basis of such convictions she had made a serious attempt to kill him. This led to her hospitalization.

The clinical history obtained at that time shows that Mary Smith grew up on a farm. When she was seven her mother died; she lived with relatives for a time until her grandmother came to keep house for her father for a few years. Mary Smith attended a country school for a few years, but left it to take over household duties. At fourteen she went into domestic service, and later worked in a store; at eighteen she married. Her first husband was fifteen years older than she, and his family disapproved of the marriage; he died three years later, leaving her with two children. During the next sixteen years she was married and divorced twice. She is said to have gone from one religious denomination to another, in search of help she could not find. But she reared and supported her two children by attending a school of design and opening up a dress shop, which prospered, ultimately employing eight girls. Both children graduated from high school and later from the state university.

After her children left home she married a neighbor, but this fourth marriage too ended in divorce, and the patient went to live first with her daughter, then with her son, and shortly after this took a position as a housekeeper to a man whom she subsequently married. Her children described this fifth husband as a kindly, gentle, if somewhat unsophisticated farmer with a good deal of native wisdom and humor. But after three years of marriage—she was then sixty-three years old—Mrs. Smith insisted that he was mixed up in liquor traffic and narcotics smuggling, that he put poison on her toothbrush and in her milk, that he had put spiders in her bed, and, finally, that he had in some way gotten hold of her son and had him tied up in a house in the country where he was being tortured. She threatened to kill her husband—he said—if he did not desist. On the day before her admission to the hospital she claimed to have been taking a nap while her husband, reading the Sunday papers, rattled them in such a way as to keep her awake. He so angered her that she picked up a hammer—it was said—and rushed at him and struck him on the side of the head. According to the patient, her husband then seized a shotgun and drove her from the house. (According to the husband, he was sound asleep when struck on the head.)

At the time of her admission to the hospital in 1936 Mary Smith was assigned to a ward for disturbed female patients. (Sexual segregation was then customary.) She was examined, "diagnosed," and given routine ward care. She appeared—it is recorded—to be "disturbed, restless and confused."

One year after her admission her physician noted on the chart that Mrs. Smith was "somewhat better, but still delusional." She was, accordingly, continued on the routine "treatment program" of the hospital for the chronically ill. It was "standard operative procedure" then; in three-fourths of the state hospitals in the United States and nine-tenths of the mental hospitals of the world it is "S.O.P." today!

Two years after admission there is another note: "The patient is delusional. Works willingly in the sewing room."

Another year passed: "The patient becomes disturbed frequently . . . is delusional, mildly paranoid. She still believes that her linen is medicated by someone plotting against her and causing her skin to itch."

Two years later: "This patient has made no essential changes since the last report of two years ago except that she seems less delusional and in somewhat better physical condition."

Another three years passed, and a note describes her as preoccupied with ideas of Unity, and occasionally showing mild excitement; later as "frequently" disturbed, delusional, and paranoid. "She believes that the linen is medicated by someone plotting against her."

Six years after her admission divorce proceedings were brought by her husband and in connection therewith she was examined by a medical board consisting of three psychiatrists who "unanimously adjudged her incurably insane."

Seven more years passed; it was now 1949. Little recorded change in her condition had occurred. She had become one of those 400,000 American citizens who sit and eat and excrete and sleep on the wards of state institutions, cared for in a routine way but untreated by any intentional method because they are regarded as incurable. Rows of rocking chairs line long, ill-lighted, ill-ventilated halls smelling of disinfectant, sweat, stale urine, and decomposing food. In such a ward, with eighty other patients, Mary Smith sat in a rocking chair, rocking and "jabbering something." Occasionally she would scramble to her feet and rush to the barred windows, shake them vigorously, and call out something loudly to imaginary people on the ground far below. She might return to her chair and soon resume her rocking, or she might stand at the window for long periods, holding to the bars and shouting hoarsely to imaginary listeners outside. (This is the picture many people have of mental illness and its proper treatment.)

In March 1949, in keeping with a radical change in hospital administration, the doctor who had been put in charge of the ward began systematic effort to become acquainted with each patient in it. Few of them paid any attention to his approach. Most of them had little or nothing to say to him. Mary Smith had always had a great deal to say, but no one had listened very long because it was a highly pitched, angry harangue which went over the same theme again and again.

But the new doctor listened, and Mary Smith talked on. It was her same old oft-recorded story. Her son had come from California. He wanted to see her but "they" wouldn't let him in. So he had to go back to California without seeing her. But he would come again tomorrow. She knew her son would not forget his mother; he never forgot his mother; he came every day. She said she could hear her son cry every night because she didn't show up at his home. She could see him down there on the grounds; but they wouldn't let him in. It was too long a trip for him to have to go to California and back every day.

With the latter statement the doctor had to agree. Her faith in her son's loyalty he had to admire. The frustration of not seeing her son he had to deplore. And after he had listened and admitted and agreed and deplored—but mostly just listened—he suggested that Mary Smith and he take a walk together and look for that son.

The doctor took her walking under the trees on the grounds and along the walks. They passed some of the individuals whom she had pointed out from her barred window, high above the ground, as her son. "Together we would introduce ourselves to the person and find out who he was and where he stayed (usually these were employees or other patients), and we would walk back to the ward without any particular comment from me," recorded the doctor.[1]

Without referring to the possibility that the mistaken identity of the people on the grounds was in part a reflection of her failing eyesight, the doctor arranged to have some spectacles fitted for her. The nurses gave her some things to read and stopped to chat with her. Soon, while she still demanded to see her son downstairs, a change seemed to be coming over her. She ceased to raise her voice so stridently. Occasionally she got up quietly from her chair and, instead of going to the windows and shaking the bars, straightened a rug. She helped some of the nurses in the bedmaking. She asked when the doctor was coming by today.

The change progressed rapidly. A month later she was being permitted for the first time in thirteen years to go out walking on the grounds all by herself. She returned regularly and safely. No one was attacked, no one was injured, no one was disturbed.

Her capacity for self-control and directed effort grew rapidly. She began to help the nurses regularly in making beds and cleaning the rooms. She helped lift some of the more helpless patients. She went downtown for a minor shopping expedition with one of the aides and was astounded by the many automobiles and traffic lights.

As her improvement continued she was considered for what has always been called in state-hospital vernacular a "parole," that is to say, permission to remain outside the hospital for a short time on a trial visit, staying perhaps in a boarding home. Some of the relatives and friends and even the doctor who had originally brought her to the state hospital opposed her "parole," reminding the new doctor that she had attempted to kill her husband thirteen years previously, and perhaps another husband before that, and that she had been incurably insane ever since, officially so declared. It was alarming, they felt, to release so dangerous a woman from the custody of the iron-barred asylum. (Let it not be concluded that these were harsh or uncaring people. They had fully adopted the view which a score of physicians had taken of this case for many years. How could they now believe the impossible news?)

So Mrs. Smith remained in official—but not actual—confinement. It was no longer an asylum for her, indeed, scarcely a hospital. It was a dormitory. She had demonstrated to the nurses that she could take good care of patients on the ward, and she began plans for obtaining such work in the community. She put an advertisement in the newspaper, made arrangements to answer telephone inquiries (by being in the front office of the hospital at certain hours), and answered the replies orally and by mail. She was allowed to meet some appointments and made a good impression.

All this time she was seeing her beloved doctor every day. Now, however, she was preparing to leave him and she wanted to take up again the life that she had left so many years before. In October 1949 she left the hospital for a prolonged stay, but continued to come out once a week to the hospital to see her doctor. Early in November she took a position as a practical nurse caring for an elderly woman. (She herself, at that time, was seventy-six.)

She became active again in the local branch of the Eastern Star, to which she had belonged many years before. She re-established broken contacts with several former friends. She began going out to movies, to concerts, and to church services. When her first patient died of cardiac failure, Mrs. Smith had made such a good impression upon several physicians concerned with that case that she immediately had four requests for her services for the care of other cases requiring home nursing.

In February 1963, eleven years after Mary Smith had left the hospital, her daughter, an intelligent businesswoman, informed us that her mother, now approaching ninety, was continuing to get along surprisingly well. Once during the decade she had returned for a few months to the hospital which had been, for so many years, her second home. She then went to live in a nursing home, spending frequent week ends with her daughter. She put on several programs at her church during the winter of 1961, knitted and crocheted presents for her friends at Christmastime, read to various sick neighbors, and visited her grandchildren frequently. "She is an excellent worker, helpful and cooperative, occasionally cantankerous and meddlesome, but one of the best-organized women I ever knew at any age," declared her daughter.

Recapitulation of the Case

The case of Mary Smith is not a unique one. Unexpected improvements and recoveries in long-hospitalized patients have often been reported and are familiar to most experienced psychiatrists. They happen now and then in every psychiatric hospital. Sometimes they occur without relevance to any detectable external changes. In this instance there are some presumptive reasons for associating the change with the person and program of a new physician and his associates. We shall examine this apparent effect carefully, because it illustrates some of the roles which a physician may play in the contest of forces determining the course of illness. More than that: we think it illustrates the advantages of the new point of view in psychiatry.

Let us review the case as it was seen originally and then as it was seen in the light of a new concept of psychiatric diagnosis and treatment. Consider first of all that Mary Smith was not a neglected patient in the ordinary sense. She was well known to the superintendent and to the medical staff and to the nurses. She had been seen and examined many times. Various physicians had studied her and a fairly elaborate case study had been made and added to over the years. The historical facts had been assembled; repeated physical examinations and psychological examinations had been made. She was "presented at staff," and, upon the basis of the findings of the case study, a diagnosis had been tendered, discussed, and finally recorded.

It was "Acute Confusional Insanity."

This diagnosis was revised, subsequently, to one of "Dementia Praecox, paranoid type," which went unaltered for a span of years. It was then changed to "Paranoia." Later it became "Schizophrenia," and still later "Paranoid State."

This is diagnosis in the old style. It was very common for patients who remained in the hospital for a period of years to have a half-dozen or more changes in the diagnostic label.

With such diagnostic conclusions staring doctors and nurses in the face, probably no one expected Mrs. Smith to recover. Recovery was not the goal of the doctors' efforts. I know this, because I was one of those doctors once; we hoped of every patient that he or she *might* be one of those rare ones who showed improvement and even "remission," but we saw the process as a malignant one, and our goal was the mitigation of severe symptoms and then the adjustment of the patient to the hospital way of life. (I speak personally of an earlier time, but I know this still applied when Mrs. Smith was there.)

Without reference to the diagnosis, the standard regimen of treatment was usually something like this:

Confinement with maximum security (homicidal threat)

Regular diet

Sedative as needed (more recently, an ataractic would have been administered instead)

Elixir of Iron, Quinine, and Strychnine, one teaspoonful before each meal to stimulate appetite

Sedative hydrotherapy tub, twice weekly, for 2 hours at 96 degrees.

Mrs. Smith was so treated—and *well* treated. The "nurses" * got her up in the morning, marched her in line to the bathroom, later to the

---

* Actually there were no nurses in the modern sense. There was one head nurse for the entire hospital (1850 patients). Then there were aides, or practical nurses—usually married couples, living on the wards with the patients. Some were kind, some were unkind. Some patients were lucky, and some were not.

dining room, and still later to the "sitting room," that long dismal corridor on which all patients sat in a line of rockers. The doctor in charge of her ward certainly passed through it at least once a day, usually accompanied by the head nurse, and on Sunday mornings by the superintendent. It is very likely that at least once during the week, and perhaps more than once, the doctor stopped to visit with her. He asked how she had been doing. He made periodic observation entries on the chart, and if the nurse said that the patient had been constipated, he prescribed a cathartic. He may have suggested some "occupational therapy"—some rag-sewing or mending. He undoubtedly had some responsibility in connection with permitting visits from her relatives or even visits to them, and giving permission for her to be taken to such events as the Christmas dance. He no doubt served as an arbiter in various incidents of altercation on the ward.

Thus the doctor's role, once the "diagnosis" had been completed, was that of presiding authority, a kindly but busy friend and general sponsor. One could speak of this as treatment of a sort; in a more modern day we put great stock in the beneficial effects of milieu treatment, i.e., the constructive and educative values of a planned, therapeutic environment. But milieu treatment has as its goal the training of the patient to *leave* the hospital. Treatment of the sort given Mrs. Smith was aimed rather at helping her to make the best of her fate, of her confinement to the asylum. The doctor and the nurses undoubtedly tried to help her enjoy life as much as possible under the circumstances. She would discover that life inside a hospital was not as terrible as people outside thought it was, a little world of its own in which she might be moderately happy in spite of her affliction. They would have to continue to confine her, but they would protect her, and they would protect her relatives and the outside world against her obtrusive and hazardous return.

A little later the doctor may have tried the effects of various physical and chemical devices. He may have prescribed hydrotherapy or vigorous exercises or (much later) shock therapy. I say he may have, because the probabilities are that after the first few months, the period to which the dubious appellation of "intensive treatment" became attached, there was no room for her on the hydrotherapy schedule and there were no aides to supervise any exercises or special treatment—especially for a patient who had remained so many months and even years without material change.

What happened with Mrs. Smith is what still happens with so many "chronic patients," the acceptance on the part of both patient and relatives, and, worst of all, on the part of physicians, of a passive resignation. "She has become a chronic," think the doctors. "It is too bad about Mrs. Smith," think her friends, "but it is good that somebody is taking care of her." "It is no use," thinks the patient.

Many words have been coined to describe this state of mind as seen in the patient, "institutionalization" being the best known. But we never have had a very good word to describe the same state of mind as it exists in the physicians and in the relatives.

And this state of mind is of the utmost malignancy. It assumes that the situation is hopeless, insofar as any recovery and resocialization are concerned. Everyone gets the idea—sometimes from the mouth of the psychiatrist—that this is the way the patient must live, the only way she knows how to live, the only way she can live. Everyone quits trying, as it were—and for all sorts of reasons *other* than scientific ones. The doctors have more recent and more interesting clinical challenges; the nurses are busy with other patients; the relatives are not always too anxious to have the patient return to their area. The patient may find secondary gains from the care she receives. But most of all—and we shall say more about this in the final chapter—everyone gives up hope. No one has any expectations that anything will make any difference. Death is patiently, helplessly, hopelessly awaited.

Now and then—as we have said—in every hospital some long-time patient, here or there among the hundreds or thousands, suddenly shows an unexpected improvement. The news spreads through the place like the pealing of a bell. The section chief and the head nurse are summoned to see the miracle. The superintendent is apprised. The relatives are notified. The good news is discussed at the doctors' lunch table. Everyone feels a slight lift. One patient has rejected the role of passive resignation and ward-level adaptation. He or she has begun to look about, to take realistic steps toward a reacceptance of reality and readaptation to the modes of the outside world. He is encouraged, of course, by the ward personnel, who are delighted and proud; they give the patient a great deal of attention, which of course furthers the process.

In the case of Mary Smith something like this happened, but under circumstances which do not permit us to describe it as spontaneous.* For after many years of a restless, unhappy, often noisy and disturbed routine, she began to change. And she changed in direct chronological relationship to the efforts of a physician to effect some change.

---

* Which, actually, it *never* is; we just don't know what happens sometimes.

What did this physician do? What were the doctor's roles in the change that occurred in Mary Smith? As we shall see, his roles were many. He gave treatment; he arranged treatment; he supervised treatment; he counseled additional treatment; he checked up on treatment. He obtained the cooperation of many people, including the patient's daughter and the patient herself. Even before all this treatment, he made a diagnosis. It was this diagnosis which determined the treatment he planned and put into effect. This diagnosis was made according to the concepts we have presented. The case study gave hints as to what forces might be strengthened, what potentialities developed, what steps one might try to get the patient to take for herself, and what measures one might persuade the environment to take.

But I submit that what the new doctor and the new regime did *differently* was to approach their tasks, their responsibilities to Mrs. Smith and to all her fellow patients, with a different attitude and hence a different *modus operandi*. By "different" I mean different from previous physicians and regimens. Attitudes are hard to describe; but they are sometimes expressed by, as well as in, procedures.

I was not there, but I am sure that the first thing which Mary Smith's new doctor did (he and the nurses and others associated with him who were to carry out the treatment program) was to make contact with her. They let it be known to her that she was *noticed*, that they were interested in her, that they were *not* satisfied with her adjustment level, and that they intended to do something about whatever it was that troubled her. They gave their attention to Mary Smith; they noticed her as a troubled human being; they listened to her story.

Making contact with a psychiatric patient is of the utmost importance. In physical illness, given a pain somewhere in the body, no one is too much offended by the doctor's manner of approach. We can put up with clumsiness, gaucherie, or even rudeness from a busy doctor if he will just give us some evidence that he is proceeding without delay toward affording us relief; our sensibilities do not matter so much.

With a psychiatric illness it is different. Loss of contact with others is the very thing the patient suffers from, and the doctor who muffs the approach can easily thereby destroy all possibility of being helpful, or at least postpone it a long time. Of course, if one does not *expect* any treatment to be helpful, there is no use in taking such pains.

Mary Smith had been noticed before, a great many times. She had had the attention of many physicians and nurses, some of whom surely made efforts to reach her. Why, then, did the notice of one particular physician after all those years get across to her clouded and troubled mind enough to arouse a flicker of hope and hence a tiny current of reciprocal relationship?

I can only say that some doctors know *how* to notice patients, intuitively perceiving the inward longings denied by the outward acts.* The tone of voice in speaking to a patient, the inflection, the facial expression and gestures, the manner of approach—these and no doubt many other subtle things combine to "reach" a patient who has been untouched by hundreds of inquiries of "How are you feeling today, Mrs. Smith?" "Well, how are things going for you?" "Do you need a cathartic, Mrs. Smith?" "Please don't shake the bars, Mrs. Smith. Your son is not here."

I think I can see this doctor strolling unhurriedly through his wards, looking seriously at Mrs. Smith when he came her way and sitting down beside her quietly. I can see him listening gravely to her "jabbering" for five or ten minutes—even longer—perhaps saying nothing himself. Perhaps he asked a few questions which indicated some credence in what she was saying, some hint that he did not regard it as total absurdity. Perhaps then he nodded, patted her hand, and strolled on. A few days later he may have asked her to tell him a little more about her son, the one she thought she heard downstairs. In some such way conjunction was made and communication was established.

The Doctor as a Listener

Listening is one of the most important tools the psychiatrist possesses. Listening has both diagnostic and therapeutic functions. What Mrs. Smith's doctor heard and what he observed as he was listening enabled him to see that further listening, while it might not edify him, would serve the purpose of benefiting her. It would enable her to reduce some of the resentment and anger and at the same time examine some of the reasons for them.

---

* The question of the interaction of certain patients with certain physicians and of patients of a certain type with physicians of a certain type has long been a matter of scientific investigation. It forms a part of careful studies in practice in The Menninger Foundation, known as the Psychotherapy Research Project. It has also been the subject of studies by Professor John Whitehorn and various of his associates. (Whitehorn, John C., and Betz, Barbara J. *Am. J. Psychiat.*, 111:321, 1954; APA *Psychiatric Research Reports*, 5:89, 1956; *Am. J. Psychiat.*, 113:901, 1957; *Am. J. Psychiat.*, 117:215–223, 1960.)

Ernst Ticho speaks of "psychotherapeutic listening." [2] He distinguishes between the listening we do in ordinary life and professional listening, the latter being a technique that has to be learned and long practiced. It has to be a listening which notes whatever the patient says; it also notes what the patient does not say, or says by means of gestures, postures, and facial expressions. We must listen with the heart as well as with the mind, and yet not become involved in a distorting excess of countertransference.

A distinguished American poet has pictured Moses coming down from the mountain with not ten but *eleven* commandments, the "eleventh commandment" being a single word: *"Listen."*

> It is not enough that one's own inner voice
> Make of one's life a lifelong monotone.
> I, me, mine, to-for-because-of me, rejoice
> A man but little, then less, less, and none.
> What does he hear for news who has only heard
> From his own island? It is a treasure of dust
> On the wind when he unlocks his word-hoard.
>
> Moses' commandment opens the world's mouth
> To utter the memory of life. One listener
> Is man multiplied, man taking in time's breath
> To be in one body ancestor and heir.
> He owes one duty thus: attention. Man
> If he means to live shall hold his whole mind
> At ready awake. With this the law began.
>
> So Moses brought the eleventh commandment down,
> Knowing his will stir, his blood hasten
> That the word be said aloud, the word be known,
> That on it all men might take hold and fasten
> On it, and hear it in all tongues: Listen.
> He lifted the tablets up before them saying
> The word that gave them all words: Listen.[3]

Years ago Mrs. Menninger and I quoted from an unassuming essay by a magazine writer because it was the clearest and most persuasive account of this commandment I had ever read. After another quarter-century I still think so, and propose to quote from it here even more extensively than in our earlier book:

Who are the people, for example, to whom you go for advice? Not to the hard, practical ones who can tell you exactly what to do, but to the listeners; that is, the kindest, least censorious, least bossy people that you know. It is because by pouring out your problem to them, you then know what to do about it yourself.

When we listen to people there is an alternating current, and this recharges us so that we never get tired of each other. We are constantly being re-created. Now there are brilliant people who cannot listen much. They have no ingoing wires on their apparatus. They are entertaining but exhausting too. I think it is because these lecturers, these brilliant performers, by not giving us a chance to talk, do not let us express our thoughts and expand; and it is this expressing and expanding that makes the little creative fountain inside us begin to spring and cast up new thoughts and unexpected laughter and wisdom. That is why, when someone has listened to you, you go home rested and lighthearted. . . .

I discovered all this about three years ago, and truly it made a revolutionary change in my life. Before that, when I went to a party I would think anxiously: "Now try hard. Be lively. Say bright things. Talk. Don't let down." And when tired, I would have to drink a lot of coffee to keep this up.

But now before going to a party, I just tell myself to listen with affection to anyone who talks to me, *to be in their shoes when they talk*; to try to know them without my mind pressing against theirs, or arguing, or changing the subject. No. My attitude is: "Tell me more. This person is showing me his soul. It is a little dry and meager and full of grinding talk just now, but presently he will begin to think, not just automatically to talk. He will be wonderfully alive." . . .

Now why does it do them good? I have a kind of mystical notion about this. I think it is only by expressing all that is inside that purer and purer streams come. It is so in writing. You are taught in school to put down on paper only the bright things. Wrong. Pour out the dull things on paper too—you can tear them up afterward—for only then do the bright ones come. If you hold back the dull things, you are certain to hold back what is clear and beautiful and true and lively. So it is with people who have not been listened to in the right way—with affection and a kind of jolly excitement. Their creative fountain has been blocked. Only superficial talk comes out—what is prosy or gushing or merely nervous. No one has called out of them, by wonderful listening, what is true and alive.

Now how to listen? It is harder than you think. I don't believe in critical listening, for that only puts a person in a strait jacket of hesitancy. He begins to choose his words solemnly or primly. His little inner fountain cannot spring. Critical listeners dry you up. But creative listeners are those who want you to be recklessly yourself, even at your very worst, even vituperative, bad-tempered. They are mentally saying as you express these things: "Whee! Hurrah! Good for you!" and they are laughing and just delighted with any manifestation of yourself, bad or good. For true listeners know that if you are bad-tempered it does not mean that you are always so. They don't love you just when you are nice; they love *all* of you.

Besides critical listening, there is another kind that is no good: passive, censorious listening. Sometimes husbands can be this kind of listener, a kind of ungenerous eavesdropper who mentally (or aloud) keeps saying as you talk: "Bunk . . . Bunk . . . Hokum."

In order to learn to listen, here are some suggestions: Try to learn tranquillity, to live in the present a part of the time every day. Sometimes say to yourself: "Now. What is happening *now*? This friend is talking. I am quiet. There is endless time. I hear it, every word." Then suddenly you begin to hear not only what people are saying, but what they are *trying* to say, and you sense the whole truth about them. And you sense existence, not piecemeal, not this object and that, but as a translucent whole.

Then watch your self-assertiveness. And give it up. Try not to drink too many cocktails to get up that nervous pressure that feels like energy and wit but may be neither. And remember it is not enough just to *will* to listen to people. One must *really* listen. Only then does the magic begin.

Sometimes people cannot listen because they think that unless they are talking, they are socially of no account. There are those women with an old-fashioned ballroom training which insist there must be unceasing vivacity and gyrations of talk. But this is really a strain on people.

No. We should all know this: that listening, not talking, is the gifted and great role, and the imaginative role. And the true listener is much more beloved, magnetic than the talker, and he is more effective, and learns more and does more good. And so try listening. Listen to your wife, your children, your friends; to those who love you and those who don't; to those who bore you, to your enemies. It will work a small miracle. And perhaps a great one.[4]

There is more to psychotherapy than listening to a patient, although that is the basis of it. There are certain conscious and deliberate efforts to comfort or reassure, or to warn or encourage, or to correct and enlighten. Much credit is given by some to the affording of insight, i.e., the helping of a patient to understand and forgive and restrain himself in the light of forgotten or unnoticed facts or beliefs which unconsciously determined false attitudes or actions. Insight helps, but insight alone will not suffice. Other devices to enhance the arrested learning and growing must also be used.

But the effective factors in psychotherapy, as perhaps in much other therapy, are largely unconscious. They are certainly unconscious to the patient—and they may be unknown also to the doctor. Of these we shall have more to say in the next chapter.

Because listening is the most important technical tool possessed by the psychiatrist, we have discussed it at some length. Mary Smith was indeed listened to: she was listened to by her psychiatrist, by her nurses, by her psychologist, and by others. And as they listened, in addition to relieving her isolation, together they accumulated data about her psychological functioning which was organized by the psychiatrist into a descriptive psychological-examination report, such as we outlined in the preceding chapter.

The case study made of Mary Smith twenty-odd years earlier was, as we conceded, adequate for the purposes of its makers. Her doctors had described her behavior adequately; they had perceived her symptoms accurately. What they lacked, presumably, was a grasp of the meaning of her illness, and hence any access point at which it might be relieved. The data they had collected were not organized in such a way as to provide an understanding of her difficulties, or of her very considerable potentialities. The doctors saw only her *reactions*, the outer aspect of her illness. These were seen by them as features of a disease, not as signals, as communications, as emergency devices being used to maintain a troubled and threatened equilibrium.

Application of the New Principles

Suppose we attempt to organize the historical and examinational data of her case in a way which *will* give us a useful understanding of the illness. Let us ask ourselves a series of questions.

First of all, *was she really ill?* Certainly her brain and her bodily organs were intact; no disease was present in that sense. But her earlier physicians would have said, "Yes," because she showed such psychopathology as delusions and disturbed behavior.

We, too, would say, "Yes." There was undoubtedly a persistent dyscontrol as we have defined it. We would qualify our answer a little, however; a part of her symptomatology was certainly dependent upon her contemporary environment, the treatment she was getting. The effects of a mustard plaster are sometimes more serious than the pain for which it was applied.

How ill was she? What degree of dysorganization was present? How great was the threat of further disintegration, total disorganization? What was the trend of the illness-recovery process?

Here again we would largely agree with her earlier physicians; they considered her severely ill, indeed "demented"; we would describe her as showing evidences of a Fourth Order of disorganization, with fluctuations, but no trend of change.

Next let us ask not, How ill was she? but, *How was she ill?* How was the dysorganization being manifested? In answer we here would list the symptoms that have already been noted: her hyperactivity, chronic excitement, delusions of being the special concern of her son, verbal and physical aggressiveness, complete impairment of social effectiveness.

Does a conventional designation exist for this clinical picture? Yes; it corresponds to what many colleagues would describe as "a chronic schizophrenic reaction with paranoid coloring." This is clumsy; we don't think it really tells us anything, but it will do for the statistical records of the hospital, which we are obliged to keep trying to use.*

---

* One thoughtful colleague comments: "I don't agree that this designation does not tell us anything. If it is accurate, it tells us at least that (1) Bleuler's first degree

But now comes the *crucial question: How can this illness, this aberrant, impaired way of living, be accounted for?* Or *can* it be accounted for? Can it be explained in a logical way? To explain a case dynamically is to discover the ways in which drives have been frustrated and derailed and deformed; to explain it developmentally and genetically is to relate present problems of adjustment to crippling experiences in childhood, the effects of which have hung on throughout the years, known or unknown. To explain it economically is to show how the manifest symptoms are the best the patient can do under the stresses which have overtaxed her coping powers and threatened a disorganization. What we are attempting is a combined viewpoint which embraces all these principles.

Here, in brief, is the formulation which suggests itself from the rather scanty information the doctor could pull together about Mary Smith:

A girl early deprived of her mother and subsequently passed on to various relatives with occasional attendance at a country school became self-supporting at the age of fourteen. She married at the age of eighteen a man fifteen years older than herself who died three years later, leaving his widow with two children. Thus an emotionally under-privileged child had the additional misfortune of losing her first major heterosexual partner. Blessed with good health, intelligence, and a capacity for hard work, she reared and supported her children adequately and established a small business. Her singular and conspicuous psychological difficulties had to do with inability to establish a continuing and constructive relationship with a male companion. Yet at the same time she had almost as much difficulty in remaining free from "entangling alliances" with men, possibly because of her great inner sense of deprivation and loneliness. Full of energy, vitality, and ambition, she repeatedly contracted marriages which restricted the activities she most enjoyed. This was particularly painful as she lost her youth, her attractiveness, her friends, her children, and finally her way of life. Resentment and anger at her increasing barrenness accumulated to the point of direct aggressive action, rationalized by delusions. A frightened and mystified husband conveyed her to the state hospital, where the confinement and the conventional methods of handling of patients continued to provoke frustration and anger with enlarging fantasies that her son would rescue her from her unhappy plight. Thus she remained, at essentially the same stage of low-level organization in which she had entered the hospital, in spite of changing regimens, for a period of seventeen years—idle, restless, disturbed, importunate, noisy, uncomfortable, and socially useless. But she still had her intelligence and her energy; *and her delusions show that she still had hope!*

criteria are met in this clinical picture, and (2) that there is thought disorganization, and (3) that the direction taken by the thought content is projective. However, it is true that this is insufficient for an adequate grasp of the patient's affliction or disturbance or the needs arising from or associated with it."

Ordinarily, this kind of preliminary formulation is re-examined, altered, and recast several times in the course of treatment as the therapist comes to know his patient better. The doctor's understanding of the meaning of the illness proceeds through a series of progressively more accurate approximations to the "true" one. But even first and crudest formulations provide helpful orientation as the doctor tries to extend his first "contact" with the patient and listens with sensitivity and understanding to the scattered confessions, associations, memories, or responses of the patient.

Let us look at her illness from the standpoint of presumptive pressures, relative pressures, pressures or forces powerful in *her* case which might not have been so dominant in another case. What was it that she could not bear?

Several things suggest themselves. In the first place, she could not bear desertion or, let us say, another desertion, or the loneliness of it. For desertion is just what she had had time after time at critical periods —desertion by her mother (death), desertion by her husband, desertion by her children in their growing up.

Secondly, she apparently could not bear an intimate relationship with a man in which she, with her long-imbued habits of self-reliance, was obliged to accept a role of subordination. The history hints that she had some aversion to physical sexuality. Certainly it was less important to her than companionship, but that companionship seems to have had to be one in which she was in charge, the provider, the arranger, the commander.

The third thing she could not bear, one might conclude from the history, was enforced idleness. She had worked from childhood. She "loved" to work. She was competent and industrious and effective. But of course in the hospital she had no outlets for this.

Planning Treatment

Could a *treatment program* be roughed out on the basis of these conclusions? Could something be done to assure her against desertion? Could some friends be found for her whom she would accept? Would it be possible to take advantage of her obvious loneliness? Perhaps her hostile and narcissistic maneuvers would break down if some opportunity were provided for transitional love attachments. Obviously she still loved her son and daughter in her way; until she could return in a realistic way to her actual son and daughter, might other sons and daughters be found upon whom she could practice, so to speak, and relearn ways of interacting with fellow human beings? Could her physician find just that right distance in his relationship to her which would console and inspire her, without alarming or threatening her?

And could work be found for her to do—useful tasks, tasks of service to others, and tasks of increasing difficulty? Were there other patients toward whom she could be helped to assume a supportive role, in which she would have some opportunity again to feel managerial and executive and—in her way—even affectionate?

One thinks next of the possibility of finding a way to employ her intelligence. So much of it had been turned into delusional formations, so little other opportunity of exercising it had developed, that it might seem to be a particularly likely avenue of access. In view of the many months and even years in which she had not been encouraged to talk by being listened to, might the mere matter of listening to her patiently enable certain discharges of affect, clarifications of the thinking process?

And so it was. The rough outlines of the treatment given to combat her loneliness, her idleness, her detachment, and her misconceptions have already been mentioned. She was listened to, she was given something to do, she was given some patients to do things for, she was given encouragement and commendation, and some of her misconceptions were patiently attacked and corrected. Her hope, in short, was exploited, her potentialities were mobilized, her special difficulties were dealt with. The effect of this program of treatment on the course of illness has already been described. We review it here only to suggest the complexity of the physician's roles in affecting the course of illness.

The way in which the doctor proceeds to carry out his many functions will vary markedly from patient to patient, depending upon the nature of the illness, the present state of emergency, and the resources available for diagnosis and treatment. In fact, it is one of his purposes in undertaking a careful case study—and this is one of the important meanings of the term "diagnosis"—that the doctor will include in his appraisal a determination regarding which of his many functions it would be useful or essential to give precedence in a particular case. But diagnosis and treatment are the primary roles of the psychiatrist, as with all other physicians. Both are transitive processes, related to the illness and to each other, continuous and interdependent.

CHAPTER XV

The Role of the Physician
(CONCLUDED)

THE INTANGIBLES

SYNOPSIS: In addition to the physician's scientific and technical functions of diagnosing and treating, the patient-doctor relation is from the outset affected by attitudinal subtleties. We describe these in this chapter as the "intangibles" of love, faith, and hope and try to demonstrate that they are crucial determinants of effective healing; indeed, that they are sublime expressions of the life instinct.

IN THE two previous chapters we have tried to show how many functions the physician must fulfill. He must be a meeter and a greeter, an observer and a listener, an examiner and a prescriber, an operator and an evaluator, an educator and a classifier, a guide and a friend. Often he must be a leader, a director, a co-worker with others in diagnosis and in treatment.

What we have proposed in this book, and tried to demonstrate, is that his most important function is diagnosis. By diagnosis we mean a way of looking at patients or people who might be patients, a way of estimating the nature and degree of their difficulties in life with an eye to assisting them—just enough and not too much—to get back on the track and to go ahead. To change his conception of diagnosis is to change not only the treatment methods of a psychiatrist but his attitude toward their use. Thus not a *vicious* but a *benevolent* circle is set up; a proper diagnosis determines better treatment methods, which effect swifter cures, which support a hopeful attitude, which alters the traditional concepts, which motivates more penetrating diagnosis, and so on around again. A change in one of these functions favorably affects all the others.

Perhaps it was evident in the case of Mary Smith that her doctor approached her problem with a certain attitude—confidence in himself and his methods, a deep respect for his patients even though they were patients, and a belief in the possibility of gaining their cooperation and furthering their recovery. Whatever the diagnostic words may have been that came from his mouth or from his pen, his diagnostic concept was that Mary Smith was afflicted with a highly undesirable but quite possibly reversible condition upon which a determined effort might have the effect of initiating a favorable turn of the curve of illness. We think this attitude, this diagnosis, and the treatment they determined contributed to the fulfillment of these expectations. "Suspect" is not the right word; we are convinced of it, we *believe* it.

But is it only a matter of faith? Is this crucial factor in the doctor's effectiveness one born of an insubstantial illusion or delusion—a simpleminded self-confidence, the easy optimism of a sanguine disposition? Or are there factors—perhaps intangible but indisputable—beyond the mechanics and dynamics and chemistry and psychology, which help to explain the greater success of some physicians and the relative lack of success of others? Is psychiatry able to tell us anything new about this ancient mystery?

Psychiatry is a branch of medicine. But it is also—in its basic dependency—a branch or application of psychology, of sociology, of ethnology, of philosophy. It derives part of its structure from these sister sciences.

In what is perhaps the most beautiful short essay ever written, a theologian and missionary listed three great and permanent goods: Faith, Hope, and Love. Of these, he declared, Love is the greatest.

Better than most of his contemporaries Saint Paul was acquainted with the sins and the suffering of mankind. "Wretched man that I am!" he cried for all human beings; "Who will deliver me from this body of death?" He did not refer here to physical death, or to that alone. He was describing the "human situation," the dilemma of all people in this vale. And for it he offered the famous social prescription implicit in his Corinthian essay.

Today, after twenty centuries, this prescription is taken very seriously in psychiatry. We would even go so far as to say that it describes the basic philosophy of the psychiatrist. Faith, hope, and love are the three great intangibles in his effective functioning. In succeeding pages we shall look briefly at each of these.

Love

The importance of love in human life has been attested by thousands of others since the time of Saint Paul, and by a few before him. But love was first scientifically examined within our lifetime by a pathologist and neurologist, Sigmund Freud. Freud learned about love from the clinical study of patients who were—not lovesick, but sick because, as it turned out, their love life was so confused and disturbed. He allowed his patients to talk, and he listened to them without interruption. He discovered some of the laws of the birth, evolution, growth, and maturity of the love life of the individual, and discovered too some of its common vicissitudes and derailments.

Furthermore, he declared for its pre-eminent importance in therapy as well as in daily life. Freud discovered and described the function of love in the constant neutralization of hostile impulses and in the maintenance of patterns of social integration, discussed earlier in this book. Love as it determines the work and effectiveness of the physician now deserves more special attention.

Psychoanalysis has shown us with great vividness how much the interference with the giving and receiving of love disrupts and demoralizes the integrative patterns of life, and makes us feel ill and act in opposition to our desires. It has shown also how important it is that someone, such as the physician, serve as a temporary or transitional love object—and hate object as well—for patients struggling to reattach or further attach themselves to their human environment constructively. Every physician who treats a patient gives him something more than "treatment"; he gives him love. This love is often tinctured with other emotions, but the devotion of the physician to his patients is love of the highest order. It is an expression of *agape*, selfless concern.

There is more to the physician's love bond for his patient than *agape*; there is usually—probably always—some actual libidinal investment as well. It is usually unconscious, and it can be discounted or even denied by such impressive designations as displacement, sublimation, countertransference, therapeutic parameter, or scientific objectivity. It can be masked by gruffness, matter-of-factness, even harshness. But it is there—the libidinal bond—and it is mutual. The patient's unconscious need for love takes advantage of the situation, unconsciously in the great majority of cases, and reciprocal needs are mutually met. Freud discovered the structure of this mutuality and called it transference. Hippocrates called it love.*

Technically transference is used to describe only the unrealistic roles or identities unconsciously ascribed to a therapist by a patient in psycho-

---

* "For where there is love of man, there is also love of the art. . . ." (Hippocrates. *Precepts*, VI.)

analytic treatment. One may speak of positive and negative aspects of or attitudes in the transference; one can say that the transference is at the moment such as to produce a positive or a negative feeling toward the analyst. But the emphasis belongs upon the fact that the analyst and the analysand are engaged in a two-party contractual relationship in which the patient makes his payment and expects a return. And a part of this mutual exchange, as we have said, is libidinal, i.e., love.

The patient does not get exactly what he originally expected from treatment. He probably expected a small miracle, and at least some prompt objective relief, or character remolding. Instead he gets evidence of the doctor's concern, he gets attention, he gets understanding, he gets enlightenment. He learns that what he thought he wanted is not what he now wants, or that it is enormously more complex than he had originally suspected. In reliving phases and incidents of his earlier life in relation to a temporary love object to whom he ascribes with impunity many roles or "as-if" identities, he reviews and revises old hates and loves and grows up to new, more adult love expectations.

While the patient is making these unconscious identifications of the physician with people in his (the patient's) past, the physician himself makes similar unconscious identification of the patient with figures in *his*—the doctor's—past. This is the countertransference phenomenon already referred to. The physician is not sick; he does not regress, as the patient does, by invitation. The doctor is supposedly able to control the temptations to infantile behavior and magical thinking which may arise. Nor does he expect the patient to recognize *his* (the therapist's) transference reactions.

The doctor's own previous experience with such love wistfulness, disappointment, sorrow, anger, and fear enables him to understand the present emotions of the patient, displaced and presently inappropriate as they are. Countertransference is, technically, not the conscious sympathetic understanding and concern of the psychoanalyst; it is the unconscious, and often unrecognized (and hence usually inappropriate) feeling and behavior on the part of the psychoanalyst. It *can* be harmful to the patient (for example, in overprotectiveness or overestimation). But controlled countertransference of a degree may also be a positive element in the success of treatment.[1]

Countertransference in the broad sense—i.e., not restricted to the psychoanalytic-treatment situation—is undoubtedly a strong element in the desire of all doctors to give treatment, of which we have spoken so often in earlier chapters. Our patients are rarely given the credit they deserve for helping us as much as they do by permitting us to treat them! The late Helmuth Kaiser,[2] formerly associated with us, composed a clever play in seven acts (published just before his death) which he called "Seven Dialogues Reflecting the Essence of Psychotherapy in an Extreme Adventure." Two psychiatrists, good friends, are brought into a clinical relationship in the following way: Following the death by suicide of a patient of one doctor, he had become increasingly depressed. He was restless, lost interest in his hobbies, and went about his work heavily and compulsively. His wife began to fear lest he himself commit suicide. She felt it quite impossible that her husband would be willing to accept treatment, but conceived the ingenious idea that perhaps his good friend Dr. T. might be willing to pretend that he was a patient and come to her husband for treatment and thereby enable them to meet and talk. The somewhat astonished Dr. T. was intrigued by the proposal and agreed to try it, with the result that the reader can anticipate—the doctor who administered the treatment was thereby cured, and both were enlightened.

This is not to imply that there are not intellectual, experimental, merciful, and economic motives in the stream of interest which a physician invests in his patient. We have discussed all that. What is being proposed here is that there are always unconscious libidinal bonds in this relationship, libidinal factors which make the doctor's practice an expression of his love, as well as an expression of his life.

Transference and countertransference can reach pathological proportions and have destructive effects as well as constructive ones; they may block rather than further the recovery process. Some physicians cannot bring themselves to let their patients get well and leave; others cannot treat some patients at all, and some patients cannot accept or interact with some physicians. The reasons for these incompatibilities may not be known or understood by either one, but they exist.

> I do not love thee, Doctor Fell,
> The reason why I cannot tell.

Transference is, by technical definition, an aspect of a patient's reaction to his *doctor*. But the same psychological phenomenon may occur in the patient's relation to other members of the therapeutic team. If the team is properly organized, this is no trouble. It can be a help. This is one of the powerful advantages of group and institutional practice. It has been studied by Reider[3] and more recently by Wilmer.

From ancient times [says Wilmer] people have journeyed to centers renowned for healing—to shrines, temples, churches, mountains, springs, villages; to Mecca and to Rome. In modern times, they seek universities, clinics, hospitals and institutions dedicated to healing. As in ancient times, the sick still make their hegira with hope, expectations, even excitement, anticipating relief, cure or miraculous recovery.

While the healing powers of ancient centers were attributed to divine intervention, modern medical centers attribute their therapeutic effectiveness to scientific treatment. The magic and mystical powers which brought relief in olden times still bring relief today and it is possible to identify a common factor through which these powers are mediated: transference to a center.

Throughout history, The Center has stood as the symbolic Mount Olympus, its spokesmen as symbolic Oracles, its very name invested with "magic."

Positive transference permits physicians with widely varying levels of training, competence and experience to speak with the authority ordinarily invested only in the famous doctors themselves. In daily brushing shoulders with these famous men, their colleagues become coated with some of the dust of greatness. The patients have trust and confidence in *all* the physicians. In the words of one patient, "These young doctors wouldn't be here unless The Center had confidence in them." What was good enough for The Center was good enough for him.

The very name of the institution is a cherished and sacred title, a powerful symbol to which much transference feeling is attached. The name not only brings heightened hopes to the patients but brings the physician himself to a greater expectancy of his own professional competence. And in this frame of mind, with reciprocal support from The Center, he commonly performs at a greater proficiency of therapeutic effectiveness than he would without "the symbol." Moreover, if the physician leaves The Center, he carries its symbol with him, almost as an amulet or charm; and in some instances as a *vade mecum* to fend off the devil on his own personal pilgrimage during his professional life. The Center's symbols are ritualized in its diplomas and certificates and its verbal power that patients pass by word of mouth: "He was trained at The Center." The physician then striving to be worthy of the Symbol may feel its power at a distance from the establishment.[4]

All this is no secret to doctors—in or out of a center. Patients all discuss these feelings with their therapists, and with others. Not all of them are able to convey their emotions as articulately as the author of this patient's "letter" to her doctor.*

I've never been in any environment before, and never will be again, where I think everyone loves me specially for no reason at all except they love everything, so that includes me too. This is somehow very much connected with watching the bird feeding stations outside the dining room and the manual arts window. People who love just one person, or people close to them, are a dime a dozen, but this place is loaded with these rare creatures like Scottie who spreads it all over the place. And Wiley, who told me some things about squirrels; Marie, Don, Steward, oh, they're all over the place.

The nicest example is Don Jones, because I've never even met him

---

* I am indebted for it to my nephew, Dr. W. W. Menninger.

but am convinced not only that he sincerely loves me, but would do so whether I were male, female, three years old or *ninety*. It's a relief and a joy to be a part of something like that, because instead of love being a burden or responsibility making me an uncomfortable jester in a spotlight, I can just luxuriate in it. It feels good to see him around the grounds from a distance. The idea is the same with the other staff members and some of the patients. Maybe I focus more on Don simply because I don't know him, so the sensation is more in a pure form, unconfused by personal knowledge or any personal interest.

The best part, of course, consists of the love I have within me for Don and the rest. It has the somewhat tremulous excitement of a brand-new happy experience, complete freedom from any strain or weight. I don't have to be apprehensive, but can just be full to the brim with it if I want to, and nobody cares. I can play around with it, test it, think about it, and splurge. Right now I daily anticipate my arrival at badminton because it's so good to see both Jay and Miss T. at the same time. Sometimes I think I should thank Miss T. before she leaves, because she has this all-inclusive, timeless kind of love thing, and wherever she goes she'll make sad people feel better.

This should perhaps somehow zero in directly to one's doctor, but that doesn't necessarily follow in all cases. Our time and relations in activities and the hospital are completely separate from the tiring job of getting better. The doctors get everything from general professional respect and intellectual admiration to the whole run of hatreds, fears, "crushes," and intense affection for the one who will ultimately help us, depending upon their individual characters and specific points of treatment, I guess.

Long before I recognized this massive love bit around the hospital I noticed it in you, and thought it was a little weird. You seemed to be over-enthused in all directions, for the whole place, every patient, little boy scouts, your family, bugs, birds, and every old thing around you. One Sunday night when you were on duty, a patient came to tell me that if it hadn't been for you, she wouldn't have made it through the day. She was apparently hovering between getting up and just staying in a heap, when you appeared and made some simple remark of "I see you're almost up" or "You're getting there" or some such thing, and in a burst of sunshine she shaped up and felt wonderful. I thought she was pretty dim to wonder so just why she'd felt better, and explained to her as if she were an idiot child that it's simply because you love her; that when you spoke to her you meant that you love her, hoped she'd soon be up and have a happy day; that you love us all and that's why we feel better. She thought that was grand, loped off full of smiles, and I dismissed her as just another stupe straightened out.

Somewhere along the way I began to connect your attitude with that of Jay, Wiley, Don, etc., and decided that what I'd told her really was true. It amused me no end, because she's a real numbskull, but apparently no more than I in this instance.

Then it became quite fun watching you love everywhere, and I really think you do. People I don't even like, you really and sincerely care about. Simultaneously, I was busy elsewhere spotting types, and the whole thing became infinitely fascinating. Norma, with whom I eat breakfast, lunch and supper, and see a lot, was a fun test for this theory. Your interest in her face confused hell out of her at first—a lot of things about you did. She's an ornery one when she's suspicious, but by the time you got through she was utterly convinced that you, for some strange reason of your own which she no longer questions, really cared about her.

It's as if the hospital has surrounding me a series of countless little doorways to love. Through you, Don, Jay, and each that I am exposed to in this manner, within this temporary security, I can go through the never-ending fields of the same thing anywhere I eventually ever go.

This patient was—as you see—articulate, grateful, and quite sure what it was that she felt. Some of her statements are true, some are not; they should not be read as objective judgments. They were all true for *her*. They reflect her emotional state, *then*. When she is *more* "well" she can be more objective in her appraisal.

The doctor and the whole therapeutic milieu [5] should aim at replacing the emotional transference judgment with an objective judgment—not through arguments, not through reasoning, not through contradiction, but through example; not through indiscriminate permissiveness or coercion but through the use of measures which increase the patient's self-confidence. Then latent powers of righting himself and maintaining his balance in spite of adversities will develop. The patient can do this if he is sure of his love relationships—loved by someone and permitted to love someone (or something!). He must be able to feel that he can love without penalty—not without price, not without cost to himself, but without punishment.

Most of us spend a lifetime finding out what love really is. It is surely little wonder that, with the start they receive in childhood and adolescence, many people reach adult life without the faintest conception of what it is, or of what it might be for them. Companionship, group membership, infatuation, exhibitionistic dominance or submission, and especially unselective sexual desire are all commonly mistaken for and called "love." This is understandable in an adolescent but not in mature adults; yet even biological scientists can be as confused on this point (e.g., Kinsey [6]) as some of our patients.

Freud first shocked and then comforted many people by saying, in substance, that no one was satisfied with his sex life, that no one's sex life was fully or always normal. It is ironic that the man who first *scientifically* described psychosexual evolution should have been characterized as salacious when actually what he showed us was that the more mature our sexuality, using the word in a broad sense, the less obtrusive is sex in the narrow sense. The so-called "genital" stage of psychosexual evolution, i.e., the stage of mature sexuality, is one in which the attraction is between personalities as a whole, not merely between parts; hence the functions of the genital organs are, in this stage, no longer the principal expression of love.

No, the life instinct is by no means identical, as some people have thought, with the procreative instinct, nor was this ever implied or believed by Freud. The world's greatest lovers have not been Don Juans and Casanovas, but Schweitzers, Gandhis, Helen Kellers, and such saints as Francis of Assisi. It is a common misconception of psychoanalysis that in some way it disrobed love and showed it to be something carnal, urging us at the same time to have no shame. This is a calumny. What psychoanalysis showed was that true love is more concerned about the welfare of the one loved than with its own immediate satisfactions, that it demands nothing, but is patient, kind, and modest; that it is free from jealousy, boastfulness, arrogance, and rudeness; that it can bear all things, hope, and endure. So said Saint Paul. So said Freud.

It is this intangible thing, love, love in many forms, which enters into every therapeutic relationship. It is an element of which the physician may be the carrier, the vessel. And it is an element which binds and heals, which comforts and restores, which works what we have to call—for now—miracles. "For some patients, though conscious that their condition is perilous, recover their health simply through their contentment with the goodness of the physician." (Hippocrates: *Precepts*, VI.)

Faith

Much more could be said about the function of love in physician-patient relationships and the illness-recovery process. Many have written on the subject, including the senior author. Somewhat less attention has been given to the role of another item of Saint Paul's triad, faith. We have discussed in this book some of the things patients believe; but what do doctors believe?

Do they, indeed, believe anything? There is a common notion, disseminated by novels and sentimental television stories, that doctors are cynical skeptics and that they regard faith and science as antithetical. This, of course, is ridiculous; all doctors who think admit that they base their work upon hypotheses, i.e., articles of faith or assumption. They like to stipulate that this investment of faith is a tentative one, that every hypothesis must be doubted *almost* as much as it is believed in, that no hypothesis is sacred and any one may be replaced at any moment, if positive disproof is discovered.

But *until then* the scientist—including the physician, *including the psychiatrist*—will put his faith in his hypothesis and live and work by virtue of this faith God, it is true, is not one of the hypotheses employed by all physicians, although by many He is.

What, then, do the doctors as a group—all doctors including all psychiatrists—put their faith in? All doctors by their actions if not by their words believe unswervingly in their usefulness to the sick man. Almost all of them believe that what they do is helpful, at least sometimes—that medical science and medical knowledge can be employed for the benefit of the individual and of the race.

How this usefulness finds its best *modus operandi* is a question which has long split medical believers into two camps. Indeed, the history of medicine may be viewed as essentially a record of the fluctuating dominance of one or the other of *two* opposing faiths.

According to one point of view, represented by the teachings of the school of Cos in ancient Greece, therapy consists in an assistance offered to nature, a working with her, as it were, on the assumption that she is wise and benevolent and that the human being is only part of her greater structure. The other great school of medical thought of that time, at Cnidus, saw nature less benignly and regarded treatment as consisting essentially in the correction of nature's blunders. These teachers pointed to nature's obvious and gross mistakes and had little respect for the *vis medicatrix naturae* extolled by the followers of Hippocrates on Cos.

One rarely hears the *vis medicatrix naturae* mentioned in medical circles today, although one daily sees it tacitly relied upon. But relied upon with what degree of avowed confidence? Does the present-day physician —let us say psychiatrist—view it as a basic reality, a faithful friend or an obsolete superstition? When one observes the skill with which nature mends wounds, corrects deformities of trees and shrubs and scarred landscapes, one wonders whether the proud march of medical science has blinded many a doctor to the quiet but incessant forces working in the direction for which, with somewhat presumptuous arrogance, he often takes the full credit and acclaim.

It is astonishing to reflect how little the present-day doctor declares his faith in or his rejection of this important concept. He would probably *claim* to be a follower, in principle, of the school of Hippocrates, especially in regard to his *own* illnesses. (Most doctors abhor taking medicines.) But it is equally probable that in practice he emulates the Cnidians. He may even repudiate the doctrine of a *vis medicatrix naturae*, or declare it to be the essence of Christian Science. Thus the problem of the doctor's relation to the concept of a natural healing power is "perhaps the greatest of all problems which have occupied the physician for thousands of years," declared the great medical historian Max Neuburger.[7] "Indeed," he continued, "one could designate it as *the* problem of medicine, since the aims and limits of therapeutics are determined by its solution. . . . Almost every physician either directly or indirectly takes a position; indeed, *must* take a position in regard to it."

The father of medicine, Hippocrates, declared his position definitely and unequivocally. "Nature is the healer of disease" reads the superscription of Book VI of his *Epidemic Diseases*. Observation of the course of illness was his constant admonition, and he and his school always had a special eye for the efforts made by the organism toward self-regulation and self-repair. Our present-day notions of ego function, the self-regulation described in an earlier chapter, were anticipated by him 2500 years ago. Hippocrates believed that nature, by her tendency toward maintaining and re-establishing an equilibrium, restored health. This was the earliest statement, perhaps, of the vital balance.[8]

Hippocrates was opposed by the Cnidians, as stated above, but his most articulate opponent lived several centuries later, Asclepiades of Bithynia (196–124 B.C.). He actually lived after Galen and it was Galen's version of Hippocrates which Asclepiades attacked indirectly. He ridiculed it as a fantasy. Asclepiades held that re-establishment of the normal depended upon the energetic attack of the physician, and treatment accorded to the Hippocratic persuasion was called a "meditation of death." This do-something philosophy was exemplified by the polypharmacy and polysurgery which gave medicine a bad name for centuries—the boiling-oil treatment of wounds, the induction of "laudable" suppuration, the violent emetics and purges, the cauterizings, sweatings, bleedings, and other tortures. All these were in the name of therapy, of course, and they all patently lack faith in any *vis medicatrix naturae*.*

---

* Galen *pretended* to be a follower of Hippocrates and gave lip service to the importance of the *vis medicatrix naturae*. But actions speak louder than words; he was in practice an "incurable polypharmacist." Neuburger once rightly defined Galenism as "the combination of extensive drug treatment with the theoretical recognition of nature as the curer. [For the Galenists] . . . the medieval talk of hygiene became more and more mere lip service. The coming into being of pharmacies made drugging even easier. No wonder that the Renaissance Galenists—Botallus, Riolan, Guy Patin or Mercurialis—were hyperactive therapists." (Ackerknecht, Erwin H. "Aspects of History of Therapeutics." *Bull. Hist. Med.*, 36:389–419, 1962.)

One can scarcely say that these vigorous and even destructive exponents of overtreatment were lacking in faith. But their faith was certainly not in nature nor in its healing powers or recovery trends. It was, rather, in some assurance of an inborn or acquired skill, knowledge, and power to combat disease. Thus even by the suffering patient, whose agonies were often increased by the measures intended for his relief, the doctor was looked up to with wistful hope and gratitude. It was often a case of "Though he slay me, yet will I trust in him." But if this medieval faith and practice seem to us barbarous and superstitious, we must remember that these doctors were doing their best. They were trying zealously, and they were acting in accordance with their faith (although they may have denied having any).

The physician as a servant of nature and nature as the healer of disease reappeared in the first half of the sixteenth century. It was the great Paracelsus (1493-1541) who spoke out "with inflaming, yet even today convincing words" of the all too greatly neglected and misunderstood healing power of nature. The organism, said he, is not (something) fixed but "a formation constantly striving up and down by a continuous creating and destroying process; it is a totality permeated by purposefulness, whose parts possess a certain degree of independence." [9] This extraordinarily modern-sounding and dynamic description was far beyond the grasp of his contemporaries, who disputed, opposed, contradicted, and ridiculed him. And it is not surprising that for all his theories and declarations of faith, Paracelsus never trusted nature enough to let her use these powers—at least in the opinion of Ackerknecht. "Though non-Galenic, his drugs are at least as numerous as those of the Galenists." [10] But surely we should not reproach Paracelsus or anyone else for not quite living up in practice to the faith he proclaimed.

A century later Paracelsus (and Hippocrates) had another worthy fellow-minded ally. Thomas Sydenham (1624-1689) was called the English Hippocrates. He conceded that "the activity of 'Nature' is not free from reproach in all cases" and that "its healing endeavors . . . are delayed, variable and misplaced," but he believed and taught that nature healed, that it "night and day watches over and provides for our welfare" and struggles purposefully and automatically toward recovery. Included in the natural healing methods of nature as he saw it were "critical excretion, removal of pathogenic materials, secretions . . . hemorrhage, skin eruptions . . . exudate," and, most valuable of all, fever.[11]

Like Paracelsus, Sydenham was opposed by most of his contemporaries. Sylvius and Tomas Willis—whose names are also famous in medicine

and known to all doctors because of their *anatomical* discoveries—adhered to the anti-Hippocratic, anti-*vis medicatrix naturae* position. Typical of their contemptuous, minimizing attitudes is this diatribe by Sylvius:

> For many [physicians] as, following the custom of the ancients, en-
> trust most of the work of curing the sick to the chimaeric nature, or to
> some I-know-not-what, and then, save for diet, which they direct some-
> how, are only spectators of the fight, which they babble of as being stirred
> up between nature and the disease: and so they are umpires of the vic-
> tory which goes sometimes to the disease and sometimes to nature. [As
> many as take this course] are actually at fault in negligence. . . . I do
> not indeed deny that sick persons can be cured, nay more, that they often
> are actually cured, although no drugs have been prescribed for them by
> physicians; but no one could easily persuade me that the same people
> are cured as quickly, safely, and easily as if suitable medicines had been
> administered at the same time.* [12]

In the early part of the eighteenth century the leading exponent of the
views of Hippocrates, Paracelsus, and Sydenham was Boerhaave of Holland. He earnestly endeavored to make therapeutic use of artificially
induced fever, fever being Sydenham's favored form of natural healing
modality.** Boerhaave was particularly impressed by the healing effects
of malaria! It was to be over two hundred years before this idea was
adapted by "modern" medicine to the cure of syphilitic encephalitis or
to the relief of arthritis and arthralgia by inducing chills and fever with
injections of foreign protein.

Boerhaave had great influence, and the doctrine of the *vis medicatrix
naturae* once more gained momentum throughout the medical world. It

---

* By the end of the seventeenth century the discoveries of Galileo, Bacon, and Descartes
had overthrown many of the Aristotelian concepts, including that of nature as a consciously purposeful, supermundane agency. The *vis medicatrix naturae* was discarded
along with the personification of good news, etc., as a superstition or a semi-religious
concept unworthy of the new positivism. But Robert Boyle, a deeply religious man,
opposed the concept for a different reason, holding that it had become a kind of idol.
He recognized a metaphysical, cosmic purposefulness, but he considered that somatic
processes proceeded according to mechanical laws. It was Boyle who coined the expression "mechanism" to replace the concept "nature." "Not a conscious purposefulness of nature, but an accidentally purposeful effect of a blind powerful mechanism is
also to be ascribed as maintaining the individual, and as necessary for the re-establishment of health." (Neuberger, Max. *The Doctrine of the Healing Power of Nature
Throughout the Course of Time.* New York: L. J. Boyd [privately printed], 1932.)
** Wrote Boerhaave: "We praise fever as the most prosperous instrument of the physician by means of which nature accomplishes the most perfect cure of a thousand
diseases, acute and chronic, otherwise incurable. . . . The physician versed in the
ways of nature, and her imitator, comes to her aid when she is unable to cope with
chronic ailments. . . . He reduces, heats, causes pains, agitates, rubs, fondles, moves,
reddens, by means of food, medicaments, his hand, in order to create a fever by his
industry; and that by skillfully directing the fever he may put languishing nature on
her feet, and break the obstinate [resistance of] the disease." (Neuberger, Max. Ibid.)

was disputed by Hoffmann, on the right, who saw the body as a machine and ridiculed the idea of nature's having wisdom, and it was disputed also by Stahl, on the left, who went beyond the Hippocrates-Galen-Paracelsus-Sydenham-Boerhaave line in his famous conception of a "life force." For Stahl the organism was something fundamentally different from a machine. For although he was impressed by the amazing automatic self-regulation of the organism, he was equally impressed by the rapid decomposition of post-mortem tissue. Deliberation over these phenomena led him to believe that living flesh does not putrefy because it is daily renewed. His concept of a life energy or living principle streaming throughout the organism, maintaining its permanence, balance, and harmonious processes and striving toward unity, is strikingly similar to the life instinct or integrative principle of Freud and others (including the authors) although put by him in more unsophisticated language than that used by leading theoretical biologists today.

And Stahl was attacked in the early eighteenth century in very much the same terms as those in which Freud's instinct theory is attacked today. He frankly admitted that his view was equivalent to assuming the existence of a soul, but held that as a physician and a chemist he was not interested in debating the philosophical ramifications of this question. He held that the continuous maintenance of the body, the defense against damage, the equalization of disturbances appearing through regulating healing actions, reflected the striving of a life principle. There is in the normal state, he believed, a *"perpetua therapia interna"* aimed at maintenance of the organism. Thus healing and defense reactions are only modifications of normal living processes (cf. anabolism and catabolism). "The vast majority of the manifestations of disease are to be conceived of as the healing endeavors of the organism." [13] *

Stahl himself raised the question and sought in vain to discover why the energy of nature seemed less efficacious in chronic afflictions than in acute afflictions. He ascribed this in part to the nature of man, which tends to error and to excess.

---

* The practical result of the philosophy of Stahl was an intelligent "expectative therapy which indeed stood in brilliant contrast to the polypragmasia of most of his medical contemporaries." Although he had many followers, Stahl had vigorous and even more numerous opponents including the two already mentioned and the philosopher Leibniz. Declared Leibniz: "If the soul had the power over a machine of being able to command it to do something it would not do of its own accord, then there would be no reason why it should not be able to command anything whatever . . . and then nature would be the most efficacious healer of all diseases and would never be disappointed of her purposes." (Neubergber, Max: op. cit.)

Stahl's influence increased in France, led by de Sauvages, who attempted the fusion of iatrophysics with Stahl's vitalism. He called the mysterious and elusive element the *primus motor*, and called the symptoms of disease which were not the immediate effects of the injurious agent "signs of defense"(!). Bordeu, Barthez, Pinel, and other French physicians continued in the Stahl tradition with various modifications of the formulation.

Argument thus continued through the centuries, back and forth and up and down, dominance passing from one position to the other and varying with countries and within countries. Each new discovery would start a wave of encouragement to one or the other view. For example, the introduction of cinchona bark gave great impetus to the medicalists; the observation at autopsies of the spontaneous repair that had occurred in aneurysms gave encouragement to Hippocratics. The discovery of autolysis and bacterial action canceled some of Stahl's argument; but the gradual relinquishing of bleeding and other useless procedures was in line with his views.

From the middle of the nineteenth century on, the great zeal for the collection of facts put an end to voluminous theoretical speculation. The blooming of pathographic anatomy (Rokitansky), the development of new physical diagnostic methods (Auenbrugger, Laennec, Skoda, and Zahli), and the growth of the new pharmacology (Schmiedeberg, Abel, and Cushny) greatly strengthened the concept of a healing power of nature by weakening confidence in mysterious drug effects. In 1845 Zehetmayer wrote these prophetic words: "The wider the testing of drugs progresses, the more enlightened, the simpler, surer, and more natural our therapy will stand out, the more definite its limits appear." [14]

And while some of us will continue to depend on the *vis medicatrix naturae*, in which we believe, we should not sentimentalize Mother Nature. She's not all good. She does some terrible things—although not as terrible as man does to her. Faith in her healing powers need not be faith in her unfailing benevolence.

Drought, the ensuing famine, floods and ensuing chaos, hurricanes, typhoons, tornadoes, and tidal waves are not kindly. Torture and butchery and waste and disease exist among the wild creatures of the earth, and in plants. And nature has to assume the responsibility for cancer and leukemia and deformities and malignant infections. In some respects man has always had to fight against nature. But to give credit where credit is due, nature also nurtures and creates and fructifies. And nature endows some organisms, among them man, with internal intrinsic healing powers.

The same sorts of disputes which have raged in general medicine for two thousand years regarding the proper placement of faith have likewise been apparent in psychiatry ever since it has had any identity as a medical specialty. There have always been the active treaters and the more patient observers; there have been chemicalists and physicalists and expectants; there have been the sadistic and the humane; there have been the moralists and the objectivists; there have been the theorists and the practical men.

No matter which of these he is, the doctor puts his faith in something. If it is too broad and vague to say that he puts his faith in nature, it is insufficient to say that he puts it in "facts"; all faith has some relation to facts, but all faith likewise transcends facts and in a sense defines them.

The doctor who puts his faith—as he thinks—chiefly in the effectiveness of chemicals and instruments, the doctor who puts his faith in moral suasion and psychological catharsis, the doctor who puts his faith in the effectiveness of education and rehabilitation techniques, the doctor who puts his faith in God—all these believe more than they admit, more than they realize, and more than they can demonstrate. Scientists unite in repudiating magic, superstition, and theory devoid of all relation to facts. But each has his faith, his scientific conscience, his belief in the validity of science, i.e., that science works.*

And the psychiatrist of today, what does he believe? In what does he place his particular faith? What does he count on for assistance in his efforts? Surely he believes in *something* within the patient that can be aroused to cooperate in the contract of healing, and he believes in a probable success for their efforts. He believes that psychiatry is a scientific discipline and obeys the laws of other sciences. He believes, too—some psychiatrists, at least, and I think the "some" are legion—in the potency of the three intangibles which we are now discussing.

---

* There is a common belief among them in the importance of the integrity of personal judgment. "This does not mean that [the scientist] ceases to listen to the opinions of other scientists, nor . . . to be influenced in his own decisions by what other scientists have said and done. It means simply this: in each instance in which a question of science is raised for him, the decision as to correctness must be made by himself, and cannot be devolved upon any other person. . . . The acceptance of the other's judgment is always conditional, regardless of the authority and prestige of the one whose decision is accepted. It is conditional upon the understanding that if the procedure were repeated by himself, the same conclusion would most likely be reached. . . . No procedure, conclusion, hunch, hypothesis, or theory is free from scrutiny. Nothing is free from scrutiny. Even the method of inquiry itself is to be examined." (Hartung, Frank E. "Science as an Institution." *Philosophy of Science*, 18:35–54, 1951.)

Time was—perhaps in places it still is—when psychiatrists put too much of their faith in words, technical phrases, magic formulas, pompous nonsense. Pirandello's scorn [15] for this is no greater than that of many a colleague:

DOCTOR: Will you let me speak? I don't work miracles, because I am a doctor and not a miracle-worker. I listened very intently to all he said; and I repeat that that certain analogical elasticity, common to all symptomatised delirium, is evidently with him much . . . what shall I say?—much relaxed! The elements, that is, of his delirium no longer hold together. It seems to me he has lost the equilibrium of his second personality and sudden recollections drag him—and this is very comforting—not from a state of incipient apathy, but rather from a morbid inclination to reflective melancholy, which shows a . . . a very considerable cerebral activity. Very comforting, I repeat! Now if, by this violent trick we've planned . . .

BELCREDI: (*suddenly*): I say, I've never understood why they take degrees in medicine.

DI NOLLI (*amazed*): Who?

BELCREDI: The alienists!

DI NOLLI: What ought they to take degrees in, then?

FRIDA: If they are alienists, in what else should they take degrees?

BELCREDI: In law, of course! All a matter of talk! The more they talk, the more highly they are considered. "Analogous elasticity," "The sensation of distance in time!" And the first thing they tell you is that they don't work miracles—when a miracle's just what is wanted! But they know that the more they say they are not miracle-workers, the more folk believe in their seriousness!

—*Henry IV*

Believing that mental illness is a reversible condition and that it is amenable to planned intervention, that nature and the intrinsic forces of recovery are on his side, the "optimistic" psychiatrist seeks a point of access to the disease process, expecting to find one. He scrutinizes the environment, the patient's life history, his physical and psychological equipment, looking not only for evidences of malfunction and maladaptation, but for the assets of the situation, the favorable factors, the potential in both patient and environment which might be exploited to effect a step up, a turning point and new direction in the course of illness.

The psychiatrist who doubts the efficacy of any such nebulous view of the healing power of nature approaches the same patient, the same environment, the same symptoms, with different spectacles. He sees some things clearer and larger than his colleagues; but some things he never sees at all; he may not even know how to look for them. For every doctor is embarrassed with a superabundance of data in every case. And the art is to select the significant ones. Significance is determined by the selector's faith, a faith which finds reciprocity in the patient's faith.

The question is often asked of psychiatrists whether religious belief helps or hinders the recovery process. There are all kinds of religious beliefs, and some patients, like some psychiatrists, put little faith in any of them. A few put much faith in forms of religion which seem (to us) esoteric and unconvincing. This makes any kind of generalization difficult if not absurd. But one is tempted to summarize it that faith in *something* is a *sine qua non* of sentient life, sometimes stretched too far and used too uncritically, but more often pathetically lacking in fiber and tone. Perhaps it is only a shibboleth that some seem to be capable of being believers, while others pride themselves on not being up (or down) to it, and prefer to be known as skeptics or agnostics.

It was Max Born [16] who said, "There are two objectionable types of believers: those who believe the incredible and those who believe that 'belief' must be discarded and replaced by 'the scientific method.' " *

We all know from the practical experiences of daily life that there is more or less credulity and more or less skepticism in each of us. But to simplify matters let us say that some are chiefly or predominantly believers—believers in a philosophy, a set of values which shapes their lives—and some are chiefly doubters. They both do great things (and some petty things). The believers dream dreams; they form ideals and set goals; they build castles in the air and schemes on paper. Meanwhile, the skeptics, who work alongside them and share their meals and their taxes and their pleasures and their sufferings, quarrel with them only in theory.

For even the most hardened skeptic, if he is also creatively given to research, must carefully nurture and work to keep alive the germinal truths which vitalize his research. "It is not easy for an embryonic truth to live, much less to develop, in the mind of its host. Before wasting on it anything but the most casual thought the host will subconsciously try to stifle it with indifference, downgrading, excuses, etc. Even if he fertilizes it with some preliminary cogitation, orientation, and experimentation the 'original thought' must overcome many dangers and 'enemies' as it

---

* Born himself believed in continuous creation and flatly disputed the metaphysical principle that everything must have a cause. It is inevitable, he said, that a monistic concept of experience has to be abandoned. "If quantum theory has any philosophical importance at all, it lies in the fact that it demonstrates . . . the necessity of dual aspects and complementary considerations." Let there be no more loose talk about the holy principle of psychological determinism. "Nature is ruled by laws of cause and laws of chance in a certain mixture."

changes, successively, from a thought to a 'notion,' then 'an idea,' a sidetracked 'conviction' or a growing 'concept,' and a prenatal 'belief.' At birth it becomes a valid belief, then after his own confirmation it is a personally known 'fact.' " [17]

It takes both believers and skeptics to make a civilization. For while they do not get along very well in theory, they work together and need each other. Believers are optimistic in a way which skeptics sometimes consider fatuous. The skeptics tend to be pessimistic; they are practical and tough-minded, as William James put it. Believers are more idealistic and tender-minded; they regard the skeptics as materialistic and short-sighted. The skeptics often regard the believers as naïve and even a bit balmy.

But in one very important respect the apparent conflicts between belief and skepticism disappear; in a real and very urgent conflict, these people are all on the same side. They are all united against a common enemy. Both believers and skeptics are people of minds, people of hearts, people who are trying to understand themselves and their fellow men and the world in which they all live. That is why some believe and why some doubt. They yearn to better the troubled world they live in. Their real opposition—the common enemy, if you please—is something else. It is the evil, the destructiveness in the world, and more especially it is the complacency of the comfortable. It is the indifference, the apathy, the hardness of heart which troubles neither to believe nor to doubt, but simply does not care.* The common enemy is not some starry-eyed idealist, nor even, as Norman Cousins [18] says, "some powerful nation or totalitarian power controlling world ideology. It is rather the man whose only concern about the world is that it stay in one piece *during his own lifetime* . . . up to his hips in success . . . [who] not only believes in his own helplessness, but actually worships it [assuming] that there are mammoth forces at work which the individual cannot comprehend much less alter or direct."

Only in the presence of some kind of belief can there be a truly moving concern for mankind. Granted that too often this concern is lacking; everyone who makes any observation of human suffering has been puzzled

---

* Cherbonnier in his beautiful essay, *Hardness of Heart*, describes the forms of idolatry indulged in by the hardhearted. He lists the hidden gods of cynicism as nationalism, humanism, communism, phallicism, promiscuity, the glorification of money, and the various euphemisms such as frugality, shrewdness, and sound economy. Cherbonnier also lists iconoclasm, existentialist despair, and a so-called state of "adjustment" and "relatedness" toward which some psychiatrists are believed to steer their patients. (Cherbonnier, E. LaB. *Hardness of Heart*. New York: Doubleday, 1955.)

by this "certain blindness in human beings." "According to one tenable view," sagely observes one of our great American psychologists, Henry Murray, "the Satanic aim is to prevent all developments in [a melioristic] direction by shattering man's faith in the existence of the necessary potentialities within himself and reducing him to cynicism and despair until the demoralization and abasement of his personality has reached a state beyond recovery and in one disgraceful debacle of genocidal fury he terminates the long, long history of his species." [19]

Public complacency was publicly deplored by Zoroaster twenty-five centuries ago; a little later Pericles and Socrates and Plato deplored it; the Hebrew prophets deplored it; * Jesus deplored it.** The Stoic ideal of imperturbability, the Epicurean ideal of tranquillity, the Buddhistic ethic, all glorify indifference to reality. "This spite against one's own existence, so utterly contrary to the spirit of the Bible, characterizes even some of the Christian mystics. 'He alone hath true spiritual poverty,' wrote Meister Eckhart, 'who wills nothing, knows nothing, desires nothing.' " [20]

This philosophy easily becomes corrupted to read ". . . who doesn't disturb the *status quo*, who lets well enough alone, who minds his own business and doesn't concern himself about things which do not concern him." Did not William Lloyd Garrison get just what he might have expected for "shooting off his mouth" all the time about the evil and horror of slavery? If Mr. Garrison didn't choose to have slaves around to beat, abuse, and exploit, that was all right. But need he try to force his views on others who chose to do differently, who happened to like what was perfectly legal and profitable and comfortable?

Slavery is so almost indescribably awful that we find it difficult today to quite believe that human beings were treated by our immediate ancestors with such savage heartlessness.[21] We flatter ourselves that such iniquity is extinct, that it was an anachronism in United States history, an inexplicable hangover from the Dark Ages, and that nothing so wicked would be tolerated today. This is a cheerful philosophy but a most fatuous and dangerous one.

Exploitation of fellow human beings did not begin or disappear with Hitler, or with the African slaves, or with Genghis Khan, or with Nero, or even with the Assyrians and Hittites. Man has grown increasingly more expert at it and able to accomplish it on a larger scale. And just as Eichmann was able to remain immune from the attacks of his conscience by

---

* "I will take away the stony heart out of your flesh."—Ezekiel 36:26.
** "And he looked around at them with anger, grieved at their hardness of heart."—Mark 3:5.

ascribing the responsibility for his misdeeds to the orders given him by someone else,[22] so all of us tend to deny our personal participation in and responsibility for what is done in our name, in our country, by our fellow citizens.

I vividly recall a dramatic moment in the visit of our psychiatric commission to the European theater of war in the spring of 1945. Some of our officers were raging at the German civilians in Weimar for declaring that they did not know what was going on at their suburban Buchenwald and deplored it as much as anyone.[23] It happened that we had a patient (an American soldier) for consideration that day, and in reviewing his background it was discovered that he had spent some time on a chain gang in the South. The same officers who had been denouncing the German citizens insisted that the man must be lying, since such prison abuses "had long since disappeared in America." I asked the prisoner if he had spent any time in a sweat box; he had, and even the recollection of it paled him. My colleagues didn't know what it was.

At this very moment millions in our world are sick, miserable, frightened, imprisoned, intimidated, exploited, starved. Some of this is deliberate; much of it is needless. Some readers will be angry that I have even reminded them that it exists; like Eichmann, they may even plead, "Not responsible." "There is nothing we can do about it; it is none of our business; I doubt if it is true anyway; it is their own fault, they are just lazy; and am I my brother's keeper?"

The political panacea to which was appropriated the idealistic title "Communism" began (and ever begins again) in part as a reaction to misery and despair, but also, in part, as a reaction to the apparent obliviousness and indifference shown to this suffering by more fortunate people. The remark "Let them eat cake" possibly did more to inspire the French Revolution than all the banners proclaiming Liberty, Equality, and Fraternity.

The comfort experienced by the supposedly indifferent is often an illusion, sometimes stupidity and ignorance, sometimes a stubborn effort at denial. But it certainly evokes bitter reactions. The Communist reaction has already been mentioned, but perhaps the equally mislabeled "Extreme Right" syndrome is similarly explicable. This is not to discount in its motivation yearnings for power, for companionship, and for attracting attention. But some of these individuals perceive clearly the danger of complacency without recognizing their own ideological relationship to the persons or movements which they so frantically fear and hate.

Even in our affluent American society mass poverty persists at a time

of general prosperity, "real poverty in the old-fashioned sense of the word
. . . hard put to it to get the mere necessities beginning with enough to
eat"—this in perhaps a fourth of our population.[24] But not only poverty
and hunger pervade the world; there are everywhere cruelty, prejudice,
crime, corruption, ugliness, despair, illness, pain.

Evil goes in many guises and is called by many names. Perhaps the
best name for it is the old-fashioned personification, the Devil.* It has
two faces—the destructiveness itself, with the suffering and loss it causes,
and the indifference to it of those more fortunate. Thus suffering and
complacency together form the common enemy of both skeptics and
believers.

Each day—certainly each decade—seems to find the world in a different stage of conflict. At one moment the good seems to be triumphant,
and we are about to say that the world has grown much better, when
our eye is caught by the threat of imminent self-destruction toward which
the nations seem to be headed. Social improvement in one part of the
world encourages us only so long as we keep our eyes away from South
Africa, or the American prison system, or the arms race.

This is not meant to imply that the recognition of evil and good,
or even the acceptance of our own responsibility for combating evil, is the
be-all and end-all of religious faith. Einstein's thoughtful and humble admiration of the "illimitable superior spirit who reveals himself in the slight
details we are able to see with our frail and feeble minds" describes an
impersonal god: "That deeply emotional conviction of the presence of a
superior reasoning power which is revealed in the incomprehensible universe forms my idea of God." [25]

But Max Planck [26] went a little further:

"Thus, we see ourselves governed all through life by a higher power,

---

* Who, according to Judaic and Christian theologians, is himself an angel, a fallen
angel, but still an angel who might be redeemed. Most of us assume that the theory
of devil possession is extinct. But in 1962 there was published in France, England,
and the United States a book entitled *Evidence of Satan in the Modern World*. It
bears an official church imprimatur and was published by the estimable firm of Macmillan. It bears such chapter titles as "Satan in the Modern World," "Satanism and
the Devices of Satan," "Lucifer and His Allies," and "The Mentality of Satan."
"Whatever may be the cause of possession—and it often seems an unfathomable
mystery—we might sum up the mentality of Satin [sic] by these three words: *pride,
contempt* for his victim, and *tenacity*." The author concedes that in the sixteenth century "many stories of demonic possession were fabrications." "The anti-Catholic
polemics of emergent Protestantism were dominated," he explains, "by satanism. The
whole movement for Protestant reform was haunted from the beginning by the shadow
of the demoniac." (Cristiana, Leon. *Evidence of Satan in the Modern World*. New
York: Macmillan, 1962.)

whose nature we shall never be able to define from the viewpoint of exact science. Yet, no one who thinks can ignore it. . . . The individual has no alternative but to fight bravely in the battle of life, and to bow in silent surrender to the will of a higher power which rules over him. For no man is born with a legal claim to happiness, success, and prosperity in life. We must, therefore, accept every favorable decision of providence, each single hour of happiness, as an unearned gift, one that imposes an obligation. The only thing that we may claim for our own with absolute assurance, the greatest good that no power in the world can take from us, and one that can give us more permanent happiness than anything else, is integrity of soul, which manifests itself in a conscientious performance of one's duty. And he whom good fortune has permitted to cooperate in the erection of the edifice of exact science will find his satisfaction and inner happiness, with our great German poet, in the knowledge that he has explored the explorable and quietly venerates the inexplorable."

The reverence for mystery, for vastness, for beauty, for inscrutable intelligence, for order and power—this is one component of the sentiment called religious. Some describe it as "the sensuous experience of God." Some reject this. "But many believers declare the statement 'God exists' to be [not meaningless but] an expression of certain mystic feelings which they experience. Here the usual verification procedures are of no relevance. To Einstein, as to Spinoza, God was a symbol embodying the harmony of the cosmos. To Tolstoi and to Schweitzer, God was whatever brought out a feeling of oneness among men. Who is to say what the 'real' meaning of the assertion 'God exists' should be? Declaring the statement meaningless, as it stands, is a challenge for greater clarification, hence further exploration of psychological or social conditions which induce people to take sides on this question. On the other hand, treating the statement as a factual proposition to be asserted or denied simply serves to polarize the controversy, to pit people against each other on what at this stage is only a *verbal* issue and what is likely to remain only a verbal issue as long as further exploration is cut off by emotional commitments to one or the other reply." [27]

There is more to the religious sentiment than reverence, even when reverence becomes actively expressed in worship. There is the matter of believing, of accepting the unprovable thing, the unlikely thing, the impossible thing—the miracle. Life itself is such a miracle. Perhaps evil, too, is a miracle—an unwanted one, but there, all the same. And so, likewise, is the persistent determination to combat evil a miracle—the urge to allay suffering, to help others, to improve our world, to seek for the highest good for all living, to plan benefits for generations we shall never see, to reach out toward the unmanifest, and to note our mistakes, to repent our sins, and to try again. And, whether or not they declare belief in it, scientists as well as saints, stiff-necked skeptics as well as worshipers, share this miracle and are impelled and sustained by it in their unending warfare against the common enemy.

Hope

Of the three great intangibles determining the effectiveness of one individual upon another, teacher upon student or doctor upon patient, we have left until the last the one which is proverbially left until the last. When Pandora opened the jar from which all the evils now in the world emerged, there remained behind one little sprite: Hope.

Perhaps we think of her most often as a consolation, a weak, wistful antidote for the multiple miseries that accompanied her. But if Hope was considered a blessing, why did she remain behind in the jar? Whether good or evil, why did she not fly out with the rest of them and go to work on poor mankind? The Pandora story is intriguing in many respects, most of all because it is the only clear mythical enunciation of the birth of Hope. Adam and Eve were led by their curiosity to discover the meaning of good and evil; Pandora was led by her curiosity to discover evil—and Hope, whatever *she* was.

Pandora herself has been the subject of much art and literature. She has meant many things to different people—the first woman (i.e., a Greek Eve), an all-gifted woman, an all-giving woman, the mother of all women, the model of curious and meddlesome women, a benevolent woman, the releaser of goods rather than evils upon the earth. In some versions Pandora even becomes Hope herself, and it is a curious fact that Pandora never had a box; Hope and the troubles were encased in a *pithos* or storage jar until Erasmus decided to change it to a box in 1508 A.D.! *

There is no question, according to the Hesiodian version, that Hope is considered one of the evils, and this was the general Greek opinion. Greek sacred literature and philosophers and playwrights presented the view that, since fate was unchangeable, hope was an illusion, "the food of exiles" (Aeschylus) and, indeed, "man's curse"! (Euripides). Quota-

---

* These comments are taken in large part from the brilliant and beautiful monograph by the Panofskys. (Panofsky, Doran and Erwin. *Pandora's Box*. New York: Pantheon, 1962.)

tions from Solon, Simonides, Pindar, Thucydides, and others say this in different ways. The Greek feeling about hope is vividly expressed in Anouilh's adaptation of Sophocles' *Antigone*,[28] where, referring to herself, the heroine cries, "We are of the tribe that asks questions, and we ask them to the bitter end—until no tiniest chance of hope remains to be strangled by our hands. We are of the tribe that hates your filthy hope, your docile, female hope; hope, your whore . . ." (Creon interrupts with "Shut up! If you could see how ugly you are, shrieking those words!")

From this one can see that it was intrepid indeed of Saint Paul, writing to *Greek* friends, to declare to them that hope, which they despised, should stand along with love. In this Paul was loyal to his Hebrew heritage (Psalms 42, Isaiah 40) as well as his Christian convictions. For while the Jews were, to be sure, people of faith, they were also at all times and perhaps above all a people of hope who, despite tribulation, trial, exile, annihilation, isolation, dispersion, torture, and slaughter, clung to the expectation that the Messiah would come and the world get better. Hence, with the spread of the Judaeo-Christian message and the military dispersion of the Jews, hope had its missionaries, and Paul was one of many.*

In general, hope has had few public defenders and many scorners. Poets and philosophers have tended either to ignore hope or to adopt (rather bitterly) the fatalistic and cynical view of the Greeks:

"Hope—fortune's cheating lottery, where for one prize a hundred blanks there be" (Cowley, 1647).

"Worse than despair, worse than the bitterness of death, is hope" (Shelley, *The Cenci*, 1819).

"Hope is the worst of all evils, for it prolongs the torment of man" (Nietzsche, *Human All-too-Human*, 1878).

What, then, is the modern notion about hope? Are we Greeks or are we Jews? Or do we ignore hope altogether? Our shelves hold many books on the place of *faith* in science and psychiatry, and on the vicissitudes of man's efforts to *love* and to be loved. But when it comes to hope, our shelves are nearly empty, and our scientific journals are silent. The

---

* This great heritage to us from the Jews is apt to be lost sight of in our admiration for the lucidity—and frigidity—of Greek rationalism. "The fundamental characteristic of Hebrew thought is its ethical optimism." In a sense the whole history of the Jews is a study of hope, hope springing out of all their discouragements and misadventures and disasters—"a hope living and powerful, ennobling and transfiguring them with ideal strength and beauty." (Goodspeed, George Stephen. *Israel's Messianic Hope*. New York: Macmillan, 1900.)

Encyclopaedia Britannica devotes many columns to the topic of love, and many more to faith. But poor little hope! She is not even listed!

The cupboard is not entirely bare. Much has been written by Christians on hope and on Messianic hope. Hope still plays a prominent role in Judaism, dramatized by the Nazi holocaust on the one hand and the Israeli triumph on the other. We are using the word "hope" in a broader sense, describing less an aspect of religious faith than the character of a certain mental set. What is the scientific view of hope?

In his three-volume examination of psychoanalytic treatment Thomas French deals extensively with hope as the activating force of the ego's integrative function. He believes that hope is an essential part of the recovery drive: "Hope is based on present opportunity and on memories of recent success." [29]

A Spanish psychiatrist, Lain,[30] in Madrid, has published an extensive monograph on *Waiting and Hope—The History and Theory of Human Expectancy.*

And there are a few contributions by non-psychiatrists.[31] For example, in a study of suicide some colleagues found that "when hope disappears through the loss of opportunities to reach life's goals, destructive drives previously subordinated to other goals become discharged . . . against the self." [32]

But in general the situation is just as Mrs. Menninger and I described it some twenty years ago: "In scientific circles there is a determined effort to exclude hope from conceptual thinking, first because of the general obloquy of admitting any psychological concepts into materialistic and fanatically empirical science; and second, because of a fear of corrupting objective judgment by wishful thinking. But all science is built on hope, so much so that science is for many moderns a substitute for religion. . . . Man can't help hoping, even if he is a scientist; he can only hope more accurately." [33]

Shortly after writing this, I became interested in hope as it appeared in young physicians who were entering upon psychiatric training. They were not quite sure what they were getting into, or why they had decided to pursue a career in psychiatry. Nevertheless, they usually seemed quite calm and resolute, confident that they would soon be expanding their knowledge and skills along this special and exciting avenue of medical training.*

---

* Perhaps the increasing popularity and respectability of psychiatry have tended to change this somewhat of recent years. Lebensohn in the Kober Lecture for 1962 puts

Behind the façade presented by these acolytes there were often tumults of conflicting voices, fearful insecurity, and bold over-self-confidence. The dramatic picture of psychiatry fascinated them, the reputed resistance to treatment challenged them, the multiplicity of methods appalled them. They were assigned to wards filled with vacant or frantic faces, turned now upon "the new doctor." It was usually long after their initiation into the uncanny world of mental illness that they could distinguish the moving process, or have the personal experience of interaction with a recovering patient.*

Nevertheless, the novitiates assailed their tasks headlong, sometimes with a *furor therapeuticus*. There was nothing mercenary or aggressive about this; they were not working for money. They were struggling to become therapeutically effective in a new kind of relationship with patients. Sometimes they would go too far, presuming or expecting or promising too much. More often, frustration or sad experience or self-depreciation would erode the confidence required for persistent effort, and the little candle of hope, which had burned for a while so brightly, would weaken, sputter, and go out.

For such men psychiatry ceases to be a vocation, a philosophy, a way of life; it becomes a dreary chore of dealing with despairing patients. It becomes a way of making a living, a branch of the medical business of routinely seeing sick people. This may be a round of monotonous office visits giving rise to such jokes as the famous one about "Who

---

it this way: "The very respectability which psychoanalysis (and psychiatry) has achieved as a professional way of life now attracts to it young men of quite a different stamp than was the case in the early twenties. In those days psychoanalysis was suspected and derided. To practice it was a risky way of earning a living. In spite of this, and possibly because of this, the early psychoanalysts were a gifted, daring, creative and dedicated group. They instilled a spirit of hope, enthusiasm and scientific promise in an area which had become static, custodial and stale. But how different today seem the bright young men who enter the field! They have only to complete their training—no small feat in itself—to be assured of instant security, automatic prestige, financial bounty, and a long waiting list of prospective patients. The course of training is hard, but the rewards are rich. And in the training process, can one doubt that the temptation is great to complete the requirements according to the book or to accept uncritically the methods and the manners of the master?" (Lebensohn, Zigmond M. "American Psychiatry—Retrospect and Prospect." *Med. Annals. Dist. of Columbia*, 31:379–392, July 1962.)

* Clifford Scott, our Canadian colleague, says of this, "This is what happens when the fear of hope disappears and is transferred into courage . . . the courage to tolerate waiting, anticipating, pining and the as yet unfulfilled hope. . . . Even when a person is most hateful, most hopeless or most helpless, the situation is never quite 100 percent, and some proportion of love is still at work unconsciously and repetitively. It may eventually grow and alter the whole situation." (Scott, Clifford, from a personal letter dated January 4, 1960.)

listens?" Or it may go on in the hospital, where hopeless physicians preside over hopeless patients.

For these men psychiatry has indeed been, as they say, oversold. People's expectations have been raised too high. The enthusiasm of inexperience only awaits the disillusionment of time. "It is enough if we bestow kindness," they say, "listen to the griping and wait for the inevitable. What can you do with such people? Hope is for fools."

Most of the young men who pass through our training programs do not go that route. Their horizons remain high—perhaps rise higher. We like to think that they have learned what limits to place upon their expectations and what guards to place upon their implied promises. But their hope should remain unextinguished and unextinguishable. They should believe steadfastly that there is no patient for whom something helpful cannot be done, but we also like them to realize that the changes which the patient desires in himself, or which the physician desires in his patient, may not be the ones which will come about. It is a responsibility of the teacher to the student, just as it is of the young doctor to his patient, to inspire the right amount of hope—some, but not too much. Excess of hope is presumption and leads to disaster. Deficiency of hope is despair and leads to decay. Our delicate and precious duty as teachers is to properly tend this flame.

We may not go as far as Martin Luther, who said that everything that is done in the world is done by hope, but we can certainly agree with Samuel Johnson that "where there is no hope there can be no endeavor."

I propose, therefore, that we examine this essential constituent of both treatment and teaching. How shall we think of hope? Is it something which *deserves* our concern as scientists? Or only as philosophers and poets? Is it only an epiphenomenon of life and the healing art? Do we, perhaps, tacitly ascribe hope to temperament, a sort of fringe benefit deriving from certain fortuitous congenital arrangements of glands and neurons? This is slight improvement upon the humoral theories of sanguinity and melancholy treasured by our forebears. If we ascribe hope, as some psychoanalytic writers have done, to recollections of maternal infallibility and recurrent oral gratifications, what combination of these experiences shall we regard as optimum? Others have seen in hope a prevailing note of fear, a counterphobic denial of the horror and despair born of self-destructive trends or of the immanence of existential doom.

More congenial to my thinking is the ascription of hope to the mysterious workings of the repetition compulsion, the very essence of which is a kind of relentless and indefatigable pursuit of resolution and freedom. I would see in hope another aspect of the life instinct, the creative drive which wars against dissolution and destructiveness. But some will say, with Freud, that this is only our speculative abstractions to supply a model for practical thinking and behavior. Our mythology, he called it.

Twenty years ago Mrs. Menninger and I submitted the thesis in *Love Against Hate* that hope was the dim awareness of unconscious wishes which, like dreams, tend to come true. We said then that thoughts and hopes and wishes

> are already correlated to the plan of action which would bring these about, even though the whole project is ultimately renounced as too difficult or too dangerous. . . . This essential identity of hoping, wishing, purposing, intending, attempting, and doing is a little difficult for the practical common-sense man to grasp, because for him it makes a great difference whether a thing is executed or only planned or only hoped for . . . There *is* a difference in the *fate* of the impulse, the degree with which it is correlated with reality, inhibited by internal fears, supported by other motives, etc.—but the motive force is the same. . . . The hopes we develop are therefore a measure of our maturity.[34]

Hope is not identical with optimism; optimism always implies some distance from reality, as Marcel points out, so that obstacles appear attenuated. The optimist, like the pessimist, emphasizes the importance of "I." But hope is humble, it is modest, it is selfless. Unconcerned with the ambiguity of past experience, hope implies process; it is an adventure, a going forward, a confident search.

But on the other hand, hope must also be distinguished from expectation, i.e., from conclusions based on observed facts. "We are saved by hope," wrote Saint Paul to some Christians in Italy, "but hope that is seen is not hope: for who hopeth for that which he seeth?"

Should we perhaps distinguish, as Schachtel [35] does, magic hope from realistic hope (and correspondingly, magic joy from realistic joy)? Magic hope is

> the mere wishful expectation and anticipation that somehow things will change for the better. Another person, God, fate, some event . . . or—quite often—the mere flow of time, the beginning of a new year, the eternal tomorrow, will magically bring fulfillment without one's having anything to do about it. . . . This 'tomorrow' of magic hope has been denounced eloquently by Camus. He sees in it man's worst enemy. . . .

Realistic hope, on the other hand, is

> based on the attempt to understand the concrete conditions of reality, to see one's own role in it realistically, and to engage in such efforts of thoughtful action as might be expected to bring about the hoped-for

change. The affect of hope, in this case, has an activating effect. It helps in the mobilization of the energies needed for activity. By activity I mean not only motor activity but also the activity of thought or of relating oneself to another person, e.g. in an attitude of loving concern.*

The person who feels hope, based, to use Hegel's expression, on *"real* possibility" in contrast to merely phantasied, magic possibility, will usually act with more sustained energy than the person who acts without this affect. Of course, there exist all degrees of transition and mixture of magic and realistic hope, as is equally true of other embeddedness- and activity-affects. We have to picture these transitions on a continuum, on one end of which the quasi-intrauterine, embeddedness-affects would be located, on the other end the pure, realistic activity-affects. The affects which we find most frequently in reality usually are located somewhere between the two extremes of this continuum, with either the embeddedness or the activity quality prevailing.

Let us then redefine hope as the positive expectations in a studied situation which go beyond the visible facts. We are not theologians, eschatologists, political scientists, economists, or others concerned with different courses of human development and process. But as physicians who make diagnoses of disease, we are presumed to have some idea about the probable effects of our intervention. We like to think this is a matter of logical, rational conclusion. But all of us who have practiced some years know how the best-laid predictions of mice and psychiatrists "gang aft agley."

And often it would seem to be this element of hope—hope in the doctor, hope in the patient, and hope in others concerned in the matter —which plays not a passive but an active role in the developments. Perhaps this is only to say that our present scientific knowledge is not sufficient to recognize or identify or properly credit all the forces working *for* recovery any more than we know in any case all the forces against which we are working. And this we know: Sometimes hope fails, and death ensues, while sometimes hope endures, and the impossible happens.

Each of us who has been in practice more than a decade has seen the "hopeless case" recover. And we have sometimes seen, or so it seemed, that a mother's or father's indomitable hope was a factor in this recovery. True, we have also seen hope deferred, making the heart sick. But recovery certainly does sometimes occur in conditions considered "irreversible" and "hopeless," without an external change that can

---

* Clifford Scott conceives of hope as the fourth step in a kind of hallucinatory gratification in a state of need. Waiting, the first step, is succeeded by anticipating, this by pining, and finally by hope. "Hope takes into account a more complex relationship to the object . . . e.g., the time necessary for the changes to occur . . . Hope is a positive balance of love which can emcompass, restitute and repair effects of hate." (Scott, W. C. M. "Depression, Confusion and Multivalence." *Int. J. Psa.* 41:497–503, 1960.)

be in any logical way related to the illness. I venture to mention some other phenomena which lend some basis to reliance upon hope. Mind you, I am offering no proofs, only some instances where expectation went beyond the visible facts.

Carl Hamburger,[36] in an extraordinary book on the *Self-Healing of Hopeless Illness*, has collected quite a few such cases in the area of general medicine. My eye fell particularly on one of a child afflicted with total bilateral optic atrophy combined with severe vascular lesions in the retina, who made a complete and totally inexplicable recovery. Both the affliction and the subsequent restoration were checked by outstanding ophthalmologists.

The reported recovery from such conditions as optic atrophy, epilepsy, feeble-mindedness, carcinoma, and advanced mental deterioration evokes curious emotional reactions in doctors, associated with tacit incredulity. We simply cannot quite concede the possibility that immutable laws can be broken. It almost angers a scientific medical man to be told that a colleague has observed an instance of something contrary to all established medical principles and precedent and pathology. Most of us are like the priest who allegedly refused to look through Galileo's telescope lest, as he said, it destroy his faith (and change his vocation!).

The skepticism of physicians comes about partly, no doubt, from habit, pride, vested interest, and intellectual laziness. But it is basically determined by the necessity in science to constantly combat wishful thinking as a basis for judgment in the physician, as a basis for exploitation in the charlatan, and as a basis for passive submission in the patient.

But it seems to occur in great waves or cycles, as we have suggested in our review of the revivals of confidence in the *vis medicatrix naturae*. Disappointment in the expected results of a drug leads to discouragement and to therapeutic nihilism—with the abandonment of both expectations and hope. Dour, pedestrian medical drudgery then plows ahead until a cry is raised, Here is a remedy! Expectations rise; hope burns brighter. The use of the remedy spreads; it is applied to all sorts of "similar" and related conditions. It becomes a panacea. Gradually, then, disappointment leads to discreditation and discreditation to discard.

When I was still in medical school, which was before arsphenamine had been introduced in this country, we were taught on the one hand that nearly all chronic disease was related to syphilis and that syphilis was essentially incurable. One professor (Post) vigorously denied this, assuring us that we could cure many patients with mercury and iodides. And certainly other physicians long before him believed that they had done so. But there was much discouragement, and the prevalent mood of medical skepticism was so great that the introduction of arsphenamine with its dramatic effect upon some stages of syphilitic infection was gingerly received. Even after its usefulness became indisputable, its effect upon brain and spinal-cord syphilis was still considered negligible. It was the persistence of Ernest Southard, Harry Solomon, and others who used it in the treatment of these "incurable" conditions which paved the way for the later victories of tryparsamide, then malaria, and finally penicillin.

Meanwhile, Sigmund Freud was working on a rational technique of doing something about the "incurable" neuroses, and Clifford Beers and Adolf Meyer, a businessman and a neuropathologist, preached to an incredulous profession and public the forgotten discovery of Brigham and Woodward and Butler and Ray that mental illness was not incurable and might even in some instances be preventable.

Reports of the successful treatment of psychiatric patients still bring uplifted eyebrows and tongue-in-cheek reactions. Even psychiatrists themselves tend to be mutually suspicious of reported successes. There are jokes about the "cult of curability" and about the medical reporting done in popular magazines, from which doctors seem to be getting their latest information. But where could such an article as "Schizophrenics in the Sun" be published, other than in *Harper's* or some other intelligent *lay* journal? This is an account by a distinguished layman of a Swedish experiment in which forty-nine patients were flown from a psychiatric hospital near Stockholm to an Italian seaside resort fifteen hundred miles away. Most of them are described as being "schizophrenics" (!) of long standing, half of them for years restricted to the hospital grounds, and four of them sick enough to require constant attendance when off of the ward. "Under the shock treatment of bright new skies and vividly strange surroundings, tears came to the eyes of a human statue; one man who had barely said a word for years began to talk; another whose mind had seemed utterly sunless laughed for joy at the sight of Rome. People long sunk within themselves began to notice and help their neighbors. After they had returned to Sweden, twenty-nine patients were chalked up as having clearly benefited from the holiday, and of these a dozen were scheduled for discharge." [37]

Such "moral treatment" is certainly not based upon conventional or recognized scientific medical principles. If things had gone wrong, poor Dr. Izikowitz might have been liable for malpractice suits, for he was certainly not using treatments which corresponded to accepted modes and practices. I am afraid we shall have to charge the doctor with having been equipped with courage, intelligence, resourcefulness, and hope.

Many other such examples could be cited.

But this curability of incurable "schizophrenic" and "senile" patients is being demonstrated all the time—every day, in fact. It is most dramatic when there has been a recent change in the personnel responsible for a group of patients, because with the new people there may come a new philosophy of treatment.

I remember a vivid personal experience. In the revolution which took place in the Topeka State Hospital in the late 1940s, one of our young graduates, distinguished for the modesty with which he masks his very considerable ability, was put in charge of nine large wards. He selected two of these for a special program. They had long been utilized as wards to which the aged and infirm were consigned.

On January 1, 1950, the population of these two wards was eighty-eight; the average age of the patients was sixty-eight. Fifty-one of them were bedfast and had been so for an average of ten years. About a score of them had no control over their excretory functions, and forty-one of them were spoon-fed at every meal. One of these patients had been on this ward for fifty-eight years; the average stay was over ten years.

Picture this ward full of long-time bedridden, incontinent, hopeless, vegetating patients. Then picture Dr. Howard Williams taking over with his therapeutic team of cheerful young nurses, aides, social workers, and psychiatric residents. Every patient became a focus of attention. The ward was transformed from a museum of dying human specimens into a hospital-home in the best sense. Music and television were brought in, cages of canaries and potted plants were placed about the dreary halls, new lighting fixtures and pretty curtains and drapes were installed. Birthday parties were held, and relatives were urged to come to these, and for week-end visits. A score of social activities were instituted with the combined aid of patients, staff members, and volunteers. The patients themselves painted a shuffleboard court on the floor of the previously sacred "sitting hall," and a ramp was constructed (by the patients!) over a short but difficult flight of steps, which enabled some of the bedfast patients to be moved into the social center. Finger painting, furniture sanding, leather-tooling, Bingo games, water-color painting, and all sorts of things were introduced.

A change in the clinical status of the patients was perceptible immediately. Three weeks after the program had been begun, one patient was discharged to cooperative and interested relatives who were delighted to have their old father rise, as it were, from the grave and return to them.

By the end of the year *only nine* of these nearly ninety patients were still bedfast, and only six of them were still incontinent. Five had died. Twelve had gone home to live with their families. Six had gone out to live by themselves, and four had found comfortable nursing-home provisions. Four of the original eighty-eight were now gainfully employed and self-supporting.

What Howard Williams did at the Topeka State Hospital had been done many times before in other places. Over a hundred years ago it had been done in New England and New York by half a dozen young pioneer psychiatrists. But time after time psychiatric leaders have built up living institutions of psychiatric care and treatment only to have them sink into oblivion with the passing of their inspirers. The morale of the workers falls, the goals and achievements are forgotten, and once more the glacier of public indifference and custodial pessimism grinds its smothering way over the landscape, obliterating hope and progress.

Just this happened in the case of every one of the individuals we have mentioned. A few years after Woodward's retirement in Massachusetts public support for his hospital failed and "the insane were once more regarded as incurable." [10]

The late Dr. Harold G. Wolff, distinguished for his research in psychosomatic medicine, contributed in the *Saturday Review* for January 5, 1957, "A Science Report" entitled "What Hope Does for Man." He cites numerous phenomena which impressed him with being results beyond the expected fact. The introduction to this article, which undoubtedly had his approval, reads thus: "Hope, like faith and a purpose in life, is medicinal. This is not merely a statement of belief, but a conclusion proved by meticulously controlled scientific experiment. A famous physician here reviews the evidence and, in the spirit of a New Year's resolution, urges people everywhere to re-examine the means by which they strive to attain their ends—and so profit in terms of health and happiness."

Some of the examples cited by Wolff had to do with somatic responses to expectations, for example, the engorgement of the stomach lining under certain conditions of perceived or anticipated threat (cf. Walter Cannon). But Wolff was most impressed by certain mass phenomena such as the difference in the death rate from tuberculosis among primitive people who were completely in despair and some who had a little more hope for relief. He was very much impressed by the findings of the group working in the Human Ecology Program at the New York Hospital, which have since been published in the study about midtown Manhattan.[38] He cites the heavy death rate of six thousand American prisoners of war captured by the North Koreans, about one-third of whom died.

> Medical observers reported that the cause of death in many instances was ill-defined, and was referred to by them as "give-up-itis." Occurring as it did in a setting of serious demoralization, humiliation, despair and deprivation of human support and affection, the prisoner became apathetic, listless, neither ate nor drank, helped himself in no way, stared into space and finally died.
>
> A recently completed study of the effects of imprisonment on Americans during World War II tells us that approximately 94,000 United States prisoners of war were taken in Europe. These men were imprisoned about ten months. Less than 1 per cent of them died before liberation. In contrast, in the Pacific theater, about 25,000 Americans became prisoners of war. They remained in prison four times as long as those captured in Europe, and suffered far more than any others the effects of threats, abuse and humiliation. Their demoralization was often extreme. Over one third died before liberation.
>
> Six years after liberation, those who survived the Japanese prison experience were re-examined. In the first place the total number of deaths in this group during these six years was more than twice the expected incidence for a similar group of persons not so exposed, and three times as great as in the group of United States prisoners of war in Europe. The causes of death included many diseases not directly related to confinement or starvation. Thus, nine times the expected number died of pulmonary tuberculosis, twice the expected number died of heart disease, more than twice the expected number of cancer, more than four times the expected number of diseases of the gastrointestinal tract, twice the number from suicide and, most striking of all, three times the expected number of deaths as a result of accidents. . . .
>
> In short, prolonged circumstances which are perceived as dangerous, as lonely, as hopeless, may drain a man of hope and of his health; but he is capable of enduring incredible burdens and taking cruel punishment when he has self-esteem, hope, purpose, and belief in his fellows.[39]

When Doctors Bartemeier, Romano, Kubie, and Whitehorn, and I went to the European Theater of World War II for my brother Will and the Surgeon-General, we arrived at the Buchenwald prison camp a few days after it had been entered by our armed forces. What I remember most vividly of that terrible place was something we didn't actually see. But we heard it at first hand. The night before we got there, our United States Army doctors had given what they called a "smoker" for the physician prisoners they had discovered and released. It was a kind of unearthly medical-society meeting. Army rations were put out as refreshment, with some wine and tobacco, incredibly relished by the emaciated but overjoyed guests. Communication in words was imperfect because of language difficulties, but the spirit was unmistakable. The members of a fraternity were reunited. And in the spirit of the fraternity, experiences were exchanged.

These doctors, prisoners along with all the others, had followed the same routines of rising at four a.m., standing in shivering roll calls, then day-long drudgery on the *Autobahn*, shivering roll calls again, and finally a cold bowl of thin soup and a crawl up onto wooden plank shelves to sleep. They were starved and beaten and overworked like all the others, with no reason to expect any other fate than the miserable death and cremation which they observed about them daily.

But now comes the unbelievable. At night, when the other prisoners were asleep, these thin, hungry, weary doctors got up and huddled together in a group, and talked. They discussed cases. They organized a medical society. They prepared and presented papers. They treated sick fellow prisoners and made plans for improving health conditions. Then they began to smuggle in materials to make various medical instruments. And finally they built, of all things, an X-ray machine! The pieces had to be located somewhere; then they had to be stolen, they had to be concealed in the prisoners' clothes; they had to be carried back to the prison on the long, weary marches after work. The guards had to be bribed or otherwise thrown off the scent.

But little by little, with the aid of some engineers and electricians among the prisoners, these doctors put together a workable X-ray machine and used it, secretly, at night, in their efforts to ameliorate the lot of their fellow prisoners. This was what dedication to medicine and humanity could do—*kept alive by hope.**

But someone who remembers may ask bitterly, what of the thousands who died miserably, for *all* the hopes they nurtured?

Even here I would not concede that hope had altogether failed. I would believe that hope had sustained them in their martyrdom, and that their hopefulness, however frail and tortured and ultimately defeated, was communicated on down through prison generations to those

---

* A colleague, Joost Meerloo, formerly of the Netherlands but now in New York City, wrote me and commented upon our report: "Unconsciously hope must be rooted in Eros. In prisons and concentration camps I experienced that when there still was the expectation to meet the beloved at home, then there was hope. The notion to be loved and desired kept the prisoners alert, or to say it paradoxically, as long as one expects that there will be somebody to sleep with in the future, hope is not gone." It is a curious thing that the symbol now used conventionally in biology to mean female sex is used all over the Orient as the sign of Eros and of hope—also of fertility!

who were ultimately freed and brought us the record of this medical miracle. Who can read the eloquent last messages of the condemned in *Dying We Live*,[40] and fail to catch a spark of hope from them?

Confirmation for the sustaining function of hope in life has recently come from a most unexpected quarter—the psychobiological laboratory. At the annual convention of the American Psychological Association in September 1956, Curt Richter [41] of Johns Hopkins reported an astonishing phenomenon. It was simply this, that when placed in certain situations which seemed to permit no chance for escape, even vigorous animals gave up their efforts and rapidly succumbed to death. This was observed experimentally in both laboratory rats and wild rats. "After elimination of the hopelessness feature," reported Richter, "the rats do not die. . . . (Indeed, the speed of their recovery is remarkable). A rat that would quite certainly have died in another minute or two, becomes normally active and aggressive," swimming vigorously fifty to sixty hours. Richter emphasized that not the restraint alone, nor the immersion, nor the exposure, nor the trimming of whiskers will explain the phenomenon. It is, he insisted, the loss of hope.

Richter added some confirmatory data from other fields and suggested an extrapolation from his laboratory observations to explain the occurrence of sudden death in rabbits, chimpanzees, foxes, raccoons, some birds, musk oxen, otters, minks, and even human beings. "Some of these instances," he said, "can best be described in terms of hopelessness, all avenues of escape appearing to be closed."

This is not an isolated observation or hypothesis. For example, from a large amount of psychosomatic investigation Engel, Schmale, and associates in Rochester, New York, consider that what they describe as "helplessness" and "hopelessness" reflect a necessary if not a sufficient condition for the development of organic disease.[42]

And then there is the Queequeg phenomenon of "voodoo death" in *Moby Dick*, which Walter Cannon and others have amply substantiated with authentic data from primitive societies. No doubt most of us can recall instances in which the loss of hope seemed to accelerate the arrival of death for a patient. There are many such stories, unconfirmed, of course, but highly suggestive, in the daily press.

Twelve days ago, Mrs. Helen E. Hopke lay in her bed fighting to stay alive to see her daughter's wedding.

Incurably ill for the past five years, Mrs. Hopke had been indirectly responsible for the meeting about a year ago of her daughter, Rose Marie, 20, and the girl's intended husband, Arthur Woodrow Hudson, 26.

Rose Marie had acted as nurse and housekeeper to her bedfast mother. While buying medicine she met Hudson, a pharmacist in a local drug store. Friends said it was the girl's first romance.

They also said all that kept Mrs. Hopke alive in recent months was the thought of the impending marriage.

The 56-year-old mother heard the couple enter the house laughing and talking about the April 4th wedding. She heard them enter the next room.

Their chatter ended in three blasts from a shotgun.

Police said Hopke, opposed to the marriage, wanted his daughter to continue to care for her mother. He became enraged at reading the wedding notice in the paper, shot the couple then turned the gun on himself.

Rose Marie was taken to one hospital where she is recovering. Her mother was taken to another.

Tuesday night, Mrs. Hopke died.[43]

All these things seem to me to support the theoretical proposal that hope reflects the working of the life instinct in its constant battle against the various forces that add up to self-destruction. It would be too narrow to regard it as a form of self-sufficiency since, as Gabriel Marcel [44] points out, there is something essentially unnarcissistic and beyond self in hope. One sees this in the hopefulness not of the patient but of the physician.

In studies of the new drugs, for example, patients who receive only placebos sometimes show much improvement. In one study that I know about, testing an excellent drug, more patients in the group which had only placebos were able to be discharged from the hospital than from the group of those who got the actual remedy (although a larger number of the latter showed marked improvement).[45] The *doctors* believed!

Whatever the explanation offered for such phenomena, to invoke suggestion or coincidence (whatever *they* are) will not suffice. There is more to it. And yet we doctors are so schooled against permitting ourselves to believe the intangible or impalpable or indefinite that we tend to discount the element of hope, its reviving effect as well as its survival function. Because of the vulnerability of every doctor to the temptation of playing God and taking the credit for the workings of the *vis medicatrix naturae*, we are necessarily extremely cautious in attributing change to any particular thing, and least of all to our own wishful thinking.

This placebo phenomenon keeps popping up all the time. It is ancient, it is popular, it is powerful. Even the advent of specific drugs and "miracle cures" has not forced it into oblivion. It remains unexplained by modern psychodynamics. All physicians, knowingly or unknowingly, employ it, know something about it, and talk privately of its accomplishments. Yet it has no scientific status.* For some members of the profession, its therapeutic use was considered a violation of medical trust.

The real case against placebos is, then, not their ineffectiveness but rather their effectiveness. They afford an easy way to gain undeserved credit and often fool the physician as much as or even more than the patient. The modern physician, looking over the struggles the profession has had in getting out of the mire of quackery and the exploitation of sufferers, looks with horror on anything harking back to it. Furthermore, no doctor likes to be deceived. Placebos obtain high percentages of positive responses, and the physicians who unknowingly dispense them in research controls may become very angry when they discover the truth.

One cannot help being amused at the length of the list of placebo devices which physicians constantly employ *on themselves* as well as on their patients, without giving much thought to the matter. Take, for example, the flavors added to various liquid drugs, the Epsom salts put into foot-soaking water, the erythema-producing substances in various skin ointments, the pink color in mouthwashes, the tincture of benzoin in steam inhalations, the use of various let's-not-name-them substances for "sterilizing" skin wounds, which leaves all pathogenic bacteria unharmed.

Some gestures in the direction of absolute honesty are themselves dishonest. Even what the doctor earnestly believes to be truth sometimes isn't, as Henderson [46] has suggested, and the patient may be misinformed and misled by the doctor's good intentions to be truthful. And those physicians who take pleasure in slaughtering hope under the impression that they are being paragons of honesty may best be compared to those surgeons of an earlier day who bravely poured boiling oil into wounds to hasten healing.**

---

* I am paraphrasing here the first paragraph of an excellent study by Fischer and Dlin. (Fischer, H. Keith, and Dlin, Barney M. "The Dynamics of Placebo Therapy: a Clinical Study." *Am. J. Med. Sciences*, 232:504–512, 1956.)
** The word placebo means "I will please," the implication being that the remedy is given to please the patient rather than to cure him. Some placebos may be dangerous to the patient, but such things are not truly placebos, which above all must conform to the basic Hippocratic axiom, "Do no harm." By the middle of the fifteenth century, "placebo" was in general use as a simple synonym for "flattery" and "flatterer," and it continued to serve that purpose through the sixteenth and seventeenth centuries. It then came to mean a courtesy designed to soothe or gratify. Its inclusion in the vocabulary of medicine is rather more recent. It made its first clearly recorded appearance there (as "an epithet given to any medicine adapted more to please than benefit the patient") in the 1811 edition of Hooper's Medical Dictionary. It could

In this chapter we have tried to suggest that the role of the physician in diagnosis and in treatment is made more complex and difficult to analyze because of great intangible forces which operate through it. For all our modern advances in knowledge, our new discoveries in physics and chemistry, molecular biology and microchemistry, light-ray uses and ultra-microscopes, we still have no explanation or real understanding of some of the most obvious and profound changes which can be induced,

---

hardly have been included much earlier. For until around the early part of the nineteenth century, when chemistry began to develop into a science capable of discerning the true nature and action of drugs, all medicines, as far as anyone could tell, were equally worthy or worthless. "The placebo can powerfully mimic the tranquilizing touch of certain ataractics. 'There is no good evidence that meprobamate (the chemical name of Equanil and Miltown) can be distinguished from a placebo in treating anxiety in psychiatric out-patients,' two clinical pharmacologists at the Johns Hopkins University School of Medicine—Victor G. Laties and Bernard Weiss—reported to the *Journal of Chronic Diseases* in a recent review of the subject. Their conclusion was largely derived from two well-controlled studies carried out in 1957. One of these, the work of Herbert Koteen, assistant professor of internal medicine at Cornell University Medical College, involved twenty-five patients, whose symptoms included anxiety, muscle tension, restlessness, and irritability. In the course of this trial, each patient consumed thirty-seven bottles of meprobamate capsules and thirty-six bottles of matching lactose placebo capsules. All were told simply that they were taking something that would help them. 'The results,' Koteen noted, 'reveal that meprobamate in the currently recommended dose had no greater effect in relieving symptoms than did the placebo.' If anything, the placebo was the more effective. An analysis of reports on the patients showed that twenty-three of the thirty-six bottles of placebo capsules produced marked improvement. For meprobamate the count was twenty-one out of thirty-seven. A team of English investigators—M. J. Raymond, C. J. Lucas, M. L. Beesley, B. A. O'Connell, and S. A. F. Roberts—conducted the other study reviewed by Laties and Weiss. Fifty-one psychoneurotic patients took part in the test, and each was given five different ataractic drugs and a placebo. In addition to meprobamate, the drugs were amobarbital (Amytal), chlorpromazine (Thorazine), benactyzine, and a preparation containing, among other things, Rauwolfia. Thirty-three patients responded favorably to amobarbital, twenty-five to meprobamate, twenty-five to the Rauwolfia preparation, nineteen to chlorpromazine, and eighteen to benactyzine. But twenty-two patients responded just as favorably to the placebo.

"Henry K. Beecher, professor of anesthesiology at Harvard University Medical School, notes in a recent report to the *Journal of the American Medical Association*, 'we have found that rather constantly thirty per cent or more of these individuals get satisfactory pain relief from a placebo.' ('Satisfactory relief' is defined by Beecher as 'fifty per cent or more relief of pain at two checked intervals—forty-five and ninety minutes after administration of the agent.') A total of four hundred and fifty-three men and women, all patients at Massachusetts General Hospital, participated in these tests. The number of patients who obtained relief ranged from a low of fifteen per cent in one study to a high of fifty-three per cent in another. Moreover, Beecher adds, the studies produced 'strong evidence that placebos are far more effective in relieving early postoperative wound pain when [the pain] is severe than when it is less so.' The impact of the placebo on clinical headache, according to a classic study conducted by E. M. Jellinek, professor of biometrics at the Yale School of Medicine, in 1946, is even more emphatic. In this study, a hundred and ninety-nine general-hospital patients were regularly given a lactose placebo upon complaint of headache. Approximately sixty per cent of the patients reported prompt relief." (Roueché, Berton. "Placebo." *The New Yorker*, October 15, 1960, pp. 85-103. Reprinted by permission; © 1960 The New Yorker Magazine, Inc.)

by pragmatic methods, in human beings. Hence we have some reason to expect more than the seen facts of a case justify. It would be most unscientific indeed to ignore—or continue to ignore—those potentially positive factors in the balance determining the health-illness process which represent intangible and invisible forces. The power of suggestion is only a reflection of the deep influences of faith, of love, and of hope—these three, and if the greatest of these is love, the least credited is hope.

Having come this far in our search for the essential intangibles of psychiatric treatment, a word of caution is in order, a demurrer of sorts. We hope the reader can share our deep respect for these intangible factors in the therapeutic efficacy of the healer. But it is possible to become too enraptured of them in a kind of trusting faith that "all's well with the world" and that now that *our* attention has been called to a problem, it will begin to diminish.*

It certainly will not do for us to forget those tangible forces working toward recovery which we discussed in an earlier chapter. True, when one sees these abused by a therapeutically determined zealot, one sometimes reacts by retreating to a kind of indifferentism or hands-off policy which in turn arouses counter-reactions. Carl Rogers [47] is only half right when he urges his students to recognize that in most if not "all individuals there exist growth forces, tendencies towards self-actualization, which may act as the sole motivation for therapy. We have not realized that under suitable psychological conditions those forces bring about emotional release in those areas and at those rates which are most beneficial to the individual. . . . The individual has the capacity and the strength to devise, quite unguided, the steps which will lead him to a more mature and more comfortable relationship to his reality."

This conviction is the cornerstone for Rogers' philosophy and the essential rationale for his "non-directive therapy." The misgivings about this position, expressed by one of us some years ago, bear repetition here. "It is the insufficiency of this philosophy as an exclusive rationale for treatment which has made it unpopular in some quarters where concern is felt about the danger that a Pollyannaish optimism would interfere with the acceptance of therapeutic responsibility for a patient. Sick

---

* Now and then I hear a colleague reporting a social observation in terms that suggest that since psychotherapy is achieved by means of words, *anything* a psychiatrist says under almost any circumstances is to be regarded as official treatment. Not only the young doctor himself, but many laymen begin to think in these terms and I wonder sometimes if that is why talks by psychiatrists to lay groups and women's clubs and even individual families are so zealously sought after by some.

individuals differ in the strength and effectiveness of their 'drive toward health.' In some people the will to live and grow flickers, fades, or even dies. What is it which prevents the 'release' in some patients of the propensities for progressive adaptation and change? It may reassure the therapist to believe that a patient if left to his own devices in a permissive setting will find the best possible solution to his neurotic predicament. But we all know of patients who under such circumstances seemed to get caught up in an even more relentless self-destructive process leading to still more failures, more suffering, more defeat. Many patients whom we see seem to have committed themselves, consciously or unconsciously, to stagnation or slow spiritual death."

Rogers and many like him, in a gentle, kindly regard for the potentialities of the individual, give insufficient credence to the self-destructive propensities of human beings. "A permissive atmosphere and a sincere respect for the worth of the individual are essential ingredients of good psychotherapy, but there are times when the most respectful and accepting thing to do for a sick person is to insist on his being confined to a closed ward, or put to work in a full activity program, or treated with a variety of more subtle therapeutic modes. One needs more than kindness and good will to be an effective therapist. One cannot simply leave it to the patient to find his own solutions. There may *be* alternative and more fulfilling resolutions for a patient's neurotic plight; the patient partially knows this when he seeks out a therapist for help, but in doing so he also says he cannot do anything more on his own to find these more successful solutions. And, of course, in a sense he is right. We must know how to bring to bear our knowledge and skills in such a way as to help him pull himself out of his quandary. To help the person come to grips with his intrinsic resistance to growth and change is a delicate art. Non-directiveness as Rogers defines it may be one of the essential tools of this art, but as the only tool it must surely be insufficient." [48]

Southard was my teacher, and above all men I have known, and entirely out of keeping with the spirit of his day, he placed great hope in psychiatry. The "high years for psychiatrists," as Southard called them, really began after his death. The public had been alerted by the literary dissemination of the discoveries of Freud and also by the growing "mental hygiene movement." Most doctors had had almost no psychiatry in their medical-school training. Twenty-five years after Southard died, we were in the midst of another world war. There was a shortage of psychiatrists. To enlist interest and recruit doctors, I visited medical schools over the country and talked at length to students, deans, and faculty members. I found that a common objection to entering psychiatry was an impression that our patients "never get well." It is such a hopeless field, they said. Penicillin and the other miracle drugs are more definite and exciting than the dreary wards of state hospitals, filled with silent, staring faces.

We can see, now, that these students had been shown the wrong side of psychiatry, its failures rather than its successes. But one thing struck me then which has remained in my mind indelibly. I perceived vividly how hopelessness breeds hopelessness, how the non-expectant, hope-lacking, or "unimaginative" teacher can bequeath to his student a sense of impotence and futility, utterly out of keeping with facts known to both of them! Surely even these misled students knew that *some* psychiatric patients recover, even if they didn't know that the vast majority do so. But, like their teachers, they adopted some of the symptoms of their patients: hopelessness and goallessness!

This experience only reinforced my conviction that hope, that neglected member of the great triad, was an indispensable factor in psychiatric treatment and psychiatric education.

The psychoanalytic treatment method was a great discovery, but this is not what changed psychiatry. It was the new understanding that psychoanalytic research gave us concerning men's motives and inner resources, the intensity of partially buried conflicts, the unknown and unplumbed depths and heights of our nature, the formidable power each of us holds to determine whether he lives or dies. It was the realization that we must encourage each individual to see himself not as a mere spectator of cosmic events but as a prime mover; to regard himself not as a passive incident in the infinite universe but as one important unit possessing the power to influence great decisions by making small ones.

Freud's great courage led him to look honestly at the evil in man's nature. Freud persisted in his researches to the bottom of the jar, and there he found hope. He discerned that love is stronger than hate, that hence, for all its core of malignancy, the nature of men can be transformed through the nurture and dispersion of love. In this way the destructiveness can be transcended.

"Ye shall know the truth and the truth shall make you free," said another wise One. For this emancipating truth Freud searched not in physics or chemistry or biology, but in the tabooed land of the emotions. From the Pandora jar of man's mind, full of harmful and unlovely things to be released upon a protesting world, there turned up—last of all— hope. Selfishness, vengefulness, hate, greed, pettiness, bitterness, vindictiveness, ruthlessness, cruelty, destructiveness, and even self-destructiveness—all these are in us. But not only those. Invisible at first, but slowly pervasive and neutralizing, came love, and then—perhaps because of it— came faith, and then hope.

Love, faith, hope—in that order. The Greeks were wrong. *Of course* hope is real, and of course it is not evil. It is the enemy of evil, and an ally of love, which is goodness.

It is our duty as physicians to estimate probabilities and to discipline expectations. But leading away from probabilities there are paths of possibility, toward which it is also our duty to hold aloft a light. And the name of that light is Hope.

CHAPTER XVI

Prevention, Endurance, and Transcendence

SYNOPSIS: *From the traditional viewpoint, much is gained by providing ever more effective therapies for mental illness. But the goals of psychiatry must go beyond cure to prevention. With this emphasis, psychiatry becomes deeply involved in the well and the sick, in social structure, mores, attitudes, and values. A broad reappraisal of the health-illness continuum in that context also has implications for the goals of treatment. These need no longer be confined to a reinstatement of the status quo ante ("recovery" in the popular sense), but might push forward toward the development of new potentialities and transcendence of previous levels of vital balance to a state of being "weller than well".*

WE HAVE ROUNDED the circle. In Chapter I we proposed taking a look at the psychiatry of yesterday and then the psychiatry of today, with a glance into the possibilities of psychiatry for tomorrow. We outlined diagnosis in a new key, viewing human beings as in a constant process of adaptation, subject to occasional major derailments. Estimating the severity and reversibility of these derailments, we said, and determining how and why they occur, might enable us to plan logical and effective intervention.

We continued then with a discussion of *organization;* after dipping deep into *dysorganization* and describing that in many phases, we returned at last to *reorganization;* i.e., to recovery and reconstitution. We described the human organization interacting with the environmental organization, noting particularly the individual's motives and his ways of coping with interferences in their expression. We described the psychological machinery for dealing with them, leaving an elaboration of the physiological machinery to colleagues versed in that area.

When the stress of adjustment reaches a certain height, we said, numerous emergency relief devices are summoned, like the firemen and police in a city. Their efforts become apparent to the outside world in diverse forms of altered behavior which often is disruptive and uncomfortable. But its purpose is essentially salvaging. It endeavors to effect a compromise between self-destructive and self-preservative forces. A strategic retreat is made under the shelter of the "symptoms." When they have done their work and served their purpose, when shifts in the balance of determining factors have resulted in a reduction of tension, the emergency measures disappear and the customary life mode is resumed.

For the pathologist and the pessimist such excursions constitute illness; for the therapist and the optimist they represent a lowering of the level of optimal degrees of healthiness. Illness and recovery are but two aspects of the same process. "As a man develops a disease, so begins at the same time a fight between the disease and the counter striving life, which seeks incessantly to overcome the new enemy . . . The moment of disease is at the same time the moment of healing." [1]

Our theory regards the two aspects of the process as representing the dominance of one or the other of the two polar drives of the personality, which are in a continuous and infinitely varied state of conflict, fusion, and defusion. The aggressive and self-destructive forces are constantly opposed by constructive, integrative, and reintegrative ones. From these derive both the automatic healing measures within the organism and the search for the assistance of benevolent and useful features of the environment, including the physician. The goal of therapeutic intervention is the expediting of the upward trend of the illness-recovery process. To accomplish this the positive factors must be identified as well as the negative or pathogenic factors, the former to be supported and the latter combated.

Psychiatric treatment has evolved through many stages—extrusion; ostracism; torture; execution; studied neglect; dreary maintenance; kindly care; mechanical, surgical, and electrical assaults of various kinds; an infinite assortment of chemical alteratives, sedatives, and stimulants; and varied programs of work therapy, play therapy, music therapy, psychotherapy. The long era of therapeutic nihilism was terminated by the discovery of arsphenamine and of psychoanalysis.

With the new knowledge came new hope. As our eyes were opened to the power of the malignant forces in the environment and to those within the personality, we had begun to find ways of combating both. New treatment methods and philosophies evolved. Young people of both sexes began to turn in increasing numbers to the acquiring of various skills in the service of assisting the recovery of the mentally ill. These workers brought to the task also the force of their personalities, their affections, their faith in psychiatry, their hopeful confidence that better things were possible.

With this great wave of faith, hope, and dedication, combined with scientific and professional growth, psychiatry ascended into hitherto untouched heights. On the one hand, mental illness was recognized and officially declared by the organized medical profession to be "the number-one health problem of our country." On the other hand, the application of new methods and a new spirit revolutionized psychiatric hospitals and changed the expectations for recovery from mental illness from very low to very high. True, there remain many cases of stubborn chronicity, especially in the partially disabled, but it is now common knowledge that the vast majority of hospitalized patients recover and return home within a few weeks or months of admission. (This assumes a modern and properly operated psychiatric hospital.)

The success of psychiatric treatment has had two paradoxical consequences. One of these was the great increase in the numbers of those seeking help. Many sufferers who had resigned themselves or who had been resigned by their relatives to despair, and many others previously not considered amenable to psychiatric treatment began to seek it. Couples in marital discord, confused schoolchildren whose potentialities were obviously greater than their achievement, misunderstood or misunderstanding employees whose joy in work had become replaced with bitterness and inefficiency, clergymen and teachers dissatisfied and frustrated in their profession, offenders whose criminal acts did not get them what they sought—all these and many other individuals began coming to psychiatrists. And although the psychiatrists have gradually surrounded themselves with many therapeutic assistants, treatment case loads continued to mount far more rapidly than additional psychiatrists could be trained.

Thus the success of psychiatry also aroused the long-cherished and wistfully protected notion of *prevention*. Better than treatment, better even than diagnosis, would be the diminution of the incidence of need. Not that anyone expects the vicissitudes and sorrow of life to disappear: accidents will continue to happen, aggressions will continue to erupt, wounds will continue to be inflicted. But might not something be done to mitigate the severity of the reaction or the frequency of the *severe* reaction? Does the knowledge of what things men cannot bear, or of what they bear only with the greatest difficulty, or of how their ability to bear stresses becomes impaired—could this knowledge give us a basis for improving life conditions and hence life itself?

Many so-intended social programs have been offered, but those in charge of public affairs, who give careful ear to public-health measures of other sorts—concerning food and water and sewage—are not inclined to take seriously the practical measures proposed for the insurance of mental health. Psychiatrists plead the importance of security and affection in early mother-child relationships, better schools, better teachers, better playgrounds and more of them. But school-board members still are inclined to regard such measures as too expensive or irrelevant. Our government still separates thousands of (Indian) children from mothers by force at an early age and consigns them to educational factories at long distances from their homes on the basis that learning English and arithmetic is more important than learning to love and to feel secure.

No one disputes the theoretical importance of stable family life, fidelity in marriage, kindness to children, and such pleasant things, but they are not thought of generally as basic to mental health. Our divorce rate rises, the battered-child syndrome appears ever more frequently, racial intolerance and bitterness increase. Psychiatrists plead for wilderness areas, not for the preservation of beauty but for the preservation of mental health. What happens? Certain commercial interests protest and one stubborn politician blocks the efforts of years with impunity. Art galleries, museums, concert halls, gymnasiums, and facilities for outdoor recreation are commended as contributing to mental health, but it is a handful of angels who keep such things going.

All these measures have been proposed time and time again; many of them have been tried—are being tried—if often halfheartedly. No one really knows what a "total push" social reform of this kind might accomplish. It would be certain to receive the denunciation of politicians and hardheaded "realists" who consider such measures luxuries to be earned by the public "if it *really* wants them" but certainly not to be providently cast before—well, not swine but "unappreciative masses." The objectors have a point; if the masses are unappreciative, if the individuals *in* the mass cannot do their part in obtaining such bonanzas, these well-intended provisions become just that—bonanzas. They do not prevent mental ill health; they further it.

On the other hand, whenever I hear economic Tories raising this point in the course of a debate on the promotion of mental health, I am reminded of the intransigent British Parliament which in one century lost the American colonies through dogged adherence to a legal principle, and in the following century let the doctrine of *laissez faire* hypnotize them into contributing to the death by starving of two million of their citizens in Ireland, lest by governmental intervention they break the economic principle and save some lives.[2]

We have daily cause to remember that even in this best and certainly most prosperous of all countries, in this best or at least best-known of all possible worlds, there is too much sorrow and too much suffering, there is too much evidence of personal and social disorganization, there is too much mental ill health. The crime rate increases steadily; vandalism spreads; suicides multiply; neighborhoods decay; hospitals remain crowded; unemployment, strikes and other labor difficulties bespeak unrest and frustration in employment and industry. Science suggests this need not be.

An old Talmudic version of the Golden Rule reads "Love thy neighbor, he *is* thyself." We must try to protect our neighbor to protect ourselves; we must endeavor to prevent his mental illness, and our own. Too many of our neighbors still need food, a few clothes, a few hours of rest from exhausting labor. But along with sustenance and garments and shelter—indeed, to learn to share these necessities of life—we must find better techniques for living together, and for living closer together, as we are going to have to. We must find better ways of joining together in mutual satisfactions and for mutual benefit, while yet retaining our individuality, our personal identity, and our inescapable personal responsibility.

We must discover better methods of controlling dangerous impulses, both within ourselves and in some other drivers whose brakes are defective. Our innate aggressiveness and destructiveness have been so infinitely multiplied in power and potential consequence by recent physical and chemical discoveries that their control has become the most important problem in the world. All of us now living are threatened, constantly and imminently.

If these things that we have been saying were known to all teachers, would our schoolrooms improve? If they were known to all school-board members, would our teachers improve? If they were known to all employers, would work losses recede and profits rise? If they were known to labor leaders, would work satisfaction increase and industrial strife diminish? If they were known to clergymen, would religion move into new roles of importance and meaning? Would this be an effective approach to prevention?

No one has shown conclusively that good results would follow. This is a faith of ours rather than proved knowledge. But we have seen many small demonstrations in The Menninger Foundation, during seminar courses to industrialists, clergymen, and physicians. We see in many of these groups the surprising phenomenon of a sudden lifting of horizons, an enlightenment, an "improvement" in the mental health of people who weren't sick! The meaning of human life, of all human behavior, of "sickness" and "health" may suddenly change.

"We have gained a new concept of man!" exclaimed two clergymen near the end of one such session. "A changed concept of man requires a changed concept of God; and if of God, then of all our world, too." Many industrialists and executives have expressed similar sentiments in other words. This is more than a simple "learning experience" (although it is *that*, too). It is an internal reorganization resulting from a shaking up, a new insight, even a bit of travail and perplexity, but it enables further advance.

And what does psychiatry offer toward the alleviation of the dreadful predicament? Should we be hesitant to contribute to world thinking what we know of human nature? Is one of our colleagues wrong to suggest that perhaps it is "not an extravagant speculation that mental hospitals will be a nucleus of future progress in man's understanding of man, for they are natural centers for study and research in human relations and will not be overlooked indefinitely"? [3]

We psychiatrists are familiar with this in another setting, that of clinical practice. Not infrequently we observe that a patient who is in a phase of recovery from what may have been a rather long illness shows continued improvement, past the point of his former "normal" state of existence. He not only gets well, to use the vernacular; he gets as well as he was, and then he continues to improve still further. He increases his productivity, he expands his life and its horizons. He develops new talents, new powers, new effectiveness. He becomes, one might say, "weller than well."

Weller than Well

Of course this doesn't always happen, nor does it happen often enough. But that it happens at all—and every experienced psychiatrist has seen it—this fact should alert us to latent possibilities, just as the bobbing lid of his mother's teakettle caught Watt's attention and curiosity. What could it mean? It violates our conventional medical expectations, so perhaps it is often overlooked and occurs more often than we know. It may contain a clue for both better prevention and better treatment.

Abraham Lincoln is a famous example of this. Many people do not know of his several attacks of severe mental illness. His law partner, Stuart, described him as a "hopeless victim of melancholy." His future wife's relatives considered him "insane." [4] According to one version, on his wedding day all preparations were in order and the guests assembled, but Lincoln didn't appear. He was found in his room in deep dejection, obsessed with ideas of unworthiness, hopelessness, and guilt.

Prior to his illness Lincoln was an honest but undistinguished lawyer whose failures were more conspicuous than his successes. This was when he was considered well—*before* his mental illness made its appearance. What he became and achieved *after* his illness is part of our great national heritage.

John Stuart Mill, to take a less well-known example, suffered an attack of mental illness in 1826, when he was twenty years old, in which he was obsessed with the thought that even if he could have everything he wanted he would still not be happy. "Although 'suicidal' for many months," writes Szasz, "[Mill] 'recovered' from this turmoil, which some might call a 'depression,' and underwent a process of profound personality reorganization. There is no way of telling how Mill managed to reorganize himself, nor was this apparently clear to him. But of the result, he could inform us." [5]

Mill wrote: "The experiences of this period had two very marked effects on my opinions and character. In the first place, they led me to adopt a theory of life, very unlike that on which I had before acted, and having much in common with what at that time I certainly had never heard of, the anti-self-consciousness theory of Carlyle. I never, indeed, wavered in the conviction that happiness is the test of all rules of conduct, and the end of life. But I now thought that this end was only to be attained by not making it the direct end. Those only are happy (I thought) who have their minds fixed on some object other than their own happiness; on the happiness of others, on the improvement of mankind, even on some art or pursuit, followed not as a means, but as itself an ideal end. Aiming thus at something else, they find happiness by the way." [6] *

Another example, most poignant to physicians, psychiatrists, psychologists, is none other than William James, who also became a great man only after he had been a very sick man. He was described as physically frail at nineteen; at twenty-three he had many presumably psychosomatic

---

* Mill went on: "The enjoyments of life (such was not my theory) are sufficient to make it a pleasant thing, when they are taken *en passant*, without being made a principal object. Once make them so, and they are immediately felt to be insufficient. They will not bear a scrutinizing examination. Ask yourself whether you are happy, and you cease to be so. The only chance is to treat, not happiness, but some end external to it, as the purpose of life. Let your self-consciousness, your scrutiny, your self-interrogation, exhaust themselves on that; and if otherwise fortunately circumstanced you will inhale happiness with the air you breathe, without dwelling on it or thinking about it, without either forestalling it in imagination, or putting it to flight by fatal questioning. This theory now becomes the basis of my philosophy of life. And I still hold to it as the best theory for all those who have but a moderate degree of sensibility and of capacity for enjoyment; that is, for the great majority of mankind."

symptoms (eyes and stomach); at twenty-five he dropped his medical studies because of his health and took many treatments in Europe. He was depressed and entertained suicidal thoughts. "He awoke every morning with a horrible dread. For months he was unable to go into the dark alone . . . he wondered how other people could live so unconscious of the 'pit of insecurity beneath the surface of life.'"

"The world owes a great deal to these personal misfortunes," wrote Norman Cameron. "James was thrown heavily upon his own resources; his incapacities and frustrations at such a time gave him an intense and intimate appreciation of the deepest philosophical and religious problems; his illness clearly 'developed and deepened the bed in which the stream of his philosophic life was to flow.'" [7]

This is a man who thereafter became one of the greatest scientists who has ever lived, certainly the greatest psychologist and perhaps the greatest philosopher that America has produced. He transcended his illness to become "weller than well."

Many other examples could be given. Indeed, from friends who heard us discuss this have come numerous suggestions, records, and illustrative biographies; especially from my friend Rudolph Treuenfels. Max Weber had written a few minor books prior to a severe depression at fifty, from which he emerged to write his masterpiece, *The Protestant Ethic and the Spirit of Capitalism*. Conrad Ferdinand Meyer was a Swiss poet whose best work followed an illness, according to one authority. Ignatius Loyola is believed by some to have experienced a severe mental illness between his undistinguished military career and his subsequent very distinguished religious period.

Transcendence of illness is something the public does not ordinarily envision. In his goodheartedness the man of the street is glad to be told that someone with a mental illness is being properly cared for or is, perhaps, even getting better. He reads with pleasure in his local newspaper that "the friends of John Smith will be happy to learn that the hospital doctors report him to be improving and he will be glad to receive letters." He may even declare with confidence that he believes that old John Smith may yet get back on the job and be just about as good as ever. But it is still hard for him to believe that people like John Smith can ever really "be the same again" or be free from the suspicion of lurking susceptibility to irrationality. This uninformed attitude leads to a cruel stigmatization which is diminishing, but which is still present in the minds of too many good people. And as for the illness experience representing a growth, a blessing, a gateway, so to speak, into a life of greater mental healthiness—this seems almost inconceivable.

The authors of this book hope for nothing more than that mental illness and recovery may be seen in this wider, deeper view. Please believe that from a total of seventy years of work with psychiatric patients we are not unaware that some do not get as well as we would wish, that some long remain susceptible to losses of equilibrium and temporary recessions. We well know how difficult it is, sometimes, for sufferers to get well —even with all the help that we can muster. But we also know that transcendence does occur. And perhaps it is not an exception but a natural consequence of new insights and new concepts of treatment!

Transcendence might happen oftener if we could more frankly acknowledge the possibility of its occurrence, expect it, and hope for it, even though we are bound to be often disappointed. Doctors occasionally see indisputable evidences of it even in medical conditions. People who have tuberculosis in younger life often become very healthy and resistant to all infections subsequently. The famous world-record miler, Glenn Cunningham, suffered as a child from burns on both legs so severe that it was predicted he would never recover sufficiently even to walk.*

No one who saw Helen Keller at the age of six could have guessed what she was to become at sixteen, or be at sixty (and eighty-three). The little college in Kansas which turned down the application of George Washington Carver had no inkling of the genius contained in the humble, shabby Negro boy, or it might have stretched its snobbish admission rules; when Christy Brown's mother observed her speechless, spastic child drawing in the dust of the floor with his toe, not even she could imagine that the little "imbecile" would become an author and an artist. These examples may be trite and well known to many, but the reader can be certain that there are thousands of unknown examples who have not been discovered or who have not yet written about their experiences.**

---

* But doctors are apt to look upon these as exceptions. A recent book of radio talks by a doctor whom I do not know concerns itself with "high-level wellness," an exhortation for "maximizing the potential of which the individual is capable, within the environment where he is functioning." Surely there is nothing wrong with this aspiration, but doctors will be suspicious if not supercilious. (Dunn, Halbert L. *High Level Wellness*. Arlington, Va.: R. W. Beatty Co., 1962.)
** But many have. I would especially commend *Very Much Alive* by Terry McAdam, *Greet the Man* by Harold Wilke, *My Left Foot* by Christy Brown, *Born That Way* by Earl R. Carlson, *If a Man Be Mad*, by Harold Maine, and *None So Blind* by Bernice Clifton. In *Minds That Came Back* (New York: Lippincott,

This chapter, written to recapitulate and round off the message of the book, may now itself need recapitulating. It can all be said to be an answer to the question put earlier, What difference does it make?

What difference does it make how we see psychiatry? Are we better off in viewing mental illness not in the old ways but as a process, as an episode of disequilibration, a degree of temporary disorganization in a life course? What difference does it make if, instead of carefully fitting these conditions with proper names and classifying them in lists of diseases, we think of them as representing one kind of human vicissitude to which we are all subject and for which some of us stand by to offer first aid in emergencies?

It makes the difference, we propose, that the new view justifies hope; an attitude of hopefulness in turn favorably affects the unfavorable condition.

This is a point of view in psychiatry which has rapidly grown along with the rapid growth of psychiatry itself in scope and in popularity. People rush for help. With and without adequate diagnosis, they are receiving many treatments and many cures, which is what one would expect. We have even begun to speak earnestly of prevention—not only to speak of it, which has often been done before, but to relate it to sociological and educational and recreational programs as a new justification for these latter. And, we have said, perhaps education, education as to the very facts we have reviewed in this book, is itself the most potent preventive measure.

What we cannot prevent we must deal with, especially the extreme and disabling attacks of mental illness which are so costly to the individual and to those about him. For these we should provide first of all accurate diagnosis, not a synthetic name for the pathology but an analysis of the factors which have combined to produce it, the internal factors and the external factors. Such a diagnosis permits us to recommend treatment measures likely to be effective.

Being realistic, we know that in spite of the best diagnosis and the best treatment some patients will not recover. This is a minority, but of all people we psychiatrists should be the last to ignore a minority. And there are some who in spite of everything will continue to need our sympathy, our patience, and our help in the hope that some vestige of inner

---

1961), Dr. Walter Alvarez has collected data on seventy-five recovered patients, some of whom illustrate our point, and in an appendix lists annotated autobiographies by many people—"cripples," "paranoiacs," "epileptics," alcoholics, drug addicts, sexual deviants, tramps, prisoners, blind-deaf people, lepers, and others.

strength will sustain them in their necessity for brave, but tortured, endurance.

Meanwhile, most of us will be dealing more promptly with our own bouts of mental illness, or getting effective help if we need it. Life resumed goes on as before, almost as well as before, sometimes even better.

But, of course, illness is not the *only* way to learn. The aspiration to improve oneself, to become "weller than well," to reach out constantly toward a more nearly perfect way of life—is this the virtue and the blessing of only a few fortunate ones? Is it given only to geniuses, or is it something latent in all of us, too easily stifled? If one reflects on the one hand how opportunities are daily discarded by millions in favor of escapism, intoxication, and chronic suicide, one tends to answer the question one way; when one observes, on the other hand, the unswerving efforts to obtain an education, acquire knowledge, improve character, and better the world in many ways, which are demonstrated by many an illustrious example, and by many unknown heroes and heroines,[8] one tends to answer the question another way.

Benjamin Franklin, that great American genius, inventor, thinker, and statesman, worked conscientiously and systematically all his life toward enhancing his mental health, toward becoming weller than well. As he later recorded it, he early

> conceived the arduous project of arrival at moral perfection. . . . But I soon found I had undertaken a task of more difficulty than I had imagined. While my care was employ'd in guarding against one fault, I was often surprised by another; habit took the advantage of inattention; inclination was sometimes too strong for reason. I concluded, at length, that the mere speculative conviction that it was our interest to be completely virtuous, was not sufficient to prevent our slipping; and that the contrary habit must be broken, and good ones acquired and established, before we can have any dependence on a steady, uniform rectitude of conduct. For this purpose I therefore contriv'd the following method. . . . I made a little book, in which I allotted a page for each of the virtues. I rul'd each page with red ink, so as to have seven columns, one for each day of the week, marking each column with a letter for the day. I cross'd these columns with thirteen red lines, marking the beginning of each line with the first letter of one of the virtues, on which line, and in its proper column, I might mark, by a little black spot, every fault I found upon examination to have been committed respecting that virtue upon that day.

The thirteen virtues Franklin listed were: Temperance, Silence, Order, Resolution, Frugality, Industry, Sincerity, Justice, Moderation, Cleanliness, Tranquillity, Chastity, and Humility. He determined to give a week's strict attention to each of the virtues successively, going "thro' a course in thirteen weeks, and four courses in a year."

I was surpris'd [he wrote] to find myself so much fuller of faults than I had imagined; but I had the satisfaction of seeing them diminish . . . After a while I went thro' one course only in a year, and afterward only one in several years . . . but I always carried my little book with me.

Something that pretended to be reason, was every now and then suggesting to me that such extreme nicety as I exacted of myself might be a kind of foppery in morals, which, if it were known, would make me ridiculous; that a perfect character might be attended with the inconvenience of being envied and hated; and that a benevolent man should allow a few faults in himself, to keep his friends in countenance.

. . . But, on the whole, tho' I never arrived at the perfection I had been so ambitious of obtaining, but fell far short of it, yet I was, by the endeavour, a better and a happier man that I otherwise should have been if I had not attempted it; . . .

It may be well my posterity should be informed that to this little artifice, with the blessing of God, their ancestor ow'd the constant felicity of his life, down to his 79th year, in which this is written.[9]

There are no doubt many colleagues who will see in such self-correction and programming not so much a "foppery in morals" as something psychopathological for which, no doubt, an impressive psychiatric designation can be found: compulsivity, narcissism, masochism. These words do not well describe, in my opinion; and they surely do not condemn. The self-discipline and aspiration of that magnificent character stand out resplendently. Not only was he the "better and happier man" for his pains, but so may thousands of others be who catch the inspiration for self-improvement and self-realization, and who possess the humility to work at it and think about it, "alert with noble discontent" down to their seventy-ninth year!

Doctors have traditionally concentrated upon pathology to the neglect of potentialities and assets to be exploited. Conceiving it to be the doctor's first business to relieve the patient's pain, align his broken bones, prescribe a cathartic, psychiatrists have too much followed this medical tradition. But mental health and its achievement must include *in the doctor* a vision of continued growth, the continuing discovery and realization of new potentialities.

"The potentialities of development in human souls," wrote William James sixty years ago, "are unfathomable. So many who seemed irretrievably hardened have in point of fact been softened, converted, regenerated, in ways that amazed the subjects even more than they surprised the spectators, that we can never be sure in advance of any man that his salvation by way of love is hopeless. We have no right to speak of human crocodiles and boa-constrictors as of fixedly incurable things. We know not the complexities of personality, the smouldering emotional fires, the other facets of the character-polyhedron, the resources of the subliminal region." [10]

Transcendence of illness is not only an individual goal, but it may be seen as a collective striving as well, the thrust of human evolution. Our colleague, Gardner Murphy, puts it this way:

> Human potentialities are given by the action of that which sleeps within us upon the unformed potentialities of the world. . . . We are provided with a complex set of organic equipment, and if it is not allowed to function, something happens to us, just as in using it we find joy. If we have tissues within us which through learning and thinking develop and enrich us, we shall in the same way find joy both in the new and in the old activities and in the process of learning and thinking. If thinking becomes a group-supported activity, we may, like the Athenians, foregather just to think, as the Icelanders foregather to play chess, or the Germans to make music. In the long run, the use of the brain, if not pre-empted entirely by the sheer process of keeping alive or keeping up with the Joneses, leads, over the centuries, to more and more exquisite cultural products. Those, according to my thesis, which supervene after ten generations of cumulative thought are just as directly and fundamentally an expression of human nature as breathing or eating. Because man has this rich potentiality for sensory, motor, intellectual experience, and has to combine all this in fresh acts of cultural creativeness, he is doing nothing more than realizing these potentialities when he writes *Macbeth* or flies a plane at Kitty Hawk. And it is not only human to invent oneself out of one world into another; it is also human to keep moving toward a destination which is not set within man's present nature but keeps changing as the nature of his environment changes. The bio-cultural reality keeps rolling up on itself.[11]

With the message of these magnificent words we draw our book to a close. We have covered a variety of themes and we have used many words and many pages to do so. But through them all has run this thread; implicit in the eloquence of William James and Ernest Southard and Gardner Murphy, it is a message which can also be put in more prosaic terms; it can even be conveyed in the language of gesture and feeling, without words. It is the assertion of hope, of faith in every individual's potential for growth and development and self-transcendence. It is a declaration of love for and of belief in one's fellow creatures.

In one form or another, each of the authors has tried to say some of these things before. This message was implicit, for example, when Martin Mayman wrote some years ago:

> Inner unrest, even turmoil, need not signify only illness, it may often signal incipient change for the better. Not all disequilibria are unhealthy; instability may indicate a condition still in flux whose direction of change may remain uncertain until a new integration is reached. Even in relatively

healthy persons there will be periods or circumstances in which positive striving may be mistaken for wasteful inner strife.

Certainly, unrest holds out at least the prospect of a change for the better, unlike the stagnation which often characterizes those patients who seem to have settled into a state of illness, who almost recoil from the prospect of change, who live their lives almost as if they were keeping themselves in a kind of protective custody, carefully putting off situations which might open up new experiences and new growth. A relatively healthy ego often welcomes (even invites) disturbance in its equilibrium; people seek stimulation and challenge, as recent experiments have shown.[12]

It was this same thought which Paul Pruyser had in mind when, tongue in cheek, he asked, "Is mental health possible?" and then answered the question by suggesting that

> mental health should be seen not as a state of rest nor as homeostatic return to a previous condition, but as a realization of values which can only be achieved through becoming as opposed to "being." Earlier we spoke of "heterostasis" and indicated how strained the traditional language of science becomes when it tries to deal with goals, strivings, purposes, expectations and the realization of potentialities. Yet we cannot evade the issue that, psychologically speaking, living is worth its cost only when it entails progressive order, increased awareness of the complexities of reality, deepened wisdom and enlarged experience. And these, we submit, may well be the product of the suffering and temporary defeat represented by a phase of illness.[13]

And it is a message which the third author of the trio would offer as his *l'envoi*, in words employed a few years ago to describe a patient's frame of mind at the termination of treatment:

> . . . Although it is true that his expectations were not met, his gains were *beyond* his expectations! He had learned to live, to love and to live, to love and to be loved and therein to live. This was his great gain.
>
> Learning this simple thing, and recognizing it to be a universal principle, of which his own personal experience is but an example, represents a beginning constructive identification of himself with the universe, with reality, with other people. No one ever gets as much love as he wants, no one gives as much love as he might. Choices can be made but choice involves the assumption of responsibility and the necessity for renunciation. But life is for living and this he has gained the courage to accept.[14]

The three of us, too, subscribe to those great lines of William James: "*Will you or won't you* have it so? is the most probing question we are ever asked. We are asked it every hour of the day, and about the largest as well as the smallest, the most theoretical as well as the most practical things. We answer by *consents* or *non-consents* and not by words. What wonder that these dumb responses should seem our deepest organs of communication with the nature of things! What wonder if the effort demanded by them be the measure of our worth as men!" [15]

It is this philosophy, this view of human life, and this understanding of mental illness and psychiatry which we want most to leave with our readers—those who know about mental illness, those who think they know nothing about it, those who have experienced and recovered from it, and those who are perhaps at this moment passing through the valley of the shadow.

We would especially impart this viewpoint to those distressed regarding a friend or relative. It is a frightening and heartbreaking experience to see the "alienation" of one we thought we knew, and it is perhaps natural to fear the worst. This horror, mixed with sorrow, anger, and guilt feelings, may be involuntary and irresistible—for a moment. But an informed intelligence, while soft-voiced, as Freud remarked, is fortunately persistent. For even though we grant the contradictory and presently inexplicable fact of cancer, and the less dramatic but no less malignant nature of some other afflictions, we do not recede from our position that the mentally ill usually recover. Mental illness is a curable condition and the mentally ill *can* be cured. The hopeless patient is a myth.

In the past ten years my brother, Doctor Will, has spoken earnestly to the legislatures of many states—Oklahoma, Ohio, Pennsylvania, Kentucky, Michigan, California, Iowa, Minnesota, Oregon, Tennessee, Texas, Wyoming, Maryland, West Virginia, North Dakota, Colorado, Alabama, Arizona, Vermont, Washington, and South Carolina. The legislators have listened attentively; they have risen to acclaim his words. In many instances they have acted upon them.

What has he told these legislators? Simply that mental illness is our pre-eminent health problem in America, that the mentally ill can be helped, that most of them can be cured, that it is less expensive and more humane to treat them scientifically than to confine them despairingly. The percentage of people helped and the rapidity of their recovery are directly proportionate to the extent to which modern concepts of psychiatric treatment are entertained and applied. This has been re-demonstrated in the Topeka Veterans Administration Hospital and the Topeka State Hospital for the past twenty years.*

This is the "news" my brother has taken to legislators and others. He has not been alone in spreading this gospel; it has other eloquent spokes-

---

* This demonstration began before introduction of ataractic drugs.

men. Yet over 80 per cent of the state hospitals of our country still fail to offer any treatment at all to the patients assigned to them and confined in them! *

This is hard for us to understand. It is hard to understand how Massachusetts in 1850 and scores of other states since then could have let a magnificent demonstration like that of Woodward, Todd, Brigham, Bell, Butler, Ray, Stedman, and Kirkbride sink into oblivion and desuetude while thousands of patients who undoubtedly could have been cured dragged out their weary lives in the dismal wards of state hospitals. Many still do.

Why is the public so willing to retain its pessimism and cling to the ancient superstition that mental illness is incurable? Why does not every heartbroken father whose son's career has been suddenly interrupted by mental illness, or every grieving mother, every saddened wife—why do not these dear relatives (and their name is legion) join together to move mountains, if necessary, in order to insure help for their loved ones?

Do people inwardly believe, still, that the mentally ill are damned and that is the end of it? Is this the negative of William James' "will to believe," a will *not* to believe? Is this incredulity born of an innate pessimism or of a fear of seeming gullible? Or is it perchance a refusal to take the responsibility which acceptance of the facts implies?

For we *can* help them. We *must* help them. They need help—that is what their illness means, no matter how disguised. It is a cry for our assistance, and we must know how to answer. We cannot plead ignorance, for we know how to do it. It is not our helplessness that has deterred us so long, but our hopelessness.

The injunction of Isaiah to "Comfort my people" rests heavily upon psychiatrists. For they must point the way, not yielding to the discouragement of asking, "Who hath believed our report?" Because *we* know that, depending upon how the particular mental illness is understood and reacted to—by the patient and by the relatives and by the community and *by the medical profession*—the future may be brighter than anything the past has held.

Where there is life there is, usually, hope. Earlier we considered giving this book the title *Where There Is Life*. But we felt that in one sense the implication was misleading; it was as if to say that *only while* there

---

* These are the figures of the study of the Joint Commission on Mental Illness and Health (1961).

is life is there hope, that hope is sustained by life. Our point is rather that life is sustained by hope—that where there is hope there is life!

Life is more than permutations in the DNA molecule as the Fifth Symphony is more than vibrating air. And mental illness is more than an aggregate of errors in body physics and chemistry. It is a universal human experience which has a salvage function in maintaining the vital balance.

APPENDIX:

Attest and Exhibits

DON'T GO, PLEASE. We have something yet to show you. It is a collection of precious documents, a review of the psychiatric nosologies of all times. Each of them represents the labors of a lifetime—the dedicated, loving efforts of a scientist, or even a whole school of them, to record what he saw and believed.

Gaze kindly upon them, dear reader; they are a noble heritage. From them grew the concepts of today. Leaf the pages and observe for yourself what the trend has been. These are not mere words arranged in columns; these are thoughts; these are views of mental illness projected by our predecessors. Each had its day, its friends, its users. Each received from those that preceded, and contributed to those that followed. In this way our science has developed.

Psychiatric nosology has often been a matter of mere listing or classification. Genera, species, types, and specific entities have been identified and described, sometimes with enormous elaborateness. From simple beginnings there have been eras of tremendous expansion, with the inclusion of many entities, and—as now—eras of return to greater simplicity, approaching our unitary concept of mental illness.

Over the course of five thousand years, two or three "entities" grew into hundreds and then thousands of mental illnesses. With the development of the modern scientific era the parabolic curve describing the number of recognized mental illnesses began to swing back again toward the baseline. The thousands became hundreds, then scores, then dozens. From almost infinity the number of recognized entities became progressively smaller, approaching unity as a limit. That is why we originally proposed to call this book "The Return to the Unitary Concept of Mental Illness."

But what does all this mean? Merely that by trying to name things and parts of things much was learned of certain aspects of mental illness. But as we came to better understanding of its nature we have been able to discard most of the fictions which we have used during the long reaches of more incomplete knowledge.

I. PRIMITIVE PSYCHIATRIC
CLASSIFICATIONS

2600 B.C.–500 B.C.

Our immediate ancestors were human beings like ourselves, with nerves and brains like ours, desires and disappointments like ours. They, too, became partially disorganized under stress and sought medical help. It is not surprising therefore that scattered through ancient records one finds descriptions of behavior corresponding in an identifiable way with clinical syndromes still seen today. Sumerian and Egyptian references to what we would call melancholia and hysteria, using these as syndrome designations, are found as far back as 2600 B.C. In the famous Ebers papyrus (1500 B.C.) senile deterioration and alcoholism are also described. The very first definite syndrome description medical historians believe to have been that of mental illness associated with senile deterioration, ascribed to Prince Ptah-hotep (*circa* 3000 B.C.).[1]

An attempt to classify mental-illness pictures—perhaps the first and at least the oldest one now known—is to be found in the Ayur-Veda (1400 B.C.), a system of medicine of ancient India. The groupings were made on the basis of seven kinds of demoniacal possession. It was believed that the enraged spirits of devils, giants, gods, or dead men entered into the person, producing the various forms of mental illness.

The philosophical formulations of the ancient Hindu literature, notably the writings of Charaka and Susruta, show clearly a tendency to link psychology with philosophy and religion, a trend which has been a great obstacle to the development of psychology and psychiatry as sciences. Susruta, whose dates are uncertain, but who may have lived about a hundred years before Hippocrates, injected an amazingly modern tone into the mystical harmony of these philosophical systems; he believed that strong emotions not only might produce mental disorders but might even be responsible for certain conditions requiring surgery.

II. Ancient Greek and Roman Classifications

460 B.C.

Hippocrates (about 460–377 B.C.) is usually credited with introducing psychiatric problems into the domain of medicine. Under his name we possess a number of writings [2] surviving from ancient Greek medicine. Collecting the names ascribed to mental illness described or mentioned in these writings, we get the following list:

1. Phrenitis (acute mental disturbance *with* fever)
2. Mania (acute mental disturbance *without* fever)
3. Melancholia (all kinds of chronic mental disturbances)
4. Epilepsy
5. Hysteria (paroxysmic dyspnea, pain, convulsions)
6. Scythian disease

Among these conditions, only one (epilepsy) retains today the same name and meaning. Hippocratic concepts of *mania* and *melancholia* were much broader and vaguer than what we call by those names. *Hysteria* described a variety of paroxysmic conditions seen in women. An interesting description of the "Scythian disease" identifies it as comparable to what is now called "transvestism," then occurring in the setting of a particular culture (somewhat like the "berdaches" among North American Indians).

Plato was a contemporary of Hippocrates and was, like most Greek philos-ophers, deeply interested in medicine. His interesting discussion of the forms of "madness" (*mania*) in the *Phaedrus* seems to be a legacy from priestly medicine.[3] Plato distinguishes a "madness given us by divine gift," and another which is the consequence of physical disease. The first includes the four varieties of prophetic, religious, poetic, and erotic inspiration. We can summarize the whole in this way:

I. Divine Madness
    1. Prophetic Madness (given by Apollo)
    2. Religious Madness, or Enthusiasmus (given by Dionysus)
    3. Poetic Madness (inspired by the Muses)
    4. Erotic Madness (inspired by Aphrodite and Eros)
II. Natural Madness, originating in physical diseases

These or similar distinctions were later incorporated in many of the psy-chiatric classifications up to the seventeenth and eighteenth centuries.

100 A.D.

Among the few ancient medical authors whose works have survived, A. Cor-nelius Celsus, who lived in the first century A.D., is of particular interest. In his treatise *De Medicina*,[4] diseases are described briefly but clearly in Latin, in the systematic order *a capite ad calcem* (from head to heels). Among diseases of the head, mental diseases are enumerated in the following order:

    1. Phrenesis (i.e., the Phrenitis of Hippocrates)
    2. Melancholia (a long-lasting depression caused by black bile)
    3. "A third kind of disease" (probably mania, but not named by Celsus. Two forms: with and without hallucinations)
    4. Delirium *ex metu* (delirium caused by fright)
    5. Cardiacum
    6. Lethargus (acute, dangerous illness with insurmountable need to sleep)

Epilepsy is described in a separate chapter as *morbus mitialis*, and hysteria is listed with the diseases of the womb.

Aretaeus, "The Incomparable," of Cappadox toward the end of the first century offered a somewhat more elaborate classification.

    1. Epilepsy ("ordinary" and "hysterical")
    2. Melancholia
    3. Mania of three types (ordinary, recurrent, and "divine")
    4. Delirium due to alcohol or drugs
    5. Senile dementia
    6. Secondary dementia

Not quite a century later, Galen (129–199 A.D.) extended the list, although he did not offer a systematic classification of mental diseases. Throughout his extant works [5] we find descriptions of a number of clinical conditions, which can be arranged in the following four groups:

    I. Humoral-pathological types: Melancholia with its manifold manifes-tations

II. Psycho-pathological types: Anoia, Moria, Paraphrosyne
III. Anatomo-pathological types: Phrenitis, Hysteria, Cardiacum
IV. Clinical types: Epilepsy, Catalepsy, Lethargy, Apoplexy, Carus

To this last group must be added malingering, on which Galen wrote a treatise; among simulated disease he mentioned feigned delirium. His is the oldest known description written from the medical point of view.

375 A.D.

During the decline of the Roman Empire, a few original minds accomplished some good works. Among them was Posidonius, a physician of the second half of the fourth century A.D. His works are lost, but since they served as a rich mine for later compilers, we are able to reconstruct the outline of his psychiatric nosology,[6] which included:

1. Phrenitis (acute meningitis)
2. Carus (sleeping-sickness)
3. Coma
4. Lethargus
5. Skotomatikon (vertigo)
6. Ephialtos (Incubus, or nightmare)
7. Epilepsy
8. Melancholia, with several subforms
9. Mania
10. Hydrophobon, *alias* Lyssa (rabies)

In the early Byzantine Empire, Alexander of Tralles (sixth century) was the most famous physician of his time. His textbook,[7] describing diseases with little regard for theoretical speculations and strong emphasis on therapeutics, mentions among diseases of the head the following:

1. Headaches, with three kinds:
   a. Cephalalgia (acute headache)
   b. Cephaleia (repeated headaches)
   c. Hemicrania
2. Phrenitis
3. Lethargus
4. Epilepsy, with three subforms:
   a. from the stomach
   b. from other parts of the body, in children
   c. from the head, in infants
5. "Paresis" (i.e., partial, incomplete paralysis)
6. Melancholia, with the following subforms:
   a. from excess of blood in the whole body
   b. from excess of blood in the head
   c. from yellow bile (patient angry, agitated)
   d. from black bile (patient sad, fearful, with delusional ideas)

Mention should also be made of the works of Caelius Aurelianus,[8] which probably date from the fifth century. Aurelianus was a member of the Methodist group of physicians and translated into Latin some of the works of Soranus of Ephesus. From his Latin versions of Soranus's treatises on acute diseases and chronic diseases the following psychiatric conditions are selected:

1. Phrenitis (an acute mental derangement accompanied by acute fever)
2. Lethargy (a state of torpor, stupor, and impaired or dull senses)

3. Satyriasis (an acute state of strong sexual desire with mental aberration, often produced by drugs)
4. Incubus (a state of continual nightmares)
5. Epilepsy (in the form of either coma or convulsions)
6. Mania (a chronic impairment of reason without fever consisting of anger, merriment, sadness, futility, fear)
7. Melancholy (mental anguish and distress with dejection, silence, animosity, longing for death, suspicion, weeping)
8. Homosexuality (seen as an affliction of a diseased mind, in both males and females)

625–700 A.D.

One of the last of the famous ancient physicians was Paul of Aegina (625–700 A.D.). His classification [9] is rather an uncritical enumeration of psychiatric disorders:

1. Headaches, with three subforms:
   a. Cephalalgia (acute headaches)
   b. Cephaleia (chronic headaches)
   c. Hemicrania
2. Phrenitis
3. Phlegmon of the brain
4. Erysipelas of the brain
5. Lethargy
6. Carus
7. Catochus, or coma vigil, catoche, catalepsy
8. Oblivion (amnesia)
9. Fatuity (loss of reason and memory)
10. Vertigo
11. Epilepsy
12. Melancholia, with three subforms:
    a. Brain melancholia
    b. Melancholia from sympathy with the general system
    c. Hypochrondriac melancholia
13. Mania
14. Demonomania (patients believed to be possessed by evil spirits)
15. Incubus (or nightmare)
16. Lycanthropy
17. Love-sickness
18. Apoplexia
19. Convulsions or spasms
20. Tetanus
21. Tremblings
22. Hysterical convulsions (or uterine suffocation)

One can see how, in the course of ten centuries, from Hippocrates to Galen and from Galen to Paul of Aegina, the number of psychiatric "diseases" had increased and become increasingly differentiated.

III. Psychiatric Classifications in the Middle Ages

864–925 A.D.

After the ruin of the ancient world, medicine flourished throughout the Islamic countries. Among the outstanding Arabic physicians, two deserve mention here.

Rhazes (864–925 A.D.), the great Persian physician distinguished in all fields of medicine and surgery, wrote among many treatises a brief one recently translated into English under the title *The Spiritual Physick of Rhazes*.[10] The author takes for granted the classical Aristotelian division of human psyche into "three souls": the vegetative, animal (or "choleric"), and rational. On this distinction he bases a summary classification of psychopathological disorders according to the "failure" or "excess" in each one of the three souls; hence, the following:

	FAILURE	EXCESS
Vegetative soul	Lack in nutrition, growth	Search for pleasure, lust
Animal soul	Lack of fervor, pride, courage	Arrogance, will to dominate
Rational soul	Lack of curiosity, interest	Excessive quest, "melancholia"

In another chapter of the same book Rhazes discusses *drunkenness*, a topic surprisingly neglected in extant Greek medical books. Rhazes speaks not only of the effects of drinking but of its psychological motivations: to dispel anxiety, to meet situations requiring particular courage and cheerfulness.

980–1037 A.D.

Avicenna (980–1037 A.D.), a Persian poet, philosopher, and physician, was the author of the *Canon of Medicine*, probably the most successful book in medical literature. It was used as a medical textbook for centuries in the Islamic as well as in the Western European world. The *Canon* gives a methodical exposition of the highly artificial system elaborated by Galen. The diseases are described in the order *a capite ad calcem*. Mental diseases are therefore included in the chapter on diseases of the head, in the following order: [11]

1. Phrenitis (action of yellow bile on meningies or brain)
2. Lethargus (action of phlegma in the same regions)
3. Coma vigil (mixture of yellow bile and phlegma in the same regions)
4. Delirium or Insania with several subforms, according to the humor (black bile, yellow bile, red bile, or putrefied phlegma)
5. Fatuitas (feeble-mindedness due to a lesion in the middle ventricle)
6. Amentia (due to a lesion of the middle ventricle)
7. Oblivio (loss of memory, due to lesion of posterior ventricle)
8. Hallucinations (or apprehensionis vitium) (lesion of anterior ventricle)
9. Mania (fury), with as a subform the mania canina (the patient is aggressive, but submissive as a dog)
10. Melancholia (due to black bile)
11. Lycanthropy (delusion of being transformed into a wolf, occurring in February)
12. Lovesickness (amor insanus, can be diagnosed by the pulse)
13. Ephialtos (alias incubus or nightmare)
14. Mollities (passive male homosexuality)
15. Hydrophobia

It is easy to see that almost all these disease entities are a mixture taken from Galen and his Greek successors, with concepts based variously on pathological anatomy (phrenitis), or on psychopathology (fatuitas, amentia, oblivio, hallucinations), or on humoral pathology (melancholia), or on clinical pictures (delirium, mania, lycanthropy, lovesickness, hydrophobia). Notable is the introduction of sexual pathology in the psychiatric nosology (possibly under the influence of the Hippocratic description of the "Scythian disease").

1225–1274 A.D.

In the medieval, Occidental world, Saint Thomas Aquinas (1225–1274), the distinguished Catholic theologian, wrote much in the field of psychology. He reintroduced the Aristotelian frame of reference, distinguishing the three "souls" (vegetative, animal, and rational) and their "faculties" (or "powers") —a framework which was used for many centuries. Thomas Aquinas did not make any systematic exposition of his ideas on abnormal psychology. Students who gathered together all references in his writings to psychiatric conditions have organized the following list of entities as he appears to have conceived them: [12]

I. Conditions of supernatural origin: hallucinations and insanity from the action of the demons
II. Conditions of natural origin:
  1. Stultitia (feeble-mindedness)
  2. Epilepsy
3. Phrenesis
4. Lethargia
5. Mania
6. Melancholia
7. Insania, Amentia

IV. PSYCHIATRIC CLASSIFICATIONS
DURING THE RENAISSANCE PERIOD

1450–1600 A.D.

During the Renaissance period (1450–1600), most physicians used classifications based on the concepts of the ancient Greek, Roman, and Arabic authors. The influence of Galen was predominant. Two independent personalities, however, Paracelsus and Platter, stand out for originality.

In France, Jean Fernel (1497–1558), was called "the French Galen." His psychiatric classification can be given as a typical instance of those of the traditionalist physicians of the Renaissance: [13]

I. Diseases of the brain envelopes
  1. Cephalalgia
  2. Cephaleia
  3. Hemicrania
II. Diseases of the brain substance
  A. Through disturbance of the faculties
    1. Frenesia
    2. Delirium
    3. Melancholia
      a. Black bile in the whole body
      b. Black bile in the head
      c. Hypochondriac melancholy
    4. Lycanthropy

    5. Mania
  B. Through deficiency of the faculties
    1. Stultitia (stupidity)
    2. Amentia (loss or absence of intelligence)
    3. Oblivio (loss of memory)
    4. Cataphora
    5. Obnubilatio
    6. Catoche
    7. Lethargy
III. Diseases of the ventricles
  1. Vertigo
  2. Epilepsy
  3. Nightmare
  4. Apoplexia

III. Diseases of the ventricles [cont.]

5. Paralysis	7. Tremor
6. Convulsions	8. Catarrh

Another typical example of Renaissance psychiatry was the work of a German physician, Johannes Schenck, who compiled a textbook [14] consisting of interesting case histories from the writings of other ancient and modern physicians and arranged in the traditional order. Mental disturbances are presented:

1. Headache	13. Convulsions
2. Drunkenness	14. Incubus
3. Vertigo	15. Melancholia
4. Phrenitis (with Galen's three subforms)	16. Lycanthropy
	17. Hypochondriac melancholia
5. Lethargy and carus	18. Mania
6. Catalepsy	19. Lovesickness
7. Sleeplessness	20. Enthusiasm (i.e., need to jump
8. Noctambulism (i.e., somnambulism)	and to dance, cured by means of music)
9. Amnesia	21. Fanaticism
10. Apoplexy	22. Vitus' chorea
11. Stupor	23. Demonomania
12. Epilepsy	

In England the Renaissance interest in mental diseases seemed to have concentrated on the concept of *melancholy*. This word had evidently taken on a very broad and vague meaning, as evidenced by Timothy Bright's *Treatise of Melancholie* (1586),[15] considered the first psychiatric book written by an Englishman. In it, melancholia was given the following subforms:

1. Natural Melancholia (resulting from excess of black bile)
2. Unnatural Melancholia (resulting from an alteration of one of the humors)
   a. from alteration of black bile
   b. from alteration of yellow bile
   c. from alteration of blood
   d. from alteration of phlegma (this subform was disputed)

"Natural melancholia" was one of the "natural humors," i.e., one of the Galenic temperaments. It included not only a sad and gloomy disposition but all kinds of vague feelings of sullenness, irritability, moodiness, and oddities in conduct. "Unnatural melancholia" was a more severe emotional or mental disorder. The worst alteration was the so-called "adustion" (combustion) of humors, which led to the most violent and disorderly passions and finally to "insanity."

Under the name of Galen is a treatise *On Melancholy*, which medical historians consider the work of a later author. It is a compilation based mostly on Galen's teaching. In it three forms of melancholy are listed:

1. *General melancholia* (resulting from an excess of black bile in the whole body)
2. *Brain melancholia* (resulting from an excess of black bile in the brain)

3. *Hypochondriac melancholia* (resulting from the ascension to the brain of vicious vapors engendered in the stomach)

The author of this treatise names other etiological forms of melancholia:

1. Constitutional melancholia
2. Melancholia resulting from a one-sided diet
3. Melancholia resulting from the "adustion" of yellow bile
4. Melancholia resulting from suppression of hemorrhoidal or menstrual flux
5. Melancholia resulting from precipitating emotional factors

Finally he describes particular clinical types of melancholia; one of them being *Lycanthropy* (the delusion of being transformed into a wolf).

The break with Galenic tradition was effected for the first time by Paracelsus (1493–1541), whose main innovation was that of introducing chemistry into medicine, although he did much speculating about the cosmic and spiritual "causes" of diseases.

Paracelsus was probably the first physician to abandon the "ideal" of classifying diseases from the head down. He attempted to group them according to their interdependence in families. His psychiatric classification is to be found in his treatise *On the Diseases Which Deprive a Man of His Reason:* [16]

I. Epilepsy
II. Mania (acute, violent mental disorders)
III. Vitus' chorea
IV. Suffocation of the intellect (all kinds of paroxysmic accidents, excepting epilepsy)
V. Wahnsinn ("insanity"), with five subforms:
    1. Lunacy (periodic disorders, rhythmed by phases of the moon)
    2. Insanity (hereditary mental diseases)
    3. Vesania (mental conditions caused by poisons)
    4. Melancholia (emotional disorders)
    5. Preternatural diseases (demoniacal possession and obsession)

Paracelsus's attempt to break with traditional Galenic medicine was a failure. But Basel, the town where Paracelsus had failed in 1527, was the home of another medical reformer, Felix Platter (1536–1614), who succeeded in a part of the reforms vainly attempted by his predecessor. He, too, gave up the old classification methods and introduced a new principle of classification which is immediately apparent in the following listing: [17]

I. Imbecillitas mentis (mental deficiency and dementia)
    1. Hebetudo mentis (idiocy)
    2. Tarditas ingenii (imbecility)
    3. Imprudentia seu Defectus judicii (feeble-mindedness)
    4. Oblivio (forgetfulness)
    5. Memoria imminuta (gross loss of memory)
II. Consternatio mentis (disturbances of consciousness)
    1. Somnus profundus (deep sleep, i.e., for instance under the effect of drink)
    2. Sopor gravis (carus, coma, etc.)
    3. Sopor cum febre or Lethargus

4. Sopor cum delirio
   a. Cataphora
   b. Coma agrypnion
   c. Typhomania
   d. Ecstasy
5. Stupor cum resolutione (apoplexia and similar conditions)
6. Stupor cum convulsione
7. Stupor vigilans (catalepsy)
8. Stupor remanente motu (with conservation of muscular attitudes)

III. Mentis alienatio (psychosis)
1. Stultitia
   a. Moria
   b. Fatuitas
   c. Infantia (silly behavior)
2. Temulantia (inebriety and other intoxications)
3. Commotio animi (violent emotions and passions)
   a. Amor animi commotionis species (lovesickness)
4. Melancholia
   a. Hypochondriasis
   b. Lycanthropy
   c. Misanthropy
5. Mania (fury)
   a. Hydrophobia (rabies)
   b. Saltus Viti (chorea)
6. Phrenitis (acute delirium with fever at the onset)
7. Paraphrenitis (acute fever preceded by fever without delirium)

IV. Mentis defatigatio (mental exhaustion)
1. Insomnia graviora (severe sleeplessness through exhaustion)

Besides these various *natural* conditions, Platter described *preternatural* ones.

v. Psychiatric Classification in the Seventeenth Century

During the seventeenth century the fight between the traditional Galenic medicine and the new, more scientific approach became more intense. Some of the psychiatric classifications (e.g., those of Robert Burton) clung to the traditional concepts, while others (e.g., those of Paolo Zacchias and Thomas Willis) followed new principles.

Paolo Zacchias (1584–1659), the greatest pioneer of legal medicine, expounded a system of psychiatric diagnosis attempting to synthesize the legal and the medical points of view. His psychiatric nosology can be summarized in the following table: [18]

I. Fatuitas (mental deficiency and insufficiency)
1. Ignorantia, or imperitia, hebetudo (dullness, mental laziness)
2. Fatuitas proper (imbecility)
3. Stoliditas (idiocy)
4. Oblivio (loss of memory, dementia)
5. Deaf-mutes (assimilated by the fatuiti)

II. Insania (mental and emotional conditions, without fever)
  A. Primary insania (mania and melancholia)
      1. Mania (acute excitement, fury)
          a. Extasis (a kind of violent mania)
          b. Lycanthropy (40-days-long psychosis, in early spring)
          c. Hydrophobia (rabies)
          d. Acute conditions resulting from snakebites or poisoning.
      2. Melancholia (chronic conditions with fixed ideas)
          a. Hypochondriasis with delusions
          b. Hypochondriasis without delusions
          c. Hallucinations without delusions
          d. Amor (lovesickness)
          e. Demonomania (possession by evil spirits)
          f. Fanatismus (people who prophesy)
          g. Lymphatismus (senseless terrors or visions)
          h. Praestigiati (bewitched people)
          i. Engastrimythi (ventriloquists)
          j. Enthusiasti (religious exaltation)
          k. Noctambuli (somnambulism)
  B. Secondary insania (symptomatic mental disturbances)
      1. Apoplexia
      2. Epilepsy
      3. Thunderstrokes
      4. Lethargy, coma, carus
      5. Suffocatio uteri, furor uteri (hysteria)
      6. Syncope, lipothymia
      7. Agony
  C. Passions: Iracundia (anger), drunkenness, etc.
III. Phrenitis (acute delirium with fever), and Paraphrenitis (fever delirium)

A quite different classification, based on the traditional Galenic concepts, was expounded by Robert Burton (1577–1640). The singular interest of the English in melancholy, previously mentioned, explains the tremendous popularity of his *Anatomy of Melancholy* (1621).[19] At the beginning of the book Burton expounds briefly a general classification of diseases, showing the place of melancholy among them:

I. Diseases of the body
II. Diseases of the head
  A. Outward: diseases of the eyes, ears, nose, etc.
  B. Inward
      1. Diseases of meninges
          a. Headache
      2. Diseases of ventricles
          a. Caro
          b. Vertigo
          c. Incubus
          d. Apoplexy
          e. Epilepsy
      3. Diseases of the nerves
          a. Cramps
          b. Stupor
          c. Convulsion
          d. Tremor
          e. Palsy
      4. Excrements of the brain: catarrhs, sneezing, rheums
      5. Diseases of the brain substance
          a. Phrenitis (frenzy)

b. Madness (mania),	Hydrophobia
with subforms:	St. Vitus' Dance
Ecstasy (enthu-	Demoniacal pos-
siasm, revela-	session or ob-
tions, visions)	session
Lycanthropy	c. Melancholy

As for melancholy itself, Burton admits that the distinction of its various kinds is "a labyrinth of doubts and errors," and he gives at least two classifications.

The anatomical classification (which is only an elaboration of the old classification of the pseudo-Galenic treatise on melancholy) includes:

1. Head Melancholy ("proceeds from the sole fault of the brain")
2. Body Melancholy ("when the whole temperature is melancholy")
3. Hypochondriacal or Windy Melancholy ("ariseth from the bowels, liver, spleen or membrane called mesenterium")

The other classification is a psychological one and comprises:

1. Love Melancholy
2. Melancholy arising from study ("the misery of the scholars")
3. Religious Melancholy

Another noteworthy classification was the work of Thomas Willis (1622–1675), the English physician so well known for his discoveries in the field of brain anatomy. Although he kept the old Galenic concept of humoral pathology, he was both a keen clinician and an indefatigable experimenter. Among his works two are outstanding: the *De Morbis Convulsivis* (1667), a complete treatise of all convulsive diseases (epilepsy, chorea, hysteria, etc.), and *De Anima Brutorum* (1672), a synthesis of neurology, psychology, and psychiatry. His classification was as follows: [20]

1. Headaches	8. Morosis (imbecility, debility,
2. Lethargus, and kindred diseases	stupidity, dementia)
(coma, carus, etc.)	9. Paralysis
3. Insomnia	10. Phrenitis and fever delirium
4. Coma vigil	11. Mania
5. Incubus	12. Melancholia, with a great
6. Vertigo	number of subforms
7. Apoplexia	13. Arthritism
	14. Acute colic pains

Laignel-Lavastine and Vinchon mention that Willis's description of acute colic pains correspond exactly to the *syndrome solaire aigu* of Laignel-Lavastine (acute pains originating in the plexus solaris). This means that Willis tried to integrate into psychiatry central-nervous-system and vegetative-nervous-system "facts."

VI. PSYCHIATRIC CLASSIFICATION IN THE
EIGHTEENTH CENTURY

In the eighteenth century the number and the diversity of psychiatric classifications increased steadily. However, in all the resulting confusion a few trends are discernible. Eighteenth-century nosologists can be put in three groups: the systematists, the rationalists, and the humanitarians.

The Systematists

In the efforts of these eighteenth-century nosographers a new and extremely important assumption gradually crept into their way of thinking. Up to the time of Sydenham, illness, however precisely it may have been differentiated into syndrome pictures, was thought of as developing from a single pathogenesis: either disturbed humoral balance or a disturbance in the tensions of the solid tissues of the body.

Medicine, and with it psychiatry, had entered a new era with the arrival of Sydenham (1624–1663) on the medical scene. Sydenham brought to medicine a freshness of viewpoint which cut through the metaphysical morass into which it had slipped and set it moving again along scientific channels. He rejected all previous speculations of the humoralists, solidists, and others and became a vigorous advocate of specificity and pluralism in the concept of disease. He believed in diseases rather than in a single kind of disorder at the root of all ailments. He revived, therefore, the Cnidian tradition, so long recessive. Sydenham captured the imagination of medical men and philosophers both and touched off an enthusiastic search for the mental "disease" which still grips psychiatry today.

Sydenham advocated the careful study of morbid phenomena, decrying the indulgence in speculation which was characteristic of so many of his contemporaries of the iatro-chemical school of medicine. He held (1) that all diseases should be reduced to certain definite species with the same care that the botanist exercised in the description of plants, (2) that all hypotheses and philosophical systems should be entirely set aside and the pathological phenomena described with the same accuracy that a painter observes in painting a portrait. Said he: [21, 22]

And in truth it is my opinion that the principal reason of our being yet destitute of an accurate history of diseases, proceeds from a general supposition that diseases are no more than the confused and irregular operations of disordered and debilitated nature, and consequently that it is a fruitless labor to endeavor to give a just description of them.

Then in the beginning of the eighteenth century there was one man who attempted a direct continuation of Sydenham's nosological work and more particularly sought to carry out Sydenham's ideas of describing the diseases in the same way as botanists described plants. This was François Boissier de Sauvages, a scholar who flourished at Montpellier and published a small book, *Traité des Classes des Maladies*, in 1731. He was himself a botanist, besides being a physician, and in his book he now sought to group the diseases in classes, orders, and genera, just as natural scientists were at that time occupied in arranging plants and animals in a perspicuous system. Such an attempt to place and group all diseases in a definite system was quite a new departure, though a few very imperfect attempts in this direction had been previously made, such as those by the Swiss physician, Felix Platter, in 1602 and the Amsterdam physician, Johnston, in 1644.

Boissier de Sauvages (1706–1767) devoted his whole life to the task of elaborating this new medical nosology. His enlarged book, published in Latin in 1763, and posthumously in French in 1770–1771, contains a revised and enlarged description of his system, with a long introduction and discussion about the principles of nosology and of classifications in general.[23] His classification comprises ten classes of diseases:

1. Vices (objective symptoms of the skin)
2. Fevers
3. Inflammations
4. Spasms
5. Disturbances of breathing
6. Weaknesses
7. Pains
8. Dementia (see below)
9. Discharges
10. Cachexia (anatomical modifications)

Conspicuous is the subdivision of Class 3 into three subgroups: inflammations of skin, mucosa, and parenchymata. It is probably the first instance of a histological classification of organic diseases. *Phrenesis* constitutes, as inflammation of the meninges, the No. 11 of order II (inflammations of membranes).

Class 4 (spasms) includes all kinds of convulsive diseases; among others, epilepsy, hysteria, and chorea.

Class 6 (weaknesses) includes, as its fifth order, the seven genera of "comas": catalepsy, ecstasy, typhomania, lethargy, sleepiness, carus, apoplexy.

Class 8 includes the bulk of mental diseases, divided into four orders and twenty-three species as follows:

ORDER I. Disturbances of peripheral, extra-cerebral origin
1. Vertigo
2. "Berlue"
3. Diplopia
4. Tintoin
5. Hypochondriasis
6. Somnambulism

ORDER II. Disturbances of instinctual and emotional life
7. Pica
8. Voracity
9. Polydipsy
10. Antipathy (includes what we call today the phobias)
11. Nostalgia
12. Panophobia
13. Satyriasis
14. Nymphomania
15. Tarantism
16. Hydrophobia (rabies)

ORDER III. Disturbances of intellectual life
17. Paraphrosyne (toxic or symptomatic delirium)
18. Dementia, or amentia
19. Melancholia (see below)
20. Mania
21. Demonomania

ORDER IV. "Folies irrégulières":
22. Amnesia
23. Insomnia

It is noteworthy that Boissier de Sauvages considers demonomania as a purely natural disease, kindred to melancholia. Melancholia itself is divided into fourteen species:

1. Ordinary melancholia
2. Erotomania (lovesickness)
3. Religious melancholia
4. Imaginary melancholia (like hypochondriasis, without physical basis)
5. Extravagant melancholia
6. Melancholia attonita (the patient remains silent, immobile)

7. Vagabond melancholia (intense need of movement)
8. Dancing melancholia (choreomania)
9. Hippanthropic melancholia (delusion of being transformed into a horse)
10. Scythian melancholia (a man's delusion of being transformed into a woman)
11. Melancholia anglica (alias *taedium vitae*, wish for death)
12. Zoanthropic melancholia (delusion of being transformed into an animal)
13. Enthusiastic melancholia (belief of being divinely inspired)
14. Sorrowful melancholia

Boissier de Sauvages' work had tremendous influence and inspired a long succession of imitators. The first of them was the Swedish naturalist Carl Linné (1707–1778).*

Linné's enthusiasm for Boissier's nosology led him to publish his own *Genera Morborum* in 1763.[24] It is obvious from comparing their nosologies that Linné meant only to revise and complete Boissier's nosology rather than to present a new one. Boissier's genera and species keep their names and distinctive marks, being only regrouped in a slightly different way. Linné distinguishes 11 classes instead of 10, and 325 genera instead of Boissier's 295. The bulk of mental diseases Linné placed under the more comprehensive name of *Mentales*, as the fifth class. This class is divided, not into four, but into three orders:

A. *Ideales* (Order III of Boissier: disturbances of intellectual life)
B. *Imaginerii* (Order I of Boissier: disturbances of sensorial activity)
C. *Pathetici* (Order II of Boissier: disturbances of emotional life)

---

* "It is difficult to judge at the present time of the amount of sensation caused by Sauvages' work at the time of its appearance, but one man at least was greatly impressed by it, namely the Swede, Carl Linné. Linné was then studying in Holland where he graduated as a doctor of medicine in 1735, the same year in which he published his 'systema naturae.' From the moment of first reading Sauvages' book he became deeply interested in this man, in whom he discovered the same capacity for systematic arrangement as in himself, and for thirty years these two men carried on an extensive correspondence, became close friends, and were mutually greatly influenced by each other, although they never became personally acquainted. In 1773 Linné commenced the correspondence by requesting Sauvages to send him his book which he had 'sought in vain throughout Sweden, Lapland, Norway, Denmark, Germany, Holland and England.' To Boissier de Sauvages he wrote 'My dull brain can only take in and comprehend that which can be conceived systematically. Anyone with a bent for method will find truths in your work which will live till distant times.' In later letters he wrote: 'You are the only systematician among physicians, you alone have broken the ice and cleared the way. You alone have thrown open the road which blind moles refuse to enter.'

"Hence, when Linné became professor of theoretical and practical medicine at Upsala, he based his lectures on Boissier de Sauvages' system.

"In reality, Linné's nosology consisted essentially in a description of symptoms, the various species of disease depending upon the various circumstances under which the symptoms appear. Such a description was very far from Sydenham's idea of giving a proper description of the diseases. That, however, a great want had been met by Sauvages' nosology is testified by the appearance of a number of imitators and successors in the following years." (Faber, Knud: *Nosography in Modern Internal Medicine*. New York: Hoeber, 1923, pp. 20–21.)

While in the frame of these three orders Boissier distinguishes three genera, Linné finds twenty-five, giving most of them the same names Boissier did.

Although Linné's classification is conceived of as a phylogenetic system, it is, in actual fact, merely descriptive; the 325 "diseases" which it recognizes are described for the most part in terms of specific symptoms and grouped accordingly. Linné's system thus contributes little to the understanding of psychiatric illnesses, but it is of historical interest because it furnished the model for many nosological attempts during the nineteenth century. In fact, the great influence of the Linnéian principles of classification on the scientific thought of the nineteenth century, with its emphasis on formal aspects and arbitrary divisions, tended to obstruct the development of psychiatric insights.

We shall mention here only a few representative names and classifications from the eighteenth-century part of this prolific era of psychiatric nosology. Among the many followers of Boissier de Sauvages and Linné, William Cullen (1712–1790) was a controversial figure. A pioneer in the field of neuropathology, he believed that mental disease was a pathological condition of the mind. In 1777 he published his book *First Lines of the Practice of Physik,* in which he describes paranoid forms of mental disorders under the term *vesaniae.* His *Synopsis and Nosology,*[25] published in 1769, was an elaborate attempt to classify illnesses according to the Linnaean principle of Classes, Orders, Genera, and Species. Mental illnesses are subdivided into four orders—comata, adynamias, spasms, and vesanias.

In the original this classification appears twice, with modifications to be mentioned; once on pages xv to xxiii, then again—with elaborations—on pages 27 to 46. The second version gives many definitions. As we print it, the classification is principally as in the first version, with some of the definitions from the second version arbitrarily transposed and interpolated by us. The spelling is not uniform in the original, and no attempt has been made by us to correct obvious inconsistencies.*

Class II. NEUROSES (injury of the sense and motion, without an idiopathic pyrexia or any local affection)

    Order I. COMATA (diminution of voluntary motion, with sleep, or a deprivation of the senses)

        Genus 42. APOPLEXIA (almost all voluntary motion diminished, with sleep more or less profound; the motion of the heart and arteries remaining)

      A. Idiopathic

        1. Apoplexia sanguinea (with symptoms of universal plethora, especially of the head)

        2. Apoplexia Serosa (with a lucophlegmasia over the whole body, especially in old people)

        3. Apoplexia Hydrocephalica (coming on by degrees, affecting infants, or those below the age of puberty, first, with lassitude, a slight fever and pain of the head, then with slowness of the pulse, dilatation of the pupil of the eye, and drowsiness)

        4. Apoplexia atrabiliaria (taking place in those of a melancholic constitution)

* Genera 1 to 41 appear in Class I. The classification is in two parts—one roman, the other arabic. A "[*sic*]" after a word indicates an exact reproduction from the book.

5. Apoplexia traumatica (from some external injury mechanically applied to the head)
6. Apoplexia Venenata (from powerful sedatives taken internally or applied externally)
7. Apoplexia Mentalis (from a passion of the mind)
8. Apoplexia Calateptica [*sic*] (in the contractile muscles, with a mobility of the limbs by external force)
9. Apoplexia Suffocata (from some external suffocating power)

B. Symptomatic

1. Of the intermittent fever	6. Epilepsy
2. Continued fever	7. Podagra
3. Phlegmasia	8. Worms
4. Exanthema	9. Ischuria
5. Hysteria	10. Scurveys [*sic*]

Genus 43. Paralysis (only some of the voluntary motions diminished, frequently with sleep)

A. Idiopathic species

1. Paralysis partialis (of some particular muscles only)
2. Paralysis Hemepligia [*sic*] (of one side of the body Vary according to the constitution of the Body—a. hemiplegia in a plethoric habit b. in a leuco pleglematic [*sic*] habit)
3. Paralysis paraphegia (of one half of the body taken transversely)
4. Paralysis venenata (from sedative powers applied either externally or internally)

B. Symptomatic species

1. Asthenic
2. Paralytic
3. Convulsive

Order II. ADINAMIAE (a diminution of the involuntary motions, whether vital or natural)

Genus 44. Syncope (a diminution or even a total stoppage, of the motion of the heart for a little)

A. Idiopathic species

1. Syncope Cardiaca (returning frequently without any manifest cause, with violent palpitations of the heart, during the intervals; from a fault of the heart or neighboring vessels)
2. Syncope occasionalis (arising from some evident cause, from an affection of the whole system)

B. Symptomatic

Genus 45. Dyspepsy (anorexia, nausea, vomiting, inflation, belching, rumination, cardialgia, gastrodynia, more or fewer of those symptoms at least concuring [*sic*], for the most with a constipation of the belly, and without any other Diseases either of the stomach itself, or of other parts)

A. Idiopathic

B. Symptomatic (from a disease of the stomach itself) (from a disease of other parts, or of the whole body)

Genus 46. Hypochondriasis (dyspepsia with languor, sadness and fear without any adequate causes, in a melancholic temperament)

Genus 47. Chlorosis (Dyspepsia, or a desire of something not used as food, a pale or discoloured complexion. The veins not well filled, a soft tumour of the whole body, asthenia, palpitation, suppression of the menses)

Order III. SPASMI (irregular motions of the muscles or muscularfibres [*sic*])

Sect. 1. *In the animal functions*

Genus 48. Tetanus (A spastic rigidity of almost the whole body. Varying according to the remote cause as it arises either from something, internal. 1 from cold, or from a wound. It varies likewise, from whatever cause it arises according to the part of the body affected)

Genus 49. Trismus (as spastic rigidity of the lower jaw)

    Species 1. Trismus nascentium (seizing infants under two months old)

    Species 2. Trismus traumaticus (seizing people of all ages either from wound or cold)

Genus 50. Convulsio (an irregular clonic contraction of the museles [*sic*] without sleep)

    A. Idiopathic   B. Symptomatic

Genus 51. Chorea (attacking those who have not yet arrived at puberty, most commonly within the 10th or 14th year, with convulsive motions for the most part of one side, in attempting the voluntary motions of the hands and arms, resembling the gesticulations of mountebanks, in walking rather dragging one of their feet after them, then lifting it)

Genus 52. Rhaphania (a spastic contraction of the jolnts [*sic*] with convulsive agitations and most violent periodic pain)

Genus 53. Epilepsy (a convulsion of the muscles, with sleep)

    A. Idiopathic

        1. Epilepsy cerebralis (suddenly attacking without any manifest cause, without any sense of uneasiness preceeding [*sic*] excepting perhaps a slight [*sic*] vertigo or Scotomia)

        2. Epilepsy Sympathic (without any manifest cause, but preceeded by the sensation of a kind of [*sic*] Air rising from a certain part of the body towards the head)

        3. Epilepsy occasionalis (arising from a manifest irritation, and ceasing on the removal of that irritation. Varying according to the difference of the irritating matter, and thus it may arise. From injuries of the head, pain, worms, poison, from the repulstion of the itch, or an effusion of any other acrid humour, from crudities in the stomack [*sic*] from pasions [*sic*] of the mind, or from an immoderate haemorrhage [*sic*] or from debility)

Sec. 2. *In the vital functions*

Genus 54. Palpitatio (a violent and irregular motion of the heart)

Genus 55. Asthma (a defficulty [*sic*] of breathing, returning by intervals, with a sense of straightness in the breast, and a noisy respiration with hissing, in the beginning of the paroxysm there is either no cough at all, or coughing is difficult, but towards the end the cough becomes free, frequently with a copious spitting of mucus)

  A. Idiopathic

    1. Asthma spontaneum (without any manifest cause or other concomitant disease)

    2. Asthma Exanthematicum (from the repulsion of the Itch or acrid effusion)

Genus 56. Dyspnoea (a continual difficulty of breathing, without any sense of straitness [*sic*], but rather of fullness and infraction in the breast, a frequent cough throughout the whole course of the disease)

  A. Idiopathic

    1. Dyspnoea Catarrhalis (with a frequent cough, bringing up plenty of viscid mucus)

    2. Dyspnoea Sicca (with a cough, for the most part, dry)

    3. Dyspnoea aerea (increased by the least change of weather)

    4. Dyspnoea Terrea (bringing up with the cough an earthy or calculous matter)

    5. Dyspnoea aquosa (with scanty urine and oedematous fat, without any signs of an Hydrothorax)

    6. Dyspnoea Pinguedinosa (in very fat people)

    7. Dyspnoea Thoracica (from an injury done to the parts surrounding the thorax or from some bad conformation of them)

    8. Dyspnoea extrinseca (from evident external causes)

  B. Symptomatic

    1. of Diseases of the heart or large vessels

    2. of swellings in the abdomen

    3. of various Diseases

Genus 57. Pertussis (a contagious disease, convulsive strangulating cough, reiterated with noisy inspiration, frequent vomiting)

Sect. 3. *In the natural functions*

Genus 58. Pyrosis (a burning pain in the epigastrium with plenty of aqueous humour, for the most part insipid, but sometimes acrids [*sic*] belchings [*sic*] up)

Genus 59. Colica (pain of the belly, especially twisting round the navel, vomiting, a constipation)

  A. Idiopathic

    1. Colica spasmodica (with retraction of the navil [*sic*], and spasms of the abdominal muscles. Varying by reason of some symptoms super-added; hence, a. Colica, with vomiting of excrements, or of matters injected by the anus; b. Colica, with inflammation supervening)

    2. Colica Pictonum (preceded by a sense of weight or uneasiness in the belly, especially about the navel, then comes on the colic pain, at first flight and interrupted, chiefly augmented after meals, at length more severe and almost con-

tinual, with pains of the arms and back, at last ending in a Palsy. Varying according to the nature of the remote cause, and hence,

a. from metallic poison
b. from acids taken inwardly
c. from cold
d. from a contusion of the back

3. Colica Stercorea (in people subject to costiveness)
4. Colica accidentalis (from acrid matter taken internally)
5. Colica meconialis (in new born [sic] children from a retention of the meconium)
6. Colica Callosa (with a sensation of structure in some parts of the intestines and frequently of a collection of flatus with some pain before the constricted part, which flatus also pass-ing through the part where the stricture [sic] is felt gradually vanishes. The belly slow, and at last passing only a few liquid foeces [sic])
7. Colica Calculosa (with a fixed hardness in some part of the abdomen, and calculi smetimes [sic] passing by the anus)

Genus 60. Cholera (a vomiting of bilious matter, and likewise, a fre-quent excretion of the same stool, anxiety, gripes, spasm in the calves of the legs)

A. Idiopathic
1. Cholera Spontanea (arising in a warm season without any manifest cause)
2. Cholera accidentalis (from acrid matters taken internally)
B. Symptomatic

Genus 61. Diarrhoea (frequent stools, the disease not infectious, no primary pyrexia)

A. Idiopathic
1. Diarrhoea crapulosa (in which the excrements are voided in greater quantity than naturally)
2. Diarrhoea biliosa (in which yellow faeces [sic] are voided in great quantity)
3. Diarrhoea mucosa (in which either from acrid substances taken inwardly, or from cold, especially applied to the feet; a great quantity is voided)
4. Diarrhoea Coeliaca (in which a milky humour of the nature of chyle passed)
5. Diarrhoea lienteria (in which the aliments are discharged with little alteration soon after eating)
6. Diarrhoea Hepattirhoea (in which a bloody ferous matter is discharged without pain)
B. Symptomatic

Genus 62. Diabetes (A chronical profusion of urine, for the most part preternatural and in immoderate quantity)

A. Idiopathic
1. Diabetes insipidus (with limpid, but not sweet, urine)
B. Symptomatic

Genus 63. Hysteria (rumbling of the bowels. a sensation of a globe turning itself in the belly, assending [sic] to the stomach;

sleep, convulsions, a great quantity of limpid urine, the mind involuntarily fickle and mutable. The following are by Sauvages [*sic*] reckoned distinct Idopathic species. but by Dr. Cullen, only varieties of the same species)

Species 1. from retention of the menses
2. from menorrhagia cruenta
3. from menorrhagia serosa
4. from obstruction of the viscera
5. from fault of the stomach
6. from too great Salacity

Genus 64. Hydrophobia (a dislike and horror at every kind of drink, as occasioning a convulsion of the pharynx, induced for the most part, by the bite of a mad animal)

Species 1. Hydrophobia rabiosa (with a desire of biting the by-standers, occasioned by the bite of a mad animal)
2. Hydrophobia simplex (without madness, or any desire of biting)

Order IV. Vesaniae (disorders of the judgment without any pyrexia or coma)

Genus 65. Amentia (an imbecility of judgement, by which people do not perceive, or do not remember the relations of things)

Species 1. Amentia congenita (continuing from a person's birth)
Species 2. Amentia senilis (from the diminution of the perceptions and memory through extreme old age)
3. Amentia acquisita (occuring [*sic*] in people formerly of a sound mind, from evident external causes)

Genus 66. Melancholia (a partial madness, without dispepsia [*sic*] varying according to the different subjects concerning which the person raves) :

1. with an imagination in the patient concerning his body being in a dangerous condition, from slight causes, or that his affairs are in a desperate state
2. with an imagination concerning a prosperous state of affairs
3. with violent love, without satyriasis or nymphomania
4. with a superstitious fear of a future state
5. with an aversion from motion and all the offices of life
6. with restlessness and an impatience of any situation whatever
7. with a weariness of life
8. with a deception concerning the nature of the patient's species

The Doctor reckons that there is no such Disease as that called Doemonomania [*sic*] and that the Diseases mentioned by Sauvage [*sic*] under that title are either,

1. species of melancholy as mania or,
2. of some disease by the spectators falsly [*sic*] ascribed to the influence of an evil spirit or,
3. of a disease entirely feigned or,
4. of a disease partly true and partly feigned

Genus 67. Mania (universal madness)
A. Idiopathic

1. Mania mentalis (arising entirely from passions of the mind)
2. Mania corporea (from an evident disease of the body)
3. Mania obscura (without any passion of the mind or evident disease of the Body preceeding [*sic*])

B. Symptomatic
1. Paraphrosyne a Veneris
2. Paraphrosyne a pathemate
3. Paraphrosyne febrilis

Genus 68. Oneirodynia (a violent and troublesome imagination in time of sleep)
1. Oneirodynia activa (exciting to wakeing [*sic*] and various motions)
2. Oneirodynia gravans (from a sense of some weight incumbent and pressing on the breast especially)

Thirteen years after Cullen's book there appeared the first edition of Thomas Arnold's *Observations on Nature, Kinds, Causes, and Prevention of Insanity* (1782).[26] Arnold took sharp issue with Cullen, Sauvages, and the "botanical nosologists." According to him, there was *one* genus in psychiatry and only one, the genus *Insanity*. He allowed for two divisions: "ideal" and "notional" insanity, and 13 species:

I. Ideal Insanity (with hallucinations or illusions)	1. Phrenitic (the old phrenitis)
	2. Incoherent (amentia)
	3. Maniacal (systematized hallucinations)
	4. Sensitive (delusions of transformation)
	5. Delusive (delusions without hallucinations)
	6. Whimsical (phobias)
	7. Fanciful (our mania)
II. Notional Insanity (without hallucinations or illusions)	8. Impulsive (impulsions, compulsive acts)
	9. Scheming (delusions of grandeur)
	10. Vain, or self-important (vanity)
	11. Hypochondriacal (hypochondriasis)
	12. Pathetic ("melancholia") 16 subspecies
	13. Appetitive (satyriasis, and nymphomania)

The Rationalists

While the systematists were elaborating nosologies, another important development in science came from the great philosophical and cultural movement called the *Enlightenment*. The publication of the famous French *Encyclopédie* edited under the direction of Diderot and d'Alembert [27] included several articles on mental diseases contributed by collaborators whose names are forgotten today (d'Aumont, Menuret). If we take in account their clear definitions and descriptions of *folie, délire, démence, manie, mélancolie,* we can reconstruct the following classification:

I. *Fatuité* ("weakness or diminution of understanding and memory")
II. *Délire* ("wrong activity of understanding and memory")
1. *Folie* ("a kind of confusion of reason")
2. *Mélancolie* ("particular delusion without fever or fury")
3. *Manie* ("universal delusion without fever, often with fury")

III. *Phrénésie* (acute mental disturbance with fever and fury)
IV. *Démence* ("paralysis of the spirit," "abolition of the reasoning faculty")

Demonomania is defined as a variety of melancholia, in which patients have the delusion of being possessed or obsessed by the devil, of being witches or of being bewitched. This condition, the author adds, may result from poisoning, phrenesis, or other organic brain damage. An instance is given of a man who suffered such a "fanatic" kind of melancholia after he had been bitten by his cat.

The *Encyclopédie* shows the rationalist trend of reducing psychiatric nosology to a small number of well-defined and clearly described types. If we translate these disease entities into their later classical equivalents, we find the following correspondences:

I. *Fatuité*	Feeble-mindedness, senile dementia
II. *Délire*	Manic-depressive psychosis, schizophrenia
1. *Folie*	Psychosis with unsystematized delusions
2. *Mélancolie*	Psychosis with systematized delusions
3. *Manie*	Any acute psychotic condition without fever
III. *Phrénésie*	Acute fever delirium
IV. *Démence*	Severe organic syndromes, stuporous states

The Enlightenment movement, although born in France, spread rapidly to other countries, including Germany. One of the last of its leaders, but one of the most famous, was the philosopher Immanuel Kant (1724–1804). Kant had a wide range of interests, from cosmogony to mental diseases. In 1798 he published a kind of compendium of philosophical psychology under the title *Anthropology in Pragmatic Regard*.[28] In it, as a rather supplementary chapter, is a short treatise on "the weaknesses and sicknesses of the soul in regard to its faculty of cognition."

Kant's ideas on mental disease are difficult to summarize because he uses many words which are obsolete in German today and have no exact English equivalents. We have attempted approximate translations of some of these. His classification was as follows:

I. Weaknesses of the Soul in Regard to Its Cognitive Faculties
  A. Partial weaknesses
    1. *Stumpfsinn:* lack of wit
    2. *Dummheit:* lack of judgment
    3. *Einfalt:* lack of comprehension
    4. *Zerstreuung:* lack of attention
    5. *Thorheit:* fact of sacrificing valuable things for worthless ones
    6. *Narrheit:* foolishness which is insulting to others
  B. Total Weaknesses
    Blodsinnigkeit: idiocy, for instance cretinism
II. Sicknesses of the Soul
  A. *Grillenkrankheit* (whimsical disease)
    1. *Hypochondrie:* Excessive preoccupation with one's body, with exaggerated mirth, wittiness, joyous laughter, moodiness. "This disease originates in a childish anxious fear of the thought of death"

2. *Raptus:* Sudden change of mood. One of its manifestations can be suicide
3. *Melancholia:* "A delusion of misery, created by the gloomy person"

B. Mania, or "the disturbed disposition" (*das gestörte Gemüt*)
   1. Amentia (*Unsinnigkeit*): "the impossibility of bringing one's representations into sufficient coherence for enabling experience"
   2. Dementia (*Wahnsinn*): systematic delusions, for instance, of persecution
   3. Insania (*Wahnwitz*): unsystematized delusions
   4. Vesania (*Aberwitz*): delusion of a man who "pretends to comprehend the incomprehensible," for instance, the quadrature of the circle or perpetual motion

Because of his emphasis on the intellectual rather than the emotional aspects of mental illness, Kant is regarded as one of the "authoritative originators of the purely formalistic, intellectual point of view which characterized German psychiatry and which influenced more than it would appear on the surface English and American and to a great extent French psychiatry throughout the nineteenth century." [29] Like Platter, he grouped symptoms in syndromes; in turn grouped syndromes without a central principle.

The Humanitarians

In the second half of the eighteenth century, as a reaction against the dry intellectualism of the Enlightenment, a trend of "sensitiveness" appeared in Western Europe. Scientists began to be concerned for the deaf-mutes, the blind, the prisoners, and the mentally ill, and to search actively for methods of improving their condition. In Italy, France, and England, efforts were made toward a more humane and at the same time more effective treatment of psychiatric patients in the asylums. The primary aim of these reformers was to relieve the misery of their patients, and they gave short shrift to refined diagnoses and classifications, contenting themselves with practical, rule-of-thumb lists embracing a small number of clinical types. Thus, there developed, in opposition to the contemporary trend toward large, systematic nosologies, a minor trend toward the simplicity of the ancient Hippocratic nosology.

In Italy, Vincenzo Chiarugi (1759–1820) instituted humane treatment of the patients in a public mental hospital in Florence. He was a good clinician, checking his premorbid observations with his autopsy findings. His classification (influenced by Cullen) was the simplest possible: [30]

I. Melancholia (partial distortion of reality in regard to one or a few ideas)
   1. True Melancholia: constant depression of spirit, restlessness, impatience
   2. False Melancholia: imaginary happiness or elation, due to erroneous ideas
   3. Violent Melancholia: delirious, with hatred directed against self or others

II. Mania (general insanity with violence and impetuous actions; disconnected speech, disorganized sequence of ideas, poor judgment, abnormal actions). There are three stages:

1. the attack: agitation, shamelessness
2. the stage of violent impulses
3. remission: decreased violence—may turn into amentia

III. Amentia (general insanity, without emotional manifestations, with deficiency of both intelligence and volition)
   1. acquired
   2. congenital

The most illustrious representative of this humanitarian trend in psychiatry was Philippe Pinel (1745–1826). From the point of view of psychiatric nosology, his work is of particular interest: he started with the elaboration of a large, sophisticated classification similar to those of Boissier de Sauvages and Linné, but later, as a result of his practical work with mental patients, he came to espouse a new, very simple and pragmatic classification.

The son of a country physician in southern France, Pinel studied successively divinity, mathematics, natural sciences, and medicine. He came to Paris in 1778, lived there as a medical journalist and translator, and had a small medical practice. He devoted many years to what he considered his masterpiece, his *Nosographie Philosophique* (1798).[31]

Pinel studied carefully the systems of Boissier de Sauvages, Linné, and their successors, and criticized them in an article of the *Dictionnaire des Sciences Médicales*. His own classification is so minutely elaborated that in bare outline it fills thirty-seven pages (eight for mental diseases) in Sémalaigne's book. In Pinel's early system most of the mental diseases are put in the fourth class, entitled *Neuroses*. Pinel gave this word the definition of "functional diseases of the nervous system," i.e., diseases without fever, inflammation, hemorrhage, or anatomical lesion. In fact, this class is a heteroclite mixture where one finds neuralgias and hallucinations as well as asthma, epilepsy, ileus, whooping cough, tetanus, and rabies.

During the Revolution, the Paris hospitals suffered a complete disorganization. At the climax of disaster, in 1793, Pinel was appointed physician in the notorious hospital of Bicêtre, where he forwarded humane reforms in the treatment of the mental patients.

Two years later Pinel was appointed physician at another hospital, the Salpêtrière, where he instituted reforms in patient care. From this crucial time on, Pinel devoted himself to formulating a simple, humane system of asylum psychiatry. He accepted a professorship in internal medicine at the Medical School of Paris. Three years after his *Nosographie Philosophique* appeared (1798), he published his *Medico-Philosophical Treatise on Insanity*,[32] expounding a new classification as simple as the former one had been complicated.

Four fundamental clinical types are distinguished:

1. Mania (all conditions with acute excitement or fury)
2. Melancholia (depressive conditions, delusions with limited topics)
3. Dementia (lack of cohesion in the ideas)
4. Idiotism (including idiocy and organic dementia)

Pinel thus departed from the disease entity tradition as revised by Sydenham and reacted against the systematic nosologies of the Linnéian school. His return to the simple Hippocratic classification was thus a strong reaction against the trend of his times, and a considered effort to advance observation through classification which permitted flexibility of concepts and which emphasized clinical description. Mania, melancholia, dementia, and idiotism were, for Pinel, more than names composing a list; they were functional categories which accumulated knowledge could expand and explain.

Meanwhile, something similar was happening in America. Benjamin Rush (1745–1813) made a very telling stroke against ponderous nosographical thought by a very different means.[33] With characteristic sweep and flourish Rush created a multitude of neologistic diagnostic labels based upon some single outstanding feature of the illness. This was done with tongue-in-cheek humor, reducing nosologizing to an absurdity. For example, Rush was able to joke freely about the scores of phobias he identified.

> Rum-phobia is a very rare distemper. I have known but five instances of it in the course of my life. . . . Doctor-phobia is complicated with other diseases. It arises often from the dread of taking physic, or of submitting to the remedies of blistering and bleeding. It might be supposed to be caused by the terror of a long bill, but this excites terror in few minds, for whoever thinks of paying a doctor's bill while he can use his money to advantage another way?

Rush comments in similar vein on "church-phobia," negro-mania, land-mania, horse-mania, dueling-mania, hunting-mania, love-mania, pride-mania, range-mania, mathematical-mania, and so forth. As Riese says, "A classification admitting of almost endless varieties approaches its own destruction; namely, individualization." [34]

For Rush, as for Pinel, a mentally ill person was a troubled individual who needed understanding and kindness more than he needed the treatment of his "disease." Their humanitarian principles were an expression of their primary interest in the person and his life situation—not in his alleged disease.

Rush did, in fact, strike out against pluralism more forcefully than did Pinel. Shryock, in a study of Rush, explains that "as enthusiasm grew for identifying all possible symptom combinations as separate entities, long lists were prepared in nosographic texts which amounted to only so many names. Rush rightly felt that these texts were most confusing, and desired some simpler scheme which would really aid the practitioner. He therefore swerved to the other extreme—from the listing of innumerable, supposed disease entities to the flat assertion that there was only one." [35] He fell back (perhaps without knowing it) on one of the monistic theories of classical tradition—the belief of the old School of Asclepiades and the Methodists, that all illness is based on patterns of tension and relaxation of body tissues.

Pinel and Rush were two of the most influential figures of modern medicine and psychiatry. But the search for the specific causes of a plurality of diseases was on, and the momentum of this search was to dominate psychiatry for another hundred years, culminating in a psychiatric nihilism from which we are only now emerging.

VII. PSYCHIATRIC CLASSIFICATION IN THE NINETEENTH CENTURY

Rapid advances were made in medical science during the eighteenth century, following the anatomical discoveries of Vesalius (1514–1564) and of Harvey (circulation, 1628). The renaissance in physics which began with

Galileo (1564–1642), the invention of the microscope by Leeuwenhoek (1632–1723), and the classification of plants and animals (as well as diseases) by Linné (1707–1778) ushered in an era of scientific progress which banished the influence of Greek rationalism and the surviving theological theories of natural phenomena.

But it was the early part of the nineteenth century before this new influence was reflected in psychiatric formulations. Mental disease then began to be regarded as the manifestation of physical pathology, and the search for specific lesions and the effort to define and isolate disease entities, parallel to bodily diseases, was assiduously pursued.

Aside from this prevalent physio-pathological concept of mental disease, there were other nosological trends, and attempts were made to classify mental diseases either on the basis of the old "faculty psychology," or on the basis of the course of the disease, or by a combination of principles.

The Anti-Nosologic Trend

In the midst of the enormous development of nosologies in this period, the unitary concept of mental disease was almost lost. One of the very few representatives of this position during the nineteenth century was a German psychiatrist, Heinrich Neumann, who courageously declared: "There is only *one* kind of mental disorder; we call it insanity." It is of historical interest to note that this crucial taxonomic question had already been raised in Thomas Beddoes' book of 1803: "whether it be not necessary either to confine insanity to one species, or to divide it into almost as many as there are cases."[36] Neumann contended that the various clinical pictures described until that time were not disease entities but distinct phases of the only and one mental disease, "insanity." "Insanity," he said, begins with a phase of depression (*melancholia*), followed by a phase of excitement or fury (*mania*); then follows a phase of either death or recovery, or—if the disease continues—a phase of "weakness and perversion" of mental faculties, taking the aspects of *Verwirrtheit* (amentia) or *Verrücktheit* (paranoia); and finally, if there is no improvement, it ends with a terminal state of mental destruction called *Blödsinn* (dementia). Neumann strove to demonstrate that all clinical pictures ever described fitted into his schema, with the exception of idiocy, which he claimed was not a mental disease.[37]

Later, among contemporary European psychiatrists, Pierre Janet (1859–1947) was one of the first to fight against the usual psychiatric nosologies. Janet used to say that a psychiatric diagnosis referred more to the fortune of the patient than to anything else: if the patient was poor, he was committed in a mental hospital as a "psychotic"; if he could afford the expenses of a private sanitarium, he was put there with the diagnosis of a "neurasthenic." If he was wealthy enough to be isolated in his home under constant watch of nurses and aides, he was simply an "eccentric individual." In his book *La Force et la faiblesse psychologiques* [38] Janet devotes a whole chapter to a sharp criticism of the current psychiatric classifications. However, Janet admits that one can distinguish between two large groups: the organic and the functional diseases. It is, he says, as with an automobile which is stopped: sometimes the car stops because one of the pieces of the machine is broken; sometimes because it is out of gasoline.

The Pragmatic Trend

The rationalist-humanitarian trend of the end of the eighteenth century discarded elaborate nosologies and contented itself, as we have seen, with simple, practical classifications of four or five items. In the first half of the nineteenth century the foremost representative of this trend was Pinel's famous disciple Jean-Dominique Esquirol.

"At the beginning of the continuous development of psychiatric science stands the outstanding personality of Esquirol," writes Karl Jaspers.[39] If ever a man deserved the name of "Father of Modern Psychiatry," it was Jean-Dominique Esquirol (1772–1840). He inaugurated the scientific use of asylum statistics for the study of the causes, course, and prognosis of mental disease. He proclaimed that "an insane asylum is a therapeutic instrument in the hands of an able physician, and our most powerful weapon against mental diseases," which he proved by laying the fundaments of collective therapy. He wrote the first really scientific textbook on mental diseases, which was also the first to have illustrations, a book remarkable for its style and for its clear clinical descriptions.[40] Esquirol defined our present concepts of illusion and hallucination, remission and intermission, dementia and idiocy. His classification is the following:

1. Lypemania (i.e., depressive states)
2. Monomania
3. Mania
4. Dementia
5. Imbecility and idiocy

Esquirol gave up the word *melancholia*, which had for twenty-five centuries designated the most confused agglomeration of mental disorders. The depressive states he called *lypemania;* all other forms of "partial insanity" he put in the group of the *monomanias.*

Esquirol's classification was adopted by most of his disciples, but they soon started to subdivide the five clinical types described by their master, so that the number of clinical conditions in the nosologies steadily increased, to the point that around 1860 the need of a totally new system was felt.

Psychiatric Nosologies Based on Traditional Faculty Psychology

A whole group of psychiatric classifications, particularly flourishing in Germany, were based on the distinction of "faculties of the mind" (mostly the threefold distinction of emotion, intellection, and volition), and of two or three basic morbid processes (e.g., exaltation and depression). By taking into account each type of disorder for each faculty, one found a number of morbid conditions, which were sometimes called "genera" and subdivided into "species," thus combining this "faculty" nosology with the type of nosologies of the systematists of the previous century.

One of the chief promoters of these nosologies was Johann Christian Heinroth (1773–1843), also famous for his contention that the origin of mental disease was sin. In his classification Heinroth distinguished only one class of mental disease: *vesania,* divided into three orders, nine genera, and thirty-six species.[41] The three orders are the exaltations, depressions, and mixtures of these two. The nine genera are obtained by taking in account, in each order, the three faculties (affectivity, spirit, will). Thus we have the following table:

	EXALTATIONS	DEPRESSIONS	MIXED ORDER
EMOTION	Wahnsinn ("insanity")	Melancholia	Wahnsinnige Melancholie (delusional melancholia)
INTELLECTION	Verrücktheit (paranoia)	Blödsinn (dementia)	Verwirrtheit (mental confusion)
VOLITION	Manie	Willenlosigkeit (abulia)	Scheue (fright)

Other German psychiatrists distinguished themselves by the great number of new words they coined, although not always expressing new ideas. An instance is given by the psychiatric nosologic system of Stark (1838).[42]

	AFUNCTION	HYPERFUNCTION	PARAFUNCTION
EMOTION	Athymie	Hyperthymie	Parathymie
INTELLECTION	Anoese	Hypernoese	Paranoese
VOLITION	Abulie	Hyperbulie	Parabulie

Numerous similar classifications were made. Some tried to simplify the nosologic system; for instance Maximilian Jacobi,[43] who distinguished only two fundamental disorders, exaltation and depression, and two faculties of the soul, *Begehrungsvermögen* (desiring, or demanding faculty) and intellect; hence, the following table:

	EXALTATION	DEPRESSION
"DESIRING FACULTY"	Tobsucht (fury)	Schwermut (melancholia)
INTELLECTION	Wahnsinn ("insanity")	Blödsinn (dementia)
MIXED FORM	Delirium	Narrheit (stupidity)

Half a century later Carl Wernicke [44] elaborated this schematic approach just introduced by Heinroth.

A similar type of classification was adopted in England by Hack Tuke (1827–1895). Tuke wrote several psychiatric books, among which is his and Bucknill's *Manual of Psychological Medicine*,[45] in which not less than three classifications were proposed: a "metaphysical," a "symptomatic," and an "aetiological."

The metaphysical classification was based on the distinction of the three main faculties of the soul:

Class I: Diseases of the Intellect
 Order 1: Incomplete development: Idiocy and Imbecility
 Order 2: Disorders after development: Dementia, Delusional Insanity, Ordinary Mania
Class II: Diseases of the Emotions or Moral Sentiments
 Order 1: Incomplete development: Moral Imbecility
 Order 2: Diseases after development: Simple melancholia or Exaltation
Class III: Diseases of the Instincts or Propensities
 Order 1: Uncontrollable propensities: Mania with homicidal or other distinct morbid impulses
 Order 2: Loss of volitional power; paralyzed will

The second or "symptomatic" classification was very simple:

1. Idiocy, imbecility, and cretinism
2. Dementia
3. Delusional insanity
4. Emotional insanity
5. Mania

The third, "aetiological," classification was the following:

I. Protopathic Insanity ("insanity or mental deficiency caused by primary diseases or defective development of the encephalic centres"). Examples: Idiocy. Insanity. General Paralysis. Epileptic Insanity, when of central origin. Senile Insanity. Idio-functional Insanity, i.e., "arising from excessive action or otherwise of the functions of the brain."

II. Denteropathic Insanity ("Insanity caused by disorder of, or developmental changes occurring in other organs than the encephalic centres"). Examples: Pubescent Insanity. Uterine Insanity. Puerperal Insanity. Rheumatic Insanity. Syphilitic Insanity.

III. Toxic Insanity ("Insanity caused by alcohol and other poisons") Examples: Alcoholic Insanity. Pellagrous Insanity.

Using essentially similar principles, but with greater simplicity, was the classification of John Barlow, a British clergyman. His *On Man's Power over Himself to Prevent or Control Insanity*, published in 1853,[46] divides all mental illness into two classes:

I. Morbid affections of the nervous system and brain (containing dementia and confusional states)

II. Morbid affections of the intellectual force, due to:
   1. Inefficiency, in which appetites or instinctive emotions are left wholly uncontrolled
   2. Misdirection, where delusions of sense are reasoned and acted upon
   3. Occultation, in which organs of thought are impaired or wanting

Barlow considered his second class of "mental derangement" to be the consequence of "neglected education, of unregulated passions, of vice, of misery and . . . of mismanagement."

The Course of a Disease as a Basis of Classification

For centuries the peculiar course of a mental illness seems never to have been a factor in the diagnosis. A patient took ill, symptoms were manifested, a state of illness was described, a diagnosis was made, and that was that. The disease was given a name, listed, and classified.

Of course, it is true that as far back as Aretaeus (first century A.D.) the fact that depression and excitement might alternate and in some way or other represent aspects of the same illness was known and recorded. Aretaeus included, among his three types of mania, one which he termed recurrent. Alexander of Tralles also recognized this excessive mood cycle. For Kraepelin this phenomenon was important enough to make the basis of another "entity."

It was not until the nineteenth century that the aspect of variable chronicity in mental illness was squarely faced—in a distinction by Benjamin Rush, in 1813, between acute and chronic mania. In 1838 Jean Etienne Dominique Esquirol introduced into psychiatry the words "remission" and "intermission."

Because of his wide influence, and his emphasis on the longitudinal observation of mental disturbance, Esquirol gave new impetus to the course concept, which before his time had been only occasionally noted. Flemming (1844) following Esquirol's lead, subclassified his types of vesania as acute, chronic, and remitted.

Bénédict-Augustin Morel (1809–1873) described for the first time in 1852 [47] what he called *démence précoce:* not a disease entity, but a particular form of evolution or course of mental disease. "Dementia" meant simply "mental deterioration," and "precocious" referred to the rapidity of evolution; thus "dementia praecox" meant exactly mental deterioration after several months or a few years of disease. This type of evolution, he said, was frequently seen in young men whose ambitions were disproportionate with their abilities.

In Morel's system, for the first time, the longitudinal view of mental disorder became a major determinant in classification, although the physical etiology basis was equally stressed.

Morel attempted to make psychiatry a branch of biology and anthropology. He also incorporated into psychiatry the field of the neuroses, which he called *délires émotifs* (emotional delusions).

One of Morel's best-known concepts is that of *hereditary insanity,* which has been often misunderstood.[48] Morel contended that degeneracy was the root of many clinical conditions, going from slight character disorders to the worst forms of criminality and idiocy. Degeneracy, he said, was often progressive: from one generation to the others its manifestations became worse, until the last generation was sterile, which automatically ended the process. But Morel was not a fatalist: he discussed ways of checking the process of degeneracy and making it reversible. In these studies are the beginnings of social anthropology and racial hygiene. The result of Morel's extensive studies is summarized in the following table: [49]

I. "Insanity" (alienation)
   1. Hereditary Insanity
      a. Nervous character
      b. Perversions of the instincts
      c. Juvenile delinquency
      d. Idiots and imbeciles (hereditary form)
   2. Toxic psychoses (alcoholism, opiumism, etc.)
   3. Insanity arising from hystery, epilepsy, and hypochondry
   4. Sympathetic (i.e., symptomatic) insanity: fever delirium, etc.
   5. Idiopathic (i.e. brain organic) diseases: progressive paresis, etc.
II. Dementia (as a terminal, incurable form of insanity)
III. "Délire émotif," i.e., phobia and other neuroses

Valentin Magnan (1835–1916), who spent his whole career as director of the admission service in the great mental hospital Sainte-Anne, in Paris, extended Morel's concept of "mental degeneracy" to the point that it covered almost the whole realm of psychiatry. Whereas Morel had excluded *délire émotif* (i.e., the neuroses) from degeneracy, Magnan incorporated them into it. There was a time when in the French asylums almost every patient was diagnosed "*Dégénérescence mentale, avec . . .*" the first label being "mental degeneracy" and the second the real diagnosis. Magnan's classification of mental degeneracy was the following: [50]

I. Idiocy, imbecility, and feeble-mindedness
II. Brain abnormities. Lack of balance between the moral and intellectual faculties
III. Episodic syndromes of the degenerates
  1. *Folie du doute*
  2. Aichmophobia (phobia of pointed objects)
  3. Agoraphobia, claustrophobia, topophobia
  4. Dipsomania, sitiomania
  5. Pyromania, pyrophobia
  6. Kleptomania, kleptophobia, oniomania (impulsion to buy unnecessary things)
  7. *Manie du jeu* (gamble-fury)
  8. Homicidal and suicidal impulsions
  9. Onomatomania (with five subforms)
  10. Arithmomania
  11. Echolalia, coprolalia, with chorea (Gilles de la Tourette's syndrome)
  12. Exaggerated love for animals, antivivisectionists' madness
  13. Sexual abnormities, perversions, and deviations
    a. Spinal form (masturbation of the idiots)
    b. Posterior spino-cerebral form (brutal, undifferentiated sexual reaction)
    c. Anterior spino-cerebral form (impulsive sexual reactions to specific, differentiated stimulants)
    d. Anterior cerebral form (ecstatic, desexualized form of love)
  14. Abulia
IV.
  A. Multiple delusions
    a. Delusions of ambition
    b. Religious delusions
    c. Delusions of persecution
  B. *Manie raisonnante* (reasoning mania). *Folie morale* (moral insanity)

It was in the work of Kahlbaum (1828–1899) that the patient's age at the time of onset and the characteristic development of the disturbance were first used systematically. Karl Ludwig Kahlbaum was one of the most gifted of the German descriptive psychiatrists, foreshadowing Kraepelin in his attempt to apply the principles of natural science to clinical psychiatry. He sought to arrive at a unitary concept of mental illness based upon Morel's nosological principles of unity of cause, course, and outcome (and, if possible, a specific lesion). Notable contributions to nosological formulations in psychiatry were his distinction between the temporary symptom-complex and the underlying personality disease, and his recognition that most of the so-called forms of "insanity" are merely pictures, or symptom-complexes.

Kahlbaum's first important publication was a book on the classification of mental diseases (1863).[51] It begins with a review of the previous psychiatric classifications, distinguishing three groups: 1. systems comprising a fairly great number of fundamental types (i.e., Boissier de Sauvages); 2. systems with a small number of such types; 3. systems acknowledging only one disease (Neumann). Kahlbaum then discusses the fundamental rules of psychiatric nosology. His first rule is the distinction between organic and nonorganic mental disease; the second rule is the distinction between "total" and "partial" insanity (the old distinction between "mania" and "melancholia"); the third rule is the taking into account the whole course of evolution of the disease, as a means of isolating specific disease entities. Kahlbaum adopts the ideas of Heinrich Neumann about the existence of a mental disease with the four successive stages of melancholia, mania, *Verwirrtheit*, and *Blödsinn*. But in contrast to Neumann he admits, besides this *Vesania typica*, the existence of other specific diseases, recognizable by their different type of evolution. Finally, Kahlbaum still retains the old systematist concept of natural classes, genera, and species of diseases.

Kahlbaum's classification of 1863 is as follows:

I. Class of the Neophrenias: "Disturbances acquired before, with, or shortly after birth, characterized by a lack of psychological content in the manifestations of life"
   1. Genus Neophrenia innata (congenital forms of idiocy)
   2. Genus Neophrenia morbosa (idiocy resulting of a somatic disease acquired before birth)
   3. Genus Neophrenia carens (idiocy with lack of one of the sensorial organs)

II. Class of the Paraphrenias: "Disturbances appearing in connection with one of the periods of transition of biological development"
   1. Genus Paraphrenia hebetica, appearing during puberty
      Species Hebephrenia
   2. Genus Paraphrenia senilis, appearing in old age
      Species Presybophrenia
   3. Genus Paraphrenia hypnotica, appearing during sleep

III. Class of the Vecordias, or Enphrenias: "Idiopathic disturbances of mental life with limitation of the extent of the symptoms, beginning after puberty"
   A. Family Vecordia dysthymia: predominance of emotional disturbances
      1. Genus Dysthymia melaena, with predominance of sad emotions
      2. Genus Dysthymia elata, with predominance of joyous emotions
   B. Family Vecordia Paranoia: predominance of intellectual disturbances
      1. Genus Paranoia ascensa, with exaltation of self-feeling
      2. Genus Paranoia descensa, with depression of self-feeling
      3. Genus Paranoia immota, without modifications of self-feeling
   C. Family Vecordia Diastrophia: predominance of disturbances of volition
      1. Genus Diastrophia
   D. Family Vecordia insania: partial disturbance without predominance of one of the various functions of mental life
      1. Genus Insania

IV. Class of the Vesanias, or Panphrenias: "Idiopathic disturbances of mental life affecting the more or less complete extent of psychic life"
   1. Genus Vesania acuta (Phrenitis)
      Species: Phrenitis primaria, Phrenitis secundaria
   2. Genus Vesania typica ("idiopathic mental disease taking its course in four stages")

Species: Typica completa
Typica simplex
Typica praeceps
B. Genus Vesania progressiva ("idiopathic disturbances of mental life with true increasing of the symptoms during the course of the disease")
Species: Progressiva completa (progressive paresis)
Progressiva divergens
Progressiva simplex
Progressiva apoplectica
V. Class of the Dysphrenias ("sympathetic and symptomatic mental disturbances, developing in connection to a specific physiologic or pathological bodily condition, characterized by a total illness of psychic life and mixture of the symptoms")
A. Family Dysphrenia nervosa (originating in disease of the nervous system)
1. Genus Nervosa excitata
2. Genus Nervosa depressa
3. Genus Nervosa epileptica
B. Family Dysphrenia chymosa (originating in disease of the vegetative system)
1. Genus Chymosa excitata
2. Genus Chymosa depressa
C. Family Dysphrenia sexualis (originating in disease of sexual organs)
1. Genus Sexualis excitata
2. Genus Sexualis depressa

Kahlbaum's book of 1863 was in his mind a preliminary report and a program of a more ambitious undertaking: a collection of publications on his clinical studies. The writing of his first contribution was delegated to his collaborator, Ewald Hecker (1871), who described hebephrenia as a pubertal psychosis terminating in rapid deterioration, thus combining longitudinal observation of the course of illness with recognition that certain disorders were associated with specific periods in the life span. Obviously it is the same condition which Morel in 1852 had called *démence précoce*.

Kahlbaum described catatonia first in 1869, and in his famous monograph on the subject (1874)[52] he described it as beginning slowly and progressing to deterioration. He introduced the terms "symptom-complex," "verbigeration," "paraphrenia," and "cyclothymia." Kahlbaum's main nosological categories embody concepts which anticipated many of Kraepelin's, but his plan, wrote Meyer, "required the digestion of too many new terms, new ideas and new facts." The fundamentals could not be understood as simply as in the form which later was given them by Kraepelin.[53]

Although Kahlbaum's ideas were not much accepted in his lifetime, they influenced deeply the prevailing concepts of German psychiatry at the end of the nineteenth century. To take the course of disease as a principle of classification was one of the nosologic principles of Kraepelin, who, on the other hand, took over from Kahlbaum the clinical pictures of hebephrenia and catatonia.

The classification of the Scottish psychiatrist David Skae,[54] director of the

Edinburgh Royal Asylum, was less organized and more elaborate, but maintained the same conspicuous simplicity: Emphasis was placed on correlating clinical pictures to stages of the physiological development and general diseases.

1. Idiocy ⎫ Moral and
2. Imbecility ⎰ Intellectual
3. Insanity, with Epilepsy
4. Insanity of Masturbation
5. Mania of Pubescence
6. Satyriasis
7. Nymphomania
8. Hysterical Mania
9. Amenorrhaeal Mania
10. Post-Connubial Mania
11. Puerperal Mania
12. Mania of Pregnancy
13. Mania of Lactation
14. Climacteric Mania
15. Ovario-Mania (Utero-Mania, Insanity of Old Maids)
16. Senile Mania
17. Phthisical Mania
18. Metastatic Mania (following sudden suppression of a discharge or eruption)
19. Traumatic Mania and Sunstroke Mania
20. Syphilitic Mania
21. Delirium Tremens
22. Dipsomania
23. Mania of Alcoholism
24. Post-Febrile Mania
25. Mania of Oxaluria and Phosphaturia
26. General Paralysis, with Insanity
27. Idiopathic Mania: a. Sthenic; b. Asthenic

R. Krafft-Ebing (1840–1902), best known for his discovery of the relationship of general paralysis to syphilis and for his studies of sex, used as one of the three major psychiatric categories "psychical degenerate states" and classified the psychoneuroses (in which he included mania and melancholia) into *primary curable* and *secondary incurable* conditions, the latter being again divided into chronic mania and terminal dementia. While not very clear or logical, this marked the most systematic application of the course principle to classification which had been undertaken up to his time.[55] (The nosology was only slightly revised during seven editions which appeared between 1880 and 1903.)

In the classification of Savage, stages in the life span were utilized as the main categories, beginning with insanities of early development and continuing through forms associated with adolescence, maturity, the climacteric, and age. This quite unique classification was the following: [56]

I. Insanity of early development:
    Idiocy, imbecility
    Epilepsy, brain diseases
    Mania, melancholia, moral perversions
II. Insanity of adolescence:
    Mania with conceit; emotional melancholia and hypochondriasis
III. Insanity of maturity:
    Mania

    Melancholia
    Dementia
    General paralysis
IV. Insanity of climacterium:
    A. In women: delusions, "persecutions," hallucinations
    B. In men: hypochondriasis
V. Insanity of age:
    Mania, melancholia, dementia

The Physiopathological Trend

The discovery by Bayle (1822) that progressive paresis was a specific organic brain disease, and by Paul Broca (1861) that certain forms of aphasia were correlated with definite lesions of the cortex, brought about numerous attempts to found a purely organic psychiatry. This trend became more and more important during the second half of the nineteenth century, to the extent that around 1880 a psychiatry based on brain anatomopathology and physiopathology was considered the only scientific one. This trend was particularly dominant in German university psychiatry, where it was introduced by Wilhelm Griesinger (1817–1868).

Although Griesinger had not worked much with mentally ill patients when he published his textbook, and although he borrowed most of his case histories from French authors, he spoke with great positiveness and enunciated what seemed to be the final principles of scientific psychiatry. From his slogan "Mental diseases are brain diseases" he deduced the necessity of organizing insane asylums on the model of neurological hospitals. Mental diseases, he said, ought to be classified according to their underlying brain lesions, but since knowledge of brain anatomopathology was as yet incomplete, one had to be content provisionally with a "functional" classification. Griesinger adopted Neumann's concept that there was *one* mental disease, "insanity," and that all clinical pictures were stages of one basic morbid process, which, however, had a few variations. In this morbid process there were two phases. In the first phase, where the disease was mostly still curable, belonged *melancholia, mania,* or *monomania.* In the second phase, mostly incurable, belonged *chronic mania* or *dementia.* From the purely descriptive point of view, Griesinger distinguished three types of reaction: depression, exaltation, weakness.

Griesinger's ideas had an enormous influence, and his textbook (1845, 1861) was a success.[57] His classification therein was the following:

A. States of Mental Depression
  1. Hypochondriasis
  2. Melancholia in a More Limited Sense
  3. Melancholia with Stupor
  4. Melancholia with Destructive Tendencies
    a. With Suicidal Tendencies
    b. With Murderous Tendencies
  5. Melancholia with Persistent Excitement of the Will

B. States of Mental Exaltation
  1. Mania
  2. Monomania

C. States of Mental Weakness
  1. Chronic Mania
  2. Dementia
  3. Apathetic Dementia
  4. Idiocy and Cretinism

General paralysis was described in the chapter on the "complications of insanity."

With his slogan "Mental diseases are brain diseases," Griesinger declared war against the survivors of the old philosophical and empirical-psychological schools of psychiatry. For him and his successors, such as Meynert and Wernicke, brain anatomy was the one firm basis of all psychiatry. Where brain lesions were not demonstrable under the microscope, they assumed the existence of vascular, nutritional, or other functional disorders of the brain.

Theodor Meynert (1833–1892), a keen student of brain anatomy, supplemented his objective findings with hypotheses on the functional opposition between brain cortex and brain stem, and the role of physiological brain disturbances. His classification, expounded in his *Textbook of Psychiatry* (1884),[58] was the following:

A. Mental disorders resulting from anatomical changes:
   1. Malformations of the skull and brain (idiocy, cretinism, deafmutism)
   2. Focal anatomical processes of the brain (deliria, palsy, localized dementia, traumatic confusion, symptomatic chorea, disposition through residuals of such processes)
   3. Diffuse anatomical processes of the brain and its membranes (dementia, general paresis, senile dementia, deliria, basal meningitis, epilepsy, etc.)

B. Mental disorders resulting from nutritional disorders of the brain:
   1. Cortical irritative processes:
     a. Irritable mood. Pure maniacal excitement.
     b. Simple melancholia, depressed mood.
     c. Simple mania. Chorea.
   2. Irritable states of subcortical sensory centers:
     a. General delusional states. Simple hallucinatory confusion. Compound hallucinatory confusion with stuporous and manic periods or developments.
     b. Irritable states of subcortical sensory and common feeling or coenesthetic centers. Hypochondriasis. Hysteria.
     c. Partial delusional states: delusions of being noticed, persecuted; megalomania.
   3. Disorders of the subcortical vascular centers and hyperesthesia. Epilepsy, hystero-epilepsy:
     a. Exhaustibility
     b. Circular psychoses.

C. Intoxications

Later Meynert modified his classification, giving an increased importance to *amentia,* a vague clinical type including much of what is today called schizophrenia.

In Theodor Ziehen's textbook (1894) the major distinction is made between psychosis with and without intellectual deficit. Those with deficit are subdivided into a group with congenital and a group with acquired defects, whereas the class of defect-free psychoses is subdivided into a group of simple and one of complex syndromes. Ziehen's classification is a clinical one, as one can see from the following table:

I. Psychoses without intellectual deficit
  A. Simple psychoses
    1. Affective psychoses, with major symptoms in the realm of affect
      a) Mania
      b) Melancholia
      c) Neurasthenia
    2. Intellectual psychoses, with major symptoms in the intellectual realm
      a) Stupidity
      b) Paranoia
        Simple paranoia

> > > Hallucinatory paranoia
> > > With flight of ideas
> > > With stupor
> > > With incoherence
> > c) Madness from compulsive ideas
> B. Complex psychoses, combining several major symptoms
> > a) Secondary hallucinatory paranoia
> > b) Post-manic and post-melancholic stupidity
> > c) Post-neurasthenic hypochondriac melancholy and paranoia
> > d) Post-melancholic hypochondriac paranoia
> > e) Melancholic-manic madness
> > f) Catatonia
> II. Defect psychoses
> > A. Congenital defect psychoses
> > > a) Idiocy
> > > b) Imbecility
> > > c) Debility
> > B. Acquired defect psychoses
> > > a) Dementia paralytica
> > > b) Senile dementia
> > > c) Secondary dementia after brain disease
> > > d) Secondary dementia after functional psychoses
> > > e) Epileptic dementia
> > > f) Alcoholic dementia

One of the most famous promotors of physiopathological psychiatry was Carl Wernicke (1848–1905), a brain-anatomist, a psychopathologist, and a brilliant clinician. Wernicke began his career with a study of aphasia (1874), synthesizing the points of view of associationist psychology, physiology of the nervous reflex arc, and brain anatomy. He considered the brain an associative organ; he considered the soul to be "the sum of all possible associations." Only the most elementary mental functions are localized in the cortex, he said; the higher ones, including consciousness, are products of the associative activity. Subcortical aphasia results from interruptions of the reflex arc and "sejunction" of associations.

On the model of this aphasia theory, Wernicke attempted to build an over-all system of organicist and mechanistic psychiatry, which he expounded in his *Textbook of Psychiatry* (1900).[59] Wernicke rejected the etiological principle as a basis of nosology: since a certain syndrome can result from many different agents, and since one morbific agent can determine many different symptoms, Wernicke acknowledged only clinical syndromes related to distinct brain areas.

Wernicke distinguished three hypothetical brain areas, those of the sensory and motor "projection fields" and the totality of association fibers between these. He also distinguished three basic types of disorder: deficit, excess, and distortion. From this he composed the following table: [60]

	PSYCHOSENSORY	PSYCHOMOTOR	INTRAPSYCHIC
DEFICIT	Anaesthesia	Akinesia	Afunction
EXCESS	Hyperaesthesia	Hyperkinesia	Hyperfunction
DISTORTION	Paraesthesia	Parakinesia	Parafunction

On the other hand, Wernicke distinguished "districts of consciousness" [61] which he assumed to be localized in different fields of the brain cortex. These functional aspects of consciousness were the consciousness of one's own body, of one's own individuality, and of the outside world. Hence this purely clinical classification of mental diseases: [62]

I. Allopsychoses (psychoses with disorientation in the outside world)
   1. Delirium tremens
   2. Korsakov's psychosis
   3. Presbyophrenia
II. Autopsychoses (psychoses with disorientation in the representation of one's own individuality)
   1. Mania (with ideas of grandeur)
   2. Melancholia (with ideas of indignity, etc.)
III. Somatopsychoses (psychoses with disorientation in the representation of one's own body)
   1. Anxiety psychoses
   2. Hypochondriac psychoses

Omnibus Nosologies

During the last two decades of the nineteenth century, a gigantic effort was made to synthesize the various nosologic approaches: the clinical-descriptive approach, the somatic approach including neurology and brain anatomy, and particularly the consideration of the course of the disease.

The name of Emil Kraepelin (1856–1926) is pre-eminent in this polyvalent effort, as an exponent of detailed description, as a logical systematizer, and as an advocate of the etiological explanatory basis of classification. Kraepelin was the product and synthesizer of the work of others. He was by no means the first nosologist to recognize the need for longitudinal study of mental illness, nor the first to associate certain forms of disturbance with age periods, nor the first to classify diseases in terms of outcome. Yet his system provided within itself an explanation of the concepts utilized, and effected a synthesis which showed their interrelationships. This fact was, as we shall see, both the strength and the weakness of his nosology. As it developed through the nine editions of his textbook, the classification became not the product of a theory but a theory itself, and one which exercised a retarding effect upon new theory and new classification demanded by new facts.

The nosological productions of Kraepelin provided the resolution of problems which for centuries had preoccupied psychiatrists. It has been said that in the twenty-seven years covered by the nine editions of his famous textbook Kraepelin unintentionally wrote a history of clinical psychiatry.[63] From a small compendium, first appearing in 1883, it evolved into the imposing two-volume work of 2425 pages in the ninth edition (published in 1927, a year after Kraepelin's death).

Kraepelin is best known for his descriptive delineation of the two major synthesized concepts: dementia praecox and manic-depressive psychosis. Following Griesinger, and taking general paralysis as a paradigm of mental disorder, Kraepelin regarded mental illnesses as organic disease entities which could be classified on the basis of etiology, course, and outcome. He divided most of the so-called acute disorders into recoverable forms and the deteriorating forms. His prognostic approach to mental illnesses was probably the most outstanding and original of his nosological innovations, and later became one of the most controversial issues.[64]

Kraepelin's formulations of disease entities represent, for the most part, brilliant syntheses of more or less isolated concepts arrived at during the preceding generation by French and German workers who had done much of the analytical spadework—the older Falret, Hecker, Kahlbaum, Morel, Moreau, Magnan, and others. Even the conception of symptom-complexes (as distinct from the underlying disease-process), and the descriptive methodology which regarded course and outcome within a unitary concept of disease-entities, had been advanced by Morel and Kahlbaum many years before Kraepelin's books appeared. In his delineation of manic-depressive psychoses, Kraepelin crystallized a years-old vague tendency of psychiatrists to associate mania with depression, a trend which had become more articulate since the description of *folie circulaire* by Falret the older, and *folie à double forme* by Baillarger during the 1850s, and the description of *cyclothymia* by Kahlbaum in 1882. Likewise Kraepelin's formulation of depression can be traced through the work of Guislain, Griesinger, Krafft-Ebing, Kahlbaum, and Hecker.

In 1883 appeared Kraepelin's modest *Compendium* of 400 pages, with the following classification:

1. Depression (simple melancholia, melancholia with delusions)
2. Twilight states (hypnosis, epilepsy, hysteria, stupor, acute dementia)
3. Excitement (melancholia activa, mania, deliria with excitement)
4. Periodic psychoses (periodic mania, periodic melancholia, circular states)
5. *"Primaere Verrücktheit"*
6. Dementia paralytica (i.e., progressive paresis)
7. States of psychological weakness
   a. Idiocy, cretinism, feeble-mindedness, *"conträre Sexualempfindung"* (i.e., homosexuality)
   b. Moral insanity, *Querulantenwahn* (litiginous insanity)
   c. Neurasthenic states, obsessions, phobias, impulsions
   d. Senile dementia
   e. Secondary weakness states (*"secondary Verrücktheit,"* secondary *Blödsinn*)

Kraepelin placed in the category of "psychologic weakness" the most disparate conditions, including homosexuality (under the influence of Krafft-Ebing) and obsessions and phobias (under the influence of Morel). He also borrowed from the French the concept of the "circular states."

This system was considerably modified in the second edition, now called a *Short Textbook*, with 540 pages, published in 1887. The new classification was as follows:

1. Melancholia
   a. M. activa
   b. M. simplex
   c. M. attonita
2. Mania
3. Delirium
   a. Fever delirium
   b. Toxic delirium
   c. Transient delirium
   d. Hallucinatory confusion
4. Acute exhaustion states
   a. Acute delirium
   b. Collapsus delirium
   c. Asthenic confusion
   d. Acute dementia
5. *"Wahnsinn"* (i.e., systema-

tized delusions)
a. Depressed
b. Expansive
c. Hallucinatory
6. Periodical and circular insanity
a. Periodical psychoses (periodical mania, p. melancholia, p. insanity)
b. Circular insanity
7. "*Verrücktheit*" (paranoia)
a. Depressive form (with many subforms, particularly delusions of persecution)
b. Expansive form (delusions of grandeur)
8. "General neuroses"
a. Neurasthenia, obsessions, phobias, hypochondriasis, compulsions

b. Hysterical insanity
c. Epileptic insanity
9. Chronic intoxications
a. Alcoholism
b. Morphinism
10. Dementia paralytica
11. Acquired states of weakness
a. Senile dementia
b. Mental weakness resulting from organic brain diseases
c. Secondary states of mental weakness
12. Developmental abnormities
a. Idiocy
b. Cretinism
c. Feeble-mindedness
d. "*Conträre Sexualempfindung*" (i.e., homosexuality)

Two years later, in 1889, the third edition of the *Short Textbook* appeared. It was slightly larger (574 pages). The classification was not much modified. It is noteworthy that *Wahnsinn* now included the depressed, expansive, and hallucinatory forms as before, plus a new form, the *catatonic*.

In 1891 Kraepelin was called to be professor of psychiatry at the University of Heidelberg. In the psychiatric clinic there the patients seemed to be of quite a different sort from those he had seen at Dorpat. This incited him to make important changes in his nosologic system. The fourth edition of his *Short Textbook* was not only enlarged (693 pages) but completely transformed. In the foreword Kraepelin stressed again the impossibility of making a sharp line of demarcation between mental health and mental disease, and between the different forms of mental disease. However, he added, the needs of medical practice demanded some kind of classification, which had to be established as scientifically as possible. The new classification he proposed was the following:

1. Deliriums (fever delirium, intoxication delirium)
2. Acute Exhaustion States (collapsus delirium, Amentia, acute dementia)
3. Mania
4. Melancholia
5. "*Wahnsinn*"
   a. Hallucinatory form
   b. Depressive form
6. Periodical mental diseases:
   a. Delirious form
   b. Manic form
   c. Circular form

d. Depressive form
7. "*Verrücktheit*," alias Paranoia
   a. Depressive form
   b. Expansive form
8. Psychic degeneracy processes
   a. Dementia praecox
   b. Catatonia
   c. Dementia paranoides
9. General Neuroses
   a. Neurasthenia
   b. Hysteria
   c. Epilepsy
10. Chronic Intoxications
    a. Alcoholism

b. Morphinism
c. Cocainism
11. Dementia paralytica
12. Acquired states of mental weakness
    a. Senile dementia

b. Organic brain diseases
13. Developmental abnormities
    a. Idiocy
    b. Cretinism
    c. Feeble-mindedness
    d. Homosexuality

In this fourth edition are a few new names: the old *Verrücktheit* ("craziness") takes the more dignified name of *paranoia*; Meynert's *amentia* appears among acute exhaustion conditions; Morel's concept of degeneracy is adopted to explain conditions where an "uncommonly rapid development" terminates in a chronic state of "mental weakness"; three subforms are listed: dementia praecox (a word borrowed from Morel), catatonia (incorporating the essential features of Kahlbaum's description), and dementia paranoides.

After three further years of intensive activity, the fifth edition of Kraepelin's book was issued (1896), now no more called a *Short Textbook*, but *A Textbook*. It contained 815 pages, with photographs, graphs, and samples of handwritings. The nosologic system was completely recast, the purely empiric clinical pictures having disappeared, and the new classification based on the origin, course of evolution, and termination of the mental diseases. Thus the following classification:

I. Acquired mental diseases
   1. Exhaustion states
   2. Intoxications
      a. Acute
      b. Chronic (alcoholism, morphinism, cocainism)
   3. Metabolic diseases
      a. Myxoedema
      b. Cretinism
      c. *Verblödungsprocesse* ("dementifying processes")
         (1) Dementia praecox
         (2) Catatonia
         (3) Dementia paranoides
   4. Insanity resulting from brain diseases
   5. Involutional diseases (involution melancholia, senile dementia)
II. Mental disease resulting from a morbid constitutional predisposition
   1. Constitutional mental diseases
      a. Periodic psychosis (mania, circular psychosis, depression)
      b. *Verrücktheit*, alias paranoia (combinatory p., phantastic p.)
   2. General neuroses: epilepsy, hysteria, fright-neurosis
III. Psychopathic conditions (degeneracy insanity)
   1. Constitutional neurasthenia
   2. Compulsive insanity
   3. Impulsive insanity
   4. *"Conträre Sexualempfindung"* (psychic hermaphroditism, homosexuality)
IV. Developmental inhibitions
   1. Imbecility
   2. Idiocy

In this fifth edition the group of dementia praecox, catatonia, and dementia paranoides has been taken away from "degeneracy," and ascribed to "metabolic diseases." On the other hand, neurasthenia, compulsions, phobias, and impulsions are ranged, close to homosexuality, in the category of conditions issuing from "degeneracy." The word "psychopathy" is equated to "degeneracy." However, by far the most important feature of this edition is the emphasis given to the two big groups of "endogenous" psychoses: the "periodic psychoses," and the *Verblödungsprocesse.*

The sixth edition (1899) gave the definitive pattern of Kraepelin's nosologic system as it became generally known, with the grouping and naming of his two big endogenous psychoses: *manic-depressive psychosis,* and *dementia praecox.* Once more, the *Textbook* was "completely recast" and now published in two volumes; one on general psychiatry, with 341 pages, and one on clinical psychiatry, with 602 pages. Kraepelin gave up the fourfold arrangement of the preceding edition and went back to a less systematic but clearer classification.

1. Infectious mental conditions (fever delirium, infection delirium and weakness)
2. Exhaustion states (collapsus delirium, amentia, chronic nervous exhaustion)
3. Intoxications: acute; chronic (alcoholism, morphinism, cocainism)
4. Thyreogenic conditions (myxoedema, cretinism)
5. Dementia praecox
   a. Hebephrenic form
   b. Catatonic form
   c. Paranoid form
6. Dementia paralytica
7. Mental disorders in brain diseases (diffused diseases, circumscribed ones)
8. Involution diseases (involution melancholia, praesenile delusions of injury, senile dementia)
9. Manic-depressive psychosis: manic states, depressive states, mixed states
10. *Verrücktheit,* alias Paranoia
11. General neuroses: epilepsy, hysteria, fright neuroses
12. Psychopathic conditions (degeneracy): neurasthenia, compulsions, impulsions, homosexuality
13. Developmental inhibitions: imbecility, idiocy

This sixth edition of Kraepelin's *Textbook* had worldwide success and marked the beginning of the so-called "Kraepelinian era" in psychiatry (1899–1920). Contemporaries had the feeling that he had brought definitive light into the chaos of psychiatric nosology. Kraepelin was promoted to the directorship of the Munich university clinic, where he attracted a brilliant team of first-class collaborators and founded the first great *Forschungsanstalt* (Institute for Psychiatric Research). The clinical material he found in the large city was different from that of the small university town of Heidelberg, hence the increased emphasis on psychoneuroses and character disorders in the *seventh edition* of the *Textbook:*

1. Infectious mental conditions
2. Exhaustion states
3. Intoxications

4. Thyrogenic conditions
5. Dementia praecox (with the hebephrenic, catatonic, and paranoid forms)
6. Dementia paralytica
7. Mental disorders in brain diseases
8. Involution diseases
9. Manic-depressive psychosis
10. *Verrücktheit*, alias Paranoia
11. Epilepsy
12. Psychogenic neuroses
    a. Hysteria
    b. Fright neurosis
    c. Expectation neurosis
13. Mental conditions of constitutional origin (*originäre Krankheitszustände*)
    a. Neurasthenia
    b. *Konstitutionelle Verstimmung* (constitutional ill-humour)
    c. Constitutional excitement
    d. Compulsive states
    e. Impulsive states
    f. Sexual abnormities: masturbation, exhibitionism, fetishism, masochism, sadism, homosexuality, etc.
14. Psychopathic personalities
    a. The born criminal
    b. The unstable
    c. Pathological liars and swindlers
    d. *Pseudoquerulanten* (pseudo-litigatory paranoiacs)
15. Developmental inhibitions: imbecility, idiocy

Epilepsy is definitively taken away from the neuroses in the seventh edition. Neuroses are put into two groups, the one supposed to be of purely psychogenic origin, and the other conditioned by a constitutional predisposition. The concept of the "born criminal," shaped by Lombroso, is introduced into psychiatry.

The eighth edition of the now world-famous *Textbook* was the culmination of Kraepelin's celebrity. It now was in four volumes, published serially from 1909 to 1915, one volume of general psychiatry of 696 pages, and three volumes of clinical psychiatry totaling 2372 pages. There were now more than 400 illustrations and 45 samples of handwriting. However, in spite of all these aggrandizements, the fundamental pattern of the *Textbook* was not basically modified. There were now 17 groups:

1. Mental conditions resulting from brain injuries
2. Mental conditions resulting from brain diseases
3. Intoxications: acute, and chronic (alcoholism, morphinism, cocainism)
4. Infections (fever delirium, infection delirium, amentia, mental weakness)
5. Syphilitic mental conditions, aside from paralysis
6. Dementia paralytica
7. Senile and praesenile conditions
8. Thyrogenic conditions

9. Endogenous conditions with evolution toward deterioration:
   A. Dementia praecox: hebephrenia, depressive form, catatonia, para-
      noid form, schizophasic form
   B. Paraphrenias
10. Epilepsy
11. Manic-depressive psychosis
12. Psychogenic conditions
13. Hysteria
14. Paranoia
15. Mental disorders resulting from a constitutional predisposition
16. Psychopathic personalities
17. Oligophrenia

Among other modifications, new subforms of dementia praecox were isolated, while a borderline group of *paraphrenias* was distinguished from paranoid dementia praecox and from paranoia. The word V*errücktheit*, now all too
obsolete, was discarded. The word *oligophrenia*, now widely used in European
psychiatry, designated the various forms of idiocy, imbecility, and feeble-
mindedness.

Kraepelin's lifelong work represents probably the greatest nosologic synthesis
ever accomplished in psychiatry. Most of the systems of his contemporaries
and immediate successors were imitations of his, or inspired from him.

As the most persuasive proponent of the biological method in psychiatry,
Kraepelin succeeded in bringing about some degree of fusion of psychiatry and
medicine, which had been the goal and ideal of psychiatric workers since the
time of Hippocrates. Perhaps his greatest contribution was the perfection,
through large-scale application, of a method of clinical research adapted from
the methods used in the natural sciences, which traced the course of mental
disorder in individual cases from its earliest manifestations on through to its
termination. He provided a systematic method of clinical investigation within
a theoretical framework, which proved a tremendous impetus to psychiatric
research in the twentieth century.

Furthermore, his application of the principle of prognosis as a nosological
criterion provided a most practical tool for the clinical worker, who is interested primarily in the fate of the patient. This was fully appreciated even by
Kraepelin's critics; Meyer said that the "most suggestive and refreshing impetus of Kraepelin's departure does not lie quite as much in the creation of
pathologically analyzed and unmistakably understood types [as] in the spirit
of emphasis of that which is medically most important. That impetus will
never be lost by one who has ever been affected by it." [65]

On the other hand, the emphasis on pragmatic considerations not only contaminated the scientific purity of his concepts but, even from the clinical
standpoint, proved to be a "two-edged sword." [66] The intimate association of
prognosis with diagnosis tended to encourage a fatalistic and dogmatic attitude
not conducive to wholehearted therapeutic efforts.

An apparent paradox in the success of the Kraepelinian system is that in
spite of its sudden and understood popularity and acceptance by psychiatric
workers in many different countries, it immediately was subjected to considerable revision and criticism. It seemed to resolve nosological problems which
had plagued investigators for centuries, but the achievement of this triumph
also seemed to expose or point up the essential weakness of the nosological

principles which had been used, even in the Kraepelinian system itself. This weakness was the lack of a scientific concept of the human personality.

AMERICAN CLASSIFICATIONS

In 1869, at the annual meeting of the American Medico-Psychological Association, which was the name of the American Psychiatric Association at that time, Dr. Charles H. Nichols called attention to certain proposals of the International Congress of Alienists held in Paris in 1867. This body had adopted for statistical purposes the following method of classification:

1. *Simple Insanity* comprehends the different varieties of Mania, Melancholia, and Monomania, Circular Insanity, and Mixed Insanity, Delusion of Persecution, Moral Insanity, and the Dementia following these different forms of insanity.
2. *Epileptic Insanity* means Insanity with epilepsy, whether the convulsive affection has preceded the Insanity and has seemed to have been the cause, or it has appeared, during the course of the mental disease, only as a symptom or complication.
3. *Paralytic Insanity*, or Dementia, should be considered as a distinct morbid entity, and not at all as a complication, a termination of certain forms of Insanity. There should be comprehended, then, under the name of paralytic insane, all the insane who show, in any degree whatever, the characteristic symptoms of this disease.
4. *Senile Dementia* is the slow and progressive enfeeblement of the intellectual and moral faculties consequent upon old age.
5. *Organic Dementia* embraces all the varieties of Dementia other than the preceding, and which are caused by organic lesions of the brain, nearly always local, and presenting, as almost constant symptoms, hemiplegic occurrences more or less prolonged.
6. *Idiocy* is characterized by the absence or arrest of the development of the intellectual and moral faculties, Imbecility and Weakness of Mind constituting two degrees or varieties.
7. *Cretinism* is characterized by a lesion of the intellectual faculties more or less analogous to that observed in Idiocy, but with which is uniformly associated a characteristic vicious conformation of the body, an arrest of the development of the entirety of the organism.
8. "Ill-defined forms," or "other forms," all the varieties of mental alienation which it shall seem impossible to associate with any of the preceding typical forms.[67]

Doctor Nichols proposed that similar statistical studies be undertaken by American psychiatrists, and, according to May,[68] a series of twenty-one statistical tables was prepared and used unofficially for several years, although never formally adopted.

In 1886 the Association of Medical Superintendents of American Institutions for the Insane (which in 1892 became the American Medico-Psychological Association and in 1921 the American Psychiatric Association) adopted the classification of the British Medico-Psychological Association, with the omission of moral insanity and with the addition of toxic insanity.

But several contemporaries continued to make new proposals. Among these was Stearns, superintendent of the Retreat for the Insane in Hartford, Connecticut, whose etiological interests in mental disease are well represented in the following classification:

A. Symptomalogical
  1. Melancholia
  2. Mania
  3. *Folie circulaire*
  4. Dementia
  5. Primary delusional insanity
B. Aetiological
  1. Epochal (physiological)
     Insanity of puberty
     Climacteric insanity
     Senile insanity
  2. Sympathetic (sexual)
     Puerperal insanity
     Masturbatic insanity
     Ovarian insanity
  3. Toxic
     Alcoholic insanity
     Syphilitic insanity

4. Neuropathic
   Epileptic insanity
   Hysterical insanity
   Choreic insanity
5. Pathological
   General paralysis
   Insanity from coarse brain disease
   Traumatic insanity
   Acute delirium (typhomania)
6. Other less frequent genera and species
   Phthisical insanity, Rheumatic insanity, Gouty insanity, Pellagrous insanity, Post Febrile insanity [69]

In 1909 the New York State Commission in Lunacy adopted a classification which had been proposed in 1905 for use of the mental hospitals of that state. The Commission was assisted in this project by Adolf Meyer, then Director of the Pathological Institute, and by Theodore Hoch and a committee of superintendents of the mental hospitals.* In addition to the classification, which was devised entirely for clinico-pathological purposes, a statistical table was prepared.**

---

* Clinico-Pathological Classification of New York State Hospitals:
  1. Brain tumor
  2. Traumatic psychoses
  3. Psychoses accompanying other nervous diseases
  4. Senile psychoses
  5. General paralysis
  6. Alcoholic psychoses (with subdivision into types)
  7. Morphinism and cocainism, etc.
  8. Infective-exhaustive psychoses (delirious types)
  9. Allied disorders
  10. Depression not sufficiently distinguished
  11. Melancholia symptomatic
  12. Depressive hallucinosis

  13. Involution melancholia
  14. Disorders allied to the depressions
  15. Paranoic conditions
  16. Dementia praecox
  17. Allied disorders
  18. Manic-depressive psychoses (first, second, third, fourth, etc., attack)
  19. Allied disorders
  20. Constitutional inferiority
  21. Hysterical insanity
  22. Epileptic insanity
  23. Imbecility and idiocy with insanity
  24. Not classified
  25. Not insane

Church, Archibald, and Peterson, Frederick: *Nervous and Mental Diseases*, ed. 9. Philadelphia: Saunders, 1919.

** Statistical Table of New York State Hospital:
  1. Alcoholic insanity
  2. General paralysis
  3. Senile insanity

  4. Epilepsy with insanity
  5. Imbecility and idiocy with insanity
  6. Not insane

(From Church and Peterson, op. cit., pp. 659–660).

At the time that this classification was adopted in New York there were about as many statistical outlines in use in this country as there were mental hospitals. Different classifications appeared in almost every textbook of psychiatry published, based on etiology, pathology, symptomatology, or psychology, depending upon the author's inclination; in addition, there were English, French, Italian, American, and German classifications, each representing different schools of psychiatry. Largely because of the efforts of Meyer and Hoch in introducing Kraepelin's teachings to this country, most of the classification systems in use here were based on Kraepelinian principles, with some modifications.

In 1913 the Committee on Statistics of the American Medico-Psychological Association proposed a standardized classification adopted by the Association's membership four years later. The official report of the Committee to the Association at its annual meeting in 1917 contained the following significant passage:

> Your Committee feels that the first essential of a uniform system of statistics in hospitals for the insane is a generally recognized nomenclature of mental diseases. *The present condition with respect to the classification of mental diseases is chaotic* [italics ours]. Some states use no well-defined classifications. In others the classifications used are similar in many respects but differ enough to prevent accurate comparisons. Some states have adopted a uniform system, while others leave the matter entirely to the individual hospitals. This condition of affairs discredits the science of psychiatry and reflects unfavorably upon our Association, which should serve as a correlating and standardizing agency for the whole country . . . your Committee has endeavored to formulate a classification that could be easily used in every hospital for the insane in this country and that would meet the scientific demands of the present day.[70]

The classification officially adopted by the American Association in 1917 was largely Kraepelinian in principle and related itself principally to hospital psychiatry, equating "psychosis" with committability.

1. Traumatic psychosis
2. Senile psychosis
3. Psychosis with cerebral arteriosclerosis
4. General paresis
5. Psychosis with cerebral syphilis
6. Psychosis of Huntington's chorea
7. Psychosis with brain tumor
8. Psychosis with other brain or nervous disease
9. Alcoholic psychosis
10. Psychosis due to drugs and other exogenous toxins
11. Psychosis with pellagra
12. Psychosis with other somatic disease
13. Manic-depressive psychosis
14. Involution melancholia
15. Dementia Praecox
16. Paranoia or paranoic conditions
17. Epileptic psychosis
18. Psychoneurosis or neurosis
19. Psychosis with constitutional psychopathic inferiority
20. Psychosis with mental deficiency
21. Psychosis not diagnosed
22. Not insane

Southard criticized this classification sharply as "based upon a deductive order derived from other considerations than those of diagnosis . . . upon certain notions of etiology." Southard took issue with the pretensions of etiological classification. But his main objection was that the list was too long for practical use.

With the beginning of the twentieth century a new principle entered psychiatric thinking and psychiatric classification in America, represented by the adjective "dynamic," a word more often used vaguely than defined specifically.* Literally the word refers to energy and implies activity, contrasted with "static" and "potential." In psychology and psychoanalysis it is used to describe theories of personality in which motivation, especially unconscious, is considered basic. Fairly representative of current usage is the following definition by Murray: "Since psychology deals only with motion—processes occurring in time—none of its proper formulations can be static. They all must be dynamic in the larger meaning of this term. Within recent years, dynamic has come to be used in a special sense: to designate a psychology which accepts as prevailingly fundamental the goal directed (adaptive) character of behavior, and attempts to discover and formulate the internal as well as the external factors which determine it." [71]

For this dynamic principle and point of view we have primarily to thank one man, Sigmund Freud. The discoveries, observations, and theories of Freud began to be accepted in psychiatric circles about 1920. Psychiatric nosology at that time was based upon directly observable phenomena, either in life or in the laboratory. Even the notion of *course* of illness and that of deterioration, introduced by Kraepelin, were judged according to external, observable manifestations. Although a continuing process tending toward recovery or decline was inferred, associated conditions (e.g., senility) rather than the process itself formed the basis of classification. Etiology was the taxonomist's Holy Grail, and incessant search for a physiological or anatomical lesion responsible for the process was the prevalent professional preoccupation.

Although the psychiatric theories of Adolf Meyer (1866–1950) are not regarded as dynamic in the sense in which the term is applied today, his ergasia theory, used as the basis for his later classification, was a revolutionary departure from the symptomatic, specific lesion bases of Kraepelin and Wernicke. His biosocial theory of reaction types was, furthermore, a bridge between the physiological orientation of the nineteenth century and the psychosocial theories of today. Meyer, for example, viewed schizophrenia as a pathological reaction to stress in the environment occurring in certain personalities. He believed that a true understanding of the patient was derived from the study of the total personality reaction in all its aspects, organic, social, cultural, and psychological.

Meyer had a tremendous influence on the development of modern concepts of mental illness. His insistence on considering all the data available in any case, his aversion to dogma and to formalized, rigid concepts, and his erudition in the history of medicine enabled him to approach the problem of classification and nomenclature with great power. He thoroughly studied all the principal nosological systems both of his own time and of the past, extracting from them only what he considered of value and integrating these concepts with his own ideas.

---

* In a book entitled *Dynamic Psychiatry* (Alexander and Ross, Univ. of Chicago Press, 1953) the term does not appear in the index, although it is used and defined by implication throughout the book.

More than any other psychiatrist, he was responsible for the introduction and dissemination of Kraepelin's system of classification in this country. In endorsing the Kraepelinian principles, Meyer, as a clinician, was much impressed with the practical implications of Kraepelin's emphasis on prognosis for the routine problems of the hospital psychiatrist working with large numbers of patients. But as a scientist, he saw the dangers in the pragmatic approach of a system of classification which, like Kraepelin's, generalized from groups of cases to the individual and which arbitrarily set up disease entities in the absence of substantiating empirical data, and subordinated empirical analysis to the practical medical problem of prognosis.*

In his formulation of reaction-types, begun in 1908, Meyer harked back to his great admiration for Wernicke's principles of classification. Meyer considered them more logical than Kraepelin's, but unnecessarily complicated for clinical purposes, and he thought that Wernicke's strictly neurological outlook tended to blind the psychiatrist to many important practical problems in his work with patients.[72]

Later on, when Meyer reformulated his "reaction-types" in terms of a theory of "ergasiology," he used modifications of Wernicke's concepts of afunction, hyperfunction, and hypofunction, substituting energy-distribution for Wernicke's hypothesis of "psychic localization." In so doing, he effected a synthesis of Kraepelin's emphasis on the stream of thought, and Wernicke's almost exclusive concern with the contents of consciousness.

This later classification was the following: [73]

1. The anergasias (reactions resulting from organic structure loss)
2. The dysergasias, the deliria ("nutritionally disorganized disorders")
3. The parergasias (previously called hebephrenia, catatonia, and paranoid)
4. The thymergasias, or "sweeping involvements, largely of pure affects"
5. The kakergasias, or minor psychoses, as "badly using oneself"
6. The oligergasias or defective developments

Meyer had many admirers, but in America few followers. In Europe, where Freud never broke through into clinical psychiatric circles, Meyer's ideas were hailed with the enthusiasm which Kraepelin's had received—ten years earlier —in America. This was furthered by the work of Eugen Bleuler (1857–1937), who managed to fuse Meyerian, Kraepelinian, and even Freudian concepts. Bleuler followed Kraepelin's general scheme of classification, but went beyond the mere description of symptoms and syndromes to analyze the particular psychological reaction types associated with the various syndromes. And, as one of the first psychiatrists to grasp the significance of Freud's theories, Bleuler emphasized in his writings the contrast between the traditional descriptive psychiatry of Kraepelin and the interpretive psychiatry which was beginning to emerge at the turn of the century. His celebrated analysis [74] of the psychology of schizophrenia revised the entire concept of the Kraepelin dementia praecox and laid the foundation for the modern concept of that form of mental illness. He pointed to the disorder in the function of association as the essential psychological symptom, and described autism, blocking, and ambiva-

---

* In the 1904–1905 annual report of the New York State Pathological Institute, of which he was then director, Meyer criticized Kraepelin's postulation of mental disease-entities. He recognized that Kraepelin's manic-depressive psychosis and dementia praecox were very important groups of cases, but he thought they should be regarded merely as paradigms and not as disease-entities.

lence as psychological derivatives of the underlying toxic or structural disorder. He introduced the term schizophrenia to emphasize the fundamental intellectual-emotional disharmony, the result of association disturbance.

In his well-known *Textbook of Psychiatry*,[75] Bleuler gave the following classification, which is essentially that of Kraepelin.

1. Organic brain diseases
2. Toxic psychoses
3. Infectious psychoses
4. Thyreogenic psychoses
5. Schizophrenia (the former dementia praecox)
6. Epilepsy
7. Manic-depressive psychoses
8. Psychopathological forms of reactions
9. Psychopathies
10. Oligophrenia

To some extent, Smith Ely Jelliffe (1866–1945) and William A. White (1870–1937) did for America what Bleuler did for Europe, but with much more Freudian emphasis. They were the first to combine biological and dynamic concepts in a classification based upon the Darwinian theory of evolution. They were also the first to incorporate Freud's theories of the unconscious into a biological conception of the psyche, which they regarded as "the end-result in an orderly series of progressions in which the body has used successively more complex tools to deal with the problems of integration and adjustment. The hormone is the type of tool at the physiochemical level, the reflex at the sensorimotor level, and, finally, the symbol at the psychic level." These three levels served, for these authors, as the major categories in a biological classification of mental illness and diseases of the nervous system organized according to the reactions of the central nervous system ranging on the phylogenetic scale from the simplest levels of functional integration to the most complex. Thus they based their classification upon the threefold division of the nervous system, the *vegetative system*, the *sensorimotor* system and the *psychical* system.

Jelliffe tended, in later years, to become increasingly interested in the interconnections between these levels, and from this work has been aptly called the father of psychosomatic medicine.[76] White, in the meantime, was more concerned with psychosocial interrelationships, and hence with crime, preventive psychiatry, "mental hygiene," etc. Both were important figures in the early development of psychoanalysis, as such, in America.

The classification of Jelliffe and White was the following:

I. Psychoneuroses and actual neuroses
    A. Psychoneuroses: hysteria, compulsion neurosis, anxiety hysteria, shellshock
    B. Actual neuroses: anxiety neurosis, neurasthenia
    C. Mixed neuroses
II. Manic-depressive psychoses
III. The paranoia group
IV. Epilepsy and convulsive types of reaction
V. Dementia praecox (schizophrenia) group
VI. Infection-exhaustion psychoses
    A. Prefebrile, febrile and postfebrile psychoses
    B. Exhaustion psychoses
    C. Typhoid fever
VII. Toxic psychoses: alcoholism, opium, cocain, miscellaneous intoxicants

VIII. Psychoses associated with organic diseases
  IX. Presenile, senile, and arteriosclerotic psychoses
   X. Idiocy, imbecility, feeble-mindedness and characterological defect group
      A. Imbecility
      B. Idiocy
      C. Psychopathic constitution
      D. Anomalies of the sexual instinct

One of White's associates and students, Edward J. Kempf (1885——), was the first in this country to attempt (in 1920) a dynamic classification of mental illness based on psychoanalytic discoveries but related to physiological processes.[77] In substance what he did was to arrange psychiatric syndromes in groups related to a hierarchical order of severity, severity of disturbance of "autonomic-affective" functions. He abandoned the word "psychosis," unhappily retaining the generic designation "neurosis." He recognized:

1. *Suppression neuroses*, characterized by either clear or vague unconsciousness of the nature and effect upon himself of ungratified cravings.
2. *Repression neuroses*, characterized by vague to total unconsciousness of the nature and influence of ungratifiable affective cravings, with efforts to prevent emergence into consciousness of the disagreeable affect associated with such cravings.
3. *Compensation neuroses*, characterized by persistent striving to develop potent functions and win social esteem, initiated by fear of impotence or loss of control of asocial cravings.
4. *Regression neuroses*, characterized by failure to compensate, and regression to a preceding more comfortable irresponsible level, permitting wish-fulfilling fancies, postures and indulgences.
5. *Dissociation neuroses*—domination of the personality by the uncontrollable cravings, despite efforts of the ego to prevent it.

This was a great advance in thinking; indeed, it was too far beyond the prevalent psychiatric usage to be grasped or appreciated. Furthermore, it was complicated by Kempf's attempt to bring in dubious interpretations of autonomic nervous system functioning, which few psychiatrists felt competent to either accept or refute. It pleased neither the neurologists nor the psychoanalysts, although it bowed to both.

Beginning as a neuropathologist, Ernest Southard had been stimulated by Wernicke's theory that hallucinations, for example, reflected irritation or damage to certain brain centers. He examined large numbers of brains obtained in the Massachusetts State Hospital system and compared their gross and microscopic abnormalities with the symptoms recorded in the medical histories. He became convinced that he could predict, from microscopic and sometimes mere macroscopic examination of the brain, what type of hallucinations the patient had had during life. His brilliance and scholarliness in this amazing demonstration almost overwhelmed the skepticism of his associates, and fired the imagination of his students. As one of the latter, I can remember well the pains of disillusionment that came with the patient accumulation of contrary and refuting evidence. Parenthetically, I might add that Southard himself had begun to distrust his early Wernickean enthusiasms, and in the clinical classification made shortly before his death, based entirely on pragmatic considerations, he placed schizophrenia near the bottom of the list in respect to the certainty of our knowledge of its nature.

Another way in which Wernicke influenced not only Southard but the whole psychiatric and psychologic world was by the systematic psychopathology already mentioned. The situation faintly resembles the building of the Mendeleyeff table of atomic weights; the various psychological functions were listed, and then the conceivable variations in the "plus," "minus," or "para" directions were considered. Clinicians began to discover the existence of symptoms which they had never observed, or to think of phenomena as symptoms which they had previously disregarded. An example of this is the hypothymia or "blunting of affect" which for a time impressed clinicians as an outstanding manifestation of schizophrenia. This was reflected in the teaching of psychiatry in medical schools and of "abnormal psychology" in universities, where for the first time a systematic approach to the analysis of pathological phenomena became possible and current.

The American Psychiatric Association came out in 1916 with an attempt to simplify and standardize the nomenclature used by American psychiatrists. The Kraepelinian concepts, so well established, were reduced to a matter of twenty-one main items. The Meyerian classification was ignored. Like Meyer, Southard had been a laboratory man, a researcher. Suddenly—shortly before his election to the presidency of the American Association—he had been confronted with the practical necessity of directing a small but active psychiatric hospital and a rapidly developing teaching program (Harvard). With his characteristic freshness of mind he approached the problem of nosology from an unexpected and exceedingly practical angle. He was concerned less with differences in the clinical pictures than with differences in the ways in which the doctors under his direction handled the problem of establishing "the diagnosis."

As a result he made the proposal that, since the classification of mental diseases was not a natural but an artificial one, it should be made as practical and as simple as possible. He believed that a classification could be set up, the chief criterion for the elements of which was the definitiveness of our knowledge of the syndrome. So he arranged the common mental disease syndromes in a descending order of definiteness in diagnostic recognition and understanding. Thus, since we had more definite diagnostic criteria for the diagnosis of neurosyphilis and psychiatric pictures associated with it than for any other condition, Southard proposed to put it (paresis, etc.) as number one in his list. The next most clearly defined by empirical data was feeble-mindedness; then the convulsive disorders, etc. He made eleven such general classes.[78]

Mental Disease Groups	*Southard's Proposed Group Names*
1. Syphilitic	Syphilopsychoses
2. Feeble-minded	Hypophrenoses
3. Epileptic	Epileptoses
4. Alcoholic, drug, poison	Pharmacopsychoses
5. Focal brain	Encephalopsychoses
6. Bodily disease (symptomatic)	Somatopsychoses
7. Senescent, senile	Geriopsychoses
8. Dementia praecox, paraphrenic	Schizophrenoses
9. Manic-depressive, cyclothymic	Cyclothymoses
10. Hysteric, psychoneurasthenic	Psychoneuroses
11. Psychopathic, paranoiac, *et alia*	Psychopathoses

Southard was fully aware that his classification was not, strictly speaking, a nosology. Like many others he revolted against the endless hair-splitting arguments as to the species and sub-species to which the illness of a particular patient might belong, to the complete neglect of the patient's treatment needs. He was combating the same thing which Adolf Meyer was combating, but in a different way.

Southard thus put classification to a new purpose; namely, that of teaching and of therapeutic assistance. It might seem as though the practical usefulness of such a classification would have immediately commended it to the entire profession. So far as I know, however, his scheme was never used anywhere. It was *never even discussed* in any meeting of the American Psychiatric Association, and it was not officially employed in any university teaching center. Southard's brilliant advance was thus even more ignored than Meyer's brilliant advance in another direction.

This then was the situation in 1918 at the end of World War I. Kraepelinism dominated official psychiatric practice. Adolf Meyer had proposed one brilliant reformulation, Jelliffe and White another, while Edward Kempf had gone still further in a radical revision, and Southard had offered a practical simplification of Kraepelinism. Any one of these classifications was better by far than the one which continued in use for almost thirty years thereafter!

The classification used by the Army in World War I and by most of the mental hospitals throughout the country was the 1917 twenty-two-item list of the American Psychiatric Association. From time to time slight modifications were made, and seventeen years later (1934) the Association approved a new, somewhat revised, and considerably extended official nosology planned as far as possible on an etiological basis (Southard's objections notwithstanding). Its chief incentive was to correct certain weaknesses of the psychiatric classification section of mental illnesses appearing in the *Standard Classified Nomenclature of Disease*, the first edition of which had been published a year earlier. The principal changes were the substitution of the etiologically-weighted term "psychoses with syphilitic meningo-encephalitis" for the old descriptive term "general paresis," the substitution of the term "psychoses with convulsive disorders" for the term "epileptic psychoses," the substitution of "involutional psychoses" for "involutional melancholia"; and the addition of a new category, "primary behavior disorders."

A condensed form of the classification adopted by the American Psychiatric Association in 1934 and by the *Standard Classified Nomenclature of Disease* in its second edition (1935) is as follows:

1. Psychoses with syphilitic meningo-encephalitis (general paresis)
2. Psychoses with other forms of syphilis of the central nervous system
   a. Meningo-vascular type (cerebral syphilis)
   b. With intracranial gumma
   c. Other types
3. Psychoses with epidemic encephalitis
4. Psychoses with other infectious diseases
   a. With tuberculous meningitis
   b. With meningitis (unspecified)
   c. With acute chorea (Sydenham's)
   d. With other infectious diseases
   e. Post-infections psychoses
5. Alcoholic psychoses

a. Pathological intoxication
b. Delirium tremens
c. Korsakoff's psychosis
d. Acute halucinosis
e. Other types
6. Psychoses due to drugs or other exogenous poisons
   a. Due to metals
   b. Due to gases
   c. Due to opium and derivatives
   d. Due to other drugs
7. Traumatic psychoses
   a. Traumatic delirium
   b. Post-traumatic personality disorders
   c. Post-traumatic mental deterioration
   d. Other types
8. Psychoses with cerebral arteriosclerosis
9. Psychoses with other disturbances of circulation
   a. With cerebral embolism
   b. With cardio-renal disease
   c. Other types
10. Psychoses with convulsive disorder (epilepsy)
    a. Epileptic deterioration
    b. Epileptic clouded states
    c. Other epileptic types
11. Senile Psychoses
    a. Simple deterioration
    b. Presbyophrenic type
    c. Delirious and confused types
    d. Delirious and agitated types
    e. Paranoid types
12. Involutional Psychoses
    a. Melancholia
    b. Paranoid types
    c. Other types
13. Psychoses due to other metabolic, etc., diseases
    a. With disease of the endocrine glands
    b. Exhaustion delirium
    c. Altzheimer's disease
    d. With pellagra
    e. Other somatic diseases
14. Psychoses due to new growth
    a. With intracranial neoplasms
    b. With other neoplasms
15. Psychoses associated with organic changes of the nervous system
    a. With multiple sclerosis
    b. With paralysis agitans
    c. With Huntington's chorea
    d. With other brain or nervous diseases
16. Psychoneuroses
    a. Hysteria (anxiety hysteria, conversion hysteria and subgroups)
    b. Psychasthenia or compulsive states (and subgroups)
    c. Neurasthenia
    d. Hypochondriasis
    e. Reactive depression (simple situational reactions; others)
    f. Anxiety state
    g. Mixed psychoneurosis
17. Manic-depressive Psychoses
    a. Manic type
    b. Depressed type
    c. Circular type
    d. Mixed type
    e. Perplexed type
    f. Stuporous type
    g. Other types
18. Dementia Praecox (schizophrenia)
    a. Simple type
    b. Hebephrenic type
    c. Catatonic type
    d. Paranoid type
    e. Other types
19. Paranoia and Paranoid conditions
    a. Paranoia
    b. Paranoid conditions
20. Psychoses with psychopathic personality
21. Psychoses with mental deficiency
22. Undiagnosed Psychoses
23. Without Psychoses
    a. Epilepsy

b. Alcoholism
c. Drug addiction
d. Mental deficiency
e. Disorders of personality due to epidemic encephalitis
f. Psychopathic personality
  (1) With pathological sexuality
  (2) With pathological emotionality
  (3) With asocial or amoral trends
  (4) Mixed types
24. Primary Behavior Disorders
  a. Simple maladjustment
  b. Primary behavior disorders in children
    (1) Habit disturbance
    (2) Conduct disturbance
    (3) Neurotic traits

The 1934 classification was never popular. Many psychiatrists felt that its use by statisticians was leading to erroneous conclusions and therefore to bad management procedures. This became very evident to my brother (then Brigadier General) William Menninger, during his Army service as chief of the Neuropsychiatry Consultants Division of the Office of the Surgeon General in World War II. He began an attempt to revise the classification of psychiatric disease pictures in 1949, which has been described in Chapter II. The confused and contradictory handling of patients in the Army hospitals resulting from the unclear nosological designations then in use forced upon my brother's attention the necessity of recasting the names of syndromes in line with clinical observations and prevailing psychiatric practice in order to avoid incorrect labeling of cases, with all the consequent injustices which followed, both to the patients and to the government.

The dynamic principle upon which my brother's classification was (in part) constructed corresponds to what Halliday calls the biological conception of etiology; namely, the reaction type. This, of course, is essentially what Adolf Meyer had proposed fifty years ago. My brother's classification differed from Adolf Meyer's, however, in several respects. It was cast on a much wider base in order to include all those conditions of behavior pathology which are now envisaged as within the field of psychiatry. It was much more pragmatic in its dependence upon empirical observation and experience.

The classification, as it was originally drawn up by my brother and his advisers had to run the gamut of military and civilian concurrences, with the result that many compromises and modifications had to be introduced. As it finally emerged, it included five main groups:

1. Acute transitory amorphous reactions of disorganization
2. Neurotic reactions
3. Personality deformities
4. Feeble-mindedness
5. Psychoses; schizophrenic, paranoid, affective, and organic

As stated in the text of our book, we consider this nosology a magnificent achievement accomplished under great difficulties. Imperfect as it was, it represented an enormous advance over those in use prior to 1945. Many years were required for the Kraepelinian system to become established, but, once established, it seemed as impregnable as the mountains. Yet in a period of two or three years following my brother's introduction of his classification in the Army in 1945, it was in general use throughout the country, in spite of initial resistance and opposition.

The official report of the APA's Committee on Nomenclature and Statistics made on May 1, 1949, follows:

In formulating its mission, the Committee was immediately faced with two areas of disagreement. In the first of these, it was considered by some members that statistics are not vitally related to nomenclature, and should be handled by a second committee. After some discussion, it was the decision of the Committee that statistics logically follow nomenclature and are inseparable from it. The Committee was therefore in favor of a sub-committee on statistics but not of a separate committee for that area. In the second disputed area, the majority of the Committee were in agreement that this Committee is charged with the responsibility for clarifying and defining concepts of various clinical entities. By this decision the Committee accepted for itself the task of writing a manual of psychiatry to accompany any nomenclature upon which it may reach agreement. These two points of discussion were settled, and the Committee's outline of its mission (as finally formulated following recirculation to members by mail) was forwarded to the Secretary on March 24, 1949.

The Committee was in unanimous agreement that the present [former] nomenclature of the APA needs extensive revision. A large portion of the first meeting was devoted to a discussion of what nomenclature needs are in various sections of psychiatry and in various sections of psychiatric practice. As a method of operating, it was decided that individual members of the Committee would be assigned to small groups, each with a group leader, and that each group would be responsible for one area of psychiatric knowledge; for example, one group was to be responsible for the nomenclature of psychoneuroses, another for that of the psychoses of unknown origin, and so on. Each group in its own area subsequently would determine what was needed in a nomenclature, and by utilizing the several nomenclature systems now extant would arrive at a satisfactory system of naming. The Committee was in agreement that any nomenclature devised must be acceptable within the framework of the Standard Nomenclature, which is now in process of revision.

The report of the Chairman of this Committee, dated December 1946, summarized 15 objections to the revised psychiatric nomenclature adopted by the Army, and subsequently by the Veterans Administration. These objections are essentially those which were expressed in 1945 against the Army's adoption of a new system of nomenclature, in 1946 against the Veterans Administration's similar plan, and since that date against any change in the present diagnostic nomenclature of the American Psychiatric Association. Since these objections were voiced three years ago, and since two large organizations have experimented with a new nomenclature in the interim period, it was felt highly important to learn from those two organizations the extent of accuracy of the predicted difficulties voiced in the objections. . . .

Reports from the Army and Veterans representatives indicated that the new systems of nomenclature have been found more satisfactory by both clinicians and statisticians. The dire prophecies of utter chaos previously expressed have failed to develop, and after three years experience with the new nomenclature, both organizations have found their modifications superior to the present APA nomenclature. Both organizations also feel that the present nomenclature can be improved further.

The statistical divisions of the Army and Veterans Administration find the new nomenclature more usable for statistics than the old. Specifically, the Army complained that under the old system there appeared to be no mutual exclusion of terms, so that reports from various hospitals were difficult to evaluate.

One repeated objection to a change in nomenclature has been that there is danger of confusing the national statistics. As a matter of fact, the national office of vital statistics [formerly in the Census Bureau and now in the Federal Security Agency] uses for classification not the APA nomenclature but the International List of Diseases and Causes of Death. The International List is standard for the statistics of this country; the United States is bound to its use by treaty with other members of the World Health Organization. Actually, the International List is much more similar to the Army and Veterans nomenclature than to the APA nomenclature. Thus, one of the major objections to a change in the APA nomenclature is again not valid, inasmuch as that nomenclature is not utilized in any statistics other than those within states. When state statistics are submitted to national coding the nomenclature has to be recoded into one which is quite similar to the Army modifications.

It was decided that as soon as a tentative nomenclature system could be devised, it would be circulated to 100 or 200 selected psychiatrists, with requests for comment on the nomenclature itself, and on the etiological, psychopathological, and other considerations involved in the system. It was the unanimous agreement of the Committee that circulation to the entire membership would be a needless expense, and would not produce more satisfactory results than circulation to a selected limited group. Such a selected group should, of course, include all psychiatric teaching centers, psychiatrists in private practice, psychiatrists in institutional practice, and physicians engaged primarily in the practice of neurology.

In view of the information collected at this first meeting the Committee felt no hesitancy in proceeding posthaste with revision of the present APA nomenclature. . . . At this meeting detailed discussion of categories, working, and definition was carried out. . . . A tentative arrangement of nomenclature by categories was drawn up, and this at the present time, along with other discussion from the meeting, is in preparation for circulation to all committee members. A great amount of detailed discussion and effort went into this two day meeting which is not necessary to report at this time, except to say that a tentative new nomenclature has been arrived at, and will be circulated to members of the Committee in preparation for a meeting in Montreal this month.

In 1951 a Standard Veterans Administration classification, an elaborated and slightly modified version of my brother's was adopted, of which an abbreviated version follows here:

I. Transient Personality Reactions
   A. Acute Situational Maladjustment
II. Psychoneurotic Disorders
   A. Anxiety Reaction
   B. Dissociative Reaction
   C. Phobic Reaction
   D. Conversion Reaction
   E. Somatization Reactions
     1. Psychogenic gastrointestinal reaction
     2. Psychogenic cardiovascular reaction
     3. Psychogenic genitourinary reaction
     4. Psychogenic respiratory reaction
     5. Psychogenic skin reaction
     6. Psychogenic reaction, other
   F. Asthenic Reaction
   G. Obsessive-Compulsive Reaction
   H. Hypochondriacal Reaction
   I. Depressive Reaction

III. Character and Behavior Disorders
  A. Pathological Personality types
    1. Schizoid personality
    2. Paranoid personality
    3. Cyclothymic personality
    4. Inadequate personality
    5. Antisocial personality
    6. Sexual deviate
  B. Immaturity Reactions
    1. Emotional Instability Reaction
    2. Passive dependency Reaction
    3. Passive aggressive reaction
    4. Aggressive reaction
    5. Immaturity with symptomatic "habit" reaction
IV. Alcoholic Intoxication and Drug Addiction
  A. Alcoholism
    1. Acute alcoholism
    2. Chronic alcoholism
  B. Drug Addiction
    1. Drug addiction (specify drug)
V. Disorders of Intelligence
  A. Mental Deficiency
    1. Primary (specify cause)
    2. Secondary (specify cause)
  B. Specific learning defects
VI. Psychoses Without Known Organic Etiology
  A. Schizophrenic disorders
    1. Schizophrenic reaction, latent
    2. Schizophrenic reaction, simple type
    3. Schizophrenic reaction, hebephrenic type
    4. Schizophrenic reaction, catatonic type
    5. Schizophrenic reaction, paranoid type
    6. Schizophrenic reaction, unclassified
  B. Paranoid Disorders
    1. Paranoia
    2. Paranoid state
  C. Affective Disorders
    1. Manic depressive reaction
      a. Manic type
      b. Depressive type
      c. Circular type
      d. Mixed type
      e. Perplexed type
      f. Stuporous type
      g. Other types
    2. Psychotic depressive reaction
    3. Involution melancholia
  D. List specific character or behavior disorder and follow by—"with psychotic reaction" (type)
  E. List type of mental deficiency and follow by—"with psychotic reaction" (type)
VII. Psychosis, Unclassified
VIII. Psychoses and other Mental Disorders with Demonstrable Etiology or Associated Structural Change in the Brain, or Both
  A. Psychoses and other mental disorders due to or associated with infection
  B. Psychoses due to intoxication
  C. Psychoses and other mental disorders due to trauma
  D. Psychoses and other mental disorders due to disturbance of circulation
  E. Psychoses and other mental disorders due to

convulsive disorder
(Epilepsy)
F. Psychoses due to disturbances of metabolism, growth, nutrition
or endocrine function

G. Psychoses with new growth
H. Psychoses due to unknown or hereditary cause but associated with organic change

The Official Current Classification

As our final exhibit attesting the confusing complexity of American psychiatric nosology, we submit the official current classification published by the American Psychiatric Association in 1952 in a *Diagnostic and Statistical Manual of Mental Disorder*. The carefully prepared booklet has the merit of containing working definitions of terms and descriptions of syndromes. It is, we are assured, shortly to be revised—let us hope in the direction of simplification.

Disorders Caused by or Associated with Impairment of Brain Tissue Function

Acute Brain Disorders

DISORDERS DUE TO OR ASSOCIATED WITH INFECTION

Acute Brain Syndrome associated with intracranial infection

Acute Brain Syndrome associated with systemic infection

DISORDERS DUE TO OR ASSOCIATED WITH INTOXICATION

Acute Brain Syndrome, drug or poison intoxication

Acute Brain Syndrome, alcohol intoxication
Acute hallucinosis
Delirium tremens

DISORDERS DUE TO OR ASSOCIATED WITH TRAUMA

Acute Brain Syndrome associated with trauma

DISORDERS DUE TO OR ASSOCIATED WITH CIRCULATORY DISTURBANCE

Acute Brain Syndrome associated with circulatory disturbance

DISORDERS DUE TO OR ASSOCIATED WITH DISTURBANCE OF INNERVATION OR OF PSYCHIC CONTROL

Acute Brain Syndrome associated with convulsive disorder

DISORDERS DUE TO OR ASSOCIATED WITH DISTURBANCE OF METABOLISM, GROWTH OR NUTRITION

Acute Brain Syndrome with metabolic disturbance

DISORDERS DUE TO OR ASSOCIATED WITH NEW GROWTH

Acute Brain Syndrome associated with intracranial neoplasm

DISORDERS DUE TO UNKNOWN OR UNCERTAIN CAUSE

Acute Brain Syndrome with disease of unknown or uncertain cause

DISORDERS DUE TO UNKNOWN OR UNCERTAIN CAUSE WITH THE FUNCTIONAL REACTION ALONE MANIFEST

Acute Brain Syndrome of unknown cause

Chronic Brain Disorders *

DISORDERS DUE TO PRENATAL (CONSTITUTIONAL) INFLUENCE

---

* The qualifying phrase "Mental Deficiency" .x4 (mild .x41, moderate .x42, or severe .x43) should be added at the end of the diagnosis in disorders of this group which

Chronic Brain Syndrome associated with congenital cranial anomaly

Chronic Brain Syndrome associated with congenital spastic paraplegia

Chronic Brain Syndrome associated with Mongolism

Chronic Brain Syndrome due to prenatal maternal infectious diseases

DISORDERS DUE TO OR ASSOCIATED WITH INFECTION

Chronic Brain Syndrome associated with central nervous system syphilis
Meningoencephalitic
Meningovascular
Other central nervous system syphilis

Chronic Brain Syndrome associated with intracranial infection other than syphilis

DISORDERS ASSOCIATED WITH INTOXICATION

Chronic Brain Syndrome associated with intoxication

Chronic Brain Syndrome, drug or poison intoxication

Chronic Brain Syndrome, alcohol intoxication

DISORDERS ASSOCIATED WITH TRAUMA

Chronic Brain Syndrome associated with birth trauma

Chronic Brain Syndrome associated with brain trauma

Chronic Brain Syndrome, brain trauma, gross force

Chronic Brain Syndrome following brain operation

Chronic Brain Syndrome following electrical brain trauma

Chronic Brain Syndrome following irradiational brain trauma

DISORDERS ASSOCIATED WITH CIRCULATORY DISTURBANCES

Chronic Brain Syndrome associated with cerebral arteriosclerosis

Chronic Brain Syndrome associated with circulatory disturbance other than cerebral arteriosclerosis

DISORDERS ASSOCIATED WITH DISTURBANCES OF INNERVATION OR OF PSYCHIC CONTROL

Chronic Brain Syndrome associated with convulsive disorder

DISORDERS ASSOCIATED WITH DISTURBANCE OF METABOLISM, GROWTH OR NUTRITION

Chronic Brain Syndrome associated with senile brain disease

Chronic Brain Syndrome associated with other disturbance of metabolism, growth or nutrition
(Includes presenile, glandular, pellagra, familial amaurosis)

DISORDERS ASSOCIATED WITH NEW GROWTH

Chronic Brain Syndrome associated with intracranial neoplasm

DISORDERS ASSOCIATED WITH UNKNOWN OR UNCERTAIN CAUSE

Chronic Brain Syndrome associated with diseases of unknown or uncertain cause (Includes multiple sclerosis, Huntington's chorea, Pick's disease and other diseases of a familial or hereditary nature)

present mental deficiency as the major symptom of the disorder. Include intelligence quotient (I.Q.) in the diagnosis.

DISORDERS DUE TO UNKNOWN OR UNCERTAIN CAUSE WITH THE FUNCTIONAL REACTION ALONE MANIFEST

MENTAL DEFICIENCY

DISORDERS DUE TO UNKNOWN OR UNCERTAIN CAUSE WITH THE FUNCTIONAL REACTION ALONE MANIFEST;

HEREDITARY AND FAMILIAL DISEASES OF THIS NATURE

Mental deficiency (familial or hereditary)
Mild—moderate—severe

DISORDERS DUE TO UNDETERMINED CAUSE

Mental deficiency, idiopathic
Mild—moderate—severe

Disorders of Psychogenic Origin or without Clearly Defined Physical Cause or Structural Change in the Brain

Psychotic Disorders

DISORDERS DUE TO DISTURBANCE OF METABOLISM, GROWTH, NUTRITION OR ENDOCRINE FUNCTION

Involutional psychotic reaction

DISORDERS OF PSYCHOGENIC ORIGIN OR WITHOUT CLEARLY DEFINED TANGIBLE CAUSE OR STRUCTURAL CHANGE

Affective reactions
Manic depressive reaction, manic type
Manic depressive reaction, depressive type
Manic depressive reaction, other
Psychotic depressive reaction
Schizophrenic reactions
Schizophrenic reaction, simple type
Schizophrenic reaction, hebephrenic type
Schizophrenic reaction, catatonic type
Schizophrenic reaction, paranoid type
Schizophrenic reaction, acute undifferentiated type
Schizophrenic reaction, chronic undifferentiated type
Schizophrenic reaction, schizo-affective type
Schizophrenic reaction, childhood type
Schizophrenic reaction, residual type
Paranoid reactions
Paranoia
Paranoid state
Psychotic reaction without clearly defined structural change, other than above

Psychophysiologic Autonomic and Visceral Disorders

DISORDERS DUE TO DISTURBANCE OF INNERVATION OR OF PSYCHIC CONTROL

Psychophysiologic skin reaction
Psychophysiologic musculoskeletal reaction
Psychophysiologic respiratory reaction
Psychophysiologic cardiovascular reaction
Psychophysiologic hemic and lymphatic reaction
Psychophysiologic gastrointestinal reaction
Psychophysiologic genitourinary reaction
Psychophysiologic endocrine reaction
Psychophysiologic nervous system reaction

Psychophysiologic reaction
of organs of special sense

Psychoneurotic Disorders

DISORDERS OF PSYCHOGENIC ORIGIN
OR WITHOUT CLEARLY DEFINED
TANGIBLE CAUSE OR STRUCTURAL
CHANGE

Psychoneurotic reactions
Anxiety reaction
Dissociative reaction
Conversion reaction
Phobic reaction
Obsessive compulsive reaction
Depressive reaction
Psychoneurotic reaction,
other

Personality Disorders

DISORDERS OF PSYCHOGENIC ORIGIN
OR WITHOUT CLEARLY DEFINED
TANGIBLE CAUSE OR STRUCTURAL
CHANGE

Personality pattern disturbance
Inadequate personality
Schizoid personality
Cyclothymic personality
Paranoid personality
Personality trait disturbance
Emotionally unstable personality
Passive-aggressive personality

Compulsive personality
Personality trait disturbance, other
Sociopathic personality disturbance
Antisocial reaction
Dyssocial reaction
Sexual deviation
Addiction
Alcoholism
Drug addiction
Special symptom reactions
Learning disturbance
Speech disturbance
Enuresis
Somnambulism
Other

Transient Situational Personality Disorders

Transient situational personality disturbance
Gross stress reaction
Adult situational reaction
Adjustment reaction of infancy
Adjustment reaction of childhood
Habit disturbance
Conduct disturbance
Neurotic traits
Adjustment reaction of adolescence
Adjustment reaction of late life

The need for a practical, usable condensation of this unwieldy list, valuable as it may be for certain kinds of statistical compilation, led to the preparation of the following summary (published in the *J.A.M.A.*, September 22, 1963).

I. Acute or chronic brain disorders with impaired brain tissue function caused by, or associated with
Infection
Intoxication (drugs, poison, alcohol)
Trauma
Circulatory disturbance
Convulsive disorder
Disturbance of metabolism,
growth or nutrition
Intracranial neoplasm
Unknown or uncertain cause

II. Mental deficiency
Chronic brain syndrome of unknown cause
Hereditary and familial mental deficiency
Mild—moderate—severe

III. Disorders of psychogenic origin or without clearly defined physical cause or structural change in the brain

  A. Psychotic disorders
    Involutional psychotic reaction
    Affective reactions
    Manic-depressive reaction
    Psychotic depressive reaction
    Schizophrenic reactions
    Paranoid reactions

  B. Psychophysiologic autonomic and visceral disorders
    Psychophysiologic skin reaction
    Psychophysiologic musculo-skeletal reaction
    Psychophysiologic respiratory reaction
    Psychophysiologic cardiovascular reaction
    Psychophysiologic hemic and lymphatic reaction
    Psychophysiologic gastrointestinal reaction
    Psychophysiologic genitourinary reaction
    Psychophysiologic endocrine reaction
    Psychophysiologic nervous system reaction
    Psychophysiologic reaction of organs of special sense

  C. Psychoneurotic disorders
    Anxiety reaction
    Dissociative reaction
    Conversion reaction
    Phobic reaction
    Obsessive-compulsive reaction
    Depressive reaction
    Psychoneurotic reaction, other

  D. Personality disorders
    Personality pattern disturbance
    Inadequate personality
    Schizoid personality
    Cyclothymic personality
    Paranoid personality
    Personality trait disturbance
    Emotionally unstable personality
    Passive-aggressive personality
    Compulsive personality
    Personality trait disturbance, other
    Sociopathic personality disturbance
    Antisocial reaction
    Dissocial reaction
    Sexual deviation
    Addiction
    Alcoholism
    Drug addiction
    Special symptom reactions
    Learning disturbance
    Speech disturbance

  E. Transient situational personality disorders
    Gross stress reaction
    Adult situational reaction
    Adjustment reaction of adolescence
    Adjustment reaction of late life

IV. Nondiagnostic terms for hospital records
    Alcoholic intoxication
    Diagnosis deferred
    Malingerer

RECENT DEVELOPMENTS IN EUROPEAN PSYCHIATRIC CLASSIFICATIONS

We have seen that a unitary trend had never totally disappeared, even during the periods where the systematists developed their elaborated classifications with their many orders, classes, genera, and species. Among the authors who recognized only one mental disease, Thomas Arnold and Heinrich Neumann are the best known. We should also mention those psychiatrists who, following at a distance the example of Hippocrates and Plato, gave extremely simple classifications of only four or five types: such were the second classification of Pinel and the classifications of Benjamin Rush, Chiarugi, Esquirol, Heinroth, and Griesinger, and Morel's first classification.

Recently in Europe there has been a new trend toward the adoption of a very simple classification of four or five items.

The Spanish psychiatrist Mira y Lopez, for instance, classifies five fundamental types of psychiatric disorders: [79]

I. *Oligophrenia;* states of mental deficit, comparable to *agenesias*

II. *Dementia:* states of mental deterioration, comparable to *degeneration*

III. *Psychopathy:* states of mental disharmony and desynchronization, comparable to *dysgenesias*

IV. *Neurosis:* states of maladjustment and conflict, comparable to milder *disease*

V. *Psychosis:* states of qualitative disturbance of the Being-in-oneself, alteration of autoscopy and reality judgments, comparable to severe *disease*

Another classification, used by several Swiss psychiatrists, is the following: *

I. Reactive conditions:

II. Developmental conditions, maldevelopments (*Fehlentwicklungen*)

III. Processive conditions (*Krankheitsprozesse*)
   A. External causes: Traumatic, physical, poisons, infection, malnutrition
   B. Internal causes: Diseases of brain, endocrine glands, other organs
   C. Hereditary diseases
      a. Prevalence of the *Anlage:* Huntington's chorea
      b. Prevalence of the interplay between *Anlage* and life-history:
         Manic-depressive psychosis
         Schizophrenia

IV. Innate conditions: 1. Oligophrenia (idiocy, imbecility, feeble-mindedness)
                        2. Psychopathies

Another system has been proposed by two other French psychiatrists, Leconte and Damey, in a little book criticizing present French psychiatric nosology (1949).[80] Leconte and Damey suggest that every patient receive a threefold diagnosis: somatic, biological, and social, which would give reliable directives toward a rational treatment.

Other attempts strive more radically toward the establishment of a purely dynamic, i.e., an anti-nosologic psychiatry, where, however, each individual case could be characterized within a practical and scientific frame of reference. The most consistent of these attempts hitherto published was the work of the French psychiatrist Henri Ey. Ey suggests reducing psychiatric classification to

---

* We have been unable to find out who introduced this classification, which is used, with slight variations, by such authors as Benno Dukor, Hans Binder, etc.

the distinction of pathology of *consciousness* and pathology of *personality*. The concepts of French classical psychiatry are arranged in the following order: [81]

PATHOLOGY OF CONSCIOUSNESS (Acute Psychoses)	PATHOLOGY OF PERSONALITY (Chronic Psychoses and Neuroses)
Manic-depressive attacks	Character disorders. Neuroses.
Acute delirious and hallucinatory states. Oneiric states	Chronic delusions. Schizophrenia Dementia
Confusional-oneiric psychoses	

It would be naïve, however, to overlook or minimize the more traditional classification systems which continue to be produced. These are especially noteworthy among neuropsychiatrists and others who have a strong belief in heredo-structural and neurological factors as causes of *all* mental illness. A good example is the work of Kleist,[82] which includes schizophrenias under progressive degenerative neurogenic diseases, but leaves the door ajar for various neurotic and psychopathic disorders to be included under the special subheadings of "Abnormal dispositions with psychogenic and autogenic fluctuations" and "Abnormal dispositions with psychogenic reactions."

The Dutchman Rümke [83] has proposed a threefold classification on the basis of presumed or demonstrated etiology, each with several subdivisions of a descriptive sort, or on the basis of the typical course of illness:

I. Mental disorders in patients with previously undisturbed development and without signs of an abnormal constitution
   a) on the basis of extra-cerebral noxious influences
II. Mental disorders mainly on the basis of disturbances in the constitution.
   a) Constitutional disorders with phasic course (e.g., manic-depressive psychosis, degeneration psychoses, some epileptic psychoses)
   b) Constitutional mental disorders with progressive course (schizophrenia, paraphrenia, unclear chronic paranoid states, paranoia, chronic hypochondria, malignant chronic compulsive syndrome, some epileptic psychoses)
   c) Constitutional mental disorders noticeable during the whole life (nervositas, neurasthenia, psychasthenia, part of the psychopathies, degeneres superieurs)
III. Mental disorders on the basis of a disturbed course of development
   a) On the basis of defective natural disposition (part of the psychopathies, oligophrenic diseases and the perversions)
   b) On the basis of disturbances in the processes of growth of the personality (mainly hereditary)
   c) On the basis of mainly psychogenetically determined disturbances in the processes of growth of the personality (neuroses, character neuroses, part of the perversions, part of the psychopathies and abnormal reactions of the personality, developmental schizophrenia (type Sechehaye)

Schneider * recognizes two large groupings with combined etiological and symptomatological subdivisions:

---

* Schneider, Kurt: "Systematic Psychiatry." *Am. J. Psychiat.* 107:334–335, 1950.

I. Abnormal varieties of sane mental life
　1. Abnormal intellectual capacity (*Anlagen*)
　2. Abnormal (psychopathic) personalities
　3. Abnormal reactions to emotional impressions
II. Results of illness and developmental defects

Somatological/etiological:	Psychological/symptomatological:
1. Intoxications	
2. Paresis	Acute: clouding of consciousness
3. Other infections	
4. Other somatic illnesses	Chronic: personality deterioration
5. Abnormal brain development	(congenital: arrested personality
6. Brain injuries	development) and dementia
7. Cerebral arteriosclerosis	
8. Senile brain diseases	
9. Other brain diseases	
10. Genuine epilepsy	
?	Cyclothymia
?	Schizophrenia

The distinction between Schneider's group I and II is based on the contention that psychogenic conditions are to be described not as illness but as "abnormal variations." True illness, according to this author, is always based on somatic changes. It is a curious thing that in this way the *boundaries* of the concept of illness no longer function as principles for inclusion or exclusion, but become in themselves new psychiatric categories or classes as it were. The class-character of the currently rather common terms "reaction type" or "reactions" is based on a similar apprehension about the limits of the concept of illness. The fact that these "reactions" are nevertheless included in the classifications suggests that many psychiatrists are willing to see certain sufferers as patients, to describe them as "ill," and yet to deny that their condition can be described as "illness."

A fairly simple classification can be found in Henderson and Gillespie's well-known textbook of psychiatry,[84] which recognizes eight or nine headings:

1. Affective reaction types
2. Schizophrenic reaction types
3. Paranoiac and paranoid reaction types
4. Psychopathic states
5. Organic reaction types
6. Epilepsy
7. Mental deficiency
8. Psychoneuroses
9. Unclassified (which may include such phenomena as *folie à deux*)

Further distinctions between psychoses, abnormal personalities, and abnormal reactions are made in the classification of Kloos,[85] for whom there are three classes, subdivided on the basis of heterogenous principles, especially an "inner" and "outer" dimension:

I. Psychoses
　1. Endogenous, i.e., of unknown, constitutional organic origin
　2. Exogenous, i.e., caused by known constitutional or acquired physical disease
II. Abnormal personalities
　1. Oligophrenia
　2. Psychopathy
　3. Neuropathy
III. Abnormal Reactions
　1. Reactions to external events
　2. Abnormal Reactions to inner events (i.e., inner conflicts), neuroses

More tentative, and less tight as a classificatory system, are the proposals by Essen-Möller and Wohlfahrt [86] for making in each case two diagnoses, one described as "reactions" and based on symptomatological considerations, and a second one which specifies etiology.

ENGLAND

The Royal Medical Psychological Association of Britain undertook, about 1930, an official revision of its standard classification of mental disorder. A Committee reviewed the classifications that had evolved in England and elsewhere since Griesinger (1845) and the first international classification (1867). The first official British classification had appeared in 1882 and was revised again in 1904, 1905, and 1906, but not thereafter.* Various English psychiatrists had published slightly differing classifications: Turner (1912), Stoddart (fifth edition, 1936), Craig and Beaton (1926), Henderson and Gillespie (1927). Henderson and Gillespie followed the general outline of Kraepelin's nosology, except that the former "disease entities" of Kraepelin were called "reaction-types" after Meyer:

1. Affective reaction-types:
   a. Manic-depressive
   b. Involutional melancholia
2. Schizophrenic reaction-types
3. Paranoiac and paranoid reaction-types:
   a. Paranoia
   b. Paraphrenia
   c. Paranoid states, with or without hallucinations
4. Psychopathic states in:
   a. Aggressive psychopathic personality
   b. Inadequate personality
   c. Creative personality
5. Organic reaction-types (toxic-infectious; metabolic diseases of internal organs; cerebral degenerative, traumatic, etc.)
6. Epilepsy
7. Mental deficiency
8. Psychoneuroses:
   a. Neurasthenia
   b. Anxiety states
   c. Hysteria
   d. Obsessive-compulsive states
9. Unclassified [87]

---

* The British classification as given by Savage, in 1907, was as follows:

1. Congenital or infantile mental deficiency (idiocy or imbecility) occurring as early in life as it can be observed:
   a. Intellectual
      (1) Without epilepsy
      (2) With epilepsy
   b. Moral
2. Insanity arising later in life:
   a. Insanity with epilepsy
   b. General paralysis of the insane
   c. Insanity with the grosser brain lesions
   d. Acute delirium (acute delirious mania)
   e. Confusional insanity
   f. Stupor
   g. Primary dementia
   h. Mania
      (1) Recent
      (2) Chronic
      (3) Recurrent
   i. Melancholia
      (1) Recent
      (2) Chronic
      (3) Recurrent
   j. Alternating Insanity
   k. Delusional Insanity
      (1) Systematized
      (2) Non-systematized
   l. Volitional Insanity
      (1) Impulse
      (2) Obsession
      (3) Doubt
   m. Moral Insanity
   n. Dementia
      (1) Secondary or terminal
      (2) Senile

The British Committee considered these classifications and those which were being used in America, Germany, Holland, Norway, and other countries, and drew up a new classification in 1932. Its simplicity commends it, although it contained no recognition of the new principle of dynamic psychiatry. It was apparently used by few and soon forgotten by most.

The same year (1932) another British psychiatrist, Edward Glover, presented to the Royal Society of Medicine a paper on the "Principles of Psychiatric Classification" which was as progressive and original as the Royal Society's official classification was reactionary and sterile. So far as we know this was the first effort made by any psychoanalyst (except Jelliffe and White and Kempf) to relate psychoanalytic theories, categories, and concepts to those of general psychiatry. Glover undertook the task of reclassifying mental disease syndromes according to principles based upon the functions of the unconscious, and particularly, as he himself emphasized, according to the nature and order of the ego modifications which occur in mental illness.

"Let us see what can be done," Glover said,* "with three . . . criteria: (a) a descriptive, clinical standard, (b) a systematic ego standard, by which psychiatry can define its relation to other psychological data, and (c) a qualitative standard which, by virtue of specific or almost specific relation to the psychoses, acts as a check on the systematic standard." Glover announced that he would borrow the term "schizophrenia" to describe "a group in which the wholesale detachment of interest from the world of objects is quite unmistakable," the term "paranoia" to describe another group in which partial de-

---

* With respect to the criterion of ego control, Glover said very succinctly, "In the simplest terms of structure the ego is regarded by psychoanalysts as an organized system of psychic impressions ultimately expressed in terms of memory-traces. From the dynamic point of view, however, it can be regarded as a psychic organ of adaptation. This organ is, one might say, bounded on one side by perceptual consciousness, and on another by instinctual impulse. Perceptual consciousness is, however, more than a boundary; it is a psychic window system. Using this system the ego not only samples the stimulations of the external world, but, provided unconscious barriers do not interfere with the view, takes measure of an inner world of instinct derivatives. These derivatives are either ideas or affects. The function of the ego as a whole is to effect a compromise between the demands of instinct and the amount of gratification possible in the external world. Strictly speaking, the external world in this sense includes the individual's own body. As, however, only a few component instincts are capable of gratification apart from an external object, we may say roughly that the ego lies between instinct and an external world of objects—in other words, environment. The 'signal' system by means of which the ego tests the success or failure of its manoeuvres is anxiety. If ego manoeuvres are unsuccessful, frustrated instinct will induce anxiety; if in its attempt to gratify instinct the ego attacks the world more than immediate human representatives will endure, an environmental embargo or threat ensues; if the original impulses are exorbitant or impossible of gratification, they frustrate themselves; and if an unconscious guilt system has been established, all impulses counter to the existing codes of the ego are frustrated from within, and the result is once more anxiety. In 1877 a German psychiatrist said that anxiety was the Alpha and Omega of psychiatry. Psychoanalysis, having traced innumerable indirect signs of anxiety in conscious and unconscious territories, is prepared to say that anxiety is the Alpha and guilt the Omega of human development. Spurred by anxiety the ego makes fresh attempts at adaptation. But there are only three main lines of action possible: (a) inhibition, repression or deflection of instinct, (b) less exorbitant demands on environment (courses which presuppose some tolerance of frustration-anxiety), and (c) a pathological distortion of the ego function. This third group is then subdivided into

tachment of interest from the world is indicated by a characteristic impairment of reality sense, the delusional system, and finally, the term "melancholia" to indicate a group characterized by still less regression and by a marked degree of inturned psychic scrutiny and exaggerated affective state.

Glover's suggestions were frequently discussed and occasionally utilized by psychoanalytically oriented psychiatrists, but they made no immediate impact upon the official nosologies of any country. Indeed, during the nineteen-thirties it would appear from a review of the literature and the programs of psychiatric associations that no one was very much concerned with nosology, regarding it as a necessary but negligible evil.

The outcome of Glover's analysis was a classification which does not lend itself well to printed listing, although Glover [88] constructed a diagram which can be approximately reproduced as follows:

I. Disorders originating from fixations in the oral period:
   A. Characterized by introjection
      1. Schizophrenic group
      2. Melancholic group
   B. Characterized by projection
      1. Psychotic character
      2. Schizoid character
      3. Asocial character
II. Disorders arising from fixations in the early anal period
   A. Characterized by introjection
      Some members of the melancholia group
   B. Characterized by projection
      1. The paranoia group
      2. Drug addictions
III. Disorders arising from fixations in the late anal period
   A. Characterized by introjection
      Obsessional neuroses
   B. Characterized by projection
      The compulsive character neuroses
IV. Disorders arising from fixations in the phallic (Glover says "genital" period)
   A. Characterized by introjection
      1. Hysteria
      2. Psycho-sexual inhibition
   B. Characterized by projection
      1. Phobias
      2. Anxiety character group
      3. Social inferiority group

two: cases in which the consequences of ego distortion are roughly limited to the mind or body of the subject (autoplastic), and cases where impairment of reality relations is an outstanding feature. The psychoses represent an extreme example of the third method. The neuroses, too, belong to the third group insofar as a degree of localized ego distortion occurs; but except in some socially unimportant respects, there is in the neuroses no grave interference with 'reality testing.' " Under the criterion of qualitative reality testing Glover is less clear, but seems to have in mind the nature of object attachment. (Glover, Edward. "A Psychoanalytic Approach to the Classification of Mental Disorder." *Journal of Mental Science* 78:819–842, October 1932.)

It is obvious that Glover's theory was better worked out than his nosology, but he deserves great credit for being the first psychoanalyst since Kempf (see above) to introduce psychoanalytic concepts into psychiatric nosology.

And so we are still in an era of nosological upheavals, confusion, and uncertainty. Were it not for the pressure of statistical reporting to public health agencies, hospitals and practicing psychiatrists would have a wide choice of classifications from which to choose in line with their own beliefs and leanings. But in the midst of lengthy and complex classification systems which represent official, semi-official, or national points of view a trend toward simplicity and sobriety has become apparent. This trend is followed only spottily, mostly in certain private clinics or hospitals, and the duties of reporting to official health boards often force their users to engage in a double system of bookkeeping, as it were, one in which to state one's beliefs, the other in which to conform.

In recognition of the prevailing confusion, and in an earnest attempt to establish an international classification of mental disorders, the World Health Organization invited Ernest Stengel of Sheffield to survey all the currently used classifications, to establish principles of classification and to ponder the prospects and requirements of an international system. In his report of 1959 Stengel [89] has presented detailed listings of numerous present-day national classifications as well as private ones, and we have liberally borrowed from his publication in these pages. We refer those readers who are interested in the details of Stengel's current cross section, especially the national classifications of Canada, France, Germany, the Netherlands, Denmark, the U.S.S.R., and Japan, to his superb monograph.

Notes

CHAPTER I

1. Cabot, Richard C.: "An Appreciation of Elmer E. Southard." Southard Memorial Number, *Bull. Mass. Dept. Ment. Dis.* 4:14–29, 1920.
2. Goolker, Paul: "The Role of Diagnosis in Psychiatry." *J. Hillside Hosp.* 5:361–367, 1956.
3. Lear, John: "Taking the Miracle Out of the Miracle Drugs." *Sat. Rev.*, Jan. 3, 1959.
4. Menninger, Karl; Mayman, Martin; and Pruyser, Paul: *A Manual for Psychiatric Case Study*, Rev. ed. New York: Grune and Stratton, 1962. By permission.

CHAPTER II

1. Pinel, Philippe: *Traité medico-philosophique sur l'alienation mentale, ou la manie.* Paris: Caille et Ravier, 1801.
2. Shapley, Harlow: *Time* 14:46–48, Dec. 2, 1929.
3. Riese, Walther: "History and Principles of Classification of Nervous Diseases." *Bull. Hist. Med.* 18:465–512, 1945.
4. Clements, Forest E.: "Primitive Concepts of Disease." *Archeol. and Ethnol.* 32: 185–252, 1932.
5. Veith, Ilza: "Psychiatric Nosology: from Hippocrates to Kraepelin." *Am. J. Psychiat.* 114:385–391, 1957.
6. Zilboorg, Gregory, and Henry, G. W.: *A History of Medical Psychology.* New York: Norton, 1941.
7. Weyer, Johann: *De Praestigiis Daemonum.* Basileoe: J. Oporinum, 1563.
8. Cullen, William: *Synopsis nosologiae methodicae.* Edinburgh, Kincaid and Creech, 1772.
9. Jackson, John Hughlings: *Selected Writings of John Hughlings Jackson*, Vol. 2. London: Hodder, 1932.
10. Riese, Walther: "An Outline of a History of Ideas in Pseudo Therapy." *Bull. Hist. Med.* 25:442–456, 1951.
11. Castiglioni, Arturo: *A History of Medicine.* New York: Knopf, 1941.
12. Whitehead, Alfred North: *Modes of Thought.* New York: Macmillan, 1938.
13. Molière: *L'Amour Médecin.* Act I, Scene 7; Act II, Scene 1. New York: Macmillan, 1922.
14. Riese, Walther: ibid.
15. Nash, F. A.: "Diagnostic Reasoning and the Logoscope." *The Lancet* 2:1442–1446, Dec. 31, 1960.
16. Warner, H. R., et al.: "A Mathematical Approach to Medical Diagnosis." *J.A.M.A.* 177:177–183, 1961.
17. American Medical Association news release, July 21, 1961.
18. Meyer, Adolf: "Objective Psychology or Psychobiology." In *Studies in Psychiatry* 2:29–36, 1925. Nerv. and Ment. Dis. Mono. Ser. No. 41.
19. *War Dept. Tech. Bull. Med.*, 203, Oct. 19, 1945.
20. Riese, Walther: ibid.
21. Trousseau, Armand: *Clinique médicale de l'Hôtel-Dieu de Paris*, ed. 5. Paris: Baillière, 1877.

22. Neumann, Heinrich: *Lehrbuch der Psychiatrie*. Erlangen: F. Enke, 1859.
23. Stengel, Erwin: "Hughlings Jackson's Influence in Psychiatry." *Brit. J. Psychiat.* 109:348–355, 1963.
24. Ey, Henri: *Études Psychiatriques*, Vol. 3. Paris: DesClée de Brouwer, 1954.
25. Llopis, Bartolomé: "La Psicosis unica." *Arch. de Neurobiol.* 17:1–39, 1954.
26. Blau, Abram: "The Nature of Childhood Schizophrenia." *J. Am. Acad. Child Psychiat.* 1:225–235, 1962.
27. Szasz, Thomas: *The Myth of Mental Illness*. New York: Harper, 1961.
28. Srole, Leo, et al.: *Mental Health in the Metropolis. The Midtown Manhattan Study.* New York: McGraw-Hill, 1962. Copyright, 1962. Blakiston Div., McGraw-Hill. Used by permission.
29. Rush, Benjamin: "Lectures on the Practice of Physic: In Shyrock, R. H.: *The Development of Modern Medicine.* New York: Knopf, 1947.
30. Norwood, W. F.: "Medicine in the Era of the American Revolution." *Int. Rec. Med.* 171:391–407, 1958.
31. Whitehead, Alfred North: *The Concept of Nature.* New York: Macmillan, 1926.

CHAPTER III

1. Engel, George: "Guilt, Pain, and Success." *Psychosom. Med.* 24:37–48, 1962.
2. Stevenson, Ian P.: "The Constitutional Approach to Medicine." *N.Y. J. Med.* 48:2156–2159, 1948.
3. Romano, John: "Basic Orientation and Education of the Medical Student."*J.A.M.A.* 143:409–412, 1950.
4. Engel, George: "A Unified Concept of Health and Disease." *Perspect. Biol. and Med.* 3:459–485, 1960.
5. Cabot, Richard: *Differential Diagnosis*, Vol. I. Philadelphia: Saunders, 1919.
6. Crile, George: "A Plea against Blind Fear of Cancer." *Life* 38:128–142, Oct. 31, 1955.
7. Davidson, Henry: "Dr. Whatsisname." *Ment. Hosp.* 9:8, Sept. 1958.
8. Bazelon, David L.: *Equal Justice for the Unequal.* Isaac Ray Lectureship Award Series of the American Psychiatric Association. Chicago: University of Chicago, 1961 (unpublished).
9. Rümke, H. C.: "Contradictions in the Concepts of Schizophrenia." *Comp. Psychiat.* 1:331–337, 1960.

CHAPTER IV

1. Kraepelin, Emil: *One Hundred Years of Psychiatry.* New York: Philosophical Library, 1962.
2. Sprenger, James, and Kramer, Henry: *Malleus Maleficarum.* (Montague Summers, ed.) New York: McKee, 1928.
3. Kraepelin, Emil: op. cit.
4. Ibid.
5. Lewis, Nolan D. C.: *A Short History of Psychiatric Achievement.* New York: Norton, 1941.
6. Tuke, D. H.: *Dictionary of Psychological Medicine.* Philadelphia: Blakiston, 1892.
7. Kraepelin, Emil: ibid.
8. *Memorial of Miss Dix.* Senate, Illinois Legislature, 15th Assembly, 1st Session, Jan. 11, 1847.
9. Grob, G. N.: "Samuel B. Woodward and the Practice of Psychiatry in Early Nineteenth Century America." *Bull. Hist. Med.* 36:420–443, 1962.
10. Ibid.
11. Ackerknecht, Erwin H.: "Aspects of the History of Therapeutics." *Bull. Hist. Med.* 36:389–419, 1962.
12. Ibid.

13. Kramer, S. N.: *History Begins at Sumer.* New York: Doubleday, 1959.
14. Dennie, Charles C., and Silva, L. C.: "The Pestilence." *Bull. Soc. Med. Hist.* 4:484–532, 1935.
15. Ackerknecht, Erwin H.: ibid.
16. Selye, Hans: *The Physiology and Pathology of Exposure to Stress.* Montreal: Acta, 1950.
17. Bean, William: "Careers in Medicine." *Arch. Int. Med.* 99:847–858, 1957.
18. Bickers, William: "Medicine—East and West." *J.A.M.A.* 181:149–150, 1962.
19. Southard, E. E.: *Shell Shock and other Neuropsychiatric Problems Presented in 589 Case Histories.* New York: Macmillan, 1922.
20. Grob, G. N.: op. cit.
21. Deutsch, Albert: *The Mentally Ill in America.* New York: Doubleday, 1937.
22. Bockoven, Sanbourne: "Moral Treatment in American Psychiatry." *J. Nerv. Ment. Dis.* 124:167–194, 1956.
23. Dain, Norman, and Carlson, Eric T.: "Milieu Therapy in the Nineteenth Century." *J. Nerv. Ment. Dis.* 131:277–290, 1960. "The Psychotherapy That Was Moral Treatment." *Am. J. Psychiat.* 117:519–524, 1960.
24. Brigham, Amariah: "Moral Treatment." *Am. J. Insanity* 4:1–15, 1847.
25. Bockoven, Sanbourne: op. cit.
26. Grob, G. N.: op. cit.
27. *See* Menninger, William C.: "Psychoanalytic Principles Applied to the Treatment of Hospitalized Patients." *Bull. Menninger Clinic,* 1:35–43, 1936.

CHAPTER V

1. Lewin, Kurt: "The Conflict Between Aristotelian and Galilean Modes of Thought in Contemporary Psychology." *J. Gen. Psychol.* 5:141–177, 1931.
2. Bernard, Claude: *An Introduction to the Study of Experimental Medicine* (1865). New York: Macmillan, 1927.
   Cannon, W. B.: *The Wisdom of the Body.* New York: Norton, 1939.
3. Menninger, Karl: *The Human Mind.* New York: Knopf, 1945.
4. Goldstein, Kurt: *The Organism.* New York: American Book, 1939.
5. Bernard, Claude: op. cit.
6. Bertalanffy, Ludwig von: "An Outline of General Systems Theory." *Brit. J. Phil. Sci.* 1:134–163, 1950.
7. Haldane, J. B. S.: *New Paths in Genetics.* New York: Harper, 1942.
8. Loeb, Leo. *The Biological Basis of Individuality.* Springfield, Ill.: Charles C Thomas, 1945.
9. Henderson, D. K.: "A Revaluation of Psychiatry." *J. Ment. Sci.* 85:1–21, 1939.
10. Cannon, W. B.: op. cit.
11. Le Chatelier, H. L.: *Recherches expérimentales et théoriques sur les équilibres chimiques.* Paris: Dunod, 1888.
12. Fechner, G. T.: *Einige Ideen zur Schöpfungs und Entwickelungsgeschichte der Organismen.* Leipzig: Breitkopf und Härtel, 1873.
13. Cannon, W. B.: op. cit.
14. Freeman, G. L.: *The Energetics of Human Behavior.* Ithaca: Cornell University Press, 1948. © 1948 by Cornell University, by permission of Cornell University Press.
15. Cannon, W. B.: op. cit.
16. Bernard, Claude: op. cit.
17. Freud, Sigmund: *Beyond the Pleasure Principle. Complete Psychol. Works Sigmund Freud.* 18:1–64. London: Hogarth, 1955. By permission of Liveright, publishers, N.Y.
18. Toch, Hans H., and Hastorf, Albert H.: "Homeostasis in Psychology." *Psychiatry* 18:81–92, 1955.
19. Maze, J. R.: "On Some Corruptions of the Doctrine of Homeostasis." *Psychol. Rev.* 60:405–412, 1953.
20. Davis, R. C.: "The Domain of Homeostasis." *Psychol. Rev.* 65:8–13, 1958.

21. Wiener, Norbert: *Cybernetics*. New York: Wiley, 1948.

22. Woodger, J. H.: *Physics, Psychology and Medicine*. Cambridge: Cambridge University, 1956.

23. McCulloch, W. S.: *Finality and Form*. Springfield, Ill.: Charles C Thomas, 1952. "Modes of Functional Organization of the Cerebral Cortex." *Fed. Proc.* 6:448–452, 1947.

24. Pi Suñer, A.: *Classics of Biology*. New York: Philosophical Library, 1955.

25. Köhler, Wolfgang: *Dynamics in Psychology*. New York: Liveright, 1940.

26. Allport, F. H.: *Theories of Perception and the Concept of Structure*. New York: Wiley, 1955.

27. Bertalanffy, Ludwig von: op. cit.

28. Allport, F. H.: op. cit.

29. Gerard, R. W.: "Neurophysiology in Relation to Behavior." In *Mid-century Psychiatry*, R. R. Grinker, ed. Springfield, Ill.: Charles C Thomas, 1953.

30. Ibid.

31. Ibid.

32 Bertalanffy, Ludwig von: op. cit.

33. Allport, F. H.: op. cit.

34. Gerard, R. W.: op. cit.

CHAPTER VI

1. Rapaport, David: "The Structure of Psychoanalytic Theory." *Psychol. Issues*, Vol. II, No. 2, Mono. 6, 1960.

2. Hartmann, Heinz: "The Mutual Influences in the Development of Ego and Id." *Psa. Study of the Child* 7:9–30, 1952.

———: "The Development of the Ego Concept in Freud's Work." *Int. J. Psa.* 37:425–438, 1956.

———; Kris, Ernst; and Loewenstein, R. M.: "Comments on the Formation of Psychic Structure." *Psa. Study of the Child* 2:11–38, 1946.

Goldberger, Emanuel: "The Id and the Ego: A Developmental Interpretation." *Psa. Rev.* 44:235–288, 1957.

Grauer, David: "How Autonomous Is the Ego?" *J. Am. Psa. Assn.* 6:502–518, 1958.

Miller, S. C.: "Ego Autonomy in Sensory Deprivation, Isolation and Stress." *Int. J. Psa.* 43:1–20, 1962.

3. Freud, Sigmund: *The Interpretation of Dreams*. New York: Macmillan, 1915.

———: *The Ego and the Id*. London: Hogarth, 1947.

———: "The Anatomy of the Mental Personality." In *New Introductory Lectures on Psychoanalysis*. New York: Norton, 1933.

4. Rapaport, David: "The Autonomy of the Ego." *Bull. Menninger Clin.* 15:113–123, 1951.

5. Piaget, Jean: *The Psychology of Intelligence*. New York: Harcourt, 1950.

6. Freud, Anna: *The Ego and the Mechanisms of Defense*. London: Hogarth, 1937.

Freud, Sigmund: *The Ego and the Id*. London: Hogarth, 1927.

———: *New Introductory Lectures on Psychoanalysis*. New York: Norton, 1933.

Goldberger, Emanuel: op. cit.

Hartmann, Heinz: "Comments on the Psychoanalytic Theory of the Ego." *Psa Study of the Child* 5:74–96, 1950.

———: "The Development of the Ego Concept in Freud's Work." *Int. J. Psa.* 37:425–438, 1956.

———; Kris, Ernst; and Loewenstein, R. M.: op. cit.

Rapaport, David: *Organization and Pathology of Thought*. New York: Columbia University, 1951.

7. Freud, Sigmund: *The Ego and the Id*, op. cit.

————: "The Anatomy of the Mental Personality." In *New Introductory Lectures on Psychoanalysis.* New York: Norton, 1933.

8. Federn, Paul: *Ego Psychology and the Psychoses.* New York: Basic Books, 1952.

Nunberg, Herman: *Principles of Psychoanalysis.* New York: International Universities, 1956.

Sherif, Musaf, and Cantril, Hadley: *The Psychology of Ego Involvements.* New York: Wiley, 1947.

Thorne, F. C.: *Principles of Psychological Examining.* Brandon, Vt.: Journal of Clinical Psychology, 1955.

Weiss, Edouardo: "History of Metapsychological Concepts." In *Dynamic Psychiatry,* Franz Alexander and Helen Ross, eds. Chicago: University of Chicago, 1952.

————: *Principles of Psychodynamics.* New York: Grune and Stratton, 1950.

9. Freud, Sigmund: "The Anatomy of the Mental Personality." Op. cit.

10. Rubinfine, D. L.: "A Survey of Freud's Writings on Earliest Psychic Functioning." *J. Am. Psa. Assn.* 9:610–625, 1961.

Holt, R. R.: "Primary Processes." *Psychol. Res. Madras* 4:105–112, 1960.

11. Murray, Henry A.: *Explorations in Personality.* New York: Oxford, 1938.

12. Freud, Sigmund: *The Ego and the Id,* op. cit.

Szasz, Thomas: *Pain and Pleasure: A Study of Bodily Feelings.* New York: Basic Books, 1957.

13. Daniels, G.: "An Approach to Psychological Control Studies of Urinary Sex Hormones." *Am. J. Psychiat.* 100:231–239, 1943.

14. Finley, C. S.: "Endocrine Stimulation as Affecting Dream Content." *Arch. Neurol. Psychiat.* 5:177–181, 1921.

15. Benedek, Therese: *Psychosexual Functions in Women.* New York: Ronald, 1952.

16. Hinkle, L. E., and Wolff, H. G.: "The Nature of Man's Adaptation to His Total Environment and the Relation of This to Illness." *Arch. Intern. Med.* 99:442–460, 1957.

17. Hebb, D. O.: *The Organization of Thought.* New York: Wiley, 1949.

18. Lilly, J. C.: "Mental Effects of Reduction of Ordinary Levels of Physical Stimuli on Intact, Healthy Persons." *Psychiat. Res. Reports* 5:1–9, 1956.

19. Penfield, Wilder, and Lamar, Roberts: *Speech and Brain Mechanisms.* Princeton: Princeton University, 1959.

20. Magoun, H. W. (ed.): *Handbook of Physiology.* Washington, D.C.: Am. Physiol. Soc., 1959.

————: "A Neural Basis of the Anesthetic State." In *Sedative and Hypnotic Drugs.* Baltimore: Williams and Wilkins, 1954.

21. Holt, E. B.: *The Freudian Wish.* New York: Holt, 1915.

22. MacLeod, R. B.: "Teleology and Theory of Human Behavior." *Science* 125:477–480, 1957.

23. Goldberger, Emanuel: op. cit.

Tanner, J. M., and Inhelder, Barbel (eds.): *Discussions on Child Development,* 2 vols. New York: International Universities, 1957–58.

Thorpe, W. H.: "Some Implications of the Study of Animal Behavior." *Sci. Monthly* 84:309–320, 1957.

Tinbergen, Nikolaas: *The Study of Instinct.* Oxford: Clarendon Press, 1951.

24. Ellenberger, H. F.: "Fechner and Freud." *Bull. Menninger Clin.* 20:201–214, 1956.

25. Clifford, W. K.: *Lectures and Essays,* 1879.

26. MacLeod, R. B.: op. cit.

27. Newman, J. R.: "A Review of E. Cassirer's Determinism and Indeterminism in Modern Physics." *Sci. American* 196:147–152, March 1957.

28. Murphy, Gardner: *Personality: A Biosocial Approach to Origins and Structure.* New York: Harper, 1947.

29. Harlow, H. F. and Margaret K.: "The Effect of Rearing Conditions on Behavior." *Bull. Menninger Clin.* 26:213–224, 1962.

30. Bernstein, Leonard: *West Side Story.* New York: Random House, 1958.
31. Margolin, Sydney: From a Menninger School of Psychiatry Forum presentation.
32. Empedocles: Fragment 16 in *The Fragments of Empedocles,* W. E. Leonard, ed. Chicago: Open Court, 1908.
33. Lilly, J. P.: "The Psychophysiological Basis for Two Kinds of Instincts: Implications for Psychoanalytic Theory." *J. Am. Psa. Assn.* 8:659–670, 1960.
34. Menninger, Karl: *Man Against Himself.* New York: Harcourt, 1938.
35. Orr, D. W.: "Is There a Homeostatic Instinct?" *Psa. Quart.* 11:322–335, 1942.

CHAPTER VII

1. Butler, Samuel: *The Way of All Flesh.* New York: Dutton, 1903.
2. Menninger, C. F.: "The Insanity of Hamlet." *J. Kansas Med. Soc.* 35:334–338, 1934. (Originally read before the Saturday Night Club, Topeka, Kansas, Oct. 18, 1890.)
3. Hartmann, Heinz: "Notes on the Theory of Sublimation." *Psa. Study of the Child* 10:9–29, 1955.
   Kris, Ernst: "Neutralization and Sublimation." *Psa. Study of the Child* 10:30–46, 1955.
   Menninger, Karl: *Love Against Hate.* New York: Harcourt, 1942.
4. Selye, Hans: *Stress.* Montreal: Acta, 1950.
5. Engel, G. L.: "Homeostasis, Behavioral Adjustment and the Concept of Health and Disease." In *Mid-century Psychiatry,* R. R. Grinker, ed. Springfield, Ill.: Charles C Thomas, 1953.
6. Freud, Anna: *The Ego and the Mechanisms of Defense.* London: Hogarth, 1937.
7. Kris, Ernst: "Notes on the Development of Psychoanalytic Child Psychology." *Psa. Study of the Child* 5:24–46, 1950.
8. Powys, John Cowper: *The Meaning of Culture.* New York: Norton, 1929.
9. Murphy, Lois B.: "Learning How Children Cope with Their Problems." *Children* 4:132–136, 1957.
   ———: *The Widening World of Childhood.* New York: Basic Books, 1962.
10. Frank, L. K.: "Tactile Communications." *Genetic Psychol. Mngr.* 56:209–255, 1957.
    Harlow, H. F. and Margaret K.: "The Effect of Rearing Conditions on Behavior." *Bull. Menninger Clin.* 26:213–224, 1962.
11. Bernfeld, Siegfried: *Psychology of the Infant.* New York: Brentano's, 1929.
    Ruesch, Jurgen, and Prestwood, A. R.: "Anxiety." *Arch. Neurol. Psychiat.* 62:527–550, 1949.
12. Baumgarten-Tramer, Franziska: "Die regulierenden Kräfte im Seelenleben und ihre psychohytienische Bedeutung." *Gesundheit und Wohlfahrt* 12:533, 1951.
13. Mirsky, I. Arthur: "Psychoanalysis and the Biological Sciences." In *Twenty Years of Psychoanalysis,* Franz Alexander and Helen Ross, ed. New York: Norton, 1953.
    ——— et al.: "Studies on the Physiological, Psychological and Social Determinants in the Etiology of Duodenal Ulcer." *Psychosom. Med.* 18:514, 1956.
14. Huxley, Aldous: *The Doors of Perception.* New York: Harper, 1954.
15. Freud, Sigmund: *Three Contributions to the Theory of Sex,* 4th ed. New York: Nervous and Mental Diseases Publishing Co., 1930.
16. Dollard, John: "The Dozens: Dialectic of Insult." *Amer. Imago* 1:3–25, 1939.
17. Freud, Sigmund: *Wit and Its Relation to the Unconscious.* New York: Moffat Yard, 1916.
18. Grotjahn, Martin: "Innocent Merriment." *Commonweal* 67:605, 1958.
19. Peto, Endre: "Weeping and Laughing." *Int. J. Psa.* 27:129–133, 1946.
20. Johnson, Burgess: *The Lost Art of Profanity.* Indianapolis: Bobbs-Merrill, 1948.
    Montagu, M. F. Ashley: "On the Physiology and Psychology of Swearing." *Psychiatry* 5:189–201, 1942.
    Ross, Helen E.: "Patterns of Swearing." *Atlas* 1:77–78, 1961.

21. Barbellion, W. N. P.: *The Journal of a Disappointed Man.* New York: Doran, 1919.

22. Sterne, Laurence: *Tristram Shandy*, George Saintsbury, ed. New York: Macmillan, 1925.

23. Stengel, Erwin: "Hughlings Jackson's Influence in Psychiatry." *Brit. J. Psychiat* 109:348–355, 1963.

24. Hollander, Raymond: "Compulsive Cursing." *Psychiat. Quart.* 34:599–622, 1960

25. Montagu, M. F. Ashley, op. cit.

26. Isakower, Otto: "A Contribution to the Pathopsychology of Phenomena Asso ciated with Falling Asleep." *Int. J. Psa.* 19:331–345, 1938.

Lewin, Bertram D.: *The Psychoanalysis of Elation.* New York: Norton, 1950.

27. Bateson, Gregory, and Mead, Margaret: *Balinese Character.* New York: Academy of Science, 1942.

28. Greenson, Ralph: "The Psychology of Apathy." *Psa. Quart.* 18:290–302, 1949.

29. Rapaport, David: "On the Psychoanalytic Theory of Thinking." *Int. J. Psa.* 31:161, 1950.

30. Sherrington, C. S.: *The Brain and Its Mechanism.* Cambridge: Cambridge University, 1933.

31. Stone, Leo: "Concerning the Psychogenesis of Somatic Disease." *Int. J. Psa.* 19:63–76, 1938.

32. Freud, Sigmund: "Formulations Regarding the Two Principles in Mental Functioning." *Coll. Papers* 4:13–21, 1925.

33. Menninger, Karl: *Love Against Hate.* New York: Harcourt, 1942.

34. Dement, William: "The Effect of Dream Deprivation." *Science* 131:1705–1707, 1960.

35. Kant, Immanuel: *Critique of Judgment*, 1790.

36. Menninger, Karl: "Chess." *Bull. Menninger Clin.* 6:80–83, 1942.

37. Hayakawa, S. I.: "Obiter Dicta: Sexual Fantasy and the 1957 Car." *ETC* 14:163–168, 1957.

38. Shaw, G. B.: *Arms and the Man.* New York: Brentano's, 1913.

39. Darwin, Charles R.: *The Expression of Emotions in Man and Animals.* New York: Philosophical Library, 1955. (See Margaret Mead's Preface to this edition.)

40. Groddeck, Georg. *The Unknown Self.* London: Daniel, 1929.

————: *The Book of It.* New York: Funk and Wagnalls, 1950.

41. Tinbergen, Nikolaas: *Social Behavior in Animals.* New York: Wiley, 1953.

42. Freeman, G. L.: *The Energetics of Human Behavior.* See Chapter V, note 14.

43. Perkins, William Harvey: *Cause and Prevention of Disease.* Philadelphia: Lea and Febiger, 1938.

44. Ibid.

45. Veith, Ilza: "The Wear and Tear Syndrome—1831." *Modern Med.* 268–278, Sept. 4, 1961.

CHAPTER VIII

1. Freud, Sigmund: *Civilization and Its Discontents.* London: Hogarth, 1930.

2. Luther, Martin: *Table-Talk.* Vol. CCCXIX, 1569.

3. *See* Bartemeier, Leo H., et al.: "Combat Exhaustion." *J. Nerv. Ment. Dis.* 104:358–389, 1946.

4. Thurber, James: "The Secret Life of Walter Mitty." In *My World and Welcome to It.* New York: Harcourt, 1937.

5. Selye, Hans: *The Stress of Life.* New York: McGraw-Hill, 1956.

CHAPTER IX

1. Prince, Morton (ed.): *The Dissociation of a Personality*, ed. 2. New York: Longmans, 1908.
2. Ellenberger, Henri: "Multiple Personalities." (Unpublished paper.)
3. James, William: *The Principles of Psychology*, 2 vols. New York: Holt, 1890.
4. Schilder, Oberndorf, Greenson, Deutsch, and others are associated in the minds of psychiatrists with the study of estrangement, depersonalization, and other disturbances in the person's sense of continuity and individuality.
   Schilder, Paul: *The Image and Appearance of the Human Body*. New York: International Universities, 1950.
   Oberndorf, C. P.: "Depersonalization in Relation to Erotization of Thought." *Int. J. Psa.* 15:271, 1934.
   Greenson, Ralph: "The Defensive Function of Some Affective States." *Bull. Am. Psa. Assn.* 8:234, 1952.
   Deutsch, Felix (ed.): *On the Mysterious Leap from the Mind to the Body*. New York: International Universities, 1959.
5. Cherbonnier, E. La B.: *Hardness of Heart: A Contemporary Interpretation of the Doctrine of Sin*. New York: Doubleday, 1955.
6. Hippocrates: *Œuvres Complètes*, Vol. 5. E. Littre, tr. Paris: Baillière, 1839–1861.
7. Fenichel, Otto: "Character Defenses against Anxiety." In *The Psychoanalytic Theory of Neuroses*. New York: Norton, 1945.
8. Freud, Anna: *The Ego and the Mechanisms of Defense*. London: Hogarth, 1937.
9. Menninger, Karl: *Man Against Himself*. New York: Harcourt, 1938.
10. Jelliffe, S. E.: "Psychoanalysis and Internal Medicine." In *Psychoanalysis Today*, Sandor Lorand, ed. New York: Covici, Friede, 1933.
11. Gittleson, N. S.: "Psychogenic Headache and the Localization of the Ego." *J. Mental Sc.*, 108:47–52, January 1962.
12. Selye, Hans: *The Physiology and Pathology of Exposure to Stress*. Montreal: Acta, 1950.
13. Brierley, M. F.: *Trends in Psycho-Analysis*. London: Hogarth, 1951.
   Isaacs, Susan: "The Nature and Function of Phantasy." *Int. J. Psa.* 29:73–97, 1948.
   Jones, Ernest: "The Relationship Between Dreams and Psychoneurotic Symptoms." In *Papers on Psychoanalysis*. Baltimore: Williams and Wilkins, 1948.
   Klein, Melanie: "The Importance of Symbol Formation in the Development of the Ego." In *Contributions to Psycho-Analysis*. London: Hogarth, 1930.
   Kubie, L. S.: "The Distortion of the Symbolic Process in Neurosis and Psychosis." *J. Am. Psa. Assn.* 1:59–86, 1953.
   Milner, Marion: "Aspects of Symbolism in Comprehension of the Not-Self." *Int. J. Psa.* 33:181–195, 1952.
   Rycroft, Charles: "Two Notes on Idealization, Illusion and Disillusion as Normal and Abnormal Psychological Processes." *Int. J. Psa.* 36:81–87, 1955.
   Winnicott, D. W.: "Primitive Emotional Development." *Int. J. Psa.* 26:137–143, 1945.
14. Winnicott, D. W.: "Transitional Objects and Transitional Phenomena." In *Collected Papers*. New York: Basic Books, 1958.
15. Harlow, H. F. and Margaret K.: "The Effect of Rearing Conditions on Behavior." *Bull. Menninger Clin.* 26:213–224, 1962.
16. Freud, Sigmund: *Three Essays. Standard Ed.* 7:123–243, 1953.
17. Freud, Sigmund: "Splitting of the Ego in the Process of Defense." *Coll. Papers* 5:372–375, 1950.
18. Greenacre, Phyllis: "Certain Relationships between Fetishism and the Faulty Development of the Body Image." *Psa. Study of the Child* 8:79–98, 1954.
19. *The Wolfenden Report*. Report of the Committee on Homosexual Offenses and Prostitution. New York: Stein and Day, 1963.
20. *New York Times*, Feb. 23, 1962.

21. Schofield, M. G.: *A Minority*. London: Longmans, 1960.
Gross, Alfred A.: *Strangers in Our Midst*. Washington, D.C.: Public Affairs, Press, 1962.
22. Paget, James: "Clinical Lectures on the Nervous Mimicry of Organic Diseases." *Lancet*, Vol. 2, 1873.
23. Andreyev, Leonid Nikolaevich: *He Who Gets Slapped*. New York: Brentano's, 1922.
24. Pope, Alexander: *An Essay on Man*, 1733.
25. Alexander, Franz: *The Criminal, the Judge, and the Public*. Glencoe, Ill.: Free Press, 1956.
26. Janet, Pierre: *La Force et la faiblesse psychologiques*. Paris: Maloine, 1932.
27. Alexander, Franz: "The Neurotic Character." *Int. J. Psa.* 11:292–311, 1930.
28. Bertschinger, Hans: "Uber Gelengenheitsursachen gewisser Neurosen und Psychosen." *Allgemeine Zeitschrift fur Psychiatrie* 69:588–617, 1912.
29. Veith, Ilza: "On Malingering." *Bull. Cleveland Med. Library* 2:67–73, 1955.
30. Menninger, Karl: "Psychology of a Certain Type of Malingering." *Arch. Neurol. Psychiat.* 33:507–515, 1935.
Szasz, Thomas S.: "Malingering: 'Diagnosis' or Social Condemnation?" *Arch. Neurol. Psychiat.* 76:432–443, 1956.
31. Bean, William B.: "The Munchausen Syndrome." *Trans. Am. Clin. & Climatological Assn.* 70:236–244, 1958.
32. Menninger, Karl: *Man Against Himself*, op. cit.
33. "A Ward-Watcher's Handbook." *Riss*, July 1962, pp. 49–53.

CHAPTER X

1. Alexander, Franz: *The Criminal, the Judge, and the Public*. Glencoe, Ill.: Free Press, 1956.
2. Butcher, Devereux: "The Bloody Flesh and Sport Business." Unpublished article.
3. *Topeka State Journal*, Sept. 15, 1946.
4. Jokl, Ernst: *Medicine and Sport*. Lexington, Ky.: University of Kentucky, 1960.
Sercl, M., and Joras, O.: "Mechanisms of Cerebral Concussions in Boxing and Their Consequences." *World Neurol.* 3:351–358, 1962.
5. Onstot, Kyle: *Mandingo*. New York: Denlingers, 1958.
6. Serling, Rod: "Requiem for a Heavyweight." In *Patterns*. New York: Simon and Schuster, 1957.
7. Hugo, Victor: *Toilers of the Sea* (*Les Travailleurs de la mer*), 1866.
8. Rose, Reginald: "Twelve Angry Men." In *Six Television Plays*. New York: Simon and Schuster, 1956.
9. Adorno, T. W., et al.: *The Authoritarian Personality*. New York: Harper, 1950.
10. Putney, Rufus: "Coriolanus and His Mother." *Psa. Quart.* 31:364–381, 1962.
11. Breuer, Joseph, and Freud, Sigmund: *Studies in Hysteria*. New York: Basic Books, 1957.
12. Freud, Sigmund: "Splitting of the Ego in the Process of Defense." *Coll. Papers* 5:372–375, 1950.
13. Lindner, Robert: "Homeostasis as an Explanatory Principle in Psychopathic Personality." *Textbook of the Annual Congress of Correction*, New York, 1943.
14. Karpman, Benjamin: "On the Need of Separating Psychopathy into Two Distinct Types." *J. Crim. Psychopathol.* 3:112–137, 1941.
Glueck, Sheldon and Eleanor: *Criminal Careers in Retrospect*. New York: Commonwealth Fund, 1943.
Healy, William: *Delinquents and Criminals*. New York: Macmillan, 1926.
Satten, Joseph, et al.: "Murder without Apparent Motive." *Am. J. Psychiat.* 117:48–53, 1960.
Maughs, Sydney B.: "Psychopathic Personality." *J. Crim. Psychopathol.* 10:248–275, 1949. "Concept of Psychopathy and Psychopathic Personality." *J. Crim.*

Psychopathol. 2:329–356, 465–499, 1941. "Criminal Psychopathology." In *Progress in Neurol. and Psychiat.*, Vol. 5, 7–10, 1950, 1952–1955.

Frosch, John, and Wortis, S. B.: "A Contribution to the Nosology of the Impulse Disorders." *Am. J. Psychiat.* 3:132–138, 1954.

Menninger, Karl: "Recognizing and Renaming 'Psychopathic Personalities.'" *Bull. Menninger Clin.* 5:150–156, 1941.

15. Riccio, Vincent, and Slocom, Bill: *All the Way Down.* New York: Simon and Schuster, 1962.

16. Gardner, George E.: "The Community and the Aggressive Child." *Ment. Hyg.* 33:537–550, 1949.

17. Makkay, E. S., and Schwaab, E. H.: "Some Problems in the Differential Diagnosis of Antisocial Character Disorders in Early Latency." *J. Amer. Acad. Child Psychiat.* 1:414–430, 1962.

Berman, Sydney: "Antisocial Character Disorder." *Am. J. Orthopsychiat.* 29:612–621, 1959.

Bornstein, Berta: "On Latency." *Psa. Study Child* 6:279–285, 1951.

Bowlby, John: "Maternal Care and Mental Health." *WHO Mngr. Ser.* 2:31–34, 1952.

Glover, Edward: "Diagnosis and Treatment of Pathological Delinquency." In *The Roots of Crime.* New York: International Universities, 1960.

Michaels, Joseph: *Disorders of Character.* Springfield, Ill.: Charles C Thomas, 1955.

Redl, Fritz: *Children Who Hate.* Glencoe, Ill.: Free Press, 1951.

18. Karpman, Benjamin: ibid.

19. Satten, Joseph, et al.: ibid.

20. Reichard, Suzanne, and Tillman, Carl. "Murder and Suicide as Defenses against Schizophrenic Psychosis." *J. Crim. Psychopathol.* 11:149–163, 1950.

21. Diamond, B. L.: "Criminal Responsibility for the Mentally Ill." *Sanford Law Rev.* 14:59–86, 1961.

22. Stengel, Erwin: "Self-Destructiveness and Self-Preservation." *Bull. Menninger Clin.* 26:7–17, 1963.

23. Greenwood, Allen: "Mental Disturbances Following Operations for Cataract." *J.A.M.A.* 91:1713–1716, 1928.

24. Leiderman, H., et al.: "Sensory Deprivation." *A.M.A. Arch. Intern. Med.* 101:389, 1958.

25. Maier, N. R. F., and Glaser, N. M.: "Studies of Abnormal Behavior in the Rat." *Comp. Psychol. Mngr.* 16:30, 1940.

26. Finger, Frank W.: "Experimental Behavior Disorders in the Rat." In *Personality and Other Behavior Disorders*, J. McV. Hunt, ed. New York: Ronald, 1944.

27. Abraham, Karl: *Selected Papers.* New York: Basic Books, 1953.

28. Bateman, J. F., et al.: "The Manic State as an Emergency Defense Reaction." *J. Nerv. & Ment. Dis.* 119:349–357, 1954.

29. Davidson, G. M.: "Manic Depressive Psychosis." *J. Nerv. & Ment. Dis.* 125:87–96, 1957.

30. Lewin, Bertram D.: *The Psychoanalysis of Elation.* New York: Norton, 1950.

31. Janet, Pierre: *Psychological Healing*, 2 vols. New York: Macmillan, 1925.

32. Schwade, E. D., and Geiger, Sara: "Impulsive-Compulsive Behavior Disorder with Abnormal Electroencephalographic Findings." *EEG & Clin. Neurophysiol.* Suppl. No. 3, 1953.

Merlis, Sydney, and Denber, H. C. B.: "The Etiological Significance of Certain Brave Wave Patterns in Nonepileptic Psychiatric Disorders." *EEG & Clin. Neurophysiol.* Suppl. No. 3, 1953.

Ervin, Frank, et al.: "Behavior of Epileptic and Nonepileptic Patients with 'Temporal Spikes.'" *A.M.A. Arch. Neur. & Psychiat.* 74:488–497, 1955.

Leffman, Henry, and Perlo, V. P.: "Metrazol and Combined Photic-Metrazol Activated Electroencephalography in Epileptic, Schizophrenic, Psychoneurotic and Psychopathic Patients." *EEG & Clin. Neurophysiol.* 7:61–66, 1955.

33. Silverman, Daniel: "Psychoses in Criminals." *J. Crim. Psychopathol.* 4:703–730, 1943.
34. Monroe, Russell R.: "Correlation of Rhinencephalic Electrograms with Behavior: A Study on Humans under the Influence of LSD and Mescaline." *EEG & Clin. Neurophysiol.* 9:623–642, 1957.
35. Woods, Sherwyn M.: "Adolescent Violence and Homicide." *Arch. Gen. Psychiat.* 5:528–534, 1961.
36. Ibid.
37. Bartemeier, Leo H.: "Concerning the Psychogenesis of Convulsive Disorders." *Psa. Quart.* 12:330–337, 1943.
Clark, L. P.: "The Psychobiologic Concept of Essential Epilepsy." *Res. Publ. Res. Nerv. Ment. Dis.* 7:67–79, 1931.
Epstein, A. W., and Ervin, Frank: "Psychodynamic Significance of Seizure Content in Psychomotor Epilepsy." *Psychosom. Med.* 18:43–55, 1956.
Freud, Sigmund: "Dostoievski and Parricide." *Int. J. Psa.* 26:1–8, 1945.
Kardiner, Abram: "Bio-analysis of the Epileptic Reaction." *Psa. Quart.* 1:375–483, 1932.
38. Woods, Sherwyn M.: ibid.
39. Epstein, A. W., and Ervin, Frank: op. cit.
40. Barker, Wayne: "Studies on Epilepsy." *Psychosom. Med.* 10:73–94, 1948.
41. Pruyser, Paul W.: "Personality Testing in Epilepsy." *Epilepsia* 3rd Ser., 2:32, 1953.
42. Goldstein, Kurt: *The Organism.* New York: American Book, 1939.
43. Fisher, Charles: "The Psychogenesis of Fugue States." Presented to the Assn. for the Advancement of Psychotherapy, May 31, 1946.
44. Bond, Earl D., and Appel, Kenneth E.: *The Treatment of Behavior Disorders Following Encephalitis.* New York: Commonwealth, 1931.
45. Boisen, A. T.: *The Explorations of the Inner World.* New York: Harper, 1936.

CHAPTER XI

1. Kraepelin, Emil: *Lectures on Clinical Psychiatry.* London: Baillière, Tindall and Cox, 1913.
2. Koff, Robert H.: "The Therapeutic Man Friday." *J. Am. Psa. Assn.* 5:424–431, 1957.
3. Menninger, Karl: *The Human Mind.* New York: Knopf, 1945.
4. Von Lerchenthal, E. Menninger: "Death from Psychic Causes." *Bull. Menninger Clin.* 12:31–36, 1948.
5. Simon, Alexander (ed.): *The Physiology of Emotions.* Springfield, Ill.: Charles C Thomas, 1961.
6. Benivieni, Antonio: *De abditis nonnullis ac mirandis morborum et sanationum causis,* Charles Singer, tr. Springfield, Ill.: Charles C Thomas, 1954.
7. Ellenberger, Henri: "Der Tod aus psychischen Ursachen bei Naturvölkern." *Psyche* 5:333–344, 1951.
8. Cannon, Walter B.: "Voodoo Deaths." *Am. Anthropologist* 44:169–181, 1942.
9. Mira, Emilio: *Psychiatry in War.* New York: Norton, 1943.
10. Barber, T. X.: "Death by Suggestion." *Psychosom. Med.* 23:153–155, 1961.
Richter, C. P.: "On the Phenomenon of Sudden Death in Animals and Man." *Psychosom. Med.* 19:191–198, 1957.
11. Mira, Emilio: "Psychiatric Experience in the Spanish War." *Brit. Med. J.* 1:1217, 1939.
12. Meerloo, J. A. M.: *Patterns of Panic.* New York: International Universities, 1950.
13. Shneidman, E. S., and Farberow, N. L. (ed.): *Clues to Suicide.* New York: McGraw-Hill, 1957. *The Cry for Help.* New York: McGraw-Hill, 1961.
14. Sayre, Joel: "The Man on the Ledge." *The New Yorker* 25:34–36, 1949.

15. Raines, G. N., and Thompson, S. V.: "Suicide—Some Basic Considerations." *Dig. Neurol. and Psychiat. Inst. of Living* 18:97–107, 1950.

Stengel, Erwin, and Cook, H. G.: *Attempted Suicide.* London: Chapman, 1958.

16. Menninger, Karl: *Man Against Himself.* New York: Harcourt, 1938.

17. Meerloo, J. A. M.: *Suicide and Mass Suicide.* New York: Grune and Stratton, 1962.

18. Menninger, Karl: ibid.

19. Friedman, Paul: "Some Considerations on the Treatment of Suicidal Depressive Patients." *Am. J. Psychiat.* 16:379–386, 1962.

20. Freud, Sigmund: "Mourning and Melancholia." *Standard Ed. Complete Psychol. Works of Sigmund Freud* 14:237–260, 1957.

21. Dickinson, Emily: "I Felt a Funeral in My Brain." *Complete Poems of Emily Dickinson.* Thomas H. Johnson, ed. Boston: Little, Brown, 1960.

CHAPTER XII

1. *New York Times*, March 30, 1962, p. 1.

2. Srole, Leo, et al.: *Mental Health in the Metropolis.* See Chapter II, note 28.

3. Schelling, F. W. J. von: *Ideen zu einer Philosophie der Natur*, ed. 2. Landshut: Phil, Kruell, 1803.

4. Hunt, Morton M.: "The Case of Flight 320." *The New Yorker*, April 30, 1960.

5. Sommer, Robert, and Witney, Gwyneth: "The Chain of Chronicity." *Am. J. Psychiat.* 118:112–117, 1961.

6. Menninger, Karl; Mayman, Martin; and Pruyser, Paul: *A Manual for Psychiatric Case Study.* See Chapter I, note 4.

7. Thwaites, R. G. (ed.): *The Jesuit Relations and Allied Documents* 13:113–115, 1896–1901.

8. Schwartz, D. A.: "Paradoxical Remission of Psychoses." *Arch. Gen. Psychiat.* 6:315–319, 1962.

Duffy, John: "Medicine and Medical Practices Among Aboriginal American Indians." In *History of American Medicine* by Felix Marti-Ibanez. New York: M.D. Publications, 1958.

9. Hayward, S. T.: "The Doctor's Place in the Patient's Hospital." *Lancet* 1:387–389, 1961.

10. Le Guillant, L.: "Une Expérience de réadaptation social instituée par les évènements de guerre." *L'Hyg. Ment.* 36:85–102, 1946–47.

11. Neuburger, Max: *The Doctrine of the Healing Power of Nature Throughout the Course of Time.* New York: L. J. Boyd [privately printed], 1932.

12. Menninger, Karl: "The Amelioration of Mental Disease by Influenza." *J.A.M.A.* 94:630–634, 1930.

13. Bartemeier, Leo, et al.: "Combat Exhaustion." *J. Nerv. Ment. Dis.* 104:358–525, 1946.

14. Menninger, Karl: *Theory of Psychoanalytic Technique.* New York: Basic Books, 1958.

15. Freud, Sigmund: *Inhibitions, Symptoms, and Anxiety.* London: Hogarth, 1936.

16. Freud, Sigmund: "Recollection, Repetition and Working Through." In *Collected Papers* 2:366–376, 1924.

17. Erikson, Kai: "Patient Role and Social Uncertainty: A Dilemma of the Mentally Ill." *Psychiatry* 20:263–274, 1957.

18. Powys, John Cowper: *The Meaning of Culture.* New York: Norton, 1929.

19. Melzack, Ronald: "The Perception of Pain." *Sci. American* 204:41–49, 1961.

Butendyk, F. J.: *Pain; Its Modes and Functions.* Chicago: University of Chicago, 1962.

20. Penman, John: "Pain as an Old Friend." *Lancet* 1:633–635, 1954.

21. Ibid.

22. Ramzy, Ishak, and Wallerstein, Robert: "Pain, Fear and Anxiety." *Psa. Study of the Child* 13:157–189, 1958.

23. Koestler, Arthur: *Darkness at Noon.* New York: Modern Library, 1946.
24. Magee, K. R., et al.: "Congenital Indifference to Pain." *J. Nerv. and Ment. Dis.* 132:249–259, 1961.
25. Browning, Elizabeth Barrett: *Aurora Leigh* (1857). New York: Oxford, 1901.

CHAPTER XIII

1. Menninger, Karl: "Psychological Factors in the Choice of Medicine as a Profession." *Bull. Menninger Clin.* 21:51–58, 99–106, 1957. Reprinted in *A Psychiatrist's World,* B. H. Hall, ed. New York: Viking, 1959.
2. Holmes, Oliver Wendell: quoted by John Terry Maltsberger in "Do We Graduate as Compleat Physicians?" *Harvard Med. Alumni Bull.* July 1959.
3. Menninger, William C.: "Comprehensive Medicine—The Role of the Physician in Present-Day Practice." *Quart. Phi Beta Pi* 49:47–54.
4. Bunyan, John: "The Jerusalem Sinner Saves; or Good News for the Vilest of Men." *Complete Works,* G. Offor and R. Phillip, eds. London, 1862.
5. Hayward, S. T.: "The Doctor's Place in the Patient's Hospital." *Lancet* 1:387–389, 1961.
6. Holmes, Oliver Wendell: "Currents and Counter-Currents in Medical Science." In *Medical Essays. 1842–1882.* Boston: Houghton, Mifflin, 1892.
7. Waring, Joseph Ioor: "The Influence of Benjamin Rush on the Practice of Bleeding in South Carolina." *Bull. Hist. Med.* 35:230–237, 1961.
8. Haggard, Howard W.: *Devils, Drugs, and Doctors.* New York: Harper, 1929.
9. Deutsch, Ronald M. P.: *The Nuts Among the Berries.* New York: Ballantine, 1961.
10. Wille, Lois: In *Chicago Daily News,* March 26, 1962.
11. Guttentag, Otto E.: "An Orientation in the Foundation of Medical Thought." *J. Med. Education* 35:903–907, 1960.
12. Freud, Anna: "Assessment of Childhood Disturbances." *Psa. Study of the Child* 17:149–158, 1962.
13. Srole, Leo, et al.: *Mental Health in the Metropolis.* See Chapter II, note 28.
14. Menninger, Karl; Mayman, Martin; and Pruyser, Paul: *A Manual for Psychiatric Case Study.* See Chapter I, note 4.
15. Ibid.
16. Reinert, R. E.: Guest Editorial. *Kan. Psychiat. Soc. Newsletter* Winter 1962–1963.
17. *Time,* February 8, 1963.
18. Lao Tzu: *The Way of Life According to Lao Tzu: An American Version* by Witter E. Bynner. New York: John Day, 1944.
19. Wilson, Robert N.: "The Physician's Changing Hospital Role." *Human Organization* 18:177–183, 1959.
    Burling, Temple, et al.: *The Give and Take in Hospitals.* New York: Putnam, 1956.

CHAPTER XIV

1. Mott, James M.: "Rapid Recovery from Long-Standing Illness." *Bull. Menninger Clin.* 14:177–182, 1950.
2. Ticho, Ernst: In a course of lectures to the Fellows in the Menninger School of Psychiatry, 1962.
3. Holmes, John: "The Eleventh Commandment." *Harper's* 213:53–54, 1956.
4. Ueland, Brenda: "Tell Me More." *Ladies' Home J.* November 1941.

CHAPTER XV

1. Gitelson, Maxwell: "The Emotional Position of the Analyst in the Psychoanalytic Situation." *Int. J. Psa.* 33:1–10, 1952.
   Heimann, Paula: "On Countertransference." *Int. J. Psa.* 31:81–84, 1950.
   Racker, Heinrich: "The Meanings and Uses of Countertransference." *Psa. Quart.* 26:303–357, 1957.
   Reich, Annie: "On Countertransference." *Int. J. Psa.* 32:25–31, 1951.
   Menninger, Karl: *Theory of Psychoanalytic Technique.* New York: Basic Books, 1958.
2. Kaiser, Hellmuth: "Emergency." *Psychiatry* 25:97–118, 1962.
3. Reider, Norman: "A Type of Transference to Institutions." *Bull. Menninger Clin.* 17:58–63, 1953.
4. Wilmer, Harry A.: "Transference to a Medical Center." *California Med.* 96:173–180, 1962.
5. Cumming, John and Elaine: *Ego and Milieu.* New York: Atherton, 1962.
6. Kinsey, A. C., et al.: *Sexual Behavior in the Human Male.* Philadelphia: Saunders, 1948. *Sexual Behavior in the Human Female.* Philadelphia: Saunders, 1953.
7. Neuburger, Max: *The Doctrine of the Healing Power of Nature Throughout the Course of Time.* New York: L. J. Boyd [privately printed], 1932.
8. Ibid.
9. Ibid.
10. Ackerknecht, Erwin H.: "Aspects of the History of Therapeutics." *Bull. Hist. Med.* 36:389–419, 1962.
11. Neuburger, Max: op. cit.
12. Ibid.
13. Ibid.
14. Zehetmayer, Franz: *Die Herzkrankheiten.* Vienna: Braumüller und Seidel, 1845.
15. Pirandello, Luigi: *Henry IV.* In *Contemporary Drama,* E. B. Watson and W. B. Pressey, eds. New York: Scribner's, 1960.
16. Born, Max: *Natural Philosophy of Cause and Chance.* London: Oxford, 1949.
17. Hench, Philip S.: "The Fragile Children of Discovery." *Saturday Rev.* 38:44–45, 1956.
18. Cousins, Norman: *In Place of Folly.* New York: Harper, 1961.
19. Murray, Henry A.: "Personality and Career of Satan." *J. Soc. Issues* 18:36–54, 1962.
20. Cherbonnier, E. L.: *Hardness of Heart.* New York: Doubleday, 1955.
21. Dumond, D. L.: *Antislavery.* Ann Arbor: University of Michigan, 1961.
    Marteilhe, Jean: *Galley Slave,* Kenneth Fenwick, ed. London: Folio Society, 1957.
22. Arendt, Hannah: *Eichmann in Jerusalem.* New York: Viking, 1963.
23. Mitscherlich, Alexander, and Mielke, Fred: *Doctors of Infamy.* New York: Schuman, 1949.
24. Macdonald, Dwight: "Our Invisible Poor." *The New Yorker,* Jan. 19, 1963.
25. Barnett, L. K.: *The Universe and Dr. Einstein.* New York: Sloan, 1948.
26. Planck, Max: "The Meaning and Limits of Exact Science." *Science* 110:319–327, 1949.
27. Rapoport, Anatol: "Letter to a Soviet Philosopher." *ETC.* 19:437–455, 1963.
28. Anouilh, Jean: *Antigone and Eurydice.* London: Methuen, 1951.
29. French, T. M.: *The Integration of Behavior.* Chicago: University of Chicago, 1952.
30. Lain Entralgo, Pedro: *La Espera y la Esperanza.* Madrid, 1958.
31. Meier, D. L., and Bell, W.: "Anomia and Differential Access to the Achievements of Life Goals." *Am. Sociol. Rev.* 24:189–202, 1959.
32. Dorpat, T. L., and Ripley, H. S.: "A Study of Suicide in the Seattle Area." *Comprehensive Psychiat.* 1:349–359, 1960.

33. Menninger, Karl and Jeanetta L.: *Love Against Hate*. New York: Harcourt, 1942.
34. Ibid.
35. Schachtel, E. G.: *Metamorphosis*. New York: Basic Books, 1959.
36. Hamburger, Carl: *Selbstheilung hoffnungsloser Krankheiten*. Jena: Fischer, 1928.
37. Littell, Robert: "Schizophrenics in the Sun." *Harper's*, September 1962.
38. Srole, Leo, et al.: *Mental Health in the Metropolis*. See Chapter II, note 8.
39. Wolff, Harold G.: "What Hope Does for Man." *Saturday Rev.* Jan. 5, 1957.
40. Gollwitzer, Helmut, et al. (eds.): *Dying We Live*. New York: Pantheon, 1956.
41. Richter, C. F.: "Sudden Death Phenomenon in Animals and Humans." In *The Meaning of Death*, Herman Feifel, ed. New York: McGraw-Hill, 1959.
42. Schmale, A. H.: "Relationship of Separation and Depression to Disease." *Psychosom. Med.* 20:259–277, 1958.
43. *Topeka Daily Capital*, April 2, 1959.
44. Marcel, Gabriel: *Homo Viator: Introduction to a Metaphysics of Hope*. New York: Harper, 1962.
45. Feldman, Paul E.: "The Personal Element in Psychiatric Research." *Am. J. Psychiat.* 113:52–54, 1956.
46. Henderson, L. J.: Quoted by Alan Leslie in "Ethics and Practice of Placebo Therapy." *Am. J. Med.* 16:854–862, 1954.
47. Rogers, Carl R.: *Client-Centered Therapy*. Boston: Houghton, Mifflin, 1951.
48. Mayman, Martin: "Toward a Positive Definition of Mental Health." American Psychological Association symposium, September 1955.

CHAPTER XVI

1. Dietl, Joseph: Quoted by Max Neuburger in *The Doctrine of the Healing Power of Nature Throughout the Course of Time*. New York: Boyd, 1932.
2. Woodham-Smith, Cecil: *The Great Hunger*. Boston: Houghton, Mifflin, 1963.
3. Bockoven, J. Sanbourne: "Moral Treatment in American Psychiatry." *J. Nerv. and Ment. Dis.* 124:293–321, 1956.
4. Clark, L. Pierce: "A Psychologic Study of Abraham Lincoln." *Psa. Rev.* 8:1–21, 1921.
5. Szasz, Thomas A.: "Human Nature and Psychotherapy." *Comprehensive Psychiat.* 3:268–283, 1962.
6. Mill, John S.: *Autobiography*. New York: Columbia University, 1960.
7. Cameron, Norman: *William James*. Madison: University of Wisconsin, 1942.
8. Menninger, Flo V.: *Days of My Life*. New York: Richard R. Smith, 1940.
9. Dunford, Katherine: "Benjamin Franklin's Bold and Arduous Project." *ETC.* 19: 335–340, 1962.
10. James, William: *The Varieties of Religious Experience*. New York: Longmans, 1902.
11. Murphy, Gardner: *Human Potentialities*. New York: Basic Books, 1958.
12. Mayman, Martin: "Ego Strength and the Potential for Recovery from Mental Illness." *Festschrift for Gardner Murphy*. New York: Harper, 1960.
13. Pruyser, Paul: "Is Mental Health Possible?" *Bull. Menninger Clin.* 22:58–66, 1958.
14. Menninger, Karl: *Theory of Psychoanalytic Technique*. New York: Basic Books, 1958.
15. James, William: *The Will to Believe*. New York: Longmans, 1903.

APPENDIX

1. Whitwell, J. R. *Historical Notes on Psychiatry*. London: H. K. Lewis, 1936, p. 14.
2. Adams, Francis. *Genuine Works of Hippocrates*, translated from the Greek. 2 vol., New York: William Wood & Co., 1929.
3. Cf. Dodds, E. R. *The Greeks and the Irrational*. Berkeley: Univ. of Calif. Press, 1951, pp. 64–101.
4. Celsus. *De Medicina*, with an English translation by Walter George Spencer. 3 vol., London: Heinemann; Cambridge: Harvard Univ. Press., 1935.
5. Daremberg, Ch. *Oeuvres anatomiques, physiologiques et médicales de Galien*, French translation. 2 vol., Paris: Baillière, 1854 and 1856.
6. Cf. Lewy-Landsberg. "Über die Bedeutung des Anthyllus, Philagrius und Posidonius in der Geschichte der Heilkunde, III." *Janus*, vol. 3, 1848, pp. 116–184.
7. Brunet, F. *Oeuvres médicales d'Alexandre de Tralles*, French translation with introduction and comments. 4 vol., Paris: Geuthner, 1933.
8. Aurelianus, Caelius. *On Acute Diseases and on Chronic Diseases*, transl. I. E. Drabkin. Chicago: Univ. Chicago Press, 1950.
9. Adams, Francis. *The Seven Books of Paulus Aegineta*, transl. from the Greek. 3 vol., London: Sydenham Society, 1844. Vol. I, pp. 350–409, 633–638.
10. *The Spiritual Physick of Rhazes*, transl. from the Arabic by Arthur J. Arberry. London: John Murray, 1950.
11. Bumm, A. "P. Vattier's Übersetzung des Abschnittes über Geisteskrankheiten in Avicenna's Canon Medicinae." *Münchener Medizinische Wochenschrift*, vol. 45, 1898, p. 632–634.
12. Kopp, Paul. "Psychiatrisches bei Thomas von Aquin." *Zeitschrift für die gesamte Neurologie und Psychiatrie*, Vol. 152, 1935, pp. 178–196. Krapf, Eduardo. *Tomas de Aquino y la psicopatologia*. Monografias de Index de Neurologia y Psiquiatria, No. 2, Buenos Aires, 1943.
13. Quoted from Sémalaigne, René. *Les Pionniers de la Psychiatrie Française*. Paris: Baillière, 1930. Vol. I, pp. 21–28.
14. Schenck, Johannes. *Observationum medicarum rariorum libri VII*. Lyons, 1644. Quoted from Laignel-Lavastine, M., and Vinchon, J. *Les maladies de l'esprit et leurs médecins du XVIe au XIXe siècle*. Paris: Maloine, 1930, pp. 33–49, 83.
15. Bright, Timothy. *A Treatise of Melancholie*. London: Thomas Vautrollier, 1586. Fac-Simile Edition. The Facsimile Text Society. New York: Columbia Univ. Press, 1940.
16. Paracelsus. *Sämtliche Werke*, ed. Strebel, Zollikofer, St. Gallen. 1949. Vol. 7, pp. 31–62.
17. Quoted from the following: Karcher, J. *Felix Platter*. Basel, 1949. Christoffel, Hans. "Psychiatrie und Neurologie bei Felix Platter." *Monatsschrift für Psychiatrie und Neurologie*, vol. 27, 1954, pp. 213–227 (psychoanalytic study). Reimann-Hunziker, Rose. "Felix Platter's Abhandlungen über die Zustande und Krankheiten des Geistes." *Schweizer Archiv für Neurologie und Psychiatrie*, vol. 62, 1948, pp. 241–260 (German transl. of excerpts from Platter's psychiatric writings).
18. Vallon, Charles, and Genil-Perrin. "La Psychiatrie Médico-Légale dans l'Oeuvre de Zacchias (1584–1659)." *Revue de Psychiatrie*, 1912, vol. 16, pp. 46–84, 90–106.
19. *The Anatomy of Melancholy*, by Democritus Junior (pseudonym). Oxford, 1628. Quoted from the edition of Floyd Dell and Paul Jordan-Smith, New York: Tudor Publishing Company, 1938.
20. Quoted from Laignel-Lavastine, M., and Vinchon, J. *Les maladies de l'esprit et leurs médecins du XVIe au XIXe siècle*. Paris: Maloine, 1930, pp. 125–161.
21. Faber, Knud. *Nosography in Modern Internal Medicine*. New York: Hoeber, 1923, pp. 8–9.
22. Ibid., pp. 20–21.

23. Boissier de Sauvages de la Croix, François. *Nouvelles classes des maladies dans un ordre semblable à celui des botanistes, comprenant les genres et les espèces.* Avignon, 1732. *Nosologia methodica sistens morborum classes, genera et species, juxta Sydenhami mentem et botanicorum ordinem.* 5 vol., Amsterdam, 1763. *Nosologie méthodique, dans laquelle les maladies sont rangées par classes suivant le système de Sydenham & l'ordre des Botanistes. Traduite du latin.* Ed. Nicolas, M. 3 vol., 1770 and 1771.

24. Linné, Carolus. *Clavis Medicinae Duplex, Exterior and Interior.* First Neapolitan ed., 1793, 124 pp.

25. Cullen, William. *Synopsis nosologiae methodicae,* Edinburgh: A. Kincaid & Creech, 1769. (First English translation under title *Synopsis and Nosology, being an Arrangement and Definition of Diseases.* Hartford: Nathaniel Patten, 1792.)

26. Arnold, Thomas: *Observations on the Nature, Kinds, Causes, and Prevention of Insanity.* 1st ed., 1782. Quoted from the 2nd ed., 2 vol., 1806.

27. *Encyclopédie, ou Dictionnaire Raisonné des Sciences, des Arts et des Métiers, par une Société de Gens de Lettres.* Paris. Vol. 4, 1754, and vol. 7, 1757.

28. Kant, Immanuel. *Anthropologie in pragmatischer Hinsicht.* 1798. Quoted from the edition of von Kirchmann, J. H., 3. Aufl., Leipzig, 1880.

29. Zilboorg, Gregory. *A History of Medical Psychology.* New York: Norton, 1941, p. 309.

30. Chiarugi, Vincenzo: *Della Pazzia in genere e in specie con una centuria di ozzervazioni.* 3 vols., Florence: Carlieri, 1793–1794.

31. Pinel, Philippe. *Nosographie philosophique, ou méthode de l'analyse appliquée à la médecine.* Paris, 1798. Quoted from Sémelaigne, René. *Aliénistes et Philanthropes. Les Pinel et les Tuke.* Paris: G. Steinheil, 1912.

32. Pinel, Philippe. *Traité médico-philosophique sur l'aliénation mentale, ou la manie.* Paris: Richard, Caille et Ravier, an IX (1801).

33. Rush, Benjamin. *Medical Inquiries and Observations upon the Diseases of the Mind.* Philadelphia: J. Grigg, 1825.

34. Riese, Walther. "Pinel." *J. Nerv. Ment. Dis.,* 114, 317.

35. Shryock, Richard H. "Benjamin Rush from the Perspective of the Twentieth Century." *Transactions and Studies of the College of Physicians of Philadelphia.* 4 Sec., vol. 14, 1946, pp. 113–120.

36. Hunter, R., and MacAlpine, Ida. *Three Hundred Years of Psychiatry—1535–1860.* London: Oxford Univ. Press, 1963.

37. Quoted from Kahlbaum, Ludwig. *Die Gruppierung der psychischen Krankheiten* . . . , Danzig: Kafemann, 1863.

38. Janet, Pierre. *La Force et la faiblesse psychologiques,* Miron Epstein, ed. Paris: Maloine, 1932.

39. Jaspers, Karl. *Allgemeine Psychopathologie.* Berlin: J. Springer, 5th. ed., 1948, p. 708.

40. Esquirol, Jean-Dominique. *Des Maladies mentales.* 2 vol. and atlas, Paris, 1838.

41. Heinroth, Johann Christian: *Lehrbuch der Störungen des Seelenlebens oder der Seelenstörungen und ihrer Behandlung vom rationalen Standpunkt aus entworfen.* Leipzig, 1818.

42. Quoted from Wernicke, Carl. *Uber die Klassifikation der Psychosen,* 1899, p. 12.

43. Jacobi, Maximilian. *Die Hauptformen der Seelenstörungen in ihren Beziehungen zur Heilkunde,* 1844 (quoted by Kahlbaum).

44. Wernicke, op. cit., p. 58.

45. Bucknill, J. C., and Tuke, D. H. *A Manual of Psychological Medicine.* London: Churchill, 4th ed., 1879, pp. 46–54.

46. Hunter, R., and MacAlpine, Ida, op. cit.

47. Morel, Bénédict-Augustin. *Traité théorique et pratique des maladies mentales.* 2 vol., Nancy and Paris, 1852 and 1853.

48. Morel, Bénédict-Augustin. *Traité des dégénérescences physiques, intellectuelles et morales de l'espèce humaine et des causes qui produisent ses variétés maladives.* 1 vol. and atlas, Paris: Baillière, 1857.

49. Ibid., *Traité des Maladies Mentales.* Paris: Masson, 1860.

50. Magnan, Valentin. *Exposé des Titres et Travaux Scientifiques. Réédition à l'occasion du Centenaire de Magnan.* Clermont: Thiron, 1935 (p. 38-40).

51. Kahlbaum, Karl Ludwig. *Die Gruppierung der psychischen Krankheiten. Entwurf einer historisch-kritischen Darstellung der bisherigen Einteilungen und Versuch zur Anbahnung einer empirisch-wissenschaftlichen Grundlage der Psychiatrie als klinischer Disziplin.* Danzig: A. W. Kafemann, 1863.

52. Ibid., *Die Katatonie oder das Spannungsirresein.* Berlin: 1874.

53. Meyer, A. *Collected Papers.* 2 vol., Baltimore: Johns Hopkins Press, 1951, vol. 2, pp. 477-486.

54. Skae, David. *Of the Classification of the Various Forms of Insanity on a Rational and Practical Basis, Being an Address Delivered at the Royal College of Physicians, London, at the Annual Meeting of the Association of Medical Officers of Asylums on* 9th July, 1863, s.l.n.d., p. 15.

55. Krafft-Ebing, R. *Lehrbuch der Psychiatrie,* 1879.

56. Savage, George H. *Insanity and Allied Neuroses.* Philadelphia: Lea Brothers, 3d ed., 1890.

57. Griesinger, Wilhelm. *Mental Pathology and Therapeutics.* English trans., London: The New Sydenham Society, 1867.

58. Meynert, Theodor. *Lehrbuch der Psychiatrie,* 1884.

59. Wernicke, Carl. *Allgemeine Psychiatrie, Krankenvorstellungen aus der psychiatrischen Klinik in Breslau,* 1900.

60. Ibid. *Grundriss der Psychiatrie in klinischen Vorlesungen.* Leipzig: Thieme, 2nd ed. 1906, p. 18.

61. Ibid. *Über die Klassifikation der Psychosen.* Breslau: Schletter'sche Buchhandlung, 1899.

62. Ibid. *Allgemeine Psychiatrie.*

63. Cameron, Norman. "The Function Psychoses," in *Personality and the Behavior Disorders,* ed. by J. McV. Hunt. New York: the Ronald Press, 1944, Vol. II, p. 879.

64. Zilboorg, G., op. cit., p. 458.

65. Meyer, Adolf. "A Review of Recent Problems of Psychiatry," in *Collected Papers.* Baltimore: Johns Hopkins, 1951, vol. 2, pp. 331-385.

66. Zilboorg, G., op. cit., p. 458.

67. Bucknill and Tuke, op. cit., pp. 45-46.

68. May, James V. *Mental Diseases.* Boston: R. G. Badger, 1922, p. 244.

69. Stearns, H. P. "Classification of Mental Diseases." *Am. J. of Insanity,* vol. 44, no. 3, Jan. 1888.

70. May, op. cit., pp. 246, 247.

71. Murray, Henry. *Explorations in Personality.* New York: Oxford Univ. Press, 1938.

72. For a critical comparison of the systems of Kraepelin and Wernicke, see Meyer's "Review of Recent Problems of Psychiatry," loc. cit., vol. 2, pp. 331-385.

73. In *The Collected Papers of Adolf Meyer,* op. cit., vol. 3, pp. 285-314.

74. Bleuler, Eugen. *Dementia praecox oder Gruppe der Schizophrenien.* Leipzig: Deuticke, 1911. English Translation: *Dementia Praecox.* New York: International Univ. Press, 1950.

75. Ibid. *Lehrbuch der Psychiatrie.* Berlin: Julius Springer, 1916. 8th ed. revised by Manfred Bleuler, 1949. English translation by A. A. Brill: *Textbook of Psychiatry.* New York: Dover Publications, 1924.

76. Menninger, Karl A. "Smith Ely Jelliffe, 1866-1945—Peter Bassoe, 1874-1945." *Bulletin of the Menninger Clinic,* vol. 9, 1945, pp. 177-178. Reprinted in Menninger, Karl A. *A Psychiatrist's World.* New York: Viking, 1959, p. 826.

77. Kempf, E. J. *Psychopathology.* St. Louis: Mosby & Co., 1920, pp. 190-191.

78. E. E. Southard. "Diagnosis per Exclusionem in Ordine: General and Psychiatric Remarks." *Jour. Lab. & Clin. Med.,* vol. IV, No. 2., November 1918, p. 20.

79. Mira y Lopez, E. *Manual de Psiquiatria.* Buenos Aires: El Ateneo, 1943.

80. Leconte, Maurice, and Damey, Alfred. *Essai critique des nosographies psychiatriques actuelles.* Paris: Doin, 1949.

81. Ey, Henri. *Etudes Psychiatriques*. Paris: Desclée de Brouwer, 1954, vol. 3, pp. 32–34.

82. Kleist, K. *Mschr. Psychiatr. Neurol*, 125, 539 (1953).

83. Rümke, H. C. "Nosology, Classification, Nomenclature." In *Field Studies in the Mental Disorders*, Joseph Zubin, ed. New York: Grune & Stratton, 1961.

84. Henderson, D. K., and Gillespie, R. D. *A Textbook of Psychiatry*, 8th Ed. New York: Oxford Univ. Press, 1956.

85. Kloos, G. "Der heutige Stand der psychiatrischen Systematic." *Med. Klin.* 46:1–7, 1951.

86. Essen-Möller, E., and Wohlfahrt, S. "Suggestions for the Amendment of the Official Swedish Classification of Mental Disorders." *Acta Psychiat. et Neurol.* Suppl. 47:551–555, 1947.

87. Henderson and Gillespie, op. cit.

88. Glover, Edward. "A Psychoanalytic Approach to the Classification of Mental Disorders." *Journal of Mental Science* 78:819–842, 1932.

89. Stengel, E. "Classification of Mental Disorders." *Bull. World Health Org.*, 21:601–663, 1959.

INDEX